"CHILDBIRTH WITH LOVE
is a true gift…"

"…It contains every question you conceivably could think of asking when you are planning or carrying or giving birth to a baby. The answers you never thought about are here as well, making the most important event of your life one of discovery and compassion."

— Liv Ullmann

"…CHILDBIRTH WITH LOVE is an especially comprehensive and helpful reference book for every couple desirous of creating a baby."

— Frank Caplan
Princeton Center
for Infancy

Berkley books by Niels Lauersen, M.D.

CHILDBIRTH WITH LOVE: A
COMPLETE GUIDE TO FERTILITY, PREGNANCY,
AND CHILDBIRTH FOR CARING COUPLES

IT'S YOUR BODY, A WOMAN'S GUIDE TO GYNECOLOGY
(with Steven Whitney)

LISTEN TO YOUR BODY: A GYNECOLOGIST ANSWERS WOMEN'S
MOST INTIMATE QUESTIONS (with Eileen Stukane)

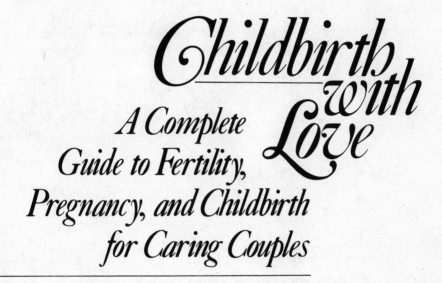

Childbirth with Love

A Complete Guide to Fertility, Pregnancy, and Childbirth for Caring Couples

Dr. Niels H. Lauersen

BERKLEY BOOKS, NEW YORK

This Berkley book contains the complete
text of the original edition.

CHILDBIRTH WITH LOVE: A COMPLETE
GUIDE TO FERTILITY, PREGNANCY AND CHILDBIRTH
FOR CARING COUPLES

A Berkley Book / published by arrangement with
G. P. Putnam's Sons

PRINTING HISTORY
G. P. Putnam's Sons edition / November 1983
Berkley trade paperback edition / September 1985

ISBN: 0-425-07390-4

A BERKLEY BOOK ® TM 757,375
Berkley Books are published by The Berkley Publishing Group,
200 Madison Avenue, New York, New York 10016.
The name "BERKLEY" and the stylized "B" with design
are trademarks belonging to Berkley Publishing Corporation.

PRINTED IN THE UNITED STATES OF AMERICA

Acknowledgments

Many couples, men and women, patients, friends, and colleagues have encouraged me to write an up-to-date, comprehensive guide for women who are planning for pregnancy in the future, women who are already pregnant, and women who want to know what to expect during labor and delivery and in the postpartum time. I know that women have been confused by all the do's and don'ts recommended during pregnancy, and worried about problems with conception and the proper management of both healthy and high-risk pregnancies. *Childbirth with Love* was written with the aim of answering an expectant mother's questions before she even has a chance to ask them. This book exists to guide a woman at all times—from her decision to conceive to the birth of her healthy baby. My hope is that *Childbirth with Love* will give a woman such a comprehensive understanding of labor and delivery that, for instance, she and her partner will realize when a delivery can proceed naturally and when intervention is necessary. Today, when women have fewer children, it is important for us to pay much more attention to every fact about pregnancy and childbirth and present a guide that confronts all questions directly and answers them honestly, but always compassionately.

My deepest gratitude goes to each and every person who has assisted in the research and preparation of this book, which was produced during long days and nights of work. Every modern treatment and suggestion was analyzed.

My most sincere thanks go to Judy Hendra for her assistance and knowledge in the preparation, editing, and perfecting of *Childbirth with Love*. Her insights, comments, and perceptions are profoundly appreciated. Without her the book would not have been presented in such a comprehensive and easy-to-understand form.

My deepest appreciation also goes to Lori Leeds, my secretary, assistant, and loyal friend, who also helped make the book possible through her advice and aid in refining the complete manuscript.

The research material was gathered by Zoë R. Graves, Lori Leeds, Maryellen Kurkulos, Kathleen H. Wilson, Carol Shiroky, and Anita Lessinger, who also helped assess and criticize some of the manuscript. My appreciation goes to each of them.

The original artwork was done by Laurel Purinton Rand, Pauline Thomas, Ellen Felten, Lynne Cooper, and Judith Lief. I also wish to thank Tom Saltarelli, Joan L. Wacks, and Alexander Marshall for photographic artwork.

Special thanks goes to Ellen Sadoff, Muki Held, Brenda Parush, Rosemary Jennings, Lynda Greenberg, Karen Kurtzberg, Elizabeth Morrison, Mona and Kent Costa, Ronni Verebay, Yanni Antonopoulos, Kathy Hendra, Sheila Weller, and John Kelly for sharing their childbirth experiences and contributing to research for the book.

Special acknowledgment goes to my agents Diana Price and Joyce Frommer for their support during the preparation of the manuscript.

I also wish to extend my gratitude to my legal adviser, Richard Allen, for his interest and advice on this project.

So many others have helped in countless ways that it is impossible to name them all, but I sincerely appreciate the efforts of each and every one of them.

I also want to extend my thanks to all my patients and their partners for the advice they gave me and for their patience during the preparation of *Childbirth with Love.*

Finally, my gratitude goes to Diane Reverand and Sara Uman, senior editors on this project, for their criticism, understanding, and professional talent. They worked hard to make the book clear and comprehensive.

I would also like to extend my gratitude to the entire staff at G. P. Putnam's Sons for their valuable assistance in the preparation of this book.

NIELS H. LAUERSEN, M.D.

To the health and happiness of
all unborn children

Contents

Introduction

A few years ago, when I began planning ahead for *Childbirth with Love*, I observed my practice carefully and decided to write a book that my own patients would find useful during their pregnancies—in other words, a book designed for this new generation of women who were having babies. Most of the women who decide to have a child today make the decision only after careful thought and equally careful planning. Yes, these women and their partners still do want children, but since they have waited until a fairly late period in their lives from the point of view of childbearing, it is more important than ever for the pregnancy to be successful and satisfying. Couples who have fewer children born later in life are naturally more knowledgeable and expect more from pregnancy and childbirth. I could see from my practice how this was changing obstetrics. Women who really cared about their pregnancies were coming into my office with questions, with a need to discuss problems, and with much more awareness of what could go wrong. They made obstetrics far more challenging for the obstetrician. They also made most of the current books on obstetrics look old-fashioned, since the research was changing so quickly that many newer topics could not be found in the standard reference texts. I know that a number of questions will be on your mind during your pregnancy and hope that this book is comprehensive enough to answer them clearly and reassuringly.

One of the fascinating aspects of pregnancy is that each woman's experience is different. We can generalize to a certain extent, but your pregnancy is nonetheless personal to you. With this in mind, I have included material on the subtle differences in a so-called normal pregnancy and several chapters on pregnancies that would not be considered normal, the "high risk" group. High risk does not mean that a child will be born with a serious handicap. Women who a few years ago would have been advised never to have a child are going through successful pregnancies today because certain problems can be isolated and treated early on. A part of this change is learning to recognize potential problems for yourself, a concept you will find continually emphasized in this book. Childbirth may be associated with more gadgets and specialized tests than it used to be, but the care you take and the environment you create for your unborn child are of preeminent importance in any pregnancy.

This new attitude toward pregnancy is what led me to choose the title, *Childbirth with Love*. We are perhaps only just beginning to realize the extent to which our environment and our actions affect our children's lives before they are born. This is not to lay an impossible burden on parents, but it is meant for us to understand that we need to care for, indeed love, our children before they are born in order to create the best possible prenatal environment for them. I am not talking about specialized equipment or knowledge beyond the reach of an intelligent, caring parent. Loving the baby from the moment of conception on is expressed by taking care of yourself and investing time and thought in your pregnancy. You will then be doing all that you can to create a prenatal environment in which your child will thrive. A child who is cared for in this way has, I believe, the best chance of a healthy and happy postnatal existence. If we are to have children only when we want them, we can indeed plan ahead, take responsibility, invest in our pregnancies. I look forward to delivering many more babies whose parents believe in childbirth with love.

☐ *Note*   For the purpose of simplicity, the author has almost consistently chosen to designate the hypothetical obstetrician in this book with the male gender pronouns—he, his, him. This gender usage should not be viewed as a political or chauvinistic choice, but rather as a means to greater clarification—making it easier to distinguish between the patient, who is always a *she*, and the obstetrician. Another factor is that currently more than 90 percent of all obstetrical specialists are men, a situation that will change, we hope, as an increasing number of women choose this profession. In this book the fetus is also referred to as *he* to make a clear distinction between the unborn child and his mother, who will always be a *she*. Of course, that is incorrect from a scientific point of view since slightly more than 50 percent of all newborns are baby girls.

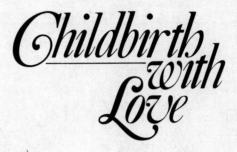

1

Planning Ahead

Nothing is more gratifying and fulfilling than the birth of a healthy child. The arrival of a first baby marks an extraordinary moment—the result sometimes of many years of planning and waiting. Some men and women will say that this is the event that finally marks their arrival into adulthood, when they stop being the sons and daughters of their own parents and become the fathers and mothers of a new generation.

Our attitudes toward having children change throughout our lives. In our teens and early twenties we usually want to avoid pregnancy. When we marry, the idea of having children remains irrelevant for many of us. We want to make a home, finish our education, become successful. The possibility of having a child is postponed for the future—something that might happen someday. We are used to thinking that our bodies are perfect, that when we want to get around to childbearing, we can always do so. Unfortunately it isn't that simple. I have treated many couples who have found that when they desire children later in life, their bodies do not function on command, because they have waited too long or they have neglected to take care of themselves in the past. If both women and men took care of their bodies from an early age and participated in their own health care, they would keep the health and strength they had when they were younger. Try early in life to get in tune with your body, to understand how your own body works. Don't take risks. However farfetched the idea of having a family may be during your teens, almost everyone, at some time in life, reaches a phase in which a child suddenly seems "the next step." Your body as well as your mind needs to be able to say yes to this. If you have used the right kinds of contraception, if you have never had venereal disease or have had the good sense to treat it immediately, and if you don't smoke or drink heavily, your body will be prepared for a child when you are ready. But you need to think about it now.

This chapter is a guide to planning ahead for a healthy child. At whatever stage of life you may be, you need to know how to protect your fertility and how to be attuned to your body.

☐ *Can You Ever Have a Child?*   Both women and men think about this at least occasionally. There have been so many stories about infertile couples that people with no intention of having a child for a while may suddenly be quite concerned about their fertility. Men or women in their thirties are probably more powerfully affected by this fear, but younger people too may feel it. The question of fertility, or rather infertility, is a real one. Some gynecologists with large practices report that as many as 25 percent of their patients come to them with fertility problems.

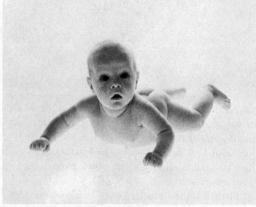

Figure 1: Will I Ever Be a Parent? Both women and men occasionally wonder about their role as future parents. *Photo by Tana Hoban, New York, N.Y.*

A number of fears, often quite unfounded, persist. Women who have been using certain kinds of contraception for a long time and who have never been pregnant often wonder if their reproductive capacity has been damaged. Other women, who have had one or more abortions, may feel guilty about the possible harm they have done to their bodies and fear they may not be able to conceive in the future. Many, many women who have had vaginal infections of some kind over the years see a horror story in a magazine that convinces them they are infertile.

Men are increasingly concerned about their fertility too, although they are sometimes more reticent about it than a woman might be. If you walk quietly into the laboratory of a medical school, you may come across a student intently examining a slide under a microscope, and if the student appears *really* absorbed, he is very possibly counting his own sperm. But older men are more likely to be concerned than younger ones, unless a young man has something in his medical history that would indicate a problem—mumps in adolescence, a childhood history of undescended testicles, varicose veins around the testicles, or DES taken by his mother when she was pregnant with him, for instance. As a man grows older, he may be afraid that his potency is decreasing or that his semen is diminishing in amount, or he may be aware of the large number of cases of infertility in which the male partner seems to be the problem.

☐ *When Should a Couple Begin to Plan a Family?* When a couple thinks ahead to childbearing, one of the most important considerations they have to take into account is their age. Unfortunately, this is inescapable. Plans to have children very often do not fit into the early years of a marriage, because both husband and wife are much more interested in finishing their education or pursuing a career, but childbearing can't be postponed indefinitely. Age affects the fertility of both men and women.

Fertility specialists often see older couples who are "subfertile." There is nothing really wrong with either of them, but the woman's ovulation patterns may be irregular, and the man's sperm count may be barely normal. Put together, these factors make conception just that much more difficult. When a couple is older they need to give themselves enough time to conceive, even if it means trying for a baby a year or two before they really want to give birth. Even for a young couple, it can take as long as a year to achieve conception.

☐ *What Is the Best Age to Have a Baby?* Ironically, teenagers, who are considered in our culture to be the most undesirable parents of all, are in their most fertile years. After a girl's menstrual period has become fully established—usually about two years after menstruation begins—her fertility is at the highest it will ever be in her lifetime. Her chances of pregnancy are increased because she is likely to have sex partners who are also fertile. A young man of eighteen or twenty usually has a very high sperm count—again, probably the highest he will ever achieve—and an aggressive sex drive as well. It is not at all surprising, then, that a teenage girl who doesn't use contraception conscientiously has a more than 50 percent chance of becoming pregnant in the first three months of a sexual relationship.

Fertility patterns have changed dramatically in the last century. Two hundred years ago, many women didn't start to menstruate until they were in their late teens, and so did not become fertile until they reached their early twenties. Only the daughters of well-off families could expect to become fertile when they were very young. This pattern changed when poor people as well as the middle class and the rich ate decently and had reasonably clean places in which to live. Better food and living conditions pushed the age of menarche (the first menstrual period) down from the late teens to the early teens, and an American girl can now expect her first period when she is eleven or twelve.

Fertility decreases very slightly when a woman is in her early twenties, but only from the unusually high point of the teenage years. In the United States, older books on pregnancy assume that a woman's early twenties are *the* proper time to have a first baby. Biologically speaking, this is a good time for a woman to conceive. A woman in her teens may be slightly more fertile, but her body is sometimes too immature to carry a child successfully. A teenager's pelvic bones may not yet have grown to their full extent to allow for the easy passage of a baby—which is why so many teenage mothers end up with a Cesarean section. Once a woman is in her twenties, her body is mature. She is probably in good shape physically and will find it easy both to conceive and to carry a baby. If her partner is about the same age, he is also highly fertile.

Unfortunately, our biological and our social arrangements sometimes do not fit one another exactly. Many American women still have their first babies in their early twenties or late teens, and may have completed their whole families by the time they are twenty-five. But an increasing number of men and women wait for a few more years before they have children.

As long as they don't wait too long, they will probably have no trouble in establishing a family. A recent major study indicates that a woman's fertility decreases really quite slowly until the age of thirty-five and then drops abruptly. Dr. Christopher Tietze of the World Population Council indicates that one in ten *previously* fertile women will be infertile by the age of thirty-five, one in three by age forty, and seven women out of eight will be infertile by the time they are forty-five. So if a woman is in her late twenties, she can reasonably assume that she is perfectly able to have a child. A few medical problems may be beginning to show themselves, but she is probably still as fit physically for a baby (and perhaps much more so emotionally) as she was in her early twenties. For many women this is the best age of all to have a child.

The maternal urge felt by so many childless women around their thirtieth birthday is prompted by the inescapable fact that it is more difficult to have a first baby after the middle thirties. If a woman's husband is slightly older than she is, his most fertile years are coming to an end as well. This is why it's really important to think and plan ahead once you are thirty or older. One of my patients who came to see me a few days after her thirtieth birthday expressed this very well. She told me how depressed she was because she was sure she could feel her eggs shriveling up in her ovaries (this was exactly how she put it). When I sympathized with her feelings and told her that if she wanted children she shouldn't wait too much longer, she replied that she and her husband were too busy and it "wasn't quite the right time to begin a family." I could only suggest that she would always be too busy and the time would never be right. "When you want something badly enough, you'll go after it, even if everything isn't perfect." Two years later I helped her and her husband deliver a beautiful, healthy son.

Ambitious couples who have waited deliberately until specifically this point in their careers to have a baby and then find it takes much longer to conceive than they thought it would, may be desperately upset by their infertility, however temporary it proves to be. If an older couple understands that conception is not quite so easy, the waiting period may become easier to bear. I always advise older couples not to delay too long before seeing an infertility specialist if they are having problems conceiving. I often recommend their going to a specialist after six months of trying rather than waiting for a year, which is the normal recommendation.

Some women in their thirties begin to develop signs of medical problems, such as hypertension or diabetes, but most women who are planning for a first baby enjoy good health at this age. If you are thirty or over, the chances are very good that you will have an easy and successful pregnancy, but a first pregnancy at this age may still be more taxing than it would be for a younger woman. The tissues are naturally stiffer, the blood flow to the uterus is diminished, the risk of giving birth prematurely is greater, and the birth itself may be more difficult. This may confound many a carefully conceived plan for the perfect pregnancy. There are women in this age group who spend the last three months of their pregnancies flat on their backs in bed instead of working, or who find it more difficult to bounce back to work immediately after childbirth. You would be wise to take account of this in making your plans.

This is particularly true if a woman is *over* thirty-five—which still does not mean that she cannot become pregnant very successfully at this age. It is very important to understand that the pregnancy *may* have more problems, and a woman should try to get herself into good physical shape before pregnancy to make the pregnancy itself easier. Her obstetrician is likely to watch her much more carefully, particularly if this is a first baby, because of the high incidence of such complications as toxemia, which is very prevalent in teenage pregnancies but also occurs when the mother is older. The amniocentesis test is now recommended for women over thirty-five, although the statistics for Down's syndrome babies only rise dramatically after a woman is forty.

An increasing number of women are giving birth successfully to first babies at an age that obstetricians only a few years ago would have considered quite abnormal, and they are enjoying their pregnancies as well. However, if a woman feels that she is fertile enough to risk waiting until she is over thirty-five, she must consider her husband's age as well. After the age of forty a man's fertility decreases significantly. There have also been studies that show that the risk of congenital malformations increases slightly if the father is over forty. Sperm quality as well as quantity changes as a man grows older, although many men father perfectly healthy children later on in life.

If this is a first baby, a woman's chances of conception after forty are decidedly slender. Ovulation tends to be irregular by that time. When a woman is forty, her eggs are also forty, which increases the risk of miscarriage and malformations of the fetus. However, a woman who has kept herself in good physical shape throughout her life can, with proper medical care, still have a child safely, even though she may need much more rest during the pregnancy than a woman of twenty would. If a previously infertile woman finds herself suddenly pregnant in her early forties, and she is healthy and wants the child, there is absolutely no reason not to go ahead with the pregnancy.

If you are now thinking of having a child and you are uneasy about your age, you will have to weigh many factors very carefully. But unless you wait for an inordinately long time, the fertility statistics are on your side. Many couples find out about their infertility in their twenties, when age is not a consideration at all. A woman who has a serious problem with her Fallopian tubes or who rarely ovulates may well have been infertile from her teenage years on. A man may have some congenital malformation that prevents him from producing healthy sperm. Fertility is not just a question of age. Nonetheless, a first pregnancy over forty would definitely place a woman in the high-risk category. She would be advised to consult a specialist in high-risk pregnancies and look for a hospital that is equipped to deal with births to older mothers.

☐ ***How Can a Man Tell if He Is Fertile?***   Assuming a man has a normal sex life with no history of prolonged impotence, there is no simple way for him to tell if he is fertile except by having his doctor take a sperm count. A man in his thirties or older who has never impregnated a woman but knows he would like to have children might be advised to have a sperm count. Sperm are definitely affected by age. After the most fertile time, at about eighteen, the sperm count decreases slowly until a man is about thirty, when it begins to drop quite sharply. A man who wants to postpone having children until well after his fortieth birthday might even consider storing his sperm.

In 25–40 percent of infertility cases (the discrepancy depends on which fertility expert is consulted) the man is discovered to be the infertile partner. The incidence of male infertility is definitely rising. But most men, like most women, *don't* encounter any problems in having children, and a man who is healthy and takes care of his body properly is doing a great deal to make sure he has healthy sperm as well.

Sperm are far more sensitive to their environment than doctors, or laymen themselves, once believed. When a man smokes, drinks, comes into contact with chemicals or pesticides, or takes drugs, these substances directly affect his sperm count and the sperm themselves. Just because the testes manufacture a constant supply of sperm, it doesn't mean you can be absolutely sure of their quality or their quantity.

☐ *Planning Ahead for Pregnancy*   A woman who has not yet had a child or even been pregnant but who looks forward to having a baby either "someday" or in the very near future, need not be afraid to check some important clues to her own fertility. This can be done very easily, even though you cannot be 100 percent sure that you are fertile until you are actually pregnant. I would strongly encourage any woman, whatever her future plans, to understand how her body works, how different kinds of contraception act on the body, and how to test for normal functioning.

You need to consider your personal medical history—what has happened in the past, what contraception you have used, how your menstrual cycle works, any serious disorders you may have had—and then test yourself to see if you are ovulating properly. If you do this conscientiously, you should have a very good picture of the present state of your fertility.

☐ *Your Personal Medical History*   It is important to think carefully about what has happened to you medically in your lifetime. If you can't remember it all, ask your mother or go through your old diaries. Then write down your medical history, so that you can furnish yourself with clues to your fertility.

The first prenatal visit always includes a work-up of your family as well as your personal medical history, so you should be prepared with this information. If there is a personal or family history of any major medical disorder, such as high blood pressure or diabetes, you should be aware that if you become pregnant, your pregnancy may need to be monitored very carefully. This does *not* mean that you should not think about childbearing, but it does mean you should consult a doctor who is skilled in taking care of high-risk pregnancies (see Chap. 6).

☐ *VD and Fertility*   In reviewing your history, try to be absolutely honest with yourself. If you have had a venereal disease in the past, this may be a significant factor when you are trying to become pregnant.

Syphilis is very rare, fortunately. Since active syphilis in a pregnant woman will seriously damage the fetus as well as the mother, a pregnant woman is routinely given a syphilis test (VDRL) at her first prenatal visit.

Gonorrhea, which has reached epidemic proportions, is disturbingly common among women in the fertile years. Unfortunately, a woman can harbor gonorrhea for a long time without realizing that her internal sexual organs may be suffering serious damage. A gonorrheal infection can travel into the uterus from the genital organs and move into the Fallopian tubes, causing infection and damage to the tubes themselves. This may also lead to a serious condition called pelvic inflammatory disease (PID), which can severely scar the tubes, cause pelvic adhesions, and quite often result in infertility. If you have had gonorrhea and were treated immediately with penicillin injections, the chance of permanent damage is less. If the disease was untreated or undetected, the resulting problems might be serious.

Gonorrhea is a common cause of infertility in women. It is so harmful that it is wise for any woman who has sexual relations with a man she does not know well to ask her doctor or a clinic to run a gonorrhea culture immediately. Even if you are tested and the results are negative, your peace of mind makes the money spent on the test a very wise investment. If you are concerned about possible damage to your Fallopian tubes from a past infection, you can arrange to undergo an X-ray of the uterus and Fallopian tubes (a hysterosalpingogram) to verify if your internal organs are in working order. The procedure for a hysterosalpingogram is described later on in this chapter.

Over 50 percent of women have had a vaginal infection of some kind in their reproductive years. These common vaginal infections, such as monilia or trichomonas, may also be sexually transmitted, but they do not threaten the internal organs. However, if you are trying to conceive right now, you should check with your doctor and have even a minor vaginal infection treated immediately. The infection may be acid enough to kill any sperm outright and so prevent conception. A herpes infection, by the way, will not interfere with conception, nor will an active case of herpes damage the conceptus or the fetus.

☐ *The Pill and Future Fertility*   Next you should take a hard look at your means of contraception over the years. If you use or have used birth control pills, there does *not*—despite stories to the contrary—seem to be a higher incidence of infertility after the use of the pill. Indeed, most women who take birth control pills will continue the same menstrual pattern after they discontinue the pill as they had before they began using it. Some women may simply find it takes a few months for menstruation to start again with regularity. Several recent studies have indicated that if a woman has taken a birth control pill with the lowest possible estrogen dose (at least less than 50 mcg [micrograms]), has been checked regularly by her doctor, and had normal menstruation before she started the pill, the chance of any permanent damage is minimal. If she plans to conceive immediately, her doctor should take her off an oral contraceptive for a few months before conception, to make sure that all the hormones are out of her body. This will prevent the slight risk of fetal abnormality or miscarriage the pill poses.

☐ *Your Chances of Conception After an IUD*   The use of an intrauterine device (IUD) can be a much more serious problem as far as a woman's fertility is concerned. The IUD was very popular in the early 1970s, when women became alarmed about the side effects of oral contraception. However, doctors did not fully appreciate the possible side effects of the IUD itself. It is now known that women who have used intrauterine devices, particularly women with several sex partners, have a decidedly higher incidence of infection as a result of using the device, and such infections can have damaging results if they are not taken care of immediately. The infection from an IUD may move into the Fallopian tubes and cause serious damage, with resulting infertility in some cases. If you had infection problems with the IUD but visited a doctor immediately, had the intrauterine device removed, and were promptly treated with antibiotics, there is probably no reason to be alarmed. Any damaging scarring of the Fallopian tubes is likely to result only if the symptoms of a serious infection are ignored. (Again, this does not mean monilia or trichomonas, which you may also be more susceptible to if you have an intrauterine device.) If you know you did have an infection at some point, but you are not quite sure whether it was monilia or something more serious, find out from your doctor what type it was and what kind of antibiotics you were treated with. There is no need to become alarmed unnecessarily, and there is certainly no reason to jump to any conclusions immediately about your fertility or infertility. But any woman who has ever worn an IUD should be aware that a "silent" infection and tubal damage is always a possibility.

An Important Note: The chances of an ectopic pregnancy (a pregnancy outside the uterus) are higher after IUD use. If you have ever worn an IUD, monitor the beginning of your pregnancy carefully. Any bleeding or pain should be reported immediately to your doctor (see Chap. 21).

☐ *Barrier Methods and Fertility*   There are no known side effects to any of the barrier methods of contraception: the diaphragm, the cervical cap, contraceptive foams, or suppositories. However, the failure rate for these methods is definitely higher than for the IUD or the pill, which is probably the reason for the rise in the abortion rate in the last few years.

☐ *Previous Abortion in Relation to Childbearing*   If you have had an abortion, you may be very concerned that this will affect your chances of a successful pregnancy. You can, however, look at the situation positively in one respect: you were able to conceive once, and so the chance of conceiving again should be that much higher. If the abortion was carried out early in pregnancy in a good clinic or hospital and under sterile conditions, it is very unlikely that any permanent harm has been done. If, however, you experienced an infection after the abortion or heavy bleeding, a tubal infection might have occurred as a result of the abortion. You should be concerned about the aftereffects of a single abortion only if complications did result from it.

If a woman has had several abortions, this might cause trauma and scarring of the cervix, resulting in an incompetent cervix. A federal study is being conducted in hospitals and clinics throughout the U.S. at this time to determine just what the long-term effect of abortion may be on a woman's future childbearing.

So-called intrauterine adhesions, in which tissues in the uterine cavity become stuck together, can also be caused by an abortion or abortions. This condition will interfere with the implantation of the fertile egg in the uterus and result in infertility. (Pelvic or abdominal adhesions that may bind the Fallopian tubes and the ovaries so that conception cannot occur can also be the result of a previous appendectomy or another abdominal operation. It is important to check your surgical history with your doctor.) So far the evidence points to the fact that women who have had multiple abortions encounter more problems in future pregnancies that are carried to term than women who have had one abortion or none. The cervix (the neck of the womb) may have been weakened, and there is a greater possibility of miscarriage and premature birth.

The back-street abortions of the prelegal days caused many women to end up with severe tubal infections that damaged their fertility permanently. Occasionally, too, a uterus was torn apart so it was impossible for a woman to hold on to a child, and miscarriage and premature delivery resulted. If you suffered serious complications in the past from an illegal abortion, do not automatically assume you are infertile, but be sure to consult a competent infertility specialist. The damage may be reversible.

The most important clue to your fertility may be your menstrual cycle. You should first ask yourself at what age you started to menstruate and when your menstruation became regular. Since the pattern of your menstruation is very important to you if you plan to have children, you should start to keep a record every month. After a few months you will probably be able to see if it follows a steady pattern (remembering that many women normally have a cycle that varies from the "average" twenty-eight-day one). If you have been skipping a month here and there, try to determine if there was any reason for it—stress, travel, or a new job, for instance. You should also note frequency and intensity of pain.

☐ **Bleeding Disorders and the Possibility of Surgery**   If a woman gives evidence of irregular bleeding or amenorrhea (an absence of menstruation), either of these certainly could interfere with the possibility of conception. Irregular bleeding can be caused by endocrine problems (difficulties in the way the hormones function)—which should be evaluated by an endocrinologist—or may be the result of noncancerous cysts or fibroid tumors growing on the uterus. The latter are very common, especially as a woman approaches the age of thirty, and may occasionally be a barrier to conception. Your doctor should inform you as a matter of course if he or she finds any fibroid tumors during a routine checkup and tell you where they are located and how large they are. Often they can be removed surgically if they appear to be preventing conception.

Irregular bleeding should not be confused with an irregular menstrual cycle. A woman's normal menstrual cycle should last anywhere between twenty-three to thirty-three days, but even for a woman whose cycle is regular, one out of every ten periods are anovulatory (without ovulation). This usually occurs when the period is a little late or if there is a long period of bleeding.

☐ **Can You Become Pregnant if You Don't Menstruate?**   Amenorrhea, which is fairly unusual in adult women, is a serious condition, but it does not mean that a woman cannot become pregnant, especially if she menstruated earlier in her life. If she has had periods before, and has suddenly stopped bleeding (and is not pregnant), there could be many reasons, which should be checked with a doctor. For instance, if a woman gains or loses more than ten pounds, this can interfere with the interaction of the brain and the hormones in the ovaries, and her menstruation will cease. Extreme tension may also cause periods to stop.

There is a long list of complex endocrine dysfunctions that can be the cause of amenorrhea.

☐ *Sports and Fertility* If you are athletic you may find that this has an effect on your periods, and they may even cease if your training program is very strenuous. Amenorrhea is a quite natural physical reaction under such circumstances since a woman who is pushing herself physically needs to carry more oxygen, and her blood count and oxygen capacity are automatically increased if she does not menstruate. By the same token, male athletes often have a lower sperm count during competitions. If you suspect that your menstruation is being affected by your athletic program and you want to become pregnant, you can decrease the amount of exercise. This should help to regulate your ovulation patterns.

If, however, your history of amenorrhea goes back to your adolescence, you should definitely see a specialist and have a thorough work-up to detect any abnormalities in your uterus or in the way your endocrine system works. Women who do not menstruate until they are twenty should also see a specialist if they want to become pregnant, because a late menarche may indicate the same problems.

☐ *Endometriosis and Future Fertility* If you have very severe pain or even moderate pain during the onset of your periods, and your menstrual cramps begin even before you start to bleed and are very painful when you do, the situation should not be ignored or passed over as "normal." If you find that you have general abdominal pain and discomfort during intercourse as well as menstrual problems, you could have a serious disorder called endometriosis. Endometriosis is a condition in which the menstrual flow (the uterine lining—the endometrium) is pushed backward through the Fallopian tubes and into the abdomen. Once there, it begins to form into tumorlike growths, which can also spread to the ovaries and the Fallopian tubes and which continue to increase in size each month under a woman's natural hormone stimulation. The result of severe endometriosis can be infertility, because the growths can become large enough to interfere with ovulation and so make conception very difficult or even impossible.

Endometriosis is often called the "career woman's disease," not because, as some doctors claim, women with a demanding job are under peculiar and "unfeminine" stress, but because the longer childbearing is postponed, the greater the chance for the endometrial tissues to spread and grow as the months pass. It is essential to treat endometriosis as early as possible, because it causes women such distress and, ultimately, infertility. It appears to be a major factor in the difficulty some women experience in becoming pregnant, particularly if they wait until later in life to have their children.

At present only one drug, Danocrine (danazol), is approved by the Food and Drug Administration for the treatment of endometriosis. This drug is very effective when taken daily for six to nine months. Birth control pills are not approved in the management of endometriosis (see Chap. 3).

☐ *Are the Internal Organs in Order?* If a woman has suffered from a pelvic infection in the past, VD, pelvic inflammatory disease, or problems after an abortion, she may be concerned that her uterus or the Fallopian tubes have been damaged. In such a case her fears can best be alleviated by checking the condition of these organs through a special test called a hysterosalpingogram, an X-ray of the uterus and Fallopian tubes. It is impossible for your doctor to tell from a routine checkup whether or not permanent damage has been done to the Fallopian tubes. If you are at all uneasy, it would be wise for you to undergo a hysterosalpingogram and put your mind at rest rather than live unnecessarily with the fear of infertility. This procedure is described fully in Chapter 3.

☐ ***Where to Start***   Obviously I have not been able to give a complete list of physical and medical conditions that affect pregnancy, and you should note down any other significant medical problems that have occurred in your life. Whether you are hoping to become pregnant immediately or not, it would be advisable for you to go over your personal medical history with your doctor at your next visit. Give him the complete history; tell him what has happened to you in the past (if you have been shy about doing this up to now), and ask him for his honest opinion of your chances of conception. If your gynecologist doesn't want to answer you and doesn't seem to understand your concern, you might want to look elsewhere for your gynecological care. You need a doctor you can completely trust and communicate with honestly.

☐ ***How Can You Tell if You Are Fertile?***   The most important thing a woman can do to confirm her fertility is to establish whether or not she is ovulating. A woman who does not ovulate regularly is not as fertile as a woman who ovulates almost every month. Ovulation is obviously vital to a woman's ability to conceive, but it is a delicate and precise occurrence, which can be affected adversely by any number of factors. The first step toward understanding why you do or do not ovulate is to familiarize yourself with the complex hormonal patterns of the menstrual cycle.

☐ ***The Menstrual Cycle***   The simplest way to find out whether you are ovulating is by examining yourself during the normal monthly cycle. From the beginning to the end of the cycle the body goes through some important and quite detectable changes.

As soon as the menstrual period starts, the hormone interaction between the brain and the ovaries begins afresh. The first day of menstruation is usually referred to as day one. At this time all the hormone levels go down to zero. If a woman has had discomfort before her period, she usually feels better now. There is a sense of relief as bleeding begins. The body feels less bloated—which has nothing to do with the bleeding per se. At this point the body eliminates its excess water and gas as the female hormones—the progesterone and estrogen hormones—decrease. The hormone levels remain at this low point for two or three days.

On the third or fourth day after the onset of menstruation the pituitary gland in the brain begins to release hormones, which, in turn, stimulate the release of the first gonadotropin hormone, the follicle-stimulating hormone FSH. (Follicles are cells in the ovaries that may develop into mature eggs.) After menstruation is over, the woman's vagina will feel relatively dry for a few days. Thick cervical mucus blocks the cervical canal, and the neck of the cervix is closed and points backward. This makes it difficult for sperm to enter into the internal organs.

As the egg follicles in the ovaries start to develop in size under the influence of FSH, the production of estrogen also increases. Estrogen is the hormone that controls the ovulation timetable. It helps to mature the egg follicles, it develops the endometrium, and it influences the cervical mucus. This heightened estrogen level reaches its highest point immediately before ovulation. By this time *one* follicle in *one* ovary has grown considerably larger than the others and has developed into a so-called Graafian follicle, a follicle capable of releasing a mature egg. The endometrium in the uterus is sufficiently developed to provide shelter for a fertilized egg, and the cervical mucus changes to encourage the penetration of sperm into the cervix. A woman's body is ready for ovulation to occur (Fig. 2).

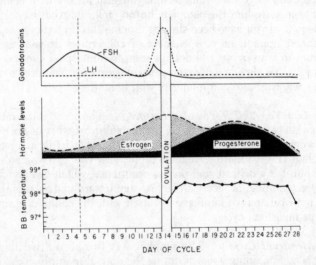

Figure 2: Hormone Variation During Menstrual Cycle: This graph illustrates the relationship between the brain hormones (gonadotropins), the ovarian hormones, estrogen, and progesterone, and their influence on the basal body temperature (BBT). The top curve illustrates the fluctuation in the follicle-stimulating hormone (FSH) and the luteinizing hormone (LH) during the menstrual cycle. The middle curve indicates the variation in estrogen and progesterone during the cycle. The bottom curve indicates the fluctuation in the BBT. Day 1 marks the first day of a menstrual bleeding. Immediately after menstruation has begun the amount of FSH increases, which in turn stimulates the estrogen production from the ovaries. The estrogen in turn will prime the cervix and increase the cervical mucus in preparation for ovulation. When the estrogen reaches a peak, it will trigger the release of LH, which will trigger ovulation. LH will increase for only one day. After ovulation, estrogen and progesterone, which are produced from the corpus luteum, will again increase, and the progesterone will cause the temperature to rise, a sign that ovulation has taken place. Thus, by observing her basal body temperature, a woman can detect her time of ovulation (which is the time immediately prior to the increase in temperature). A doctor can also use the BBT to determine if the hormone-producing corpus luteum is adequate for pregnancy. If the temperature drops during the last two weeks of the menstrual cycle, it might be an indication of inadequate progesterone production.

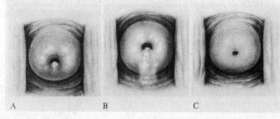

A   B   C

Figure 3: The Cervical Mucus: The cervical mucus changes throughout the menstrual cycle. The position of the cervix and the openness of the cervical canal (the connection between the vagina and the uterus) changes as well during the cycle. Immediately after a menstrual period, the cervix is pointed backward and there is no cervical mucus, or only a minimal amount (A).

A few days before ovulation, the cervical mucus will increase in amount. At the same time the cervix begins to point forward and the cervical opening widens in order to facilitate sperm penetration (B). By examining herself, a woman can feel the increased amount of mucus. This is the point where a woman is most fertile.

After ovulation, as the progesterone level in the body increases, the mucus becomes smaller in amount. The cervical opening closes and the cervix again points backward (C). This makes it impossible for sperm to penetrate the cervix.

Reproduced by permission of Little, Brown and Company, Inc., from Progress in Infertility *(Boston, Mass., 1968).*

At this point in the menstrual cycle a woman's vagina will feel much "wetter" than it did earlier. In fact, the amount of cervical mucus increases ten times over the middle of the cycle. The cervical secretion becomes thin and slippery, and if a woman traps some mucus between her fingers, she will find it stretches out in a long, thin ribbon. This extraordinary stretching ability is called *spinnbarkeit*, and the more pronounced it is, the higher the estrogen level and the greater the chance of ovulation. This thin cervical mucus allows the sperm to penetrate easily into the cervix and move up into the Fallopian tubes to meet the mature egg. If a woman examines herself internally at this point by inserting a finger in her vagina, she will be able to feel the increased wetness and a distinct change in her cervix. The cervical canal now points forward and is open to attract sperm (Fig. 3).

The increased mucus and the open cervix are sure signs that ovulation is about to take place. A woman may feel some other symptoms too. Sometimes a mild backache or a dull cramping will accompany ovulation, while a few women experience quite severe abdominal pain. This pain, *mittelschmerz* (a German word meaning "pain in the middle of the month") is unpleasant but not dangerous in any way, and it does not affect your ability to conceive. *Mittelschmerz* may cause some slight vaginal bleeding as well as pain, which can be alarming, but this is only the result of ovulatory fluid and a small amount of blood spilled into the abdomen as well as the changing contraction patterns of the uterus. Although some women find this time of month very trying, you can look on the unpleasant side effects of *mittelschmerz* in a new light: at least it will sharply remind you that you are ovulating.

You may have much pleasanter associations with the middle of your menstrual cycle. The peak estrogen levels usually increase a woman's feeling of general well-being; her skin will be clearer and her energy level higher toward the middle of the month. Often sexual pleasure is heightened around the time of ovulation, and women experience an increased desire for sexual relations and a heightened enjoyment of lovemaking.

Any sign of ovulation that you experience should be very reassuring if you are planning to have a baby in the near future or simply want to know that you are ovulating regularly. (If you are perfectly in tune with your body, as some women are, you may even be able to feel whether you are about to ovulate from the right or the left ovary.) Try to check yourself every month for a few months by doing a simple internal examination, and note down your ovulation pattern.

As the estrogen level increases a day or two before ovulation actually occurs, it results in a feedback mechanism to the pituitary gland, and this decreases the level of the FSH. The estrogen level has now reached a point at which the egg and the other changes in the body are ripe for ovulation. The estrogen then triggers the brain to release the luteinizing hormone (LH), which acts in a rapid surge to release the mature egg from the Graafian follicle. This is the precise moment of ovulation. As the egg is released from the ovary, the fimbriated (fringed) ends of the Fallopian tube next to the ovary reach up to catch the egg and guide it into the tube. Once it is safely in the tube, the cilia (fine, hairlike projections in the walls of the Fallopian tubes) slowly move the egg farther up toward the uterus (Fig. 4).

After the mature egg is released from its follicle, the cells in the ruptured Graafian follicle rapidly transform themselves into hormone-producing cells of another type. These cells in turn begin to grow together into a small cluster

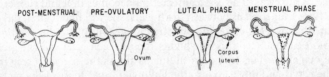

POST-MENSTRUAL   PRE-OVULATORY   LUTEAL PHASE   MENSTRUAL PHASE

Ovum   Corpus luteum

Figure 4: The Menstrual Cycle: This drawing illustrates the ovaries, Fallopian tubes, and the uterus during various phases of the menstrual cycle. Immediately after menstruation (postmenstrual) the uterus is beginning to rebuild and the ovaries are at rest. As the follicle-stimulating hormone (FSH) increases, it will stimulate the development of follicles inside the ovaries. These follicles and the enlargement of the ovaries will in turn increase the estrogen level, which will prime the uterine lining and change the cervical mucus in preparation for ovulation and for permission of sperm penetration. One of the follicles will supersede the others and become the Graafian follicle, which contains the mature ovum, or egg. The Graafian follicle with its mature egg will protrude on the surface of the ovary as the fimbriated end of the Fallopian tube reaches down in preparation to catch the egg during ovulation (preovulatory).

During ovulation the ovum will be caught by the fimbriated ends and led into the Fallopian tube, where conception may take place.

After ovulation, the fimbriated end of the Fallopian tube will release its grip on the ovary, and the cells from which ovulation occur will transform into the corpus luteum (luteal phase). The corpus luteum will produce the progesterone and estrogen that are necessary to change the uterine lining in preparation for conception. If conception does not occur, the corpus luteum will disintegrate and will decrease the level of estrogen and progesterone, triggering the release of prostaglandins, which will cause the uterus to contract and menstruation to occur (menstrual phase).

called the corpus luteum (the yellow body). It is a descriptive name for this cell group because the corpus is distinctly yellow, even to the naked eye, and a gynecologist operating on a woman who has just ovulated can detect this immediately by checking the ovary. Once the moment of ovulation is over, the cells in the corpus luteum begin to produce quantities of progesterone, the second female hormone or the "hormone of pregnancy," as it directly translates from the Latin words "pro" and "gestare." A woman can detect that her progesterone level is increasing by the change in the cervical mucus. If she examines herself, she will see that the wetness and the thin slimy mucus that were quite obvious before ovulation have vanished and the vagina feels almost as dry as it did at the beginning of the cycle. The thicker secretions produced by the higher progesterone level in the second part of the cycle act as a cork or as a diaphragm would, blocking the neck of the cervix and preventing bacteria and/or other microorganisms from entering into the uterus and possibly interfering with the implantation of a fertilized egg. The cervical canal closes once again and points backward to repel sperm, as it did at the beginning of the cycle (Fig. 3).

In the second part of the cycle, progesterone acts to prepare the uterus for a possible pregnancy. The endometrium becomes more vascular to facilitate the implantation of a fertilized egg, and the uterus itself relaxes, the natural uterine contractions decreasing. This is to ensure that the egg will implant itself in the endometrium and not suffer any damaging jolts from the uterine contractions. The higher progesterone levels in the last two weeks of the menstrual cycle make a woman feel less energetic than she had been a few days earlier, and she may be hungrier, particularly for sweets. Estrogen and progesterone combine toward the end of the cycle, and this in turn has an effect on the pituitary gland, causing both LH and FSH production to decrease. The estrogen presence, combined with progesterone, results in an increased binding of sodium, and water retention is increased. The change in hormonal levels is the reason for the bloated, tired, headachy feeling a woman often has before her period begins.

If a woman does not become pregnant, the corpus luteum begins to disintegrate at the end of the menstrual cycle. This results in a sharp drop in the progesterone and estrogen levels on the twenty-seventh day of a twenty-eight day cycle, and menstruation begins on the next day. If a woman *is* pregnant, the corpus luteum continues to function, and the high level of progesterone it produces helps to prevent miscarriage and contributes to the characteristic symptoms of the first few months of pregnancy.

☐ **The Basal Body Temperature**   The basal body temperature (BBT) is a valuable aid in establishing ovulatory patterns. You do not need to go to a doctor to find out how to take your BBT. You can use an ordinary thermometer if you like, although the special ovulation thermometer available at the drugstore is more accurate in measuring the slight temperature changes involved. Taking the BBT is a simple and inexpensive way to find out if you are ovulating normally, and it is used successfully all over the world by women who are trying to conceive.

The BBT will be of value only if it is taken every day at exactly the same time of day. Take your temperature as soon as you wake up in the morning, before you even get out of bed to fetch a cup of coffee or go to the bathroom. The theory behind the BBT curve is that a woman's body maintains a certain tempera-

A Sample Basal Body Temperature Chart

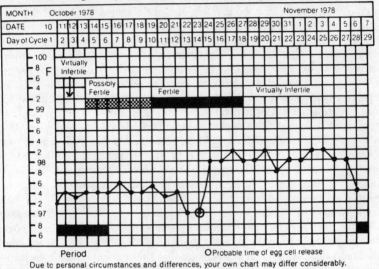

Period   O Probable time of egg cell release

Due to personal circumstances and differences, your own chart may differ considerably.

Figure 5: Basal Body Temperature (BBT) Chart: Note that the basal body temperature is low for the first twelve to thirteen days after menstruation. It then drops immediately prior to ovulation. After ovulation, progesterone will be produced in the corpus luteum in the ovary and will result in an increase in the temperature of approximately 1 degree. If the temperature remains high for more than two weeks, a woman might be pregnant. If it drops, menstruation will usually occur within one day. The bar indicates the fertile days. A woman is fertile a few days prior to ovulation and possibly one or two days after ovulation. She is virtually infertile a few days after the BBT has increased and up to the beginning of menstruation. Fertility is possible seven to eight days prior to ovulation, which is particularly important if a woman has an irregular cycle and cannot determine the exact time of ovulation.

Courtesy of Mademoiselle; *copyright* © 1978 *by The Condé Nast Publications Inc., New York, N.Y.*

ture at the same time and the same place every day as long as she is at rest. As soon as she gets out of bed and begins to walk around, her physical activity naturally increases her temperature, and the BBT will be inaccurate. If you take your temperature every morning and write it down on a temperature curve (Fig. 5), you will begin to notice a definite pattern after two or three weeks. (A rectal temperature is considered to be slightly more accurate, but some people prefer to take their temperature orally, and this is quite adequate for the purpose.) The normal temperature during and after menstruation is about 97.5 degrees Fahrenheit. Immediately after ovulation, the increased progesterone level will result in an increased body temperature of about one degree. This means that within one day after you ovulate, your BBT will rise from 97.5 to 98.5. This rise in temperature clearly indicates that ovulation has occurred. You can check yourself further by examining the cervical mucus, which will feel dryer and thicker once ovulation has taken place. The high progesterone level in the last two weeks of the menstrual cycle keeps the BBT at approximately the same temperature until menstruation begins.

You may see some small natural fluctuations in temperature all through the cycle, but you should not have any difficulty in distinguishing a regular pattern and making up your own BBT chart. Take your BBT for at least two to three consecutive months to make sure you ovulate every month; you can then establish your basal body curve and use it to determine the best time for conception. If you find it difficult to interpret your BBT or you seem to have unaccountable irregularities in your ovulation patterns, take your BBT curve to your doctor. In a normal twenty-eight-day cycle you should ovulate the thirteenth or fourteenth day after the onset of the first day of menstruation.

☐ *You Seem to Be Fertile: What Should You Do Next?*   If you are healthy and fit, your menstrual cycle is regular, ovulation signs all appear normal, and you have never had any serious medical problems, you probably don't need to do anything except see your gynecologist regularly and take care of yourself. Simply assume you are fertile until proven otherwise.

☐ *You Think You May Have a Problem: Could You Have a Sluggish Thyroid Gland?*   If you feel that your ovulation patterns are abnormal or you have irregular menstrual bleeding, you should definitely have your thyroid function tested. The thyroid gland produces hormones that closely interact with the brain hormones and can seriously upset the ovulation cycle. If a woman's thyroid hormones are low, there are other symptoms too: fatigue, decreased sex desire, hair loss, and a weight gain that has nothing to do with eating habits. Your doctor can take a blood test and put you on a thyroid medication that will not only make you feel better but will increase your chances of conception, because the thyroid hormones interact intimately with the pituitary hormones. A family history of thyroid problems is also a decided indication for a routine thyroid test even if you have no symptoms.

☐ *The Problem May Be Stress*   Emotional and physical stress, as well as travel, job change, and various other factors, can definitely alter the menstrual cycle. There is a close and delicate relationship between your emotions and the brain hormones that govern ovulation. If a woman is tense or under unusual stress, the hormones are not released, the ovaries do not function properly, and ovulation does not take place. Stress also affects the delicate transmittal signs from the pituitary to the ovaries which trigger menstruation. A woman who is tense or upset emotionally may find that her periods become irregular, or they may even stop altogether. Some researchers have speculated that stress may also alter the transport time a fertilized egg usually takes to travel down the Fallopian tube and into the uterus. If this time is speeded up or slowed down, it may prevent the egg from being implanted in the uterus and impede a successful conception.

Menstrual irregularity caused by stress is not at all uncommon. Some women who regularly take their basal body temperatures report that ovulation is often suppressed when they are under severe pressure or are experiencing marital difficulties. If you think the stresses of your job or your relationship or anything else may be affecting your ovulation pattern, look very carefully for ways to ease the tension you are under, especially if you hope to become pregnant soon.

☐   **What Is the Best Contraception for You Right Now?**   When you choose any form of contraception, be sure you know what it does to your body, and particularly what it will do to your fertility. Get to know all the pros and cons of the contraception so you can monitor yourself to be certain that nothing goes wrong.

Contraception needs change with age. If a teenager decides she is ready for sex, she should also be ready to assume the responsibility of obtaining contraception. Recent extensive studies in California (the Walnut Creek studies) have indicated that *birth control pills*—as long as a woman takes the lowest possible combination of hormones, less than 50 mcg of estrogen in connection with progesterone—are much safer than was previously assumed. The early forms of the pill used years ago contained a much higher amount of estrogen, and many of the adverse side effects reported in the last decade were undoubtedly due to that. Studies from Great Britain as well as the United States now indicate that the birth control pill is probably the safest form of contraception for a healthy young woman as long as she does not smoke excessively or have high blood pressure or diabetes.

There is one beneficial effect of the pill that a woman should be aware of: it does help to control endometriosis, a condition that often makes women infertile. While taking the pill, it is important for a woman to see her doctor twice a year and have her blood pressure checked, because one of the recognized side effects of the pill is an increase in blood pressure. If a woman does have increased blood pressure from the pill, this may be a forewarning of increased blood pressure in pregnancy too, which is known as pregnancy-related hypertension or toxemia of pregnancy. Many women will be reassured to know that pill use is not associated with increased incidence of twins or fetal abnormalities as long as there is a reasonable time between stopping the use of the pill and conceiving. In general, the birth control pill seems to be a very effective and safe contraceptive for a young woman, and will not interfere with her future fertility.

The *intrauterine device* (IUD) does seem to be associated with a higher incidence of pelvic infections, especially among women who have several sex partners. For this reason, young teenagers who are sexually very active are not the best candidates for intrauterine devices. Later in life, a woman who has only one sex partner and no history of pelvic infections and who, furthermore, is sensitive to her body, can use an IUD. However, if she experiences pain or bleeding while using the IUD, she should immediately have the device removed. Since women who have borne children seem to tolerate the device better than women who have not, the IUD may be a very good form of contraception for spacing childbearing.

The *diaphragm* has gained in popularity, mostly because women are nervous about using the pill and the IUD. The diaphragm is an excellent means of contraception if a woman is willing to use it conscientiously. Furthermore, it decreases the possibility of contracting venereal disease. The diaphragm is probably best suited to women who are married or are dating one steady partner; the problem with a diaphragm is that it is all too easily left behind in a dresser drawer just at the moment it is needed. The abortion rate is definitely higher among young unmarried women who use a diaphragm, and an abortion *may* affect a woman's future fertility.

The *cervical cap*, which is widely used in Europe but still hardly known in the

United States, may prove to be more efficient than the diaphragm. It shields the cervix more tightly than a diaphragm, and it does not have to be removed after each sexual intercourse. In the near future we will probably see a great rise in the use of the cervical cap worldwide. Other than the possibility of contraceptive failure, the diaphragm and the cervical cap have absolutely no adverse effects on a woman's fertility.

Some women use *contraceptive foams* or *foaming tablets,* such as Encare Ovals or Semicid. These contraceptives are widely available in drugstores and are often used by teenagers and young adult women. Contraceptive foams do prevent the spread of gonorrheal bacteria, but the failure rate with both these means of contraception is very high. Considering the possible adverse side effects of an abortion, the birth control pill might be the best choice for a young woman.

The *condom* is a very important method of contraception. Since a condom considerably lowers the risk of a man transmitting VD, it would be extremely sensible for a woman who is having intercourse with a man she does not know well to insist on his using a condom.

☐ *How to Plan Ahead for Pregnancy*   I began this chapter by saying that it is vital to plan ahead for pregnancy even if you believe pregnancy to be far in the future for you. Whatever you do now will affect the way you will function in the months or years to come: your bodily functions, your fertility, even your ability to control your life ten years from now. You should be as certain as possible that you will be happy in the future over the choices you make now. American women today have so few pregnancies that they demand every one be as nearly perfect as it possibly can be. Your means of contraception, your sex partners, and your health habits all have an important bearing on a good future pregnancy and childbirth.

2

Planning for Pregnancy

In the past a first pregnancy often occurred "by accident," and family planning was used to space childbearing and decide the timing of a second or third birth. Today we should rephrase the term "family planning" and instead use the phrase "planning a family." By this we mean planning ahead years in advance for the first pregnancy by taking care of our bodies and monitoring our fertility so that childbearing will be possible when a couple is ready. "Planning a family" also means making careful preparations in the months just prior to conception by evaluating and changing health habits and environment. This modern interpretation of family planning is a new concept and an extremely important one if you care not only about having a child but having a healthy one as well.

The emphasis of the first chapter of this book is on planning for childbirth even if you are not quite sure that you ever want to be pregnant. My concern that women and men should not abuse their bodies and not make the wrong choices in their lives is great because, sadly, I see so many couples who have done just this in the past and now bitterly regret it. Every woman must educate herself about her body and her fertility and learn to protect herself. Every woman and man should act on the assumption that they are going to have children at some time in their lives, no matter how they feel about parenthood when they are twenty.

When a couple finally make the decision to have a child, they begin on the second stage of "planning a family"—the important few months before conception actually takes place. For years I have encouraged my patients to regard this as a crucial time, a time to take a close look at their health, their family history, and their environment at home and at work. People who want to have a child are highly motivated to change anything in their own lives they feel may affect their unborn baby. The environment before your child's conception is not going to be perfect, however hard you try, but there are many effective changes prospective parents can make to prepare for a successful pregnancy months before conception. In fact, my own experience and the weight of recent research on conception and pregnancy indicate that it is vital to use these months sensibly.

The purpose of this chapter is to help you both plan ahead to assure that the first moments of the pregnancy itself occur under the best natural conditions.

☐ *What Is the Best Weight for Conception?*   If you are beginning to look ahead to pregnancy, consider first your weight and nutrition. A woman's ideal weight varies quite considerably according to her bone structure and ethnic background, but a healthy woman usually reaches a time in her early twenties when her weight stabilizes at a level that is right for her. Ideally, a woman will not gain or lose any significant amount of weight after she is twenty-five.

The standard actuarial weight table, which, unfortunately, has not been revised since 1960, is included here to give you a rough guide to your proper weight.

DESIRABLE WEIGHTS FOR WOMEN OF AGES 25 AND OVER*

Height (with shoes on)—2-inch heels		Weight in Pounds According to Frame (in Indoor Clothing)		
		SMALL FRAME	MEDIUM FRAME	LARGE FRAME
Feet	Inches			
4	10	92– 98	96–107	104–119
4	11	94–101	98–110	106–122
5	0	96–104	101–113	109–125
5	1	99–107	104–116	112–128
5	2	102–110	107–119	115–131
5	3	105–113	110–122	118–134
5	4	108–116	113–126	121–138
5	5	111–119	116–130	125–142
5	6	114–123	120–135	129–146
5	7	118–127	124–139	133–150
5	8	122–131	128–143	137–154
5	9	126–135	132–147	141–158
5	10	130–140	136–151	145–163
5	11	134–144	140–155	149–168
6	0	138–148	144–159	153–173

* For women between 18 and 25, subtract one pound for each year under 25.
Data from the Metropolitan Life Insurance Company, 1960.

The table is only a rough guide, because the women in the study were wearing shoes and full indoor clothing. Even taking this into account, the recommended limits are slightly higher than doctors today would consider desirable. Unless you have been very heavy or very thin all your life, you will probably be able to judge your ideal weight without relying on a chart. The ideal weight for you is the weight at which you feel best. Being too heavy or too thin upsets the regularity of a woman's menstrual cycle, especially if she is extremely underweight; it also affects her energy level and her emotions. If you are not satisfied with your present weight, try to recall a time in your life when your weight was steady, your menstruation was regular, and your energy level high. Base your desired weight loss or gain on what you weighed then.

Pregnancy may well be one of the most stressful physical events of a woman's life. This is why it is important for her to plan ahead and be physically fit before pregnancy begins. After conception she will be too busy coping with the extra physical and emotional demands of the first trimester of pregnancy to worry about dieting or strenuous exercise. In the first three months of pregnancy both the maternal blood volume and the pulse rate begin to increase, and a woman's lung capacity also expands, changing her respiration rate. These physical changes, as well as the burden of the higher hormone levels, contribute considerably to the exhausted feeling women often experience during the first trimester. A healthy, physically fit woman is better prepared to cope with these sudden demands on her body than an under- or overweight woman who never exercises.

A woman who is seriously underweight is not only lacking in energy but is probably undernourished as well. (See Chapter 15 for more information on the effect of underweight on pregnancy.) Before she becomes pregnant she should try to build up her weight and her general health by a diet of nutritious, high-energy foods.

Likewise, a woman who is obese (defined as 20 percent above the standard weight for height) may also be in for a difficult time during pregnancy. Obesity may result in an abnormal sugar level, which can lead to a large birth weight and problems in labor (there is a higher Cesarean rate for obese mothers). A high sugar level means that a woman's body may not produce enough insulin, which results in a prediabetic condition, with its increased incidence of congenital malformations. If you are overweight, try to reduce your weight before pregnancy—for your sake and for the baby's. Dieting during pregnancy can be dangerous, because the body will compensate by obtaining its energy from the body fat. This in turn will result in the production of ketone and acidosis, which can poison and even kill the baby. A steady calorie intake is essential all the way through pregnancy to ensure the proper growth of the fetus. There is some new research to indicate that during pregnancy a woman's body metabolizes so efficiently that it will convert even so-called useless calories into nutrients for the baby. A woman who severely cuts down on her calorie intake when she is pregnant is, in effect, starving her baby as well as decreasing her own energy level and her ability to cope with the physical and emotional stress of pregnancy.

Researchers now believe that severe anemia or nutritional deficiencies may diminish a woman's resistance to toxins and infections in the critical first trimester of pregnancy. While it is very helpful to give women nutritional advice and supplements during pregnancy, this should ideally begin long before a woman becomes pregnant if she has not had a lifelong history of good nutrition. Ask your doctor for a glucose-tolerance test if you suspect that you might be diabetic or have a blood count taken if you think you may be anemic.

The chapter on nutrition in pregnancy will give you some guidelines to follow in planning your diet even before pregnancy. Eating properly is so important to a good pregnancy outcome that changing your eating habits before conception and reaching a comfortable weight is among the most valuable preparations you can possibly make in planning ahead for childbirth.

☐ *Vitamins Before You Conceive*   Most doctors place very little importance on vitamin supplements. Medical textbooks usually indicate that the average American diet contains enough vitamins for general good health. Such thinking may soon have to be revised. First of all, who really has a proper diet, when so many modern foods are superrefined and artificially prepared? Second, a significant and conclusive study was recently conducted in England and Northern Ireland on the benefits of prenatal vitamin supplements.

This recent British study indicated that good nutrition at the time of conception and immediately after plays an important part in preventing at least one group of serious birth defects affecting the brain and spine. These are the so-called neural tube defects, such as anencephaly (missing brain) and spina bifida (open spine). A group of 178 women who had already borne children with neural tube defects, and whose chances of bearing a second child with the same abnormalities are 5 percent higher than those of the general population, were given an iron and multivitamin supplement comparable to two prenatal vitamin supplements daily, starting at least 28 days before conception. They continued to take the vitamin supplement until the time of their second missed period, when neural tube development in the fetus is almost completed. Their pregnancy outcome was compared with that of another group of 260 women who had also previously given birth to neural tube defective children but who had not received the vitamin supplement. The study found that only one child in the group of mothers receiving vitamin supplements had a neural tube defect, in comparison with 13 defective children among the women who did not receive vitamins (exactly the 5 percent increase normally predicted for these mothers-at-risk). This is the first study to indicate the importance of vitamins and iron intake before a child is conceived!

It is difficult from this preliminary study to determine what substances in the vitamin supplement were most effective in preventing neural tube defects, but there have been several observations from other researchers that pyridoxine—vitamin B_6—could be a very significant compound in reducing congenital malformations. Vitamin B_6 acts mainly on the central nervous system, and thus it seems obvious that a higher blood concentration of B_6 before conception would prevent fetal neural tube abnormalities. It is also interesting that women who take vitamin B_6 as part of a vitamin B-complex supplement during the early months of pregnancy have less morning sickness and seem, in general, to have better pregnancies. A recent study made in Japan has also indicated that infertile women who take vitamin B_6 may have a subsequently higher conception rate than infertile women who do not. Vitamin B_6 given in 100–300 mg doses often results in a more regular menstruation pattern, which increases chances of pregnancy.

I would highly recommend to any woman who wants to become pregnant that she increase her daily intake of multivitamins, including extra B vitamins, or take one or two prenatal vitamins or one multivitamin with extra vitamin B_6 (100–300 mg daily). A man may also benefit considerably by taking vitamins, particularly vitamin B_6, before he fathers a child. This is especially important for men who regularly smoke or drink, because smoking and alcohol deplete the body of necessary vitamins. (Vitamin B_6 depletion has been linked to a lower sperm count.) In this respect, it is interesting that the old health beliefs still persist despite changes in the ways modern foods are produced. Men still are convinced that they get extra B vitamins from beer, and beer drinking is popularly supposed to enhance a man's virility! Unfortunately, commercial beers today are produced in such a way that the vitamin content of hops is almost totally destroyed by the steam-heating process. Thus there are no *B* vitamins in *beer*; quite the opposite, beer drinkers need extra vitamin *B* supplementation. If you don't like pills, eat *bananas* instead.

☐ *Exercise*   People should always be concerned about their physical condition, but it is even more important when a woman plans to conceive. Since pregnancy puts an enormous physical strain on the body, a woman who wants to have a child should begin a regular exercise program in the months preceding conception if she is not already actively engaged in sports. In this chapter I have already recommended that overweight women try to reduce their weight to a sensible level. However, we all know it is difficult to lose weight on a diet alone, and exercise will help reduce weight and build up the body at the same time.

This is not a book on sports medicine, and I will not presume to give you a list of the best forms of exercise. Simply exercise in any way that gives you the most enjoyment and the most pleasure, and develop a program that is realistic and attainable.

One of the most important aims of any prepregnancy exercise program is to increase muscular strength and the lung and heart capacity, so the body will be able to handle a pregnancy without putting an unbearable strain on its physical limits. A woman who is in reasonable shape is less likely to suffer from muscle fatigue and backache and runs less risk of developing complications such as toxemia. And if your body is in good physical condition, labor and delivery will be much easier for you.

Now that so many of my patients exercise regularly, more and more women have told me that they experience less premenstrual tension and fewer menstrual problems. Women who were previously infertile sometimes notice that their ovulation and menstruation becomes more regular as their bodies become trimmer, and it is easier for them to conceive. On the other hand, women who participate in serious exercise or competitive sports will often find that the additional body stress results in the cessation of ovulation and menstruation. This is nature's intention; the lack of menstruation avoids loss of blood and increases a woman's blood count. Dancers and marathon runners in particular commonly experience prolonged amenorrhea. If you find your exercise program disturbing your ovulation and menstruation, this is a signal to slow down and give your body a chance to return to its normal patterns and prepare for conception.

☐ **The Environment and Your Unborn Child** We now know that many environmental and other factors influence the development of an unborn child. Only twenty years ago, scientists still by and large held the comforting theory that the placenta filters out most toxic substances before they reach the fetus via the mother's bloodstream. This idea has been totally discredited. It is now clear that environmental agents, such as drugs, alcohol, tobacco, radiation, and chemicals, have a negative effect on the conception and development of a healthy fetus. Desirable and undesirable substances reach the baby through the mother's body when she is pregnant.

At the moment of conception, egg and sperm combine to pass on a genetic heritage to a new human being. Both egg and sperm must be healthy in themselves for conception, implantation, and embryonic development to proceed properly. A defect in either the egg or the sperm will result in infertility, an early miscarriage, or a defective child. Men as well as women have an important responsibility toward their unborn children. Sperm are vulnerable to industrial pollution, radiation, chemical exposure, and the father's own health habits.

Unfortunately, many environmental factors are outside our individual control. New parents cannot hope to shut themselves off from the world entirely to ensure a perfect baby. People have to go to work, they have to breathe whatever air is available, they usually have to eat food regardless of where it is grown or what has been added to it. But a man and a woman can do a great deal, even so, to give their children a good beginning in life. Before you conceive a baby, take a close look at your health habits, your environment—your workplace and where you live—and begin to make changes in your lives if this seems necessary. If a man and a woman are healthy at the moment of conception, they will be doing all that is within their power to create a healthy child.

☐ **The Vulnerable Sperm** The male reproductive tract is very sensitive. Substances pass through the body and collect in the reproductive tract to be eliminated later, which means that a number of common toxic substances, such as lead or industrial chemicals, will pass into a man's sperm and may damage it. The damage may take several forms: (a) some sperm are killed outright, and the sperm count is lowered; (b) normal sperm movement is inhibited or changes; (c) the sperm are improperly formed; or (d) the sperm cells carry genetic abnormalities.

Sperm are composed of cells that have a high fat content. The fat cells of the body suffer from a poor blood supply, and toxic agents, including carcinogenic substances, may become concentrated in them over a period of time. Many chemical agents and other toxins are suspected mutagens as well as carcinogens. Mutagenic substances can damage the genetic material in the sperm cells, sometimes so severely that a conception will not survive the earliest stage of life. If the sperm cells experience some milder genetic damage, they may fertilize the egg, and a child with a visible birth defect may result, or the genetic alterations in the sperm cells may be so slight that the child appears normal in every way except for the potential he or she has for passing down the defect through succeeding generations.

While many birth defects appear to be quite random, recent scientific interest in the role of the sperm at conception has begun to indicate that miscarriages and congenital malformations are perhaps more often due to sperm abnormalities than to abnormalities of the egg. Researchers are now testing the male partner in marriages in which the wife has suffered repeated miscarriages. One researcher recently concluded that in these cases the father's semen shows a lower sperm count and more abnormal sperm than usual.

One day men will probably expect to have a semen analysis done as part of their regular medical care, just as they have a blood or urine test done now. Many men may find the idea distasteful at first, but perhaps they will feel different after they understand its purpose. The condition of a man's semen is a good indication of his general health and an irreplaceable method of warning him—in time, one hopes—of his exposure to hazardous substances that threaten his own health and his unborn children's future.

☐ *Smoking Before Conception*   When a man smokes tobacco heavily, the nicotine and the other chemicals damage his lungs and strain his heart; they also become stored up in the reproductive tract and directly affect his sperm. This may result in a lowered sperm count, or the sperm may lose motility or become damaged. The same is true of men who smoke marijuana heavily. Some recent tests at Columbia University linked a decreased sperm count, reduced sperm motility, and an increase in the number of abnormal sperm with daily heavy use of marijuana. The doctor who led the group of experiments was particularly concerned about marijuana's subtler effects in the form of long-term chromosomal damage. In addition, tetrahydrocannabinol, the active ingredient in marijuana, lowers the testosterone levels in the blood and so decreases the efficiency of the male hormonal system, rendering the male less virile.

If a man cannot stop smoking before the conception of his child, he should definitely try to stop smoking when the child is born, for his family's sake as well as his own. (The same advice obviously applies to women smokers in nonsmoking households.) A recent study in Japan found an unusually high level of lung cancer in women who were nonsmokers themselves but had smokers in their home environments. Researchers concluded that women who lived with heavy smokers were up to 50 percent more likely to develop lung cancer than women who had nonsmoking husbands. And a small child's lungs are still more vulnerable to the atmosphere in the home or anywhere else.

A woman should try to stop smoking well before she becomes pregnant, or better still, never begin at all. Heavy cigarette smoking over a period of years has been linked to an increased incidence of insufficient placentas, a condition that often leads to premature birth or fetal growth retardation because the placenta develops abnormally large areas of dead tissue and is unable to support the growing fetus with an adequate supply of oxygen. A woman can give up cigarettes several months before becoming pregnant and still run the risk of giving birth prematurely.

The risks of smoking during pregnancy are fully discussed in Chapter 17. They include a greater likelihood of miscarriage, fetal distress, low birth weight, and premature birth especially among older mothers.

Furthermore, both partners may find that they enjoy sex far more if they give up cigarette smoking. Tobacco tends to reduce male and female sexual desire by acting as a vasoconstricting agent and so decreasing the amount of blood reaching the sex center in the brain. Both men and women have reported an increase in sexual desire and enjoyment of lovemaking after they stopped smoking. This alone seems like an excellent preparation for conception.

If you are trying to become pregnant and you use marijuana fairly heavily, you may be unwittingly disturbing your ovulation pattern. Marijuana will block the brain hormones needed to induce ovulation.

☐ *Alcohol*   A man who drinks heavily reduces his sexual ability considerably. Large amounts of alcohol can decrease a man's sperm count, damage his sperm mobility and motility, and lower his male hormone levels. Chronic drinkers often suffer from periods of impotence or, at the very least, have a decreased desire for sex. While one or two drinks may have an aphrodisiac effect by depressing the part of the brain that controls fear and tension, three or four drinks may simply depress the brain completely and bring sedation or sleep instead of arousal. This decreased sex drive is found in both men and women who drink heavily.

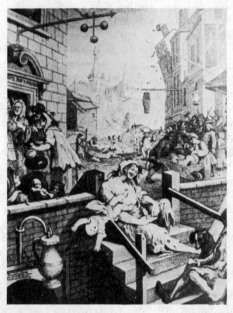

Figure 6: This famous picture, *Gin Lane* by Hogarth, is both interesting and scary. Note that the woman on the stairs is so drunk she is dropping her baby. Try to eliminate alcohol even before conception.

For the expectant mother, chronic alcohol use is a serious problem. Women who drink heavily during pregnancy run a distinct risk of permanently damaging their unborn children. The fetal alcohol syndrome (FAS) is now said to be the third major cause of congenital mental retardation in the United States, affecting thousands of children each year, who are born with both physical and mental disabilities (see Chap. 18).

While the serious birth defects seen in FAS babies are the result of months of chronic alcohol abuse, researchers think that the amount of absolute alcohol that may cause slight mental or physical growth problems prenatally could be rather small. In addition, women who drink fairly heavily often have poor eating habits, and doctors suspect this is often a contributing factor in FAS births, because the babies are malnourished as well as directly affected by the teratogenic effects of the alcohol. If you have a drink or two or smoke an occasional cigarette at the time you become pregnant, you probably have nothing to worry about, but if you do drink every day as a matter of course, the period before pregnancy is a good time to reduce your alcohol consumption.

☐   *Prescription and Nonprescription Drugs*   Look carefully at your daily use of over-the-counter remedies or your normal prescription drugs. If you have a chronic condition that requires constant medication, you will have to discuss this fully with your doctor before you become pregnant. But if you have a long-standing prescription for tranquilizers or you are using antibiotics to clear up an infection, you should stop using prescription drugs on a daily basis before you become pregnant. For instance, Valium, the most frequently prescribed tranquilizer in the United States, has been associated with a higher incidence of cleft lip and palate in the fetus, while tetracycline, a commonly used antibiotic, may accumulate in the fetal skeleton and stain a child's permanent teeth. Chapter 19 gives a full discussion of drug use and the possible side effects of different drugs during pregnancy. Even if you are fully aware that drugs have been linked to various degrees and kinds of fetal damage, and you certainly intend to watch your drug use after you become pregnant, it may be two or three weeks after conception before you even suspect you are pregnant. One Valium is very unlikely to do any damage to a pregnancy in the implantation stage, but there may be some real cause for concern if the drug use was linked to a specific ailment and you were required to take a routine dosage over a period of weeks. Since you certainly don't want to spend the rest of your pregnancy worrying about something you took in the first weeks, you should always tell your doctor that you are trying to become pregnant if you need medical treatment that involves drugs.

Over-the-counter drugs are routinely taken by American women with very little thought as to their possible hazards during pregnancy. The labeling on common drug products very rarely covers recommended doses during pregnancy and, in fact, generally implies that it is perfectly safe for a pregnant woman to take cold remedies or extra-strength aspirin with the same frequency that she would if she were not pregnant. This is an aspect of pregnancy that needs further study, especially in the light of some recent findings on heavy aspirin use in the later months of pregnancy (see Chap. 19). Obstetricians are now asking their pregnant patients to check with them if they use over-the-counter remedies for a period of time—to fight off a bad cold, for instance. If you routinely use aspirin or some other common remedy before you become pregnant, report your over-the-counter drug use to your doctor. This is nothing more than a sensible precaution, since he is quite unlikely to advise against their use altogether. You will want to plan ahead now and try to limit your general use of nonprescription drugs. Prepregnancy and pregnancy are good times to break bad habits, and rushing off to the pharmacy at the slightest sign of discomfort is one of them.

☐   *Chronic Illness and Pregnancy*   When a woman has a chronic disease, such as diabetes, hypertension, or a thyroid disorder, her drug use is in a quite different category from the woman who has a regular prescription for Valium.

She may still need to control her illness during the pregnancy, but the powerful drugs that are used in the treatment of various chronic diseases have to be used with very great care. Warfarin, for instance, which is given as an anticoagulant in cases of clotting disorders, has been linked to facial deformities, blindness, and mental retardation in 20 percent of infants exposed to it prenatally.

It is vital for a woman who takes prescription drugs for a chronic illness to discuss the whole matter thoroughly with her doctor well before she plans to become pregnant. She may be able to switch to an alternative drug that has been shown to have fewer teratogenic effects, or she may find that the risks connected with her current drug therapy are low enough to make a successful pregnancy possible. The later chapter on drugs in pregnancy has a much fuller discussion of the effects of various prescription drugs on the fetus.

Women who were once advised to avoid pregnancy or to seek a legal abortion if they did become pregnant are now being helped through their pregnancies by recent research and the work of perinatologists (a new breed of young physicians who specialize in research and management of high-risk pregnancies). For instance, women with juvenile diabetes rarely carried a pregnancy successfully until a few years ago. Newer research has now shown that the majority of congenital malformations in babies born to diabetic mothers are due to abnormalities in the first trimester and even before the woman becomes pregnant. If a diabetic mother can bring her blood sugar level under strict control before she becomes pregnant and keep it from fluctuating outside normal limits in the first trimester, she will decrease the possibility of congenital malformations in the fetus considerably. Erratic blood sugar levels later on, in the second or third trimesters, have been shown to have a far less harmful effect on the final pregnancy outcome. Early planning is therefore essential in a diabetic pregnancy.

Diabetes is only one of the more common chronic conditions that affect women of childbearing age. A woman may have an inactive thyroid condition or suffer from hypertension or collagen disease, and in all these cases, current research and new methods of high-risk management are helping women to give birth who would have been involuntarily childless in the past. A major step forward has been the establishment of perinatology as a special branch of obstetrics. This development means that more specialized care is becoming available for women who otherwise would be unable or afraid to have children (see subhead "Special Care: The Perinatologist," in Chap. 6). If your pregnancy will need such special care, I urge you to arrange to see a perinatologist several months before you make plans to conceive. If your doctor does not recommend a perinatologist to you, ask him about such a consultation. The possible inconvenience of traveling to a perinatal center or major hospital is definitely outweighed by the benefits to you and your baby.

Further material on high-risk pregnancies can be found in Chapter 24. This brief section is here to alert you in advance and to urge you to plan ahead carefully if you know you have a chronic medical problem. Your choice of an obstetrician and a hospital will be extremely important, since obstetricians are not by any means always competent to handle difficult pregnancy cases. I would strongly recommend that you look for a perinatologist or a doctor who is a specialist in your particular disorder and consult him well in advance. He will help you prepare yourself physically and be able to advise you realistically of your chances for a successful pregnancy.

An Important Note: Men who suffer from chronic conditions, such as epilepsy, are now being alerted to the possible hazards of drug use at the time of conception. For instance, there has been some recent evidence linking the use of the drug Phenytoin to malformations in the offspring of fathers receiving anticonvulsants for epilepsy. The drug was found present in human semen in concentrations about equal to the unbound fraction of the drug in serum. A man who is under a routine regimen of drug therapy and who wants to have children should consult his doctor well ahead of time to find out whether the drugs he is taking are linked with birth defects.

☐ *Genetic Counseling*   This is an area in which research is moving very quickly. (See Chapter 22 for an analysis of the major genetic diseases and the tests that are presently available to couples at risk.) Certain fatal genetic disorders, such as Tay-Sachs disease, are already detectable prenatally through the amniocentesis test. In other cases the parents' carrier status can be ascertained through special testing. Genetic counseling and/or a simple blood test to detect your carrier status is recommended if:

(a) you are both black and want to detect your carrier status for sickle-cell anemia;
(b) you are both descended from Jewish families who came from eastern Europe (Tay-Sachs disease);
(c) you both come from families of eastern Mediterranean descent (Cooley's anemia).

Genetic counseling is strongly advised if:

(a) two or more previous pregnancies have ended in miscarriage;
(b) there is a family history of particular genetic diseases (hemophilia or Huntington's chorea, for instance);
(c) a previous child suffers or suffered from a genetic disease (including anencephaly or spina bifida, which are partly due to genetic causes).

Professional genetic counseling is available from medical specialists and also from organizations, such as the March of Dimes, which will help you draw up an accurate family history and refer you to medical help if this seems appropriate. Even though you may feel that you do not want to know about your chances of being a carrier but suspect you may be one, I would urge you nevertheless to take advantage of any available screening techniques, however inadequate they may be. My general rule in advising prospective parents who ask me about genetic counseling is: *Whenever a couple is in doubt about the possibility of inherited genetic disease, genetic counseling should always be considered.* Unfortunately, many genetic diseases appear spontaneously, and a couple will not have a previous family or personal history to alert them beforehand. In addition, many genetic diseases are not detectable prenatally through amniocentesis or fetoscopy, and a genetic counselor may only be able to inform you of the chances of your passing on a genetic ailment to your children.

☐ *Other Precautions to Take Before Becoming Pregnant*   There are many other conditions that may harm a conception, some of which you may be aware of and others that may be unknown to you. Certain practical precautions can be taken before conception to avoid potential birth defects, and it is important for you to familiarize yourself with the available tests or other precautions you can follow to protect your child.

☐ *Rubella Vaccination*   If you have not been exposed to rubella (German measles) at any time in your life—as far as you know—you should arrange to have a blood test taken to determine the level of antibodies in the blood—your rubella titer. You may well have had a mild case of German measles as a child, but your mother failed to diagnose it correctly; sometimes a slightly elevated temperature and a faint rash can easily be confused with some other childhood ailment. Even this mild case may have given you an immune response and caused your body to develop antibodies to the disease, and the chance of the disease recurring is then almost nonexistent. If the rubella titer reveals that you do not carry antibodies, have a vaccination against rubella immediately, unless you are already pregnant. You should make absolutely sure that there is no chance of your contracting rubella in the first three months of pregnancy. A slight attack of German measles may hardly affect you at all, but there is a very high risk that your unborn child will be born with brain damage or will be deaf or blind.

Since rubella vaccine is live, your doctor will instruct you after the vaccination to wait for at least three months before you conceive, in order to allow your immunological system to integrate the vaccine. *These three months are essential!* Should you become pregnant before the three months are up, the live virus itself will affect the fetus, and you may be faced with the possibility of an abortion.

If you are already pregnant and discover you do not have an immunity to rubella, take steps immediately to protect yourself. Avoid large groups of children and family and friends who you know have been exposed or have a suspicious viral ailment.

The same precautions hold true for other vaccinations, such as *measles, mumps,* and *flu shots.* If you have been traveling in Africa, Asia, or South America and have been given a live virus injection against *yellow fever, cholera,* or *typhus,* it is also extremely important to wait for three months before trying to conceive.

☐ *Should You Get Rid of Your Cat Before Conception?*   Toxoplasma is a parasite found in the intestines of cats, cattle, sheep, and pigs. It induces a common disease in humans called toxoplasmosis, which many of us have had without even being aware of its mild symptoms. Unfortunately toxoplasmosis can severely damage fetal development (see Chap. 25). If a pregnant woman catches toxoplasmosis, the chance of brain malformation and blindness for the baby is very great. One common way to contract this viral disease is by eating underdone red meat or pork. (Fortunately most people cook pork until it is well done, but there is a national mania in the United States for rare steak.) Since the baby is at risk in the first few weeks after conception, reeducate your palate once you plan to conceive if you find out that you have never had toxoplasmosis.

Whether or not you have had the disease can be learned by having your doctor run a blood test in advance of your planned date of conception. The toxoplasmosis titer will measure the level of antibodies in your blood and determine whether you are fully protected. There is no vaccine available, so if you are vulnerable, you must be very careful throughout the pregnancy. If you do develop a viruslike condition once you become pregnant, and your doctor cannot exclude the possibility of toxoplasmosis, he will take another titer. A much higher titer at this time will indicate a strong possibility of active toxoplasmosis, with about a 40 percent chance that the fetus will be affected. If your titer remains the same, your doctor can rule out the possibility of toxoplasmosis and look for some other reason for the infection.

Your cat is a potential carrier of toxoplasmas if it eats wild prey of any kind or you feed it raw meat. The virus will be excreted with the cat stools and passed on to humans when the litter box is emptied. You do not have to give up your cat if you can persuade another member of the family to empty the litter box and make sure that he or she has thoroughly washed hands before coming into contact with you. A true house cat is quite unlikely to carry the virus, but you should still take all precautions and should wash your hands after you feed or pet the animal. Pregnancy is not a time to take in a stray cat, however lonely or unloved the animal may appear to be.

☐ *Viruses and Pregnancy*   Other viral diseases besides rubella and toxoplasmosis may adversely affect the developing fetus. Pregnancy outcome can be critically affected if a viral infection invades the fetus during the vital periods of development. Maternal viral infections may lead to a miscarriage or stillbirth or may be responsible for severe developmental defects. Common viral diseases besides rubella are *measles, mumps, herpes zoster, herpes simplex, influenza A strain, cytomega lovirus, Coxsackie,* and *chicken pox.*

Be sure to check all your previous vaccinations and your general health history well before you become pregnant, to take advantage of any of the available vaccines, including an *influenza shot.* Even the briefest of encounters with the flu may be significant during pregnancy, especially if it occurs in the first trimester. A high body temperature resulting from a known or unknown viral disease may also adversely affect the developing fetus. Recently three researchers from the University of Seattle found a close correlation between birth defects and high body temperatures in expectant mothers; a significant number of women in their study who had borne children with birth defects reported that they had suffered from *fevers of more than 102 degrees* in the first four months of their pregnancies.

The incubation stage for most viral diseases is about one to two weeks, which makes it possible for a woman to contract a viral disease during preconception and show overt symptoms only after the baby is conceived. As you plan ahead, make sure that you and your immediate family are properly immunized against preventable viral diseases. Do not visit a friend's or relative's house where some member of the family is ill with a viral disease or has any undiagnosed complaint with flulike symptoms. Call ahead and check first before visiting, even if this seems rude. Do not visit if someone in the house is ill and you do not know what the ailment is. The same precautions hold true for men. Research has indicated that if a man is suffering from a viral disease (particularly hepatitis) at the time of conception, this can affect the sperm adversely and result in congenital malformations. If either person is ill with a virus, pregnancy should be avoided until both are free from flu or a viral infection.

☐ *How Long Should You Be Off the Pill Before Conceiving?* It is important to give the body enough time to resume its normal ovulation pattern. You would be well advised to stop taking the birth control pill two or three months before you try to conceive. Although the hormones in the pills might be excreted in only a few days after the pill is stopped, you still want to give yourself plenty of time for this to happen.

There have been several recent studies—the latest a survey of seven thousand postpill births by the Harvard School of Public Health—which show that there is a slightly increased risk of fetal deformities if a woman conceives immediately after stopping the pill. The Food and Drug Administration decidedly recommends that a woman intending to have a child stop using oral contraceptives and use some other form of contraception for three months before becoming pregnant. This is a sensible precaution in view of the small but potential hazard involved.

If a woman becomes pregnant accidentally while she is still on the pill, she should be concerned about abnormalities in the fetus, but since each case is different, she should have genetic counseling if she decides to continue the pregnancy.

☐ *Warning on Spermicides* According to a recent study, women who use spermicides—foams, foaming tablets, or the diaphragm with a spermicidal jelly—run an increased risk of bearing a child with a serious birth defect if they conceive while using the spermicide or if the spermicide is used near the time of conception. This is a surprising and frightening new discovery. Although the studies are not conclusive, one can no longer say that a woman who becomes pregnant while using a spermicide is quite safe in continuing the pregnancy. A woman would be well advised to stop using any spermicide for a full two months prior to attempting conception.

☐ *Stress and Conception* No one can honestly say it is easy to avoid stress. Unfortunately it is a part of the way we live. But if a woman is placed constantly in stressful situations, her emotions can affect her body adversely. The same is most certainly true for men, as heart attack statistics confirm. A man who is under extreme stress may become temporarily infertile. A pregnant woman who is under stress will involuntarily decrease the blood supply flowing to the uterus and the placenta, which will result in an undernourished child or, in extreme cases, a miscarriage or premature birth. Stress definitely deprives a baby of a proper maternal environment. In planning ahead, try first to put your life in order and learn to relax. Meditation and deep-breathing exercises may be one way to do this, regular exercise may be another.

☐ *X-Ray and Conception: Avoid It* When a woman of childbearing age undergoes a diagnostic X-ray for the pelvic or abdominal areas, a simple rule should always be followed. Allow the X-ray to be taken only in the first ten days of your menstrual cycle—unless, of course, your life is in danger and a diagnosis must be made. This ten-day rule has been devised by radiologists to protect a conceptus from exposure in the preimplantation stage, when the fertilized egg is most sensitive to the possibly lethal effects of radiation.

The reproductive organs of both men and women are extremely sensitive to the mutagenic effects of ionizing radiation. Men, women, and children should *always* have protective shielding over the gonads during any X-ray that puts the ovaries or the testes in the direct line of the X-ray beam, unless it is *impossible* to take the X-ray with the shielding in place. Heavy exposure to ionizing radiation has been definitely linked to reproductive damage, and the testes seem to be more vulnerable to a lower radiation dosage than the ovaries are. The so-called safe level of radiation exposure is still very much in dispute, and a wise doctor will be very careful about exposing his patients to any X-ray procedure unless it is really necessary.

☐ *The Work Environment*   A pregnant woman at work is so commonplace now that it is difficult to remember a time (not so long ago) when a woman resorted to all kinds of subterfuges to avoid being fired by the fourth month. Most women make a few adjustments to guard against becoming overtired and carry on with their work lives quite normally right up to delivery; and companies are now gradually changing their policies to accommodate pregnant women workers. Women benefit financially and emotionally by staying at work, and as long as they take some sensible precautions, the baby is usually fully safeguarded.

Unfortunately not all work environments are suited to the pregnant worker or to a woman who wants to conceive. Some women work at jobs in which they may endanger their unborn children or even their chances of conception, not through any fault of their own, but because the conditions of the job itself are hazardous. Certain large companies have deliberately excluded potentially fertile women from higher paying jobs that would bring them into contact with materials or substances suspected of causing reproductive damage, and have relegated their women workers to jobs that pay less, often against the will of the workers. This is now a subject of great public controversy, and several lawsuits have been pressed on behalf of such excluded women workers in different industries.

The situation is complicated by our present lack of knowledge about the teratogenic effects of most of the substances in our environment. In a few cases we can be quite sure that a worker is endangering her unborn child—if she works in close contact with heavy exposures of lead, mercury, or ionizing radiation, for example. Many other substances have been shown to produce genetic abnormalities in laboratory animals but do not have a similar effect in humans—at least so far as researchers can see. The whole situation is very much complicated by the unknown effects of combinations of substances that the work environment may contain. Often, too, for reasons that are still quite mysterious, a known hazard may damage one pregnancy and not another, even though both women concerned have been equally exposed. This complex situation often makes it very difficult for a doctor to advise a woman on her best course of action during or before pregnancy, especially when personal and financial factors are taken into account.

We do know that work in certain industries poses particular risks to the fetus. Even in the early 1900s, doctors observed a high number of miscarriages and birth defects among women who worked with lead pigments in the pottery and paint trades and were able to link the adverse conditions of the women's workplaces with their inability to bear healthy children. The list of hazardous substances has grown since that time; the Occupational Safety and Health Administration (OSHA) now lists twenty-four substances used in the chemical industry alone that may cause miscarriages and birth defects. But women who work in industry are not the only ones at risk. Thousands of young women are employed as anesthesiologists, operating room nurses, X-ray technicians, dental assistants, laboratory technicians, airline flight attendants, and beauticians—some of the other jobs that may be hazardous to conception and pregnancy. Anesthetic gases, for instance, have been linked to an increased incidence of miscarriage and birth defects among the children of operating room nurses and women anesthesiologists.

Men are as adversely affected as women by the hazards of the workplace and may prove to be even more vulnerable. The wives of male operating room personnel, for instance, have been shown to have a higher risk of miscarriage than the operating room nurses or female anesthesiologists who are directly exposed to anesthetic gases. Sperm can be damaged by radiation, lead, anesthetic gases, pesticides, certain other chemicals, and radar, and may be susceptible to other substances such as heavy metals. Thousands of men may be jeopardizing their fertility by working under adverse conditions. (Industries have not yet excluded men from jobs with reproductive risks.) In 1977 an extraordinary situation was uncovered by a group of workers which caused a great deal of concern among fertility researchers. These men, who worked in a California plant manufacturing the chemical DCPB, compared notes one lunchtime and found that none of them had fathered a child since they had been employed at the plant. Several of them then had a semen analysis and discovered they were either sterile or definitely subfertile. This action by the men led to the eventual banning of the manufacture of DCPB by the federal government, but it was too late to save the fertility of the workers themselves.

If either of you works under conditions that threaten your fertility, you may be able to take certain precautions before trying to conceive, or it may be possible to persuade your employer to take them on your behalf. A worker who is regularly exposed to ionizing radiation should always wear a film badge for dose monitoring, and the badge should be read quarterly. When planning for pregnancy, look up the records of your personal dose exposures to check that you are within a reasonably safe level, and ask for a monthly badge reading, to make sure that your exposure does not go beyond the safe limits during the sensitive period of conception. A woman must also check herself regularly in the same way throughout her pregnancy. If either of you works in a hospital operating room, you should be aware that the hospital administration has an obligation to protect you by installing a special ventilation system. Such systems have proved to be very effective in reducing the amount of gas in the operating room atmosphere.

☐ *Will the Conditions Improve?*   It is to be hoped that in the future, employees will be sufficiently alarmed about the hazards of the workplace to compel their employers and the government to change their working conditions if necessary and protect their unborn children. But for now, if you or your mate is employed in an industry you fear is endangering your fertility, try to find out as much as possible about the experiences of your fellow workers, and discuss these fears with your doctor. If you think the situation is serious and your employer is reluctant to act to protect you, report the matter to your union or request an on-site inspection from the Occupational Safety and Health Administration, the government agency that is responsible for employment safety. In a very hazardous situation, a man or woman who wants children should look for other employment if this is at all feasible.

☐ *Fear of Flying*   Airline flight attendants tend to have irregular ovulation patterns because of the peculiar stress of their jobs. If they want to conceive, they often find it difficult, and if they do conceive, they have a rather high rate of miscarriage. A new and even more serious concern about flying has recently emerged. Now that airplanes, in order to save fuel, are flying in higher altitudes above the earth's ozone layer, frequent passengers as well as personnel have less protection from the dangers of atmospheric radiation. Flight attendants, cabin personnel, and passengers ought to take this increased hazard into consideration before they plan for pregnancy.

An airline flight attendant who wants to conceive should probably request a ground job or take short domestic routes for the period before and after conception, and most airline companies will make the necessary accommodations. As more women move into the work force and become valuable assets to their companies, employers will become more flexible about women's special needs before and during pregnancy. Remember, you need to avoid hazardous conditions for at least three months before the planned date of conception.

☐ *Household Chemicals*   When a couple look ahead to pregnancy, they may be tempted to completely redo the house, knowing that they will have other things to take care of during the pregnancy itself. Household chemicals and decorating supplies should be used with care at all times but particularly just before or during a pregnancy. Heavy cleaners containing large quantities of organic solvents have been linked to miscarriages and birth defects, according to a study from Finland, where one woman miscarried after her husband used heavy concentrations of organic solvents in their home. Try not to do any cleaning or house decorating that involves highly toxic substances at about the time you plan to conceive. Be careful, too, once you are pregnant, or suspect you are pregnant. In the early months you are more sensitive than usual to fumes of all kinds, and women have been known to faint while painting or using household cleaners. The effect on the fetus is also unknown. It is probably better to paint the house or finish the heavy cleaning two or three months before you become pregnant.

If you are planning to move, as so many people do when they decide to have a child, take the same precautions in redecorating and cleaning your new home. I would advise a couple to move to a new house several months before conception rather than wait for the period of pregnancy, when the physical strain of moving is much greater. It is also wise to make major changes in the house before conception. If that isn't possible, it would be better to wait until after the baby is born.

☐ *Chemical Exposures and Conception*   The American College of Obstetricians and Gynecologists (ACOG) now recommends that patients discuss their lifelong exposure to certain substances, such as chemicals, with their doctors. As we have already seen, conditions in the workplace or at home can significantly affect a man's or a woman's future fertility, but parents may be exposed in other ways as well. Recently I delivered a child who died quite suddenly, when he was five days old, from a congenital abnormality of the heart. The child's father had been in Vietnam in the late sixties and was exposed to Agent Orange, the powerful chemical defoliant that has been linked to miscarriages and birth defects. The congenital abnormality suffered by the child was a typical birth defect caused by the mutagenic effects of this defoliant, which contained dioxin, a highly toxic substance.

Agent Orange was particularly toxic because it was used in unusually high concentrations, but miscarriages and birth defects from chemical spraying have been reported recently from other areas besides Vietnam. In the late 1970s women in small towns in Oregon and New Jersey suffered an unusually high incidence of miscarriage after the herbicide 2,4,5,T was sprayed on local crops or woodlands, and similar reports have come from England as well. The story of Love Canal has shown us that people may unwittingly expose themselves to chemical hazards in their homes, schools, and recreation areas.

In 1976 an abnormally heavy rainstorm brought to the surface of the canal thousands of leaking drums containing chemical waste. Afterward, toxic-chemical air concentration was approximately a thousand times greater than in the surrounding neighborhoods, and the poisoning of air and ground soil blighted local pregnancies. The level of miscarriage soared to two to three times that of a normal population, and the number of birth defects increased. The birth defects suffered by Love Canal children vary: one child was born with three ears, other children have suffered from blindness, many others from epileptic seizures. Fortunately some of these conditions improved after the children were moved far away from the Love Canal area.

The Love Canal story is frightening, but what is even more frightening is the estimate that there are more than twenty-five hundred toxic-dump areas throughout the United States. It is quite possible for a major spillage to occur at any of those places, resulting in a similar threat to the population and an increased rate of miscarriage and congenital malformation in the surviving children.

☐ *It's Your Turn*   Pregnancy is different today compared to years ago. A couple may now postpone giving birth to a child until they are older, and may plan to have only one or two children in order to give their children the very best possible start in life. Part of this caring for your family takes the form of preparation before you conceive a child. Examine your lifestyle. Get into good physical shape, eat properly, be aware of your environment, and take some sensible precautions. These preparations for conception will considerably increase your chances of having a happy, healthy, and successful pregnancy and a child you will both love and treasure.

3

Fertility and Infertility

☐ *Mind and Body*   Pregnancy not only changes the way a woman's body looks, it changes the way a woman thinks about her body. When a woman is pregnant, she is sharing her body with another human being, and however close she feels to her unborn baby, this extraordinarily intimate relationship evokes some unique emotions. Many women find this new perspective thrilling, but some women are overwhelmed or alarmed by the changes in their bodies and their feelings. In my own experience, a woman who is naturally sensitive to the way her body functions outside of pregnancy and is at ease with herself physically, will find it much easier to make the complex physical and emotional adjustment demanded by pregnancy and delivery, and will move through the pregnancy without abnormal strain or stress.

Your body is yours, and it is important for you to understand fully how it functions and how your organs look and feel. As an immediate practical consideration, a thorough knowledge of your sexual organs and the way they work will help you considerably when you and your partner plan for conception. To begin with, you can determine whether your body is in proper working order and whether you are ovulating regularly, as discussed in Chapter 1. Also, if you have an increased understanding of your physical functions, your doctor will be able to discuss any problems with you much more openly and fully.

☐ *The External Sex Organs*   A woman's external genitalia are technically only the vulva, although some books describe the anus and the pubic hair as part of the external genitalia.

The *vulva* is not one specific organ but comprises the *labia majora* (the large lips), the *labia minora* (the small lips), the *clitoris*, and the vaginal and urethral openings. The labia majora are the outer portion of the vulva, the area that first comes to your attention when you look in the mirror. The main function of the large lips, which are covered by pubic hair, is to protect the vagina and keep dirt and sweat from entering into the vaginal opening. Because they contain numerous fat cells, they also help to maintain a correct temperature in the vagina. The vaginal environment is very sensitive to changes in moisture and temperature.

The labia minora, the small lips, are visible between the large lips on a mature woman. They vary greatly in size from woman to woman and may be very prominent in some cases. Just as the size of a man's penis will vary according to his heredity, the appearance of an adult woman's labia minora is also partly genetically determined. At first, when a girl is very young, the labia minora are tightly covered by the labia majora, but as a girl passes through puberty and her estrogen production increases, this in turn stimulates the growth of the small lips, which begin to protrude through the large lips.

The small lips are folds of delicate and sensitive skin, without pubic hair growth or fat cells. They act as an initial protective covering for the vagina and also function during sexual intercourse. During intercourse blood rushes to the small lips, enlarging them in the same way as the sudden rush of blood to the penis creates an erection for the man. This enlargement of the small lips causes a tighter grip around the penis, increasing a couple's sexual pleasure and keeping the vagina snug around the shaft of the penis. Since the labia minora are completely closed in the midline, where they come together, they give increased covering to the vaginal opening and help to keep the sperm inside the vagina after intercourse. When a woman who is trying to conceive is afraid of losing the semen after ejaculation, she can pinch the small lips together to prevent any leakage of sperm, and if her buttocks are already placed on a pillow, this will help to tilt the vagina so that the sperm will stay inside the vaginal opening.

The clitoris is located at the tip of the vulva where the small lips come together. When a baby girl is born, the clitoris is snugly covered by the clitoral foreskin, the fold of skin called the *prepuce*. This will usually loosen as a young girl grows up. The clitoris is, of course, a source of great sexual pleasure to a woman, but it is unique among the sexual organs of both male and female because it plays no role in human reproduction other than increasing a woman's desire for sexual intercourse.

Inside the upper part of the opening of the vagina is the urethral opening, the opening to the bladder. Unfortunately the urethra is placed close enough to the vagina to allow infections to be easily pushed into the bladder during sexual intercourse, and this often happens during pregnancy when the enlarged uterus presses on the urethra and distorts it. A pregnant woman would be well advised to urinate immediately after intercourse to avoid cystitis, an unpleasant and painful bladder disease.

☐ *The Vagina*   If a woman gently pulls her labia apart, she will be able to see into the outer part of the vagina or at least up as far as the area of the hymen, about one inch inside the vaginal opening. The vagina is a muscular tube connecting the uterus to the vulva which allows free passage for the menstrual blood to leave the body and the sperm to enter up into the cervix and the internal sexual organs. This tube has amazing abilities. During intercourse the muscles in the vaginal wall automatically tighten around the penis and may be so tight under some circumstances that it is difficult for the man to withdraw. During childbirth, however, the muscles in the vaginal wall relax to allow for the passage of the baby down from the uterus and through the vaginal opening to the outside. The vagina could theoretically accommodate a baby weighing as much as fifteen pounds.

☐ *The Internal Sex Organs*   A woman's internal sexual organs are linked together by a complicated series of events that occur during the menstrual cycle and make conception possible. Each organ must function fully for this cycle to be successful. The *uterus* is the largest of the internal sexual organs and is used to its full capacity only during pregnancy, when it provides housing for the growing fetus. This hollow, muscular organ looks rather like a pear, with the larger end up and the lower, smaller end, the *cervix*, pushed down into the upper end of the vagina. Inside the cervix is a small opening that connects the uterine cavity, the area in which the fetus develops, with the vagina. The uterus is normally about three inches long in a nonpregnant woman. Each month the *endometrium*, the lining of the uterus, grows under hormone stimulation, and is normally shed during a woman's menstrual period. If a fertilized egg implants itself in the endometrium, the lining remains in the uterus and will thicken and become more vascular as the pregnancy develops.

In its upper, outer corners, the uterus extends into the *Fallopian tubes*, the muscular contours leading from the uterus into the ovaries. These organs are named after the famous Italian physician, Dr. Gabriel Fallopius. Each tube is about four inches long and about a quarter of an inch thick at its thickest part. The tubes are essentially divided into three parts, each with its own function as far as the mature egg and the sperm are concerned. The portion of the tube reaching into the uterus is the *isthmus*, which is so called because it is the narrowest part. If the egg is fertilized, it moves through the isthmus and into the uterus for implantation. The middle part of the tube is the *ampulla* portion, where egg and sperm cells meet and fertilization of the egg will occur within twenty-four hours of a woman's ovulating. The Fallopian tubes are an environment extremely favorable to sperm, and sperm can often stay alive in the tubes for three or four days after they have been ejaculated into the internal organs, ready to fertilize the egg at the exact point of ovulation. A fertilized egg will stay in the ampulla area for five to seven days before it begins its final journey into the uterus.

At the outer ends of each tube are the fingerlike fringes called the *fimbriated ends*. The fimbriae are minute tubes that not only look like but function as if they were thousands of tiny fingers. They "catch" the egg by reaching down toward the point of ovulation in the ovary and surrounding the mature egg just as it is released; this prevents it from being lost in the abdominal cavity.

The *ovaries* are named after the *ova*, the egg cells, which are stored in each ovary. The ovaries are placed next to the fimbriated ends of the Fallopian tubes and on either side of the uterus. These pinkish-gray egg-shaped organs are about one and one-half inches long, one inch wide, and about one-half-inch thick. When a girl is born, she already has perfectly formed ovaries, with all the eggs she will ever need in her reproductive life span, and hundreds of thousands more that will never be used but will disintegrate gradually when she passes through menopause. A woman has as many as one-half million eggs, each one capable of being fertilized. Unlike a man, who is continually producing new sperm

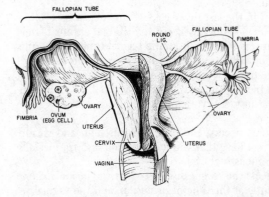

Figure 7: Female Reproductive Organs: A section of the female organs shows the connection between the vagina, the cervix and the uterine cavity; the relationship of the uterus and the Fallopian tubes; and the close proximity of the ovaries to the Fallopian tubes.

cells throughout his lifetime, a woman is unable to replenish her store of eggs, and as she matures, her eggs also grow older or can become damaged. When a woman is forty her eggs will be the same age, and this is why there is an increased chance of chromosomal abnormalities when a woman gives birth to a child later in life.

The ovaries produce hormones that are vital to a woman's reproductive life. The tissue around the egg cells is responsible for estrogen, the first female hormone that a young girl secretes from her ovaries and that controls her secondary sex characteristics: her breast growth, her new body shape, and the changes in the appearance of her external sex organs, as well as the onset of ovulation. A second hormone, progesterone, is produced from the *corpus luteum,* a yellowish collection of cells remaining after expulsion of the fertilized egg. This, the "hormone of pregnancy," ripens the endometrium after ovulation occurs and in this way regulates the menstrual period and the menstrual flow; it also acts to protect the fertilized egg once conception is established.

☐ ***Ovulation: How Can a Woman Tell When She Is Ovulating?***   Ovulation occurs only once a month, approximately fourteen days before each menstrual period begins. If a woman has irregular menstruation, ovulation still takes place two weeks before the first day of her period. However, it is difficult then to predict ovulation by using the calendar method, and a woman should examine herself carefully for signs that she is about to ovulate, by testing her cervical mucus, or establishing her own ovulation chart by using the basal body temperature method. There is a full explanation of how to do this in Chapter 1.

☐ ***The Use of the BBT as an Aid to Conception***   You will need to take your temperature first thing in the morning over a period of weeks to work out your ovulatory pattern. The way to do this is fully described in Chapter 1. The basal body temperature (BBT) curve is a very useful way to establish your probable time of ovulation, especially if you have an irregular menstrual pattern. But remember, if you want to conceive, the period just before your temperature jumps one degree is the time of ovulation. If you wait until after the rise in your BBT to try to conceive, as some misguided women have done, it is already too late. There is a possibility of conception if you have intercourse at the time of ovulation or one or two days before, because the sperm can stay alive in the Fallopian tubes for up to seventy-two hours.

The higher progesterone level in the last two weeks of the menstrual cycle— or the first two weeks of pregnancy—normally keeps the BBT at approximately 98.5 degrees. If you notice your temperature dropping several times during this period, it may be an indication of an inactive corpus luteum, and this can result in miscarriage. When the progesterone level decreases, the uterus may respond by cramping and squeezing out the egg. The BBT is thus a valuable tool in indicating the time of ovulation and in identifying problems of conception.

Important Note: When pregnancy occurs, the BBT remains high and steady. This is the first indication you will have that you are pregnant and is especially helpful if you have an irregular menstrual cycle.

A final test for ovulation reflects the recent discovery that the inside *alkaline phosphatase* decreases significantly at the time of ovulation, and the vaginal secretions become more alkaline. If a special litmus paper that changes color according to the level of acidity is inserted into the vagina, a woman can easily tell whether her vaginal secretions have changed and she is about to ovulate.

☐   *How Does the Egg Pass Through the Fallopian Tube?*   One of the commonest causes of infertility in women is a defect in the Fallopian tubes. The complicated procedure for the *in vitro* fertilization (the so-called test-tube baby) is the most sophisticated treatment devised so far for women with hopelessly damaged or defective tubes, but it will be available only to a very few couples for a long time to come. The irreplaceable function of the Fallopian tubes in conception is the reason that their protection from pelvic infections of any kind is of paramount importance.

The journey of the egg from the ovary through the Fallopian tube and into the uterus is extremely complicated, and so many things can go wrong that one is constantly reminded of what an incredible phenomenon conception is. First of all, there must be free mobility between the ovary and the outer portion of the Fallopian tube for conception to occur. Immediately before ovulation the ovary twists round so that the mature follicle (the Graafian follicle) points the egg toward the fimbriated end of the Fallopian tube. The fimbriated end then grasps down around the ovary at the site of ovulation and catches the egg. This prevents the ovum, or egg, from dropping into the abdomen and out of the sexual organs. Once the egg is safely inside the tube, the *cilia*, the tiny hairlike organs on the inside of the tube, move the egg slowly toward the uterus. The egg now begins its seven-day journey through the tube, sustained by nutrition from its surrounding egg white (the cytoplasm). If there is an obstruction in the Fallopian tube—if a past infection of the tube has damaged the delicate cilia or if endometriosis or some other disease has caused scarring and blocked the free mobility between the ovary and the fimbriated end—proper ovulation will *not* occur; the egg will be lost and conception will not take place.

☐   *How Long Does It Take to Become Pregnant?*   A young healthy couple who are having regular intercourse and are not using contraception have a statistical probability of achieving pregnancy three or four times a year. This means that even the most fertile couples have only a 25 percent chance of conceiving a child every month. The most fertile couples are generally the youngest, which is evident from the following estimates of the average possibility of conception each month using four age groups. A woman in her early twenties is considered to have a 20–25 percent probability of conception in any given month. A woman in her late twenties has a 15–20 percent chance. If a woman is in her early thirties, her chances go down to 10–15 percent, and a woman in her late thirties may have a less than 9 percent probability of conception each month.

Using the same age groups, the probability of achieving a conception *within one year* is about 95 percent for the youngest group of women, about 85 percent for a woman in her late twenties; 75 percent for women in their early thirties; and 65 percent for the oldest group, the women in their late thirties.

These averages are posited by a fertility expert from Princeton University, Dr. Charles Westoff. He has also calculated the *average* time it will take women in the different age groups to become pregnant. The oldest group will take an average of 12 months; women in their early thirties, 9 months; women in their late twenties, 6 months; and women in their early twenties, 4 months.

These are only averages and may not reflect the speed or the delay you personally experience in becoming pregnant. If it takes you longer than the "average" woman in your age group, it does not mean that you are infertile; it may only mean that it is taking you slightly longer to become pregnant. There are natural variations from one couple to another and all kinds of variables from month to month that have nothing to do with your fertility. Some of the variables include your professional and social lives, your general health, the frequency of intercourse, the positions you use for intercourse, even your emotions at mid-cycle. Because you fail to conceive during the first or second month you try, this does not decrease your chance of becoming pregnant in the next month. Your statistical chance of conception continues to be the same whether this is month one or month twelve. Even though the majority of women become pregnant fairly quickly, the minority of couples still have an excellent chance of conception; it may simply take them longer, because the mathematical probability of conception isn't quite so favorable in their case.

The length of time a couple has been trying to have children is not the decisive factor in determining their infertility or fertility, and although many fertility experts recommend that a couple seek professional help after one year of trying to conceive, the year's lapse *may* not mean anything at all. One infertility expert has reported that in his practice 20 percent of couples become pregnant between the time they get in touch with his office and the date of their first appointment. This is heartening if you consider that couples usually wait at least a year before they consult a specialist.

One clue to your chances of an early conception might be your hereditary pattern. Conception patterns are often passed down from mother to daughter, and you may learn a great deal about your own fertility from talking with your mother about her pregnancies. Remember, though, that if your mother was in her early twenties when her children were born, and you are now in your thirties, the age difference should be taken into account.

☐ *Infertility: How Common Is It?*   Although 40–50 percent of couples achieve pregnancy in the first few months of trying, 10–15 percent of couples who want to have children will still not have conceived after two years. Once again, this may be sheer probability rather than a definite indication of infertility, but after two years you should take action if you have not done so before. Of course, your age is an important factor. A new French study has suggested that women may become relatively infertile at a younger age than was hitherto supposed. While women were believed to have a good chance of conception up to the age of thirty-five, the new research conducted by French scientists showed a rapid decline in fertility in the thirty-one to thirty-five-year-old age group, with a lesser decline thereafter. The study found that 75 percent of women under the age of thirty could be expected to conceive in one year, whereas only 61 percent of women between thirty-one and thirty-five would conceive in the same time period. The number dropped to 53 percent after thirty-five.

A young woman under twenty-five has about a 7 percent chance of being infertile, but by the age of forty, one out of every three women is unable to have a child. A woman in her thirties does not have many fertile years left. There are no equivalent figures for male infertility, but once again, it is partly determined by age; a man of fifty generally has a lower sperm count than a man of twenty, although the natural decrease in his sperm count may not prevent him from having children if enough of his remaining sperm are healthy.

☐ *When Should You Start To Get Help?* First study your own body. Examine your medical history for clues to your fertility. (Chapter 1 will offer you a guide.) Make sure that you understand exactly how the ovulation and menstruation patterns work, and go over your own ovulation pattern with your partner. Pooling your facts in discussion will help both of you understand better what is involved in conception and may, indeed, help you arrive at a solution. It may be that a simple adjustment in your personal lives is all that is indicated. Some couples, for instance, don't have sexual relations often enough in the month to make conception likely, or they may be temporarily exhausted from work or personal stress, or one of them may have a low-grade infection that can prevent conception. Fertility specialists see many couples who are not biologically infertile; they simply need help in organizing their personal lives or in solving a simple health problem. If the problem seems more complicated than an inability to detect the proper time for intercourse, or your menstruation is so irregular that you find it difficult to predict ovulation, this is the time to look further.

The conventional wisdom is for a couple to see a specialist if they have failed to conceive after one year of trying, but fertility specialists themselves vary in adhering to this rule. Some of them like to see an older couple after only six months of trying, since their chances of conceiving are already reduced because of their age. Some doctors definitely recommend that a younger couple make an appointment once the year is up; others do not. One well known authority, Dr. Sherman J. Silber of St. Louis, Missouri, advises a couple to take action once they are alarmed by their continued infertility and not to adhere inflexibly to the calendar. He suggests that a year may not be long enough for a normal couple to achieve conception. My advice is to act promptly once you are aware of a problem that you cannot solve. Ask your gynecologist to recommend a fertility specialist and make an appointment. Both of you should go to the first consultation. Even if the male partner seems to have no medical history indicating a problem with his fertility, a medical examination and semen analysis by a fertility expert is *essential*. In many infertility cases, both partners are subfertile and need simultaneous treatment. The full cooperation of both partners is necessary for success to be achieved.

☐ *What Could Be Wrong?* This is in no way an exhaustive discussion of the complex factors in human infertility. However, a check list of the most common problems is a useful guide to the exploratory questions a fertility specialist will ask on your first visit.

☐ *Ovulation Patterns* Many women have irregular ovulation patterns. You can establish whether or not this is true for you by keeping a careful record of your menstruation and taking your basal body temperature for a few months (see Fig. 5). A menstrual pattern that swings crazily from month to month probably indicates that a woman is ovulating improperly. She may be ovulating late in the cycle or skipping ovulation altogether in some months. A woman's past menstrual history is significant here. If the menarche was delayed beyond the middle teens or if her periods have always been irregular, either may indicate a long-standing hormonal imbalance. A woman's physical appearance may corroborate these findings. When there is excessive hair growth on the face or arms or a few hairs around the nipples, a doctor should suspect increased male-hormone production. The upper line of the pubic hair should also be checked. If, instead of a straight upper line, the hair reaches up in a point against the navel, this may also indicate that the male-hormone level is higher than it normally is in women. Excessive hair growth on the body is an indication of a condition called Stein-Leventhal syndrome in which the ovaries are slightly enlarged and produce more male as well as female hormones. This dysfunction results in irregular menstrual cycles.

When ovulation problems are present, a doctor will treat the patient with a drug to lower the male-hormone level or with a fertility drug such as Clomid. Clomid is a mild fertility drug that works by competing with the body's own estrogen production. It can occasionally do this so effectively that a young woman will have the sensations of menopause, with hot flashes and other symptoms. When the Clomid is stopped, it will result in a tremendously increased rush of estrogen, which will stimulate the production of the follicle stimulating hormone (FSH), so the follicle will ripen properly and release the egg at the correct point in the cycle. The medication is taken for five days, starting on the fifth day of menstruation, and will result in ovulation three to five days after the termination of the drug. Intercourse can then be timed to coincide with ovulation. Seventy percent of women who do not ovulate at all can be induced to ovulate with Clomid. In cases in which Clomid proves ineffectual, a very potent drug called Pergonal may be used. The use of Pergonal increases the risk of twins and also frequently results in multiple births of three or more babies. For this reason it should never be taken except under the care of a top fertility specialist.

Irregular menstruation may also be due to a thyroid dysfunction. Your doctor should take a blood test and analyze it for the presence of T3 and T4, an iodine uptake. Many women whose thyroid function is in the lower normal value will find it very difficult to conceive. This is because the thyroid triggers the brain to release LH and FSH, which in turn trigger ovulation. Many of my patients who have had borderline low thyroid functions and were given a small amount of thyroid medication, such as 50 mcg or 100 mcg daily of Synthroid have conceived after just a few months of medication. Be sure to have your thyroid value checked and have your deficiency treated with thyroid medication, even if it is a low-normal value.

A Note: A recent study from Japan has indicated that women who were given vitamin B_6 in an experiment had a subsequently higher level of conception. A woman who wants to conceive can take two or three vitamin B_6 tablets daily (at least 50–100 mg) or a B-complex vitamin with extra vitamin B_6. This often results in a more regular menstruation pattern and will increase her chances of pregnancy.

☐ *Defective Fallopian Tubes* Many women suffer from a defect of these important internal sex organs. Tube scarring is usually the result of a past infection, whether the woman was aware of it or not. A hysterosalpingogram, an X-ray of the uterus and Fallopian tubes, or a laparoscopy is needed to establish whether the Fallopian tubes are blocked or scarred.

A hysterosalpingogram is a delicate procedure and should be done only at a reputable hospital or at a clinic skilled in infertility analysis. Since this test can be painful, a woman might want to take a pain-killer or tranquilizer before undergoing the X-ray. A water-soluble dye is introduced with a syringe into the uterine cavity via the vagina and flushed through the tubes. The contours of the uterine cavity and tubes will show up clearly on an X-ray film or fluoroscope, enabling a doctor to see any abnormality in either organ. If there are no obstructions in the Fallopian tubes, the dye will flow freely out through the tubes on both sides and surround the ovaries. Often the test will flush out small obstructions in the tubes and thereby possibly solve a woman's inability to conceive. When she has no other discernible infertility problem, a woman is 50 percent more likely to conceive within six months of undergoing a hysterosalpingogram.

☐ *Laparoscopy* If there is reason to suspect the presence of adhesions around the ovaries and Fallopian tubes, a laparoscopy may be recommended after a hysterosalpingogram has failed to aid conception. Peritubal adhesions, which can be caused by severe pelvic infections or endometriosis, may interfere with the free mobility between the ovaries and the fimbriated ends of the Fallopian tubes during ovulation and thus prevent the egg from entering into the Fallopian tubes. During the laparoscopy a woman is given a general anesthetic, and a periscope is inserted through the navel to allow the doctor to inspect the uterus, Fallopian tubes, and ovaries for adhesions or abnormalities. If adhesions have occurred, surgery may be needed to correct the problem. Unfortunately scarring is often densest at the delicate fimbriated ends of the Fallopian tubes. Scarring in this area is hard to treat surgically, and the procedure called salpingostomy, in which the fimbriae are surgically reopened, does not have a very high success rate. When the scarring is present at the canal that joins the tube to the uterus (the interstitial portion of the oviduct) and a blockage results, a microsurgeon can usually open up the obstruction and restore the patient's fertility.

☐ *Endometriosis* Endometriosis, which is described in Chapter 1, is a common cause of infertility in women. Perhaps 20 percent of infertile women suffer from this damaging condition. The buildup of the endometrial tissue outside the uterus over the years results in painful periods and eventually infertility, because scarring results on the ovaries and on the Fallopian tubes. A laparoscopy will establish whether a woman's infertility is the result of the condition.

If you think you have any symptoms of endometriosis, however mild, see your doctor immediately. Early treatment is vital. The condition can now be treated effectively with a drug called Danocrine (danazol). The recommended dose is three to four tablets of 200 mg daily taken for at least six months. Microsurgical techniques can be used if necessary to clear up residual scarring after treatment by Danocrine has destroyed the misplaced endometrial tissue.

□ *Testing the Male Partner*   The most important test in determining male fertility is the semen analysis. This will establish the sperm count by measuring the number of sperm present in a tiny amount of the semen specimen and using the results to calculate the total number of sperm in the ejaculate. A sperm count of 60 million sperm per cubic centimeter is considered normal; under 20 million is rather low. The motility of the sperm is perhaps more important than the sperm count itself. The sperm are examined under a microscope to determine what percentage are moving or not moving and how well sperm movement is proceeding. Sperm capable of fertilizing an egg proceed at a good or even rapid pace and aim straight forward; sperm that cannot hold their course or that do not have adequate motility are incapable of fertilization. The quality of the seminal fluid is then checked for proper chemical functioning. Finally, the structure of the sperm is examined. Abnormally shaped spermatozoa are incapable of fertilizing an egg, and their motility is usually so poor that they will not be capable of penetrating into the Fallopian tube.

Because the sperm count can vary according to environmental or health factors, which may change from day to day, a good infertility specialist will usually take several samples to determine a proper analysis. If a man's sperm count is very low, it does not mean there is no hope for him to father a child. He should see a urologist, a specialist in male fertility, who can treat many of the conditions that prevent fatherhood. A man who has a hormonal imbalance, for instance, can be treated with thyroid, pituitary, or male hormones (testosterone). Very commonly, infertility is due to varicocele, a cluster of varicose veins in the testes, which overheats the testicles and kills the sperm. This condition can fairly easily be corrected by surgery. Sometimes a very delicate microsurgical procedure is needed to remove an obstruction in the epididymis, the minute tube that transfers the sperm into the testes, or the testes themselves are reconstructed by using special microsurgical techniques. Such techniques to solve male infertility problems are increasingly intricate and successful.

□ *Microsurgery*   If an extensive infertility work-up is required in your case, go to a top infertility specialist. Doctors who are old fashioned in their methods or who neglect to examine both partners thoroughly will not help solve your infertility problems if they are complex. Remember, too, that you always have the right to a second opinion if a specialist recommends surgery. If surgery is indicated, you should seek out a doctor especially trained in microsurgical techniques, who will probably be affiliated with a large university medical center.

☐ ***Psychological Effects of Infertility***   Infertility can be traumatic and may have severely depressive effects on both partners. However, after proper counseling and a full comprehension of their problems by the couple themselves, many fertility problems can be overcome, and many couples are eventually helped to achieve pregnancy. The news of a long-delayed pregnancy makes for one of the happiest moments in a couple's life—some couples would say *the* happiest.

4

Conception

About 200 million sperm are released in an ejaculation, yet only one is needed to effect fertilization. In the few hours leading up to a successful conception these millions of sperm are filtered through a woman's sexual organs until a few hundred reach the vicinity of the newly ovulated egg, and the one successful sperm penetrates the inner membrane of the ovum. Nevertheless this is not a senseless obstacle race but a complex progression involving the sexual organs, a woman's hormonal balance, and extraordinary persistence of the sperm themselves. Because the ovum is capable of being fertilized for only a few hours after it is released from the Graafian follicle in the ovary, nature provides a mechanism for ensuring a steady flow of sperm through the cervix and into the Fallopian tube, with a few sperm finally reaching the egg at the appropriate moment.

The newly ovulated egg can live for only 24 hours if conception fails to take place; optimally, it should be fertilized within 6 or 8 hours. The sperm cells, however, can survive for up to 72 hours in the uterus and Fallopian tubes. This makes conception impossible if intercourse takes place more than 24 hours after ovulation. On the other hand, conception can occur if intercourse has taken place up to three days before ovulation.

Very large numbers of sperm are released in the first moment of ejaculation and move quickly into the cervical mucus. This is not necessarily a welcoming environment for the sperm. For most of the ovulatory cycle the cervical mucus is dense, an impenetrable and effective barrier against microorganisms—including sperm—and any sperm that are ejaculated at an unfavorable time will usually fail to get through. However, in the few days before ovulation the mucus changes to encourage penetration. It liquefies, it becomes clearer and more transparent, and the molecules inside the mucus are rearranged, encouraging the sperm to move in one direction through the cervix rather than lose themselves in a random pattern. These changes favor the penetration of normal active sperm and discourage the entry of immobile or irregular sperm past the cervical barrier.

As the sperm move into the cervix, they are at first unable to pass through the cervical mucus. For the first few minutes after ejaculation, millions of active sperm bounce off the mucus barrier, apparently unable to penetrate it. Finally their efforts are rewarded, and several sperm at different points of the mucus plug make separate entryways and begin to move through the mucus. Other sperm follow them in an almost single-file progression. The successful sperm then swim in a forward direction through the passageways in the cervical mucus and up into the uterus. Sperm that do not have good propulsion are simply left behind in the vagina to die.

In about thirty minutes the sperm, now reduced by many millions, travel about four inches through the uterus and into the Fallopian tubes. Although conception will take place in only one of the tubes, the sperm enter both. Here another natural barrier exists to prevent the sperm moving too quickly through the tube before the egg itself is released. During a woman's fertile period the opening to the tube becomes a filter, allowing only a few sperm through at a time into the Fallopian tube. A large number of the remaining sperm are thus held back permanently and fail to reach the site of fertilization in the ampulla portion of the tube.

The rapidly diminishing number of sperm move up vigorously through the tube under their own swimming power and with the aid of the Fallopian tube itself. The natural contractions of the tube are increased by the hormonal changes at the time of ovulation, assisting the journey of the sperm and the egg. The sperm have the more difficult voyage of the two because they are swimming upstream to reach the ampulla area and the fertile egg, but the uterine cramping will aid their journey, making it possible for the sperm to reach the Fallopian tube in five to ten minutes.

One of the most important reasons for the delay of the sperm in reaching the egg is the fascinating and still mysterious process called capacitation. Unless the sperm undergo capacitation they are unable to digest their way through the enzymes protecting the cumulus oophorus—the cloudlike structure surrounding the newly ovulated egg. Surprisingly, sperm are equipped with the proper digestive substance to attack the cumulus oophorus only if they remain outside the male reproductive tract for a few hours before attempting fertilization. Sperm that swim too quickly up the Fallopian tube are actually incapable of penetrating the egg. Apparently, capacitation involves the removal of a material coating from the head of the sperm, the acrosome. This facilitates the so-called acrosome reaction, in which the outside membranes of the acrosome create an opening in the outer layers of the egg through which the enzymes enclosed in the sperm head can escape and penetrate the cumulus oophorus. Capacitation appears to result in the destabilization of the sperm membranes, the first step toward the successful penetration of the outer layers of the ovum.

Researchers now believe that capacitation may have another important function as well. They have noticed that sperm metabolize sugar faster and move more rapidly after their incubation period at the entry to the Fallopian tube. The removal of the coating on the acrosome may add some motility-stimulating factor at this vital point, with the extra thrust given the sperm possibly enabling it to pierce the zona pellucida cleanly without the use of enzymes. The sperm's

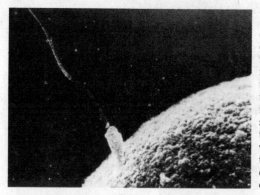

Figure 8: Conception: One sperm has reached the surface of an ovum. The head and tail are clearly visible. Note how the surface of the ovum is irregular. Before a sperm can enter the ovum, the sperm must penetrate the cumulus oophorus, the outer surface of the ovum. After the sperm has broken down this tough outer layer, the sperm head will enter the ovum and part of the tail will disintegrate. Only one sperm is needed to achieve conception.

entry into the inner portion of the egg is so clean and narrow that enzyme activity does not seem to be indicated.

☐ *Penetration of the Ovum*   First of all, the tiny number of sperm, perhaps as few as a hundred, that finally reach the vicinity of the ovum encircle the egg and attempt to penetrate it. The sperm attach the cumulus oophorus first, using their acrosomes as a means of access. These release chemicals that enable the sperm to digest their way through the cumulus oophorus and reach the zona pellucida. The penetration of this tough outer membrane of the egg cell is still a mysterious process. To avoid damage to the egg, the successful sperm must cut an extraordinarily narrow slit in the membrane to gain entry to the delicate inner egg cell.

Before researchers experimented with *in vitro* fertilization, it was generally believed that several hundred sperm were needed at the site of fertilization to enable the one sperm to fertilize the egg successfully. The theory was that numerous spermatozoa were required to "soften" the cumulus oophorus and the zona pellucida. We now know that one sperm waiting at the site of fertilization, arriving in the ampulla while the egg is still capable of fertilization, is capable of penetrating the egg by itself. If there were some way we could make sure that one healthy sperm reached the egg at the right time, the number of sperm in a man's semen would become irrelevant.

When the first sperm has penetrated through the zona pellucida, an extraordinary event takes place. A very fine but yet to be understood mechanism exists in the egg cell. As soon as one sperm cell has passed through the perivitelline space—the space between the zona and the egg cell itself—and attached itself to the membrane of the egg cell, the membrane of the egg fuses with the membrane of the sperm. The sperm head literally disappears inside the egg cell. Immediately the membranes surrounding the egg cell become an impenetrable barrier and repel the rest of the sperm. Because of this phenomenon, most human conceptions will result in only a single birth. Very occasionally, two or more sperm will succeed in entering one egg cell, and a multiple birth with identical siblings will occur. More frequently, two or more eggs are released and fertilized simultaneously. This results in the birth of fraternal twins, or siblings, who may be of the same sex or of opposite sexes.

Once the successful sperm has penetrated the membrane of the egg cell, the sperm nucleus is released into the egg cytoplasm, the part of the cell external to the membrane containing the nucleus of the egg itself. Cell division begins immediately. The 46 chromosomes in the ovum pull apart. Half of them form the so-called female pronucleus, which, after another 12 hours, fuses with the chromosomes in the head of the sperm, the male pronucleus. This forms a single 46-chromosome nucleus, the basis of the cell-division process that will go on for many months to form the new human life. The single cell divides 24 hours later, the two cells then divide again, and further divisions continue steadily while the egg is being transported along the Fallopian tube and into the uterus for implantation.

□   *Can You Choose Your Child's Sex?*   Human beings have been trying for centuries to predetermine the sex of their offspring—generally in favor of male children. Different beliefs about the way the sexes are conceived have resulted in different practices. In ancient Greece, philosophers believed that both men and women produced semen, and the sex of the child would be determined by the strengths of the male and female semen: strong paternal semen would result in a boy, strong female semen would produce a girl. The Talmud declared: "If a woman emits her seed first, she bears a male child, and if a man emits his seed first, she bears a female child."

There was another pervasive theory: that a child's sex depended on the temperature at the time of conception. Aristotle, the Greek philosopher, taught that because the male child was thought to inhabit the warmer part of the womb, a higher temperature favored the birth of boy children; and the physician Galen determined that because the right testicle is warmer than the left, semen from the right testicle was likely to produce a boy. This became the basis of many folk practices down through the centuries, and a woman who desired to conceive a male child was directed to pinch her husband's right testicle or right ear during intercourse. In some cultures the mother's thoughts during the period of procreation were said to influence the sex of the unborn child. The Japanese writer Temba encouraged a woman who wanted a male child to concentrate her thoughts on manly pursuits, such as hunting. Some Arab tribes believed that if a couple had intercourse with their heads facing the sun, a male child would most certainly be conceived.

□   *How to Make a Boy or a Girl*   Modern theories of sex selection are based on three concepts: (1) the different properties of the male and female sperm; (2) the acid/alkaline balance in the female sexual organs; and (3) the timing of intercourse. Couples have traditionally used douching or timing of intercourse or a combination of both, and many couples say they have been successful, while others declare the procedures to be useless. What truth is there in any of these approaches to sex preselection?

Female and male sperm do have different characteristics. The female sperm, which carries the X chromosome, is larger than the male sperm, which carries the Y chromosome. Since the male sperm are smaller, they seem to move faster. This gives rise to the belief that if intercourse takes place precisely at the time of ovulation, the smaller, faster sperm (the male sperm) will reach the ovum first. Conversely, if intercourse takes place a day or two before ovulation, the slower moving, denser female sperm will survive the male sperm and fertilize the ovum.

The larger female sperm is also said to live longer. This has not been proved, particularly since so many millions of sperm are involved in conception that it would be very difficult to calculate the chances of any one group. Men seem to release male and female sperm in equal numbers.

The female sperm is also believed to survive the acid milieu of the vagina better than the male sperm because it is larger and heavier. Therefore intercourse several days before ovulation occurs, at a time when the vagina still has an acid environment, is said to favor the conception of a female child. The practice of douching with an acid substance such as vinegar should, theoretically, increase the chances of the female sperm's surviving and deter male sperm. However, one writer on pregnancy has pointed out that the normal acidity of the female vagina is so pronounced that an acid douche is unlikely to have an effect, and that in any case the mucus in the cervix is not influenced by vaginal douching.

The conception of a male child is theoretically facilitated by an alkaline environment in the vagina. This is said to be increased when the woman has an orgasm. The theory that a female orgasm creates an alkaline environment in the vagina does have some validity. But the changes in the vagina are so rapid when orgasm occurs that this may have litttle barrier effect on the fate of the sperm.

However, a recent book entitled *Your Baby's Sex: Now You Can Choose*, by Dr. Landrum B. Shettles and David R. Rorvik, has proposed a complete regimen of timing intercourse and douching which Dr. Shettles claims has had great success among his own patients. Although many obstetricians are skeptical about the practicality of his recommendations, you might want to try his program, bearing in mind that I am not guaranteeing results. There are two separate procedures—one to produce a girl and one for a boy. The regimen, Dr. Shettles declares, must be followed strictly in each case.

☐ *How to Have a Girl* (*Shettles' Method*)

1. Abstain from intercourse for two or three days before ovulation.
2. Have frequent intercourse in the first stage of the menstrual cycle, to lower the man's sperm count and to increase the predominance of the longer-living female sperm.
3. Increase the acidity of the vaginal environment by preceding intercourse with an acid douche of two tablespoons of vinegar to one quart of water. An acid environment in the vagina is said to kill male sperm.
4. For the same reason, the woman should avoid orgasm, because it increases the alkalinity of the vagina.
5. The man should try to deposit the sperm at the mouth of the cervix to encourage the slower-moving female sperm. This can be achieved by shallow penetration at the time of male orgasm and the use of the male superior position.

☐ *How to Have a Boy* (*Shettles' Method*)

1. Intercourse should be carefully timed to coincide as closely as possible with the moment of ovulation.
2. A couple should not have intercourse during the woman's monthly cycle until the day of ovulation. This is to ensure the highest possible sperm count and give the faster-moving male sperm an advantage over the slower female sperm.

3. The alkalinity of the vagina should be encouraged with a douche of two tablespoons of baking soda to one quart of water.
4. For the same reason, a woman should experience orgasm, either simultaneously or before the man's.
5. The man should attempt to deposit his sperm above the neck of the cervix, so they enter into the uterus, where the environment is alkaline. Vaginal penetration should be deep, and the man should enter from the rear position.

☐ *Artificial Methods of Sex Selection by Centrifugation* Experimental work has been done in animal studies to increase the conceptions of female breeding stock, without much success so far. A method involving preselection of sperm and artificial insemination has been recently evolved by a doctor in the United States who claims a high degree of accuracy. This preselection process involves the separation of the sperm by centrifugation and can apparently be used only if a couple want a boy. After centrifugation the sperm are allowed to settle, and the lighter male sperm can be removed from the top of the test tube. Several couples who consulted the doctor have given interviews praising his services, but whether this method will ever be widely available is unknown at this time.

☐ *Amniocentesis: The Best Method?* The only sure method of sex determination at this time is the amniocentesis test, which will establish the sex of the fetus through the investigation of its chromosomal pattern. Theoretically, if the child is not of the desired sex, the parents could seek an abortion. Sex determination is *not* the purpose of amniocentesis, and a doctor is unlikely to perform amniocentesis for that purpose if he is an ethical physician.

☐ *Implantation of the Egg* Three or four days after fertilization the developing embryo is already changing its nature. The embryo's capacity for synthesizing protein is now similar to that of the adult human. The embryonic genes begin to function. By the fourth day after fertilization the embryonic cells begin a process called differentiation, in preparation for the conceptus implantation in the uterus. Differentiation, the great unsolved mystery of development, enables the single fertilized egg to develop all the complex tissues of the adult human— tissues of the bones, the brain, the internal organs, and the new ovaries or testes.

In order to survive, the embryo must not travel too quickly through the Fallopian tube and into the uterus. At ovulation the uterus is a favorable environment for sperm but an unfavorable one for the fertilized egg, and several days of progesterone action is required to prepare the uterus for implantation. So the journey of the newly fertilized egg is a gradual one, taking about four days. The contractions of the tube and the sweeping action of the cilia move the egg slowly toward the uterus, while the egg itself is continually dividing and multiplying cells. By the time the egg enters the uterus, the stages of cell cleavage have produced the hundred-cell organism called the *blastocyst*. This is the stage of development at which the inherited chromosome structure comes into play. Consequently a conceptus with a severe chromosomal abnormality will not survive the blastocyst stage and will die at about the time of implantation.

By the end of the first week of pregnancy the human conceptus has entered the uterus and lost its zona pellucida. As the blastocyst enters the uterus, electrical charges will usually result in the fertilized egg's adhering to the endometrium in the upper portion of the uterus. Blood vessels develop to provide nourishment for the developing placenta, which has its own cellular structure. The placenta now takes over the feeding of the tiny conceptus, which, until this time, has been supplied by nutrition from the egg white surrounding the egg cell. If any abnormality exists inside the uterine cavity—such as a large tumor or polyps—it may prevent implantation, and the course of pregnancy will end.

The timing of the arrival of the egg in the uterus is crucial to successful implantation. The so-called transport time is so delicate and precise that if it is slowed down by injury to the lining of the Fallopian tube or disrupted by emotional stress, the sequence of development may be seriously disrupted and the egg will fail to implant.

☐ *Ectopic Pregnancy*   Sometimes, if the passage in the tube is obstructed or abnormal, the fertilized egg may become impeded in its journey and implant itself in the tube instead of in the uterus. The egg can survive in this strange environment for a few weeks after fertilization and will continue to add new cells. Finally the conceptus will become large enough to strain the Fallopian tube and cause the tube to burst, resulting in severe abdominal hemorrhage. An ectopic pregnancy usually becomes a medical emergency after the pregnancy has gone beyond the sixth week. (See Chapter 20 for a full discussion of ectopic pregnancy.)

☐ *Test-Tube Baby*   Human offspring produced artificially from conception to birth in the laboratory still exist only in the world of fiction, although perhaps not for many years longer. Over fifty years ago the English writer Aldous Huxley invented a society of the future in which sex no longer had a direct connection with procreation and children were born and reared without parents. Babies in his *Brave New World* are conceived from surgically removed ova exposed to sperm in a test tube and then reared in containers in the laboratory until time for the decanting process—the new way of being born. So far we have reached only the first stage of this fantasy in real life with the successful conception of the children we know as "test-tube babies."

The birth of Louise Joy Brown in 1978 was the culmination of years of patient research into *in vitro* fertilization. Louise, born by Cesarean section in a hospital in Oldham, England, was the first human being to be conceived outside her mother's body. Because her mother, Leslie Brown, had such severely damaged Fallopian tubes that she could not conceive normally, Louise's conception was effected in the laboratory by the *in vitro* fertilization techniques perfected in the pioneering work of Mrs. Brown's doctors, Robert M. Edwards and Patrick Steptoe. Louise's birth has been followed by that of other children in India and Australia, and a number of American "test-tube babies" have been conceived and delivered. Doctors are presently working with infertile couples in several *in vitro* fertilization clinics throughout the U.S., and the success rate of this method has greatly increased.

Many of the techniques of *in vitro* fertilization were first developed during research into animal breeding. Veterinarians now commonly implant desirable embryos from prize cattle into surrogate mothers, and frozen cattle ova are shipped all over the world from top breeding farms. Fortunately the purpose of human *in vitro* fertilization is not, at least so far, the production of "superior" embryos. It enables women who were once considered to be hopelessly infertile because of scarred or defective Fallopian tubes to bear their own children. A woman who has seriously damaged, blocked, or absent Fallopian tubes but who still has functioning ovaries and a competent uterus would be a candidate for this new treatment. So far the clinics have worked only with couples of which the man is fertile, although, theoretically, the procedure could just as well be performed with donor sperm.

☐ *The Procedure*   The media, perhaps confused by Huxley's book, hailed Louise Brown as the world's first "test-tube baby." This would suggest that Louise was conceived and developed outside her mother's body. The correct term, *in vitro fertilization*, indicates the limits of the procedure. The ripe ovum is removed from the mother's ovary and fertilized by the father's sperm in a glass container (*in vitro* is the Latin phrase for "in glass"). After two days, during which normal cell division takes place in an incubator in the laboratory, the embryo is injected into the mother's uterus through the vagina. If the embryo successfully implants itself into the mother's womb, the pregnancy continues naturally without any further intervention.

Drs. Steptoe and Edwards worked for many years to perfect the complicated and delicate techniques required at each stage of an *in vitro* fertilization. What happens in nature must be replicated with great skill in the laboratory in an effort to bypass the Fallopian tubes by artificially performing their functions.

First the mother's ovum must be removed at the precise moment of ovulation when the Graafian follicle is ready to burst and push it out of the ovary. The mother's hormonal levels are closely monitored to determine the exact time of ovulation, and the doctor is able to locate the mature egg-containing follicle during surgery, inserting a laparoscope through the anesthetized patient's abdomen. The ripe egg is then suctioned out of the ovary with a fine needle and placed in a petri dish containing blood serum and nutrients to nourish the egg. Several hours previously a sperm sample from the father has been collected and placed in a dish with a chemical solution and allowed time to capacitate (to mature). The sperm are then introduced into the dish that contains the ovum, and the dish is placed in an incubator at body temperature to allow fertilization to occur. When the egg is fertilized, it is removed into another container, which holds a solution to aid the process of cell division.

Approximately two days after fertilization the embryo has reached the eight-cell stage and is ready for reimplantation into the mother's uterus. The timing of this stage must, once again, be very precise. The environment inside the uterus should be at the proper point of receptivity, and the embryo must have reached the right stage of development for implantation. The tiny embryo is introduced into the uterine cavity through a slender tube passed through the vagina and cervix. If the timing of the procedure is correct, the fertilized ovum will attach itself to the uterine wall and the normal course of pregnancy will follow.

The success of Drs. Steptoe and Edwards raised the hopes of many women and posed some puzzling ethical and legal questions as well. Theoretically it is now possible for a woman who does not have a uterus to hire a surrogate mother to have her baby grow and develop inside her womb. The mother's ovum could be fertilized by the father's sperm in the laboratory and then implanted into the surrogate mother's uterus. Or an egg from another woman could be fertilized and implanted into the uterus of the legal "mother" if a woman's own ovaries were inadequate. It would also be possible for a woman who possesses some superior genetic characteristic to pass on her genes through reimplantation techniques. In any of these cases a court might find it very difficult to decide between the rights of the two "mothers."

The moral questions surrounding the destruction of ova in unsuccessful *in vitro* fertilization attempts are also unresolved and thorny. One case has already been tried in New York City which involved the destruction of a fertilized ovum. A woman successfully sued her gynecologist, who, she claimed, had "destroyed her baby" by refusing to allow a fertilized ovum to be implanted in her uterus.

So far *in vitro* fertilization has proved too delicate and difficult to perform except in clinics with very skilled doctors. However, a number of physicians are being trained in this method, and it will be more available in the future. Another technique presently being developed may have a wider application because it is simple to perform. This is a lower tubal transfer method in which the egg cell is removed from the follicle at the point of ovulation and then injected into the lower portion of the Fallopian tube to bypass an obstruction. Fertilization can then take place normally through intercourse. This is a more natural approach and, it is hoped, will have a higher success rate. Of course the last few centimeters of a woman's Fallopian tube must remain undamaged for this procedure to succeed.

5

The First Signs of Pregnancy

The first overt signs of pregnancy occur within two weeks from the time of conception, although you may be confused by such symptoms as swollen breasts or fatigue because they mimic premenstrual syndrome.

Many women say they know immediately when they become pregnant, although others go through several months before they realize that pregnancy has occurred. However, a woman in tune with her body will usually know as soon as she has missed her period. Although there might be a few days of uncertainty around this time, she will usually begin to feel bloated and tired and be aware of an increased fullness of the breasts. This can be unsettling, especially if she is looking forward eagerly to become pregnant. The easiest, cheapest, and most immediate way to confirm pregnancy is to take your *basal body temperature* for a few days. If you are pregnant, the BBT will remain steadily at its high point of 98.5 degrees.

At about the time of the missed period the breasts of a pregnant woman are quite obviously larger and heavier. If she looks at her breasts carefully, she will see that the surface veins are more visible and the areola, the brown area around the nipple, has darkened in color. These changes in the breasts are caused by the increased progesterone level in the first week of pregnancy. A woman will feel tired and bloated, her appetite may increase and she may have unexpected cravings for sweets, or she may suffer from acne or skin rashes.

If a woman who has missed her period feels any of the above symptoms, she should immediately make an appointment with an obstetrician to confirm the pregnancy, or she might use the home pregnancy test.

Since our environment is increasingly polluted and since we are continually exposed to alcohol, tobacco, and medications—all of which may damage the fetus in the first trimester—it is very important for a woman to detect pregnancy at an early stage. It is equally important to be physically and emotionally prepared for pregnancy before conception takes place, as discussed in Chapter 2. There is often a natural conflict in a woman's mind between wanting a pregnancy and a fear of having it confirmed, and those feelings may sometimes become overwhelming, even when the pregnancy is planned. Your partner may sense the conflict in you and may be experiencing some conflicting emotions himself about becoming a parent. This is a very important time to discuss your feelings and make plans together.

Once you have missed the due date of your period by a few days, get in touch with your doctor and arrange for an initial examination and a pregnancy test. An early doctor's visit and a few other sensible precautions will significantly cut down the risk of abnormalities in the fetus.

☐ *How Soon Should a Woman See an Obstetrician?*   There is no exact rule, but it is advisable to see a doctor as soon as possible to have some important blood and urine tests performed. Medical abnormalities that could have an adverse affect on your pregnancy should be made known to your doctor at the beginning of the first office visit. An early visit also means that you can both discuss the questions and concerns you naturally have as a newly pregnant woman.

Since the first three months of pregnancy are the most important—during this time the vital organs and the limbs and brain structure of the fetus are being formed—it is essential that you are immediately seen by a doctor, given an examination, and placed on a proper diet with supplemental antenatal vitamins. If proper care and nutrition are not given in the first trimester, your child will begin at a disadvantage. These first weeks are probably the most crucial time of any pregnancy, and you need to look after yourself and the baby right from the beginning. Don't wait for a definitive diagnosis of pregnancy to begin your pregnancy. Be in tune with your body and begin caring for the baby and yourself as early as possible.

☐ *What Symptoms Should You Look For?*   Several quite definite symptoms will lead a woman to suspect she has conceived. These clinical signs are clear indications of pregnancy, and if you experience any of them, you should immediately be aware of the possibility of a successful conception.

☐ *The Missed Period*   *Pregnancy should be immediately suspected if a woman who normally has a regular menstrual pattern suddenly skips a period, particularly when she has not been using any form of contraception.*

The absence of menstruation *can* occasionally be deceptive under certain circumstances. It is possible for a woman who is trying to conceive to delay her period through her own desire to become pregnant. The menstrual-ovulatory cycle is under the control of the hypothalamus gland in the brain, from which the FSH and LH releasing hormones are secreted. These hormones are naturally stimulated by the brain to release their secretions of FSH and LH, which in their turn cause the ovaries to produce hormones and prime a woman's body for ovulation. If a woman becomes tense or anxious or even overly optimistic about becoming pregnant, these stresses may block the release of the brain hormones and prevent ovulation and the initiation of menstruation. This very fine interaction between the brain and ovulation is seen in all mammals and is particularly striking in certain animals; the brain hormones of rodents are so sensitive to visual and other stimuli that female hamsters, for instance, will ovulate as soon as they see a potential mate, and a female rat will ovulate when she smells the male. The close connection between the brain and fertility is also demonstrable in human beings. A woman who wants to become pregnant sometimes blocks the release of the ovulatory hormones and temporarily stops menstruating. But it would be misleading to say that the absence of menstruation is *not* an important symptom of pregnancy. If you are trying to conceive, you can look for some other unmistakable signs that will be evident around the time of the first missed period.

☐   *Can a Woman Experience Bleeding in a Normal Pregnancy?*   About one-third of all women who become pregnant experience some vaginal bleeding about the time of their expected menstrual period for the first two months after conception or at other times in the first two months. This bleeding is easily distinguished from the normal menstrual period, and a woman who observes her body carefully will suspect some abnormality immediately. The normal period begins with a light flow, becomes heavier, and then ceases once an expulsion of dark blood appears. Occasional bleeding during pregnancy is quite different in appearance and quantity. There will be spotting or slight staining rather than a decided flow of blood, while the blood itself is much lighter in color—pink rather than dark red—and bleeding will occur at unexpected times. These characteristics distinguish occasional bleeding from the normal period, even though it is sometimes accompanied by abdominal symptoms that may at first appear to be ordinary menstrual cramps.

One type of occasional bleeding in pregnancy is known as implantation bleeding. Conception usually takes place about two weeks after the onset of the menstrual period. In the week after conception the fertilized egg travels through the Fallopian tube and enters the uterus, where it will implant itself. During implantation the blood supply from the uterine lining extends into the fertilized egg to provide it with nutrition, and at this stage of the egg's development some slight bleeding, known as implantation bleeding, may occur. This is experienced as a brief show of light-colored blood, which a woman may notice a few days before she normally expects to begin menstruation. It is not a universal phenomenon. Many women do not experience implantation bleeding and instead simply become aware of a complete absence of menstruation a few days later.

Another sign of implantation is an attack of severe menstruationlike cramps. This may occur immediately after implantation takes place and is the result of hormonal changes in the uterus and the beginning of the womb's expansion. Some women who are aware of the possibility of pregnancy become alarmed by this cramping and think a miscarriage is pending, but fortunately it is usually not the case. If cramping does occur, it is advisable to decrease the level of physical activity, to give the uterus a chance to heal and increase its blood supply. Sometimes the cramping is associated with implantation bleeding, but quite often it is experienced by itself. Cramping may continue for several weeks at the beginning of a normal pregnancy without any particular cause for alarm, but it is a reminder to slow down and rest for these crucial first few weeks.

Approximately a few days after the first missed period a woman may experience slight staining and bleeding for a different reason. Bleeding sometimes occurs at about this time because the progesterone hormones secreted by the ovaries are beginning to diminish in amount and new progesterone production from the placenta has not reached a level high enough to relax the uterus. This scanty, light-colored bleeding can be expected to last for a few days. Again, during this phase, a woman who is bleeding slightly should stay off her feet, rest as much as possible, and avoid sexual intercourse. The uterus is sensitive to irritation because of the low progesterone level, and uterine stimulation can lead to increased cramping and possibly to a miscarriage. Consequently your doctor may advise complete bed rest until the bleeding has stopped and the uterus has healed properly. This type of bleeding is occasionally mistaken for menstruation, but its character is quite different from that of a regular menstrual period and an alert woman will recognize its unusual nature.

Sometimes occasional bleeding will continue at intervals throughout the first trimester or even beyond it. A woman may experience very slight bleeding two, three, or even four months after the last menstrual period before conception, for reasons that are unclear. It could be due to a slight decrease in the progesterone level—which would make the uterus more sensitive—but it could also be a type of biorhythm regulated from the brain or the uterus itself. Scanty bleeding, occurring as it does at four-week intervals, may naturally be mistaken for menstruation, especially by a woman who is less aware of her body or is not happy about the idea of being pregnant. This type of periodic bleeding does seem to indicate an increased possibility of miscarriage, and a woman should be careful not to exert herself physically during the time of her normal menstrual period for the first four months of her pregnancy. Avoid sexual intercourse if you are spotting or bleeding slightly and rest completely for a few days.

If this occasional bleeding is associated with cramping, your obstetrician may want to evaluate your progesterone level to make sure that it is sufficiently high to safeguard the proper development of the pregnancy. Some doctors treat their patients with an injection of HCG (human chorionic gonadotropin)—which in turn probably stimulates progesterone production—or with natural progesterone suppositories. The recommended dose of progesterone suppositories to prevent miscarriage is a 25- or 50-mg suppository daily. This should not have any adverse effect on the fetus, since natural rather than synthetic progesterone is used. You might have difficulty in finding a pharmacy to dispense progesterone suppositories, but at least one company, Caligor, Inc. at 1226 Lexington Avenue, New York, N.Y. 10028, is manufacturing them in the United States.

In general, if a woman experiences occasional bleeding in the first months of pregnancy, there should be no reason to suspect a congenital malformation of the fetus. But there is more cause for concern if cramping and bleeding occur simultaneously for several days together or recur over a period of weeks. This would definitely indicate a need to monitor the pregnancy carefully; a congenital abnormality of the fetus will often lead to miscarriage in the first trimester. It may be advisable to seek genetic counseling to evaluate the health of the fetus and determine whether the pregnancy should be allowed to continue.

☐ *Another Sign of Pregnancy: Breast Changes*   A woman's breasts normally become fuller and more tender as menstruation approaches because of the increase in the levels of the estrogen and progesterone, the female hormones. When conception occurs, the production of these hormones continues to rise instead of decreasing with the onset of menstruation, and one of the first signs of pregnancy is continued breast engorgement and tenderness, sometimes accompanied by a tingling feeling in the breasts and increased sensitivity in the nipples. These subtle changes in the appearance of her breasts may be a woman's first clue to the successful conception of her baby.

The breasts naturally continue to increase in size as the breast glands develop during pregnancy, and this becomes so pronounced in time that a woman will need to buy a larger, heavier bra to give her breasts more support. In the later months the milk-secreting glandular tissue increases its blood supply, the blue veins beneath the skin become more apparent, and the pigmentation of the nipples darkens even further. A number of small elevations, which look like pimples, appear in a circle around the periphery of the areola. These small round oil glands, called Montgomery's glands, begin to be noticeable during the first few months of pregnancy. Later in pregnancy the breasts may become so engorged that stretch marks become apparent; this usually happens simultaneously with the appearance of stretch marks on the abdomen.

☐ *Nipple Discharge in Pregnancy*   Once the blood supply to the breasts increases and the breast glands begin to develop later on in pregnancy, you may, if you gently massage your breasts, notice a yellowish watery fluid, the colostrum, being secreted from the nipples. This can occur at any time during pregnancy. During the latter part of pregnancy, colostrum leaks from the breasts spontaneously, and by the end of the pregnancy it increasingly resembles breast milk. Nipple secretion is not necessarily a sign of pregnancy; after childbirth and breast-feeding a woman may experience some nipple discharge for more than a year without being pregnant again.

☐ *Temperature Is a Sign of Pregnancy*   One of the first signs of pregnancy is the continued elevation of a woman's basal body temperature (BBT) at the time of the unexpected period. If you suspect you may be pregnant, take your temperature for a few days as soon as you wake up in the morning. When the temperature reading remains steadily around 98.5 degrees, the possibility of pregnancy is very high. The BBT method is, indeed, one of the least expensive and fastest ways to verify a pregnancy and one you can very easily do yourself (see Fig. 5).

☐ *Frequent Urination: Another Sign of Pregnancy*   Increased frequency of urination is commonly experienced even before a woman misses her first period. Apparently the elevated hormone levels of early pregnancy change the sensitivity of the bladder and the urethra, making them more easily irritated and stimulating the urinary reflex. This change in urination continues throughout pregnancy, and as the baby and the uterus grow, the baby will begin to rest right on the bladder and prevent it from filling sufficiently. A woman will need to urinate more frequently as a result. Complete bladder control may become difficult in the later months, and some women say this embarrassing problem is the hardest part of the final weeks of pregnancy.

☐ *Fatigue May Be a Sign of Pregnancy*   Women often complain of being unaccountably tired in the first weeks after conception. You may experience a sense of utter exhaustion, which is not cured by a good night's sleep or careful eating habits, and some women feel so generally debilitated that they are certain they are ill. A normally energetic woman may go to bed long before her normal bedtime and still oversleep the next morning or find herself exhausted in the middle of the day, without knowing what is wrong with her or why she suddenly needs so much extra rest.

This change in energy patterns is very common and very understandable when you consider the increased progesterone level in early pregnancy. We know that progesterone in the normal menstrual cycle increases a women's body temperature and also the sensation in the brain tissues, making her feel temporarily very tired. Birth control pills that contain a high level of progesterone, or progesterone injections, result in the same sensation of fatigue. This is also what happens in the early weeks of pregnancy.

Unfortunately the real reason for these natural changes in sleep patterns and fatigue levels are sometimes misunderstood by the pregnant woman and her doctor. Women may go to their doctor certain they are suffering from anemia or from the beginnings of a cold or flu, and a doctor may prescribe antibiotics or other medication without thinking to ask the patient if there is any possibility of pregnancy. Any drug he prescribes might be dangerous to the fetus in the early stages of gestation, and even if no damage is done, a woman who discovers she is pregnant a few week later will be extremely anxious about the baby's development for the rest of the pregnancy. Learning to recognize the real reason for your sudden feelings of exhaustion will prevent an unfortunate misdiagnosis by your doctor. Remember: fatigue in early pregnancy is an important symptom and a natural way for your brain to control your physical function and encourage you to slow down and get plenty of rest and sleep in the first few months of fetal development.

Your mate should understand the reason for your increased level of fatigue and your need for additional rest and sleep in the first few months of pregnancy. Husbands of my patients often ask me what has happened to their normally energetic wives to make them so lacking in vitality. Sometimes they think their partners are using pregnancy as an excuse to take a holiday from their usual responsibilities. If a husband understands how his wife feels, and how important rest is, it will be easier for him to be supportive.

☐ *Cravings: Sweets or Pickles?*   The first sign of pregnancy may be the sudden onset of some strange eating habits. A woman will begin to crave a particular food, sometimes to the point of mania. Some women have an overwhelming desire for anything sweet, or sometimes the taste buds demand bitter substances—pickles or anchovies, perhaps. One of the brighter sides of pregnancy is the stories women tell about their food cravings. One woman told me she became so obsessed with yogurt that she stored gallons of it in the refrigerator because she was so afraid she would run out of it once the store had closed. Other women seem to crave less healthy foods. A patient of mine who had always loved chocolate became absolutely addicted to it and used to visit the local skating rink daily, not to skate but to consume hot chocolate in amounts that would have made anyone but a pregnant woman horribly sick.

The reason for these sometimes bizarre changes in eating habits is, once again, the increased progesterone level in early pregnancy; and for exactly the same reason, women often find themselves wanting more sweet food just before menstruation begins. Once you are pregnant and your progesterone level rises even higher, these cravings become exaggerated. (Interestingly, a woman who rather enjoys one particular food when she is not pregnant will find herself increasingly craving the same food when she is pregnant.) The desire for a certain food increases as pregnancy develops so long as the progesterone levels continue to remain high. Later on, most women develop a strong general urge to eat in addition to their food cravings. This increased appetite is partly due to the progesterone level and is partly also a natural response to the extra nutritional needs of pregnancy. You may find yourself suddenly getting up at 2 A.M. to fix yourself a sandwich, driven by an uncontrollable urge for food, and feeling as guilty as if you were a little kid caught raiding the refrigerator in the middle of the night.

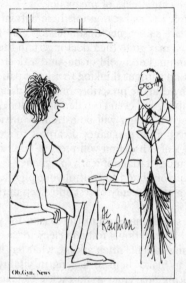

Figure 9: Reproduced by permission of the artist, Al Kaufman, and Ob.Gyn. News, Rockville, Maryland.

Ob.Gyn. News

"It's all in my mind? Constipation?"

Unfortunately some women don't have such pleasant associations with food in the first months of pregnancy. A common first symptom is an immediate decrease in appetite. This begins with a bloated feeling after a normal meal, which fails to go away as the food is digested, and a woman gradually cuts down on her food intake because her stomach feels so uncomfortable. This increasing sense of fullness can develop into a general feeling of malaise, a complete lack of interest in food, and can even lead to nausea and vomiting—the classic symptoms of morning sickness.

☐ *Morning Sickness*   Nausea and occasional vomiting in pregnancy are popularly referred to as morning sickness, although a pregnant woman may feel sick at any time of the day. Years ago women regarded morning sickness as an inevitable side effect of pregnancy, and folk remedies to counter it were commonly passed down from mother to daughter. Poor eating habits and a general

lack of fresh foods probably contributed to the prevalence of nausea in pregnancy in the past. Now nutrition and health habits have changed, and young
women eat better and have a higher vitamin intake than they used to. The vitamin content of a women's diet is significant, because pregnant women whose
intake of vitamin B_6 is particularly low seem to have an increased tendency to
morning sickness. Many of my patients don't seem to experience morning sickness to any significant degree—quite the opposite, in fact. This might be because I generally urge my patients to prepare their bodies for pregnancy by
eating well and taking extra vitamins, particularly vitamin B_6.

There are probably psychological as well as nutritional reasons for the recent
decrease in morning sickness. Psychologists believe that women who are unin-
formed or fearful of the consequences of pregnancy, or who don't want to be
pregnant, express these tensions by vomiting; in a sense, the mother is attempting to get rid of the fetus by expelling it from her body. In the past, doctors frequently saw a serious condition called *hyperemesis gravidarum*, in which the
pregnant woman vomits constantly and ends up in a state of dehydration. The
classic treatment for hyperemesis gravidarum involved bed rest in the hospital,
in a quiet room where no family, especially the husband, was allowed to visit.
Complete peacefulness in the hospital usually cured the condition and reinforced the psychiatrists' view that hyperemesis was emotionally induced.

Years ago tensions and conflicting emotions at the beginning of pregnancy
must have been experienced by many, many women. Before better health care
and modern obstetrics changed so dramatically the mother's chance of surviving childbirth, women faced not only the prospect of a difficult delivery but the
very real possibility of dying in childbirth. Without efficient birth control
methods, children were often unplanned and unwanted. Even twenty years ago
the natural-childbirth movement in America was still in its infancy, and a
woman usually went into delivery without any preparation—other than the scare
stories told her by her mother and neighbors. Fears of the unknown would certainly increase tensions and exacerbate the malaise normally experienced at the
beginning of pregnancy. We can presume that women who were tense, fearful,
and apprehensive in the past were much more likely to fall victim to severe
morning sickness. Modern women are more relaxed, reassured, and confident
about their pregnancies, and far better prepared—much less susceptible therefore to morning sickness than their sisters were years ago. Education, openness
about sexuality, and excited expectations about pregnancy are some of the
causes that have helped reduce the incidence of hyperemesis gravidarum.

Morning sickness often starts a few days after the first missed period and then
gradually disappears seven to eight weeks later, or when a woman has passed her
three-month mark. The level of HCG in the blood happens to increase at the
same time as morning sickness typically begins and is at its highest eight weeks
after the missed period. This seems to indicate a possible link between nausea in
pregnancy and the levels of HCG and to suggest that the HCG, which is secreted from the brain and the placenta, is one of the causes of morning sickness.
Studies have certainly shown that injections of HCG often make a woman feel
more nauseated. After the first three months of pregnancy are over, a woman
who has felt really unwell for the previous two months will suddenly wake up
one morning and find herself free from the persistent queasy sensations and the
desire to vomit. This happens to be exactly the time when the level of the HCG

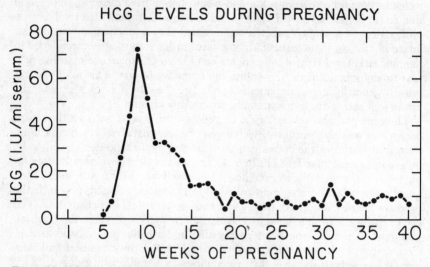

Figure 10: *HCG Levels During Pregnancy:* Human chorionic gonadotropin (HCG) increases sharply from the fifth to the tenth week from the last menstrual period, the time when the pregnant woman typically begins to experience episodes of morning sickness. After the third month or twelfth week of pregnancy, morning sickness often disappears, apparently coinciding with an abrupt drop in HCG. This pattern suggests a connection between HCG and the common discomforts of early pregnancy.

decreases dramatically. Consequently it seems very likely that morning sickness has a real physiological explanation as well.

If you wake up feeling nauseated, you may not feel like eating breakfast. Don't worry; as the day goes on, your appetite will probably pick up so you feel sufficiently well enough by the evening to enjoy a normal dinner. If you experience this pattern, don't try to eat a full meal at the times you feel sick but just nibble on something starchy and drink fluids. You can then compensate by eating more when you feel better. A woman who is vomiting in the morning should take her prenatal vitamins at night or at some time in the day when her stomach feels fairly settled.

Nausea is often brought on by the environment at home or at work. Women differ in their intolerance of common foods and other substances in early pregnancy. You may suddenly find that the smell and taste of coffee or fried food makes you vomit, or you may become immediately nauseated when someone at the office lights a cigarette. Some women are simply more sensitive to smells in general. If you discuss your particular aversions openly with your family or co-workers, you will probably be able to eliminate or cut down on your exposure to substances you find upset you. These precautions will be necessary only for a brief time. The episode of morning sickness lasts for a few weeks, and after that the smell of coffee or tobacco will suddenly have no ill effects at all on your stomach.

Often one of the first signs of the onset of vomiting and nausea is increased salivation. Many women find the amount of saliva they normally excrete increases considerably in early pregnancy and sometimes a woman will produce up to three to four quarts a day. Increased salivation begins two to three weeks after the first missed period, and may continue right up to the end of pregnancy, when it usually disappears promptly. You can relieve your need to salivate by using frequent mouth washes or by sucking on candy or peppermints.

☐ *Excessive Vomiting*   Some women are so nauseated that they can't eat at all. Occasionally a woman will vomit so violently and continually that she begins to lose weight. This can be very dangerous in pregnancy. A woman who is fasting will begin to metabolize her own body nutrients and burn up her own sugar, which will result in an increased production of ketone. Her body may become increasingly acidotic, a state that is directly harmful to the fetus.

If you have symptoms of hyperemesis gravidarum, drink an excess of fluids to help wash out the extra acid from the system, and see your doctor as soon as possible. He may try medication first, and if the condition cannot be controlled at home, he will have you admitted to the hospital, where you will be given intravenous fluids to help keep a steady body balance and avoid ketone development. Usually after a few days in the hospital a woman starts to feel better and begins to eat properly again. When severe morning sickness is treated promptly, the baby will be unaffected, but if you keep the problem to yourself and fail to tell your doctor in time, the situation may become serious enough to affect your pregnancy adversely. It could even result in the death of your baby.

An attack of vomiting can occasionally be so violent that it causes extraordinary stress to the body, and a woman may find blood in her vomit as a result. Vomiting increases the acidity of the stomach, possibly triggering a mild attack of gastritis, which in turn can result in some ulceration of the stomach. This ulceration is usually not severe enough to be dangerous; the best cure is to drink quantities of liquids and eat small portions of food frequently to neutralize the acids in the stomach.

☐ *How to Treat Morning Sickness*   The best treatment is prevention. If you are planning ahead for pregnancy, increase your vitamin B_6 intake by eating foods rich in vitamin B and taking a vitamin supplement. Multiple vitamins with extra folic acid, vitamin B, and iron are important prior to conception to decrease the risk of possible congenital malformations. In addition, a high vitamin B_6 intake fortifies the nervous system and may decrease your susceptibility to morning sickness. Good nutrition seems to be a key factor in preventing nausea in pregnancy. If you do experience morning sickness, try to eliminate from your home or place of work the substances that make you nauseated, eat small meals at frequent intervals, and drink plenty of fluids. Remember, it is important to keep the body balanced; once this is achieved, the body will usually cure itself.

There are a few other simple steps you can take to keep morning sickness to a minimum. Put dry crackers or dry toast next to your bed each night and nibble on them *slowly* when you wake up in the morning. Don't even try to sit up until your stomach feels fairly settled. If you move around or get out of bed suddenly, this may trigger an immediate attack of nausea and perhaps lead to vomiting.

Dry foods with plenty of carbohydrates—bread, cereal, crackers, and toast— are good for the feeling of nausea at any time of the day. If you find that you become sick in the middle of the morning or afternoon, learn to carry crackers in your purse to nibble on whenever a nausea attack threatens. The best general rule is never to go without food for very long. Nausea definitely becomes more insistent when the stomach is empty because there is a higher concentration of acid present in the digestive system. Small frequent meals or snacks throughout the day will help keep the stomach functioning and decrease the queasy sensations. It is sometimes hard to eat in early pregnancy, but going without food only increases the unpleasant bloated feeling and the tendency to nausea.

☐ *Bendectin and Morning Sickness*   In some instances patients do not seem to be able to overcome morning sickness by natural means alone. This may be the result of a variety of factors, some psychological, some physical. There are women who have an unusually high level of HCG in their blood, and this seems to make them particularly vulnerable to nausea.

The only drug approved by the FDA specifically for the treatment of morning sickness was called Bendectin. Bendectin received much negative publicity in the United States and Europe in the early eighties, but it is important to note that it contained only two ingredients: 10 mg of pyridoxine (vitamin B_6), which is certainly known to be safe in pregnancy, and 10 mg of doxylamine succinate. Doxylamine is an antihistamine that has been tested and thus far has been found to have no harmful effects on the fetus. Previously Bendectin also contained dicyclomine hydrochloride (Bentyl), an antispasmodic drug, which was subsequently associated with limb reduction in some animal studies and was consequently removed from Bendectin.

In the fall of 1980 the FDA held extensive hearings on the safety of Bendectin and concluded that the available information did not demonstrate an increased risk of birth defects with its use, although it did recommend caution in prescribing the drug. In spite of the FDA hearings, litigation against Bendectin continued, and the manufacturers decided in June 1983 to halt production of the drug, leaving obstetricians without a specific medication for acute cases of nausea and vomiting.

In my opinion, a woman who is suffering from morning sickness should first try to change her eating habits, avoid foods or odors that upset her, get more rest, drink sufficient amounts of fluids, and increase her vitamin B intake. If these precautions do not control the nausea and vomiting, or the vomiting becomes so severe that she is unable to function normally, or she becomes dehydrated, her doctor could prescribe Compazine suppositories, a drug that has been around for many years and has been used extensively to relieve nausea among pregnant and nonpregnant women. If a pregnant woman is still vomiting uncontrollably, her obstetrician may advise her to go into the hospital for a short time to break the cycle.

☐ *Does Morning Sickness Depend on the Sex of the Child?*   Popular beliefs once held that a woman experienced morning sickness only if she was carrying a female infant. When she carried a boy, according to many cultural traditions, the presence of the male child would make her pregnancy an exceptionally happy one, with joyful emotions and abounding good health. These beliefs were in part a reflection of the strong preference for male children, but there may have been some physiological truth involved. One theory was that the male hormone produced in the gonads of the male fetus stimulated the well-being of the mother. Although this has never been scientifically corroborated, one is tempted to believe that there is still some truth to the old stories. People couldn't have been wrong generation after generation. So many factors influence morning sickness, however, that it is impossible to come to any definite conclusion.

☐ *Do Men Have Morning Sickness as Well?* Yes, they do. Many instances have been recorded of men's lives changing in sympathy with their wives' experiences during pregnancy. Men commonly gain weight, crave particular foods, or suffer back pain, and some husbands vomit or feel queasy in the first months of the pregnancy along with their wives. The husband of a patient of mine suffered such severe stomach pains during his wife's pregnancy that he consulted several physicians and underwent extensive testing, but no cause was found for his suffering. He was treated with an antacid throughout the whole of his wife's pregnancy, and his stomach pains disappeared only after the delivery. In a few instances men have vomited and their partners have not! In these cases we can be sure the husbands are not suffering from a hormonal imbalance!

☐ *Abdominal Changes as a Sign of Pregnancy* Usually you will not see any outward changes in the abdomen in the first few months of pregnancy, and most women don't even show (put on visible weight) until they are approximately twenty weeks from their last menstrual period—in other words, four and a half months pregnant. Once you reach that point, you may feel as if your abdomen has blown up and become huge overnight! But even earlier than twenty weeks, some weight gain is normal, and your clothes will feel tighter around the waistline, although the extra weight will not be enough to change your external appearance.

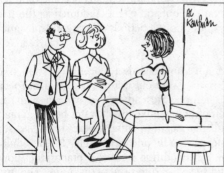

"What do you mean I'm pregnant?"

Figure 11: Reproduced by permission of the artist, Al Kaufman, and Ob.Gyn. News, Rockville, Maryland.

Among the minor changes in the abdomen which you may notice by the middle months of pregnancy is the development of a dark streak running down its center from the navel to the middle of the pubic bone. This line is the result of the increased pigmentation that naturally occurs during pregnancy and is part of the same pigmentation changes that appear on the areola. The dark streak will persist for several months after the baby is born and may remain as a faint but permanent reminder of pregnancy. In the second trimester the navel, which is ordinarily regressed, becomes level with the rest of the abdominal wall, and may protrude later on, pushed forward by the increasing pressure of the uterus. If this happens, the navel will immediately return to its normal appearance after the baby is born. You may also find that the tip of your breastbone, the xiphoid bone, which is attached to the middle of the ribs by a small joint, is being pushed upward in the last trimester by the pressure of the baby, and you may be able to feel a V-shaped bony bump in the V-shaped area between the rib cage. Finally, some women notice the appearance of stretch marks on the abdomen in the last trimester. The reason that stretch marks are common in some women and not in others is still unknown; it may have something to do with a woman's skin type.

☐ *Quickening: Another Sign That the Pregnancy Is Progressing*   By the end of the first three months the fetus is already active. The fetal limbs are tiny, but the minute hands can already make a fist, and the baby will twist its feet and curl its newly formed toes. By the end of another four weeks the mother begins to sense these fetal movements, which are stronger now and more complex as the fetal muscle development continues. Quickening, the sensation of fetal movement, begins somewhere between the sixteenth and the twentieth week. The first experience of quickening has been compared to the faint fluttering of bird wings, and it is so faint in the first few weeks that the mother may be only half aware of the new feeling in her abdomen. Sometimes a woman in her first pregnancy mistakes these early movements of the fetus for ordinary gas pains and only a few days later will suddenly understand their real meaning. Quickening marks an emotional turning point in pregnancy; the fetus, which up to this time was almost an abstraction, is now recognized as having a life potentially separate from that of its mother. The realization that the fetus is alive is often the beginning of a woman's love for her baby.

Later on in pregnancy, as the baby grows, fetal movements become quite violent. Bumps appear and disappear on the outside of the abdomen as the baby kicks out a fist or foot, and the baby goes through periods of energetic movement and quiet periods of rest.

☐ *Are You Pregnant?*   Am I or am I not? has always been a question asked in hopeful anticipation or apprehension. Every culture has had its own special methods for detecting pregnancy. Hippocrates advised a woman who had missed her period to drink a solution of honey mixed with water before going to bed. If she was pregnant, she would soon begin to suffer severe stomach distortion and pain; if not, she would sleep soundly and peacefully. In the Middle Ages a woman who wanted to know her condition went to a practitioner popularly known as a "piss prophet," who specialized in urinary diagnosis. The urine of a pregnant woman was said to have special properties: one expert taught that the pregnant urine would float milk, another said it would coat an iron needle with black spots. And according to Hebrew teachings, a woman who found her feet sinking deeply into soft ground was said to be pregnant.

☐ *Pregnancy Tests*   The most conclusive evidence of pregnancy is, naturally, a pregnancy test. As soon as you even suspect pregnancy, it is advisable to see a doctor and have the pregnancy confirmed. This can now be done early in a pregnancy through the development of more advanced testing methods than were available a few years ago: the urine pregnancy tests, which can detect pregnancy approximately ten days after the missed period, and the even more sensitive blood tests, one of which will pick up the change in hormonal levels before the missed menstrual period.

☐ *The Rabbit Test*   The early pregnancy test popularly known as the "rabbit test" was devised by Aschheim and Zondek in 1927 and was used in many places right up to the 1960s. Testing was initially performed on mice, but a Dr. Friedman adapted the test to immature female rabbits, and it became famous.

All pregnancy testing involves the detection of a special hormone, HCG, human chorionic gonadotropin. HCG is produced early in pregnancy by the trophoblast (the early form of fetal development), starting about two days after the fertilized egg implants itself in the endometrium. Production of HCG increases after implantation, at first slowly and then very quickly. The older tests took longer and were much less sensitive in picking up the HCG than the testing methods we use today.

In the rabbit test, a urine or blood sample was injected into a young female rabbit. If the woman was pregnant, the HCG in the urine or blood serum stimulated the rabbit's ovaries and blood spots or hemorrhagic follicles appeared on the ovaries. These changes were detected when the rabbit was killed and exmained 48 hours after the injection. In yet another test, the frog test, a woman's urine or blood was injected beneath the skin of an adult female frog. When the test was positive, the frog began to produce eggs and a batch would appear at the bottom of the cage only four hours later. A negative test meant that the frog's ovaries were not stimulated to begin producing eggs.

Research has now progressed a long way from the days when laboratory animals were sacrified to verify pregnancy. Modern pregnancy tests are performed on blood or urine and identify the level of HCG early in a woman's pregnancy. After HCG production begins—about one week after conception—the HCG level continues to rise in the early weeks of pregnancy, reaching a high point approximately six to eight weeks after conception; but an accurate test can be taken long before the peak level is reached. The modern tests vary greatly in their sensitivity: one very intricate test picks up the presence of HCG in the blood even before the woman misses her period; the popular urine tests are capable of diagnosing pregnancy within one month after conception.

☐ *Urine Pregnancy Tests*   The urine pregnancy test usually performed in a laboratory or in a clinic or doctor's office was developed to detect the presence of HCG in urine. Because of the relatively low level of HCG immediately after the time of the missed period, the less sensitive urine tests will not accurately detect a pregnancy until approximately ten days after the missed period; only at this point does the HCG level begin to rise rapidly enough to ensure an accurate reading.

The urine test is based on the principles of immunology. Antibodies are specially prepared to react with the HCG hormone and are placed on a slide or in a test tube. When a urine sample is added to the HCG antibodies, a certain reaction will occur, depending on whether a woman is pregnant or not. In the slide test, the HCG containing urine from a pregnant woman will bind to the HCG antibodies and, to the naked eye, the resulting sample will look milky white, without any granules. If the patient is not pregnant, and there is no HCG present, the reaction is different: the antibody HCG will bind to label HCG, and the test results will look like sour milk, with clusters of granules. This popular type of urine pregnancy test is so simple that it can be performed in a doctor's office or clinic and will yield a quick result: one drop of urine on the slide, and two minutes later a positive or negative reading can be taken. However, this is a less sensitive test than the one that is now performed in laboratories in which the urine is settled for two hours in a test tube. If the test is positive, a red ring develops at the bottom of the tube, giving a definite prognosis of pregnancy.

Because of the concern about the well-being of the fetus in the first few weeks of pregnancy, these simple urine pregnancy tests have gained great popularity in the last few years. Most emergency rooms and doctors' offices have the urine slide test available; otherwise a laboratory can be used for the more sensitive test.

An Important Afterword: If the result of your urine test is negative, you cannot be certain that you are *not* pregnant. The test may have been done too early for enough HCG to build up and give a positive result. Have a second test done a week or two later if you still think you may be pregnant because of physical symptoms you have observed.

☐ **Blood Tests** These have recently gained in popularity. The blood pregnancy tests are much more sensitive than those using the woman's urine because they are read from special gamma counters using the so-called radioimmunological techniques. One of the blood tests is based on the detection of the beta subunit of HCG, one of the subunits of human chorionic gonadotropin. A radioimmunoassay test, in which a blood sample is tested in the laboratory to check the beta subunit, is based on the following techniques. First a serum is added to the anti-HCG. If the woman is pregnant, her HCG binds to the anti-HCG instead of the radio-labeled HCG. The bound hormone is separated from the free by accepted methods. Because the blood HCG is bound to the antibody instead of the radio-labeled HCG, the counts at the bottom of the tube will be low. Low counts indicate pregnancy. If the patient is not pregnant, the radioimmuned HCG that has been added to the substance will bind to the anti-HCG, and the resulting level of radio-labeled HCG at the bottom of the tube will be high, indicating no pregnancy.

Another blood test that has been developed to detect pregnancy is the so-called receptor assay. The receptor assay blood pregnancy test detects very small levels of human chorionic gonadotropin and, moreover, can also be used very early in pregnancy, before conventional urinary pregnancy tests can pick up the presence of the hormone. These blood tests may even show a positive pregnancy result a few days before a missed menstrual period.

☐ **How Good Is the Home Pregnancy Test?** A great number of over-the-counter pregnancy tests have recently appeared on the American market, several years after such tests were freely available in Europe. The various tests are basically the same and work the same way even though the brand names are different, and most of them have been fully tested in various university laboratories. If the instructions are followed carefully, the test should be as accurate as those performed in clinics or doctors' offices. But it is very important to remember that these tests do not claim to be accurate unless they are made at least two weeks after the expected date of menstruation (that is, four weeks after conception presumably has occurred). If the test is taken before that time, the amount of HCG present is insufficient to give a positive reaction.

The package instructions for the test must be read carefully and followed explicitly to get an accurate reading. The home pregnancy tests are based on the same methods as those used in the laboratory: a few drops of urine are placed in a test tube containing the testing chemicals, water is added, and the tube is shaken up and then allowed to rest in a special holder for at least two hours. The test must remain undisturbed or the results will be inaccurate. If the test is positive, a brown ring will appear, reflected in a small mirror underneath the test tube; if it is negative, the ring will not appear. A positive test taken at the correct time will usually be accurate—about 97 percent accurate, according to one manufacturer. But if the test shows a negative result, a woman should definitely take it again a few days later if meanwhile she has not started to menstruate. There is about a 20 percent chance that a negative test may be wrong, and a belief that you are not pregnant could have serious consequences.

Women understandably like the idea of a home pregnancy test; it is much more pleasant to test yourself in the privacy of your own home than to wait around in a clinic or doctor's office to have a test made. In fact, I would urge a patient to use a home pregnancy test; it really is better to be safe than sorry, and an early diagnosis is valuable.

6

How to Choose an Obstetrician

It can be as difficult to track down a sensitive and competent obstetrician as it is to find a good gynecologist. Sometimes a woman does not give this important decision much thought. She uses her gynecologist as an obstetrician without considering if his standards of practice really meet her needs, or she may be so excited about being pregnant that she doesn't make the proper effort to choose a doctor carefully. A woman should, however, think about what she expects from her obstetrician and the hospital with which he is affiliated.

Increasing publicity over injudiciously prescribed medications, the large number of Cesarean sections performed, and the rigidity of hospital policies toward natural childbirth have led women to act for themselves instead of uncritically accepting old-established policies. Now that they are more aware, a great number of informed women are determined to find competent obstetricians who can fulfill their particular needs and care for them with respect; physicians who, furthermore, are associated with hospitals they trust. Such women are pioneers in the development of better doctor-patient relationships. It is to be hoped that their example will be followed by other women who want to deliver their children in institutions with the most modern approach to natural childbirth but with the backup facilities to manage any obstetrical problems.

When you begin your search for an obstetrician and a hospital, you must first establish your own standards for obstetrical care. Are you interested in using a birthing room? Do you want rooming-in or a central nursery for the baby? Would you prefer to have a drug-free birth? Discuss these and other issues with your partner; he should be fully involved in the planning at this stage. You must also consider the practical matter of how much you can or are willing to pay for care. Once you have reached some conclusions, you are ready to begin your search for the best obstetrician for you.

☐   ***What to Look For***   There are some basic rules when it comes to choosing the right obstetrician. While I cannot provide you with the name of the obstetrician who will suit you best, I can give you some guidelines that will help you choose for yourself. Choosing an obstetrician and a hospital are very serious decisions; they involve your own health and happiness and the care of your unborn child as well. Be as critical in your search for an obstetrician as you would be in any other important area of your life. This is, first of all, a personal decision for the two of you, but there is also a business side to selecting the right doctor. Since you are the ones paying for medical care, you should try to obtain the very best care for your money.

It is particularly important for a woman who is pregnant for the first time to see a doctor who is informed about the latest trends in obstetrical care and who has time to answer questions that may not seem important to him but are very important to her. A doctor who is hurried or cold or unsympathetic probably will not support a woman's emotional needs or gain her confidence. You will usually be able to determine this at the first visit. If the obstetrician rushes through the physical exam and does not take time to evaluate your past medical history thoroughly, or the office seems to be disorganized or unfriendly, you should probably look elsewhere immediately. You should have an obstetrician who does not resent the time he spends with his patients and their families and who is organized enough to find your files when you call him with a problem.

Your first impression of a doctor's personality is important. A peremptory or autocratic doctor will probably expect you to obey him unquestioningly, especially if he is an older man who regards his patients as little girls who are unable to make a rational decision for themselves. Not so long ago an obstetrician expected deference from his patients even when he ignored their questions or openly humiliated them. Today an obstetrician who behaves arrogantly or inconsiderately toward his patients is not going to be in practice for long!

You should have an obstetrician who will offer superior care and technical competence. For obvious reasons this is vitally important. Pregnancy and birth are critical times. You should not have to suffer years later from some mistake a fully competent obstetrician could have avoided. This is not the place to describe delivery-room emergencies, but you may be sure they do happen, and in an emergency an obstetrician must work very fast. You will want skill and experience from your doctor. But an obstetrician should also fill your specific emotional and psychological needs, and here you will have to evaluate your priorities for yourselves. One couple may be so concerned about safety or technical competence that they will consider only a doctor with great experience and outstanding qualifications and not care if they do not feel at ease with him. You may value understanding and sympathy above a long list of distinctions. If that is the case, the doctor you choose should be someone you can easily relate to, someone who makes you feel comfortable and secure. The same considerations must be taken into account in evaluating the hospital. Obstetrical practices vary widely from one hospital to another, and you should make sure, well in advance, that you will not be made miserable by rigid hospital rules or poor nursing care, or upset because the hospital seems *too* casual about the way the obstetrical unit is run.

☐ *The Second Time Around* If you are in your second pregnancy, you probably already have an obstetrician, the man who delivered your first baby, and you may want to use him again if you were satisfied with the care you received. There is a natural tendency for a woman to stay with the same obstetrician, and later on she may use this obstetrician as her regular gynecologist. When it is a successful one, this kind of doctor/patient relationship can build into a wonderful partnership that is very satisfying for both people involved. Unfortunately some women who have gone through a first pregnancy may not be at all happy about the care they received and may still go back automatically to their doctor, making the same mistake again out of laziness or because they are too busy to search for another doctor. This kind of situation can be compared to a bad marriage in which the suffering partner does not make a decision to

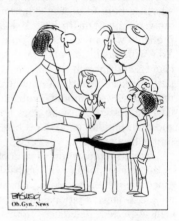

Figure 12: Reproduced by permission of the artist, B. Kusia, and Ob.Gyn. News, Rockville, Maryland.

"Maybe you're just accident prone!"

change the relationship but simply continues to suffer. Review the experience of your first pregnancy before returning to your obstetrician. If you have doubts about the way he handled the pregnancy or you really did not care for his approach, evaluate some other obstetricians before using him again.

☐ *How to Find a Competent Obstetrician Who Cares* When it comes to choosing your obstetrician, it is always important to have some alternatives. Never settle for the first doctor you see; carefully evaluate other available physicians, and do not follow your sister-in-law's or your friends' recommendations uncritically, because your needs may be different from theirs.

Being pregnant should be one of the happiest events in your life. The search for a good obstetrician who will treat you the way you deserve can begin by discussions with friends, neighbors, and family about their pregnancies. This means, of course, friends and family you trust, people who really care about you, people whose advice you respect. Often a woman who has given birth recently is the best source, but before accepting any recommendation you should be fully confident that the woman cared as much about her pregnancy as you do.

There are some useful exploratory questions you can ask to help you make a preliminary evaluation of the doctors your friends recommend. Did your friend, for instance, have natural childbirth? Did she need medication or did the doctor insist on it? How did the doctor respond to her? Her husband? Did another doctor, in fact, deliver the child? Did he do a Cesarean section without an imperative indication? The answers to these questions alone will furnish you with plenty of clues to the doctor's care and his attitude to his patients. When you have collected extensive information about the doctor/patient relationship experienced by your friends or family, compile a short list and begin your actual evaluation. This may seem like a long and tedious process, but you should not compromise your own high standards. This time of your life is simply too important! Do not take short cuts, and never choose an obstetrician for reasons of convenience; the doctor whose office is two blocks away may have the worst record for unnecessary Cesarean sections in the entire area.

If you have recently moved to a new town, the evaluation process is very much the same. Instead of a trusted friend, ask your neighbors or your colleagues at work for a recommendation. It may require some patience before you can put together your short list, and you will need to use your intuition about the women you approach in evaluating their experiences. If you do not feel at ease talking to neighbors or people at work, you can always call the administrative office at a local hospital and ask for the names of two or three obstetricians whom you can then investigate. The process will be quicker if you clearly specify what age physician you would prefer and whether you are interested in a doctor in solo or group practice. A visit to the hospital might almost be better than a telephone call, and any connections you have with a hospital, however tenuous, should be exploited. Nurses, doctors, and health-care personnel at a hospital soon get to know the capabilities of the different doctors they work with. A last resort would be to contact the American Medical Association or the American College of Obstetricians and Gynecologists and ask them for the names of doctors in your area. This is a longer process, because you will need to do more initial evaluation.

☐ *How About Your Gynecologist?*   If you are already seeing a competent gynecologist who does obstetrics as well, you may want to stay with him. There is no guarantee, however, that an excellent gynecologist will be a brilliant obstetrician. You may be quite taken aback, in fact, by the way he conducts obstetrics as opposed to gynecology; it is not unheard of for a sympathetic gynecologist to suddenly become authoritarian and rigid when he has an obstetrical patient. Your best policy is to contact a friend who has used him as an obstetrician or try to ask pregnant women in the waiting room how they like his care. Once you have some reassuring responses, you can go ahead and use him as an obstetrician with confidence.

☐ *If the Hospital Comes First*   Sometimes a couple have heard such positive reports about a hospital in their locality that they want to give birth there and nowhere else. It may be the only hospital in the area that offers a birthing room, for instance, or it may have an outstanding neonatal unit. If the choice of the doctor is secondary to the hospital, check with the hospital itself and get a list of obstetricians associated with the hospital. Then investigate them to the best of your ability until you find a doctor you particularly like.

☐ *How to Examine Your Obstetrician's Qualifications*   After you have found several obstetricians and are ready for your final choice, the second phase of the investigation begins. This means, first of all, looking closely at the qualifications of the names on your list. Many doctors who call themselves specialists in obstetrics are not board-certified obstetricians. They may have conducted hundreds of deliveries and have valuable practical experience but may not have taken the required courses to qualify them as true specialists—in other words, as board-certified physicians.

While many fine doctors are not board-certified and still give excellent care, they are not governed by the rules of the American College of Obstetricians and Gynecologists (ACOG) and may use procedures that do not reflect the board's latest recommendations. A specialty board such as ACOG constantly keeps in touch with its members regarding new developments in the field and also requires that all members attend a certain number of postgraduate classes to keep them abreast of new theories and practices. To become board-certified, a doctor must go through a rigorous resident's training lasting four to five years after he has received his initial medical degree and must pass several difficult examinations that have a high failure rate. Passing his boards indicates that a physician is a top professional in his specialty, and several studies have shown that specialists in various fields of medicine who hold board certification provide a significantly higher standard of medical care than noncertified physicians.

You may find a doctor who is described as "board-eligible" instead of "board-certified." "Board-eligible" simply means that a doctor has met all requirements but has not yet passed the board examinations.

Although many fine doctors are practicing obstetrics without passing the boards, it is possible for a general practitioner to conduct obstetrics and to call himself a specialist without having the experience to handle difficult obstetrical cases. I recently heard of one woman who developed profuse bleeding in the seventh month of her pregnancy and then, in the middle of the crisis, discovered that none of her doctors was qualified to do a Cesarean section to save her life. Instead, a board-certified specialist had to be called in especially to handle the case. The woman and her husband were so angry with her original doctors that she never returned to their care. At the same time they were angry with themselves for not examining their doctors' qualifications more rigorously.

It is easy to ascertain an obstetrician's qualifications by going to the public library or to the offices of your local county medical society and looking up his name in the *Directory of Medical Specialists.* The directory will list his birth date, the medical school he attended, the hospital in which he was a resident, and his board certification. When the term "board-certified" or "board-eligible" does not appear in a doctor's biography, you will have to make up your own mind about how important this is to you. If you do not have access to a directory, call up a doctor's secretary and ask in which specialty he holds his boards. Be suspicious if she refuses to answer you; she may be covering up for her employer.

You should note the medical school and the hospital the doctor attended during his training. Some medical schools have such a national reputation that you will recognize one immediately if it is listed in a doctor's biography. The quality of teaching even in a famous medical school can be uneven, but attendance at a prestigious school usually means the doctor has had excellent basic medical training. But do not pass over an obstetrician just because he did not attend one of the top schools. A less venerable institution may still offer solid medical teaching, and some of the younger schools are now competing fiercely with the older schools. In any case, the hospital in which the physician was a resident is probably more important, because this is where he really learned to practice obstetrics. If you recognize the hospital and you know that the obstetrical department at this particular institution has an outstanding reputation, this is excellent insurance that the doctor is highly educated in his profession. Better still, if the hospital is noted for its progressive attitude toward obstetrics, you will directly benefit from the knowledge and attitudes your doctor learned during his training.

The medical directory gives the name of the hospital with which a doctor is currently affiliated. Always request this important information from his doctor's secretary if you do not use a directory. A physician's skill is often indicated by his hospital affiliation, and the most competent physicians are generally affiliated with the best hospitals. If you live in a major urban area, the most desirable hospitals are usually the large medical centers associated with medical schools, even though their physical appearance may be less appealing than the "country club" look of some of the smaller, more suburban hospitals. This is not to say that some small hospitals are not run extremely efficiently, with extensive backup facilities such as a blood bank or an anesthesiologist constantly on call. Remember that the hospital facilities reflect the care you receive as well as the doctor's standing within his profession.

One of the advantages of the larger hospitals is that the physicians' standards are constantly monitored by the hospital administration or by specially appointed boards of physicians who supervise their colleagues' performances and criticize unnecessary treatment or surgery. (This, unfortunately, does not eliminate all unnecessary Cesarean sections at such institutions.) Hospital care is so important that I urge you to look at the hospitals in your area at the same time as you search for an obstetrician. I have known couples who began with one doctor and then tried to change physicians midway through the pregnancy because they were so horrified by what they saw during a hospital tour.

☐ **Solo or Group Practice?** Traditionally, an obstetrician practiced alone or perhaps with a partner with whom he shared the office. Obstetricians now often prefer to ease the physical burden of obstetrics by joining together in a group practice. This is becoming so popular that it may be the only choice in some areas. If there are a variety of practices in your city, you need to decide whether you want to go to an obstetrician in solo practice who will guarantee to deliver you himself, or use a group of doctors who will rotate your care according to their schedules.

Contrary to the popular belief that a solo doctor offers the best medical attention, several recent studies have indicated that obstetricians who are members of a group often give a patient better quality care. There are valid reasons for this. In a group practice, doctors tend to compete with one another, they have time to go to meetings and postgraduate classes to expand their knowledge, and the physical stress of being constantly on call is mitigated. In evaluating a group practice, look carefully at the qualifications and the reputation of the senior partner. If he is an accomplished physician, there is a good chance that he scrutinized his partners carefully before accepting them into his practice. Ask about the way the group is run. In some practices each obstetrician prefers to see particular patients and follow each one through her pregnancy and delivery. The patient naturally receives better care if the doctor in a group practice knows her well, but you can still be sure of seeing the same doctor during pregnancy and at the hospital only if you choose a solo obstetrician.

Many women prefer the security of continuous care, and it is very reassuring for a couple who know their doctor well to have him present during the stress of labor and delivery. A doctor who gets to know his patient and her husband personally is aware of what has happened throughout the pregnancy and may even know some hidden factors about the patient that can be important to the management of the pregnancy or delivery. This naturally gives a patient an increased sense of confidence.

☐ ***Should You Choose a Female or Male Obstetrician?*** First of all, do you have a choice? Perhaps not right now; the great majority of fully certified obstetricians in this country, unlike those in some countries in western Europe, are males. Recent data from ACOG indicates that only 9.4 percent of all board-certified obstetricians are women. But this small proportion does not reflect the recent rise in the number of women obstetricians in training, and the situation will soon change rapidly. Women make up 60 to 70 percent of the residents currently training in obstetrical departments in the larger university centers, which certainly indicates that in the future women patients will have many more women obstetricians to choose from.

Female doctors who train at the better medical schools and hospitals are as well qualified as any male. They may even prove to have the advantage over a man in obstetrics because they often have a better understanding of a woman's psychological and emotional needs during pregnancy and delivery. Their patients may trust them more and respond to them better just because they are women. After all, it is bound to ease fear and tension during an internal examination when you know that the doctor who is examining you knows exactly how the procedure feels. There are certain pregnant patients who would particularly appreciate a woman physician.

When it comes to choosing a doctor, gender may be an important factor in your final choice, but it is still more important to find a physician who is competent and caring, someone you can trust. I am sure the increasing number of women physicians will have a great impact on the way women's health care in general will be practiced in this country. Male physicians will be strongly influenced by the women doctors they work with, and the male bias in medicine will largely be eliminated. All of us, as a result, will be more alert, more caring—to put it simply, *better doctors.*

☐ ***Calling the Physician*** By now your original doctor-evaluation list has probably been shortened to two or three names. Your next step is to call the doctors' offices. If you are given a first obstetrical appointment date that is weeks away, this may indicate that the doctor is simply too busy to care for you properly during your pregnancy. The first months of a pregnancy are the most critical months for fetal development, and a pregnant woman should have some vital blood tests taken during the early weeks to detect any abnormalities. If you cannot get an early appointment even when you state that you are newly pregnant and need obstetrical care, or you do not like the way the doctor or his assistant treats you over the phone, call another doctor instead. Making an appointment does not, of course, bind you to that particular doctor. Your first visit should be an exploratory one; it will give you a chance to evaluate the doctor's manner, the way he runs his office, and his philosophy of care.

☐ *Are the Most Expensive Obstetricians the Most Highly Qualified?* Before you make an appointment you should find out how much a doctor charges. Most obstetricians charge a flat fee that includes prenatal care, attendance at the delivery, and a schedule of postnatal visits. The American insurance industry is quite benighted about pregnancy care, which, despite its vital importance to two human lives, is taken more lightly than a tonsillectomy. Most insurance companies pick up only a fraction of the full cost for the obstetrician, so you are probably going to end up paying most of the obstetrical bill yourself.

Some people still believe that if they pay more they get better quality care. This does hold true in some instances. Today, however, when marketing and advertising of brand names is so pervasive, we all know that price is no longer an assurance of quality. The same realization certainly applies to obstetricians. A physician's price depends on all kinds of nonmedical factors: the city in which he practices and the rent he pays for his office, for example. An office in Beverly Hills or on Park Avenue is likely to be more expensive than a medically equivalent one in Columbus, Ohio, or San Antonio, Texas. A physician who charges twice as much as another obstetrician may do so only because he caters to the super rich. So the answer is: No, the most expensive obstetricians are not necessarily the most highly qualified.

A recent evaluation of specialists hired and paid for by hospitals showed that these women and men, who are often eminent in the fields of research, generally charge their private patients much less than some of the less well qualified doctors in private practice. Look closely at a doctor's fees and do some careful financial calculating before you select your obstetrician. It might be advisable to bring your husband or partner with you to the first visit to be sure that all of your medical and financial questions will be answered. Remember that two heads are always better than one.

☐ *Can You Change Your Obstetrician?* After a woman has begun to see one doctor, she usually develops some feeling of ethical responsibility toward him and finds it difficult to change even if something has happened to upset the relationship. This is a natural feeling, but it should not prevent her from changing her doctor. It is your right to change doctors at any time. An obstetrician can surprise a patient by prescribing medications in the first trimester that make her feel uneasy or by suddenly indicating a different delivery technique from the one she initially thought he used. Sometimes it is just a question of two incompatible personalities. Many very competent obstetricians find that they constantly lose and gain patients. The doctor/patient relationship is like any other—no one can ever guarantee that it will always work out perfectly. I have occasionally lost patients who decided to seek care elsewhere because they found it too difficult to travel to my office or because we disagreed over the approach to some particular problem.

☐ **Special Care: The Perinatologist**   A perinatologist is a specialist in the management of high-risk pregnancies and deliveries (see Chaps. 2 and 23). In addition to his regular residency training, he must have an additional two years of training that is concentrated exclusively on the latest research and management of high-risk pregnancies.

The larger medical centers and the university hospitals are now hiring perinatologists in greater and greater numbers. A perinatologist on the staff of a hospital is an assurance to you, whether you use him or not, that the hospital is offering all its patients the highest standard of care. This is a very demanding and dedicated specialty. A perinatologist often earns less than a doctor in private practice who is just taking care of normal pregnancies. The total cost to you, however, is likely to be considerably higher if a pregnancy is a complicated one. A high-risk patient will probably need to be seen by the perinatologist frequently, and special tests will be required to monitor the pregnancy constantly. Usually an insurance company will take account of this and will make a larger reimbursement if the pregnancy is marked high-risk.

If there is any reason to believe that your pregnancy will be difficult, I would strongly recommend that you consult a perinatologist, even if it is only for an initial evaluation. Ask your gynecologist or internist to refer you to a perinatologist at your nearest university or hospital or larger medical center, or call the department of obstetrics at an appropriate institution yourself and ask for the names of the perinatologists on their staff.

A perinatologist is usually affiliated with a major hospital, which you will need to use for labor and delivery whether you like some particular aspects of its care or not. The safety of you and your baby must come before any other consideration in a high-risk pregnancy, and only in a large perinatal center will you find the technology and specialized medical care needed to deal with complicated obstetrical cases. There are humanizing forces at work here too. Some hospitals are now looking beyond their birthing rooms and their family-centered care for normal birth and are trying to rethink their approach to high-risk patients. This is a positive step forward and a sensible one as well. Women who have high-risk pregnancies occasionally spend weeks in the hospital before they deliver, and any steps to relieve the tension of that period are beneficial to the patient.

If you are referred to a large hospital or perinatal center outside your immediate area and you are not scheduled to arrive there before the birth itself, you and your husband may be quite anxious about arriving at the hospital in time. But let me assure you that a first baby never simply "falls out." Naturally, you should be ready to leave immediately for the hospital once labor begins. It is comforting to know that the trip to the hospital may be the only time in your life that you can hope to beat a ticket for speeding!

☐ **A Footnote on the Future of the Obstetrician**   A few years ago it was fashionable to say that obstetricians were a dying breed. Far from it! An increasing number of medical students are currently interested in obstetrics and gynecology. This should increase the geographic distribution of gynecologists and obstetricians, so that women who do not have adequate care now will receive it in the future. At the same time, obstetrics itself is changing and is attracting more highly trained and qualified doctors. As more women postpone childbearing and more pregnancies become high-risk, specialized medical and surgical training will be needed for doctors to understand the new challenges of obstetrics.

There will definitely be more doctors by the end of the century, which should benefit patients. We can expect less waiting time in doctors' offices, more competition, and therefore better service: more time spent with patients and more choice for the consumer.

7

The First Visit to the Obstetrician

Since the first visit to an obstetrician is an exploratory one, it is important for a couple to think ahead and talk over their plans for the pregnancy and birth before they enter the doctor's office. If you and your husband know what you are looking for in an obstetrician, the first visit will be more productive for you and the doctor. The best way is to write down a list of questions for the doctor beforehand. If he is a good obstetrician, you can expect him to meet your queries honestly, openly, and without resentment. Most obstetricians anticipate questions and are fully aware of the selection process couples go through before making their final choice. If the doctor is evasive or objects to being questioned, eliminate him from your short list and set up another appointment elsewhere. A doctor who resents questions at the initial visit is not going to change as your pregnancy progresses.

Your mate should also go along with you to the first appointment if possible. His reaction to the obstetrician is important, especially if he plans to be your labor coach during birth. In addition, both of you will have questions during the pregnancy, and your husband's previous acquaintance with your doctor will be invaluable. The time when the man's only function was to pay the medical expenses is long gone. Pregnancy and childbirth are increasingly an experience shared by both parents, a change of emphasis that the medical profession is, belatedly, beginning to recognize. After all, pregnancy begins at the moment of conception, an intimate act between two people who love each other, and continues through nine months of preparing and caring for a new life. This process involves not only a man's physical presence in conception but his emotional and physical support in pregnancy and delivery.

☐ *A New Emphasis in Pregnancy*   In the "old days" obstetricians were primarily concerned with one factor—the delivery of the baby—and prenatal care was confined to checking the patient's weight and general health and screening for such obvious complications as toxemia and diabetes. Recently the philosophy of care has changed completely. Today we know how important it is to have proper nutrition and to avoid anything harmful at the very beginning of pregnancy. An early evaluation by your doctor is essential because the initial visit yields some vital information he needs in the first weeks of your pregnancy.

☐ **Establishing Communications**   A first visit to any doctor usually begins by establishing your complete medical history. I prefer to do this myself rather than delegate it to the nurse, because I feel I get to know my patients better. You will be asked a number of routine questions, which will be kept as part of your permanent medical records. This is a vital part of the initial obstetrical work-up, because your medical history furnishes your doctor with important clues to your general health and pregnancy status.

☐ **Medical Health History**   A complete medical history includes a *family medical history* of both parents and a *personal medical* and *obstetrical history* of the patient.

Family History It is a good idea to review both your and your partner's family health history before you come in for the first visit, because valuable information is often overlooked during the actual interview. A history of heart disease, diabetes, twin gestation, and cancer among members of your immediate family should be noted and, if necessary, discussed with the obstetrician, as should any history of inherited disorders or congenital malformations in either of your families. The latter might require some personal research, since the death of a family member in childhood could have been the result of a genetically transmitted disease. If there is a known or suspected genetic disorder in either of your families, your doctor can then arrange for a consultation with a specialist in genetic diseases (see Chap. 8).

Personal History The personal medical history includes a list of the diseases you had in childhood and a previous or existing medical condition that requires medication or other treatment, such as diabetes, hypertension, asthma, or cardiac problems. A serious preexisting medical condition would place you in the high-risk category and would demand special attention. Any allergic reactions to medications should also be noted down on your medical records as well as any medications you take regularly. If you do take medication on a steady basis, discuss the subject with the obstetrician on the first visit. Taking prescription drugs during pregnancy is discouraged unless there is a compelling medical reason for continuing their use. Even then, your obstetrician may recommend changing to another drug if your current prescription poses a risk to the fetus.

Always check with your obstetrician before refilling a prescription or taking a nonprescription medication when you are pregnant. Just because a drug is generally considered safe, this does not mean it is safe in pregnancy, even if it can be bought over the counter. (Chapter 19 discusses the effects of some common prescription and nonprescription drugs on the mother and on the fetus.) Be sure to tell your other doctors or your dentist you are pregnant before you begin on any course of therapy or if you are advised to have an X-ray. If necessary, ask them to consult with your obstetrician before prescribing treatment.

☐ *Ob-Gyn History*   A complete gynecological and obstetrical history is included in this initial work-up. You will be asked to describe your menstruation pattern; any significant dysmenorrhea or premenstrual pain; the date and nature of any previous spontaneous or elective abortions; and any previous pregnancies and their outcome, including birth weight, length of gestation, and whether the baby was born vaginally or by Cesarean section. With a history of two or three previous spontaneous abortions, genetic counseling is usually considered advisable.

Although you may be reluctant to answer some of the questions in this preliminary work-up—for example, if you have to reveal a previous elective abortion or a venereal disease—your doctor must have all the relevant information to make a proper assessment of your pregnancy. You would want your doctor's decisions to be based on complete medical information and an accurate personal history. Remember, the information given your doctor is confidential. Troubling or embarrassing information about your past medical history is not made available to anyone outside the hospital. When you do have a medical problem, or you are concerned about something in your medical history, don't be shy about difficulties and don't try to cover anything up. Even if you have a medical problem that could lead to a high-risk pregnancy, it can usually be handled successfully if you are knowledgeable about your difficulties and are monitored carefully.

After the physician has obtained your history and has made sure that all the initial problems have been discussed, you will be asked to go to the examining room.

☐ *The Physical Examination by the Nurse*   Once you are in the examining room, the nurse will ask you to undress completely and put on a loose-fitting examination gown. Then she will ask you to empty your bladder to obtain a urine specimen. The urine will be examined for traces of sugar and protein to test for borderline diabetes, any kidney abnormality, and toxemia. If the sample does contain sugar, the doctor will be informed and a glucose tolerance test (GTT) will be scheduled. If you are a borderline diabetic or you develop the form of diabetes known as gestational diabetes in the course of pregnancy (see Chap. 24), you may be referred to a high-risk specialist for further care.

The nurse will note the date of your last menstrual period. She will then ask you to stand on the scale. Your weight at the first visit should be more or less the one it was prenatally. Next, the nurse will take your blood pressure to make sure it is normal. A woman with high blood pressure at the beginning of pregnancy might be suffering from what is known as chronic hypertension. With this condition there is often a problem of an insufficient blood supply to the placenta and consequently delayed fetal growth. Again, the pregnancy might be considered high-risk and the patient might have to be seen by a specialist and placed on blood-pressure medication, or at least expected to rest more during the gestation period.

As you can see, the initial early screening is very important in establishing valuable information about your health and the pregnancy.

☐ *The First Physical Examination*   The doctor will then see you for a complete physical examination, during which you will continue to wear the examination gown. First, your doctor will look at your eyes and skin color. Increased thyroid function often causes a slight protrusion of the eyes. Poor skin color, with dark rings under the eyes or a pale color inside the eyes, is a common sign of anemia. Skin color is generally a useful clue to your general health. Subsequently the doctor will examine your neck to make sure there are no swollen lymph glands present and to detect any enlargement of the thyroid gland. If abnormalities are found, he should discuss them with you and perhaps order further testing. A thyroid test should be done in the case of a thyroid abnormality. Enlarged lymph glands are usually a sign of infection, but a blood test should be taken to make sure there is no serious abnormality in the blood, such as leukemia or Hodgkin's disease, which can be picked up by checking the white blood-cell count.

☐ *Lungs and Heart Examination*   Next, the doctor should examine you with the stethoscope. He will listen to your lungs to make sure that there is no sign of asthma and that both lungs are completely clear of fluid. If you had asthma in the past, your doctor should always be informed; however, if he finds your lungs to be completely clear and you are not taking asthma medication, he will presume that your lungs are generally healthy. A patient with a history of tuberculosis or one whose initial examination is doubtful might be sent for a chest X-ray. Chest X-rays, however, are no longer part of routine procedure and should not be ordered except in the case of a serious cardiopulmonary disease. (X-rays should always be avoided if possible during pregnancy.) A Mantoux test or tuberculosis skin test has replaced routine chest X-rays and can be made if you have a history of the disease or are living in an area where there is tuberculosis or some chance of contracting the disease.

Next, the obstetrician will listen to your heart. During pregnancy more blood than usual circulates through the body, creating an increased load on the heart. Consequently, particularly in mid-pregnancy, a woman often develops a heart murmur quite unexpectedly. Don't be frightened if routine heart examinations in the past have never shown a murmur to be present and then one is found during pregnancy. It is probably what is known as a "functional murmur" and is not dangerous. However, if you have had heart disease in the past or there are signs of heart disease, the doctor should examine you carefully at the beginning of pregnancy, send you for an electrocardiogram, and either talk with your present cardiologist or send you to a specialist for a further examination. Always inform your doctor of a history of such ailments as rheumatic heart disease. During labor and delivery you may need to be placed on penicillin or other antibiotics if you have or have had heart disease in the past.

☐ *Breast Examination*   The doctor will examine your breasts carefully. During pregnancy the breasts enlarge naturally. This means that if you have a tendency to fibrocystic breast disease, a benign condition that induces sore, tender breast lumps, there could be considerable soreness in the early months. A malignant tumor is rarely found in a pregnant woman, but occasionally a woman who has never had a routine breast examination will have some abnormality that should be examined further. Sometimes women have aberrant breast tissue that reaches inside the armpits, which can enlarge during pregnancy as the breasts grow, and cause pain in that area. That is why your doctor will examine you for the presence of enlarged lymph glands or breast tissue underneath the armpits.

The first visit is often a good time to discuss breastfeeding. Your doctor might suggest special breast massages to encourage successful breastfeeding (see Chap. 32).

☐ *The Abdominal Examination*   The doctor will now ask you to lie down and will carefully examine your abdomen to make sure there is no enlargement of the liver or other mass in the abdominal area. Anything he discovers should be evaluated immediately to find out exactly what it is. Scars indicating a previous Cesarean section or other abdominal surgery should also be carefully noted in your medical records. With a previous Cesarean section, the type of incision is important in the future course of the pregnancy, and this subject should be discussed early in the current pregnancy. If you are using a new doctor, you should insist that he send for your records to ascertain what kind of incision was made in the uterus during the previous Cesarean section. (See Chap. 31.)

An evaluation of the size of the abdomen will be made at every routine examination to check whether or not the uterus is the correct size for your gestational age. A uterus that is unusually large could be a sign of twins or of a disease known as gestational diabetes; if it is too small, it is an indication of poor prenatal growth, a condition known as intrauterine growth retardation.

☐ *The Pelvic Examination*   Next, your doctor will sit down at the foot of the examining table and ask you to put your feet in the stirrups. He will then shine a light against the vulva to detect any abnormal discharge or the presence of venereal warts or other surface abnormalities. Any problems should be checked and evaluated and treated if necessary. Symptoms of hemorrhoids, which often become chronic during pregnancy, should also be looked for at this point. The doctor will then insert the speculum in order to open the vagina and inspect the cervix. This does not have to be unpleasant or uncomfortable if he first gently inserts a finger in the vagina and follows with the closed speculum (naturally it should be heated and at body temperature) inserted gently into the vagina up against the cervix and then opened. In early pregnancy this maneuver can easily be performed without any discomfort; as pregnancy progresses, it might become more painful, since the growing baby pushes against the vagina.

During the speculum examination the cervix will be examined for any sign of inflammation, as well as for blueness—a common sign of pregnancy. The doctor will also examine the cervix to make sure that it is properly closed. A previous abortion, or multiple abortions, could have damaged the cervix, leading to a higher risk of miscarriage. The incompetent cervix will then need special attention. If you have had a previous abortion or abortions, your doctor might ask you to refrain from sexual intercourse for several weeks until he is sure that the pregnancy is well under way. Remember: anyone who has had several abortions or several uterine manipulations in the past, should take it easy at the beginning of the pregnancy and perhaps stop having intercourse for a few weeks to make sure that the placenta implants itself firmly into the uterus. The same is true if you have fibroid tumors or any other uterine abnormality. (These topics will be further discussed in the chapters on high-risk pregnancy and serious problems during pregnancy.)

☐ *Tests During First Examination*   Certain tests are performed during this initial examination. One is a routine Pap smear, which will be taken unless you have had one done recently. It is rare to find the beginning signs of cancer in a pregnant woman, but it is always important to make sure that no early signs of cancer are present at any time. The culture for gonorrhea is not routine, but some doctors take it routinely or when they have a patient at particular risk. It is important to exclude gonorrhea, because it could affect the baby's eyes and enter into the child's bloodstream during delivery.

If you have any obvious discharge, the doctor will take a swab and examine it under a microscope. Many women do suffer from yeast infections (monilia) in pregnancy because of the natural changes in metabolism, which increase the blood sugar. When a yeast infection is present, a vaginal antiyeast medication is safe to use during pregnancy. A persistent vaginal infection is a nuisance, because it often infects the labia, which can become irritated and sore.

After this part of the examination is over, the doctor will gently remove the speculum. Again, this should not cause you any pain.

☐ *Internal Examination*   The doctor will now insert one or two fingers of one hand into the vagina and rest the other hand on the outside of the uterus. During this part of the examination he will feel the cervix, the mouth of the womb, to make sure it is sufficiently long to secure the pregnancy. He will also look for a characteristic softening and increased motility of the cervix—the Hegar's sign. Although there is not much enlargement of the uterus in very early pregnancy, one can feel both the uterus and the cervix softening slightly.

The size of the uterus, even at this very early stage, is important. Enlarge-

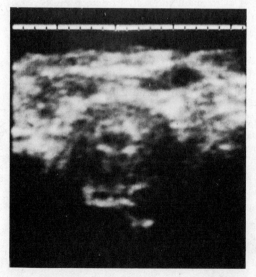

Figure 13: Ultrasonography of the Abdomen: The circular mass in the middle of this picture represents the uterine wall. A small open circle is seen inside the lighter surrounding tissue. This is the so-called pregnancy ring, often the first sign of pregnancy, which can be seen when the patient is six to seven weeks after her last menstrual period.

ment, however slight, should bear a direct relation to the date of your last menstrual period. If it does, we say that the patient's dates and the physical examination correspond. This usually assures the doctor that the woman is right about her dates. It also makes it easier for him to calculate the exact due date, which is important for a number of reasons, including the possibility that your pregnancy may exceed its due date by several weeks. (See Chapter 25, "Serious Complications During Pregnancy.") There are no audible signs of pregnancy at this point, but by the fourth month, when the uterus has grown outside the pelvis, it is possible to hear the fetal heartbeat with a special stethoscope. An ultrasound machine, the Doptone, can detect the heart rate at 12 to 14 weeks; otherwise the fetoscope can detect the fetal heartbeat at 18 to 20 weeks of gestation.

As the examination of the uterus continues, the doctor will look for any fibroid tumors, which are commonly found in women past thirty. If tumors are present, he will try to locate their exact position and will then discuss the problem with you. He might even decide to send you for an ultrasound examination to make sure of their size and position. (Most tumors are harmless and do not affect pregnancy, but, depending on location and size, they can cause prematurity and other problems.) His hand will then slide alternatively to both sides of the uterus to examine the ovaries, since he wants to be sure there are no ovarian cysts or other ovarian abnormalities. If all appears normal, this will mark the end of the internal examination.

☐ *When Is an Internal Examination Necessary?*   If you ever experience a contraction of the uterus (sign of premature labor), you should see your doctor immediately. He will probably examine you internally to rule out premature dilation of the cervix as a result of either premature labor or incompetence of the cervix. A woman with a previous history of premature birth or an incompetent cervix (an incompetent cervix is one that is incapable of holding onto the pregnancy) will be routinely examined at frequent intervals to detect any cervical changes. With a clear case of incompetent cervix, the doctor might place a Shirodkar suture around it to prevent premature cervical dilatation. (See Chapter 25, "Serious Complications During Pregnancy.") In certain other high-risk situations—for example, if you have fibroid tumors—your doctor might also feel the need to examine you internally more frequently than he would the low-risk patient. Normally, if everything is going well, the next internal examination usually takes place at the thirty-sixth week, or four weeks before the estimated due date. After this the doctor will examine you internally at weekly intervals to determine whether the cervix is beginning to soften and dilate. He can then pretty well tell whether or not you will deliver within a few days of the estimated date of birth.

☐ *Blood Tests During the First Visit*   Once your obstetrician has completed the initial physical examination he will know whether or not extra blood tests are needed or if you require only the routine tests, which include a complete blood count, blood type and antibodies, a VDRL blood test, and a rubella test. Some obstetricians and clinics will suggest additional blood tests: tests to establish carriers of sickle-cell anemia or Tay-Sachs disease, an alpha fetoprotein blood test, or other special tests that they feel are necessary in individual cases. (See Chapter 22 on Genetic Counseling for information on special genetic testing.)

☐ **Blood Count** A blood count to ascertain the hematocrit and hemoglobin levels should be taken at the first visit. This will determine whether or not you are anemic. A mild degree of anemia is very common among young women, whether they have good diets or not, and especially so in women whose menstrual flow is abnormally heavy. The extra demands of pregnancy often deplete a woman's iron stores even further, which is why doctors routinely prescribe iron and vitamin supplements during pregnancy. If you are diagnosed as anemic at the beginning of pregnancy, your physician may elect to double up on your prenatal vitamin supplementation or recommend extra iron supplementation. Later on he may schedule another blood count to evaluate your condition further. If a woman is extremely anemic, it is very important for additional blood tests, such as hemoglobin electrophoresis, to be obtained immediately to evaluate the cause of the anemia and to treat it appropriately. In such a case an obstetrician may decide to arrange for the patient to consult a hematologist or treat the patient himself with special therapy.

Sometimes anemia has a genetic origin. An anemic woman of southern Mediterranean origin may have an unsuspected case of thalassemia minor, a form of anemia commonly found among Greeks and southern Italians. When a black or Hispanic patient is anemic, her physician will usually order a further test to determine the presence of the sickle-cell trait. A positive diagnosis of either thalassemia minor or the sickle-cell trait will require special treatment, frequent follow-up visits, and repeated tests throughout the pregnancy (see Chap. 24, "High-Risk Pregnancy"). But more often than not, anemia is due to iron deficiency rather than a genetic factor.

☐ **Blood Type** During the initial visit your doctor should obtain a blood sample to determine your blood type and test for the presence of antibodies. A record of your blood type is important, because you might need a matched blood transfusion after a miscarriage or a difficult delivery. At the same time, the blood test will determine whether or not you are what is known as Rhesus (Rh) positive or Rhesus negative. Most women—about 85 percent of the population—are Rhesus positive, because they carry the Rhesus factor in their blood; the other 15 percent are Rhesus negative, because the factor is absent. This makes no difference to the Rhesus-negative woman's general health, but it does mean that the fetus is at risk in certain situations if the woman's mate is Rhesus positive. What is known as Rhesus disease rarely affects the baby of a first pregnancy, but there is a possibility that some of the Rh-positive blood of the fetus may enter the mother's bloodstream during delivery and create maternal antibodies to foreign fetal blood. Once antibodies develop in the Rh-negative mother, they become permanent, and there is the possibility of their attacking an Rh-positive child in the second pregnancy, with potentially fatal results. Fortunately an Rh-negative woman can be given a specially prepared gamma globulin serum called Rhogam at the time of delivery to prevent the formation of antibodies. As an added precaution, a repeat blood analysis should be done at the twenty-fourth and the thirty-second week of gestation to exclude the possibility of a spontaneous immunization occurring during a first pregnancy, which is rare but not unheard of.

☐ *Rubella and Toxoplasmosis Antibodies*   A simple blood test will establish whether or not a woman has an immunity to German measles. If she is not sensitized to rubella, she will be advised to stay away from young children, the most common carriers of the disease, or from any area where there is known to be a German measles outbreak.

Some physicians perform a toxoplasmosis antibody test at the first visit. A full explanation of toxoplasmosis and its effect on the fetus can be found in Chapter 2 and Chapter 24. Many women already have antibodies by the time they become pregnant. If you do not have antibodies, you should observe certain precautions, even though toxoplasmosis is a rare disease in pregnancy (see Chap. 2). At present there is no vaccine available against the toxoplasmosis virus, although one might well be developed in the future.

☐ *Consultation*   After completing the physical examination and the routine tests the doctor will usually meet with the couple in his consultation room. The consultation after the initial physical examination offers a chance for the doctor to discuss with you, and preferably your mate as well, any problems discovered during the examination. One of the reasons why women are asked to bring their partners with them for the first visit is that any difficulties may be discussed jointly. That would include problems arising out of the woman's medical history or the medical history of both families which might, for instance, make genetic counseling advisable. Also, the initial consultation is a good time for you to ask your questions and for the obstetrician to give you recommendations on general health care and discuss any general health habits that have a bearing on the pregnancy. Finally, he will outline the schedule of revisits and possibly elaborate on his philosophy of labor and delivery. If you find you are in a high-risk category, your doctor might use this time to recommend a specialist who will be able to care for your pregnancy.

☐ *Why Are the Revisits Necessary?*   Revisits are necessary even in the normal pregnancy, because the urine test, blood pressure check, and weight check should be done at least once a month during pregnancy. You need to be sure that you are not developing gestational diabetes, a kidney abnormality, high blood pressure, or the early symptoms of toxemia. The weight check is valuable because a steady weight gain is usually a sign that the fetus is progressing normally. A patient who does not gain sufficient weight may cause her baby to develop intrauterine growth retardation, a condition in which the baby is too small—and which can result in birth defects such as learning disabilities, deafness, and even blindness. On the other hand, a dramatic gain in weight late in pregnancy is often a symptom of toxemia, a condition that requires special care or even early admission to the hospital. Usually there is no need for the full internal examination at each visit. Your obstetrician will simply examine your uterus to estimate fetal growth and check your vital signs and weight.

Every routine visit is important. Most pregnancies go well, but one of the reasons they do go well is proper prenatal care. You can, of course, expect more frequent visits to your doctor if he finds some unexpected difficulty.

☐ *Diet and Weight*   Eating properly during pregnancy is so important that your doctor will undoubtedly discuss your diet with you thoroughly at the first visit. The result of your physical examination will of course be an important factor.

If you are underweight or anemic, the doctor should recommend a more nutritious diet and prescribe extra iron and vitamin supplements. If you are overweight, he will probably encourage you to increase or maintain your protein intake and restrict your intake of sugars. Dieting in pregnancy can be dangerous, and even overweight women are now expected to gain almost twenty pounds. Unless your obstetrician is very old-fashioned, he is unlikely to suggest that you restrict your weight gain to twenty pounds or under, as he might have done a few years ago. Twenty-four to twenty-seven pounds is now considered an ideal weight increase, and more than that is still quite acceptable for most normal women. If you sense from the first visit that you are going to have a constant battle over weight, that alone would be good reason to find another doctor, since there is no valid reason for automatically placing every woman, whatever her weight, height, or general health, on a restricted weight schedule. An adequate supply of calories is *essential* during pregnancy.

☐ *What About Prenatal Vitamins?*   Some obstetricians feel that prenatal vitamins should not be prescribed until the fourth month, because vitamin supplements increase a woman's morning sickness. This is based on a misconception, since morning sickness has been attributed in part to a lack of pyridoxine (vitamin B_6), one of the substances in prenatal vitamins. In addition, the tired feeling you may experience in the first trimester makes extra vitamins a necessity, especially when fatigue is combined with a decrease in appetite. If you are already taking vitamins, mention it to your doctor. Vitamin supplementation is essential for a good pregnancy, but you should be careful not to take too much vitamin A (see Chap. 16). If your obstetrician is unable to make a first appointment for a week or two, ask him to prescribe a vitamin supplement by calling your pharmacy. A vitamin, iron, and mineral supplement is an important contribution to your baby's good health.

☐ *Drinking and Smoking During Pregnancy*   Obstetricians now generally discourage pregnant women from drinking alcohol, especially during the first trimester, although an occasional glass of wine or beer is unlikely to have much effect on fetal development after the first three months. A woman who regularly drinks more than two ounces of pure alcohol a day (the equivalent of four glasses of wine or two ounces of gin or Scotch) may be compromising fetal growth and nervous-system development, while a heavy drinker definitely runs the risk of giving birth to a child with fetal alcohol syndrome (see Chap. 18). All women are encouraged by their doctors to give up smoking whether they are pregnant or not, but a pregnant woman who smokes more than an occasional cigarette is endangering her baby's health as well as her own. If you smoke, your obstetrician will undoubtedly urge you to give it up completely or at least cut down your cigarette consumption during pregnancy.

☐   **Work and Pregnancy**   Although pregnant women are usually able to work and carry on their normal activities up to the baby's birth, a few cautions may be in order. Your doctor will ask you where you work and what you do. He will want to know how much you sit or stand, whether the atmosphere and working conditions are hazardous in any way, whether you have to lift anything heavy, and how often you can take rest periods during the day. A knowledge of your working environment is important because it may affect your pregnancy, although most women continue working quite normally up to due date. Your doctor will also want to know your partner's occupation, since environmental factors at his job could indirectly affect the child's health.

☐   **Exercise and Pregnancy**   Although I encourage my patients to continue their normal lives during pregnancy, I do warn them against taking on too much activity. Pregnancy is not a time to adopt a new sport because you feel you need more exercise, and your normal routine of tennis or jogging should be cut down as the pregnancy advances. It is not true that every expectant mother can and should jog four miles a day, hold down a full-time job, and do everything at home without help. Pregnancy is not a sports event; you don't have to "prove" yourself by becoming a superwoman. The most difficult part of pregnancy is often the period after birth. If you don't take enough rest before the baby is born, you will be totally exhausted afterward. Overdoing to the point of physical exhaustion is asking for trouble.

☐   **What to Ask Your Doctor**   Many women have firm views on how they want to give birth. You may feel strongly about having a drug-free birth or at least being given the minimum of drugs; you may have read about the benefits of an epidural anesthetic; you may or may not want fetal monitoring; you may feel that routine "prepping" is degrading; or you may or may not want an episiotomy. These are subjects you should bring up on the first visit.

Many physicians now feel that drug-free childbirth is beneficial to the patient and the baby; depending on the hospital's policy, they may not do routine prepping procedures; in a few cases they may feel that an episiotomy is unnecessary. But your doctor is responsible for your health care. If he deals with you honestly, he is likely to suggest you plan a drug-free birth, if that is what you want. However, he should make it clear that he will use medication if something goes wrong, bearing in mind that the course of pregnancy and labor can be unpredictable, even in the healthiest woman. A good doctor is not carrying out his professional responsibilities if he suggests otherwise. When my patients ask me how I plan to deliver their babies, I usually recommend taking classes in prepared childbirth and using their husbands as labor coaches; I encourage them to look forward to a drug-free birth. At the same time, I always tell a couple I will have pain-relieving medication available in case it becomes necessary.

Look for flexibility and patience in your obstetrician. Make sure you agree on your fundamental approach to pregnancy and childbirth, but credit him with skill and experience at the same time. A couple's relationship with their obstetrician is quite different today from the way it was in the 1950s and 1960s. Doctors are (rightly) required to inform their patients what labor and delivery will be like, what medications might be used at the birth, and how they approach prenatal care. Except in cases of emergency, most decisions are made jointly by the expectant parents and their obstetrician.

☐ *How Often Should You See Your Obstetrician During Pregnancy?* After the first visit early in a pregnancy, a doctor likes to see a patient every three to four weeks until approximately the twenty-sixth week if everything appears normal. As long as your pregnancy continues to progress well, the next group of visits will be scheduled at three weekly intervals until you reach 32 weeks of gestation. After 32 weeks you will be asked to return every 2 weeks; then, in the last 4 weeks before delivery the doctor will expect to see you for a weekly visit so that your condition as you approach delivery can be evaluated carefully. However, if you are a high-risk patient you will be expected to see your doctor at much more frequent intervals than a low-risk woman would, although the number of visits varies from individual to individual. You might be seen by your obstetrician and a high-risk specialist at a university hospital. You might also be admitted to the hospital on a few occasions for testing.

I know routine visits often seem tedious and boring, but I assure you that it is never a waste of time to go to an obstetrician, even for a woman who feels perfectly healthy and would rather not spend the time. It is only through regular visits that your doctor can monitor the pregnancy closely enough to detect an abnormality in you or the baby before it becomes serious enough to harm the pregnancy. At the same time, you need to educate yourself and learn to distinguish worrying symptoms from the normal side effects of pregnancy. An alert, knowledgeable woman often detects a problem that needs to be brought to the attention of her doctor days or even weeks before her next scheduled appointment, thus preventing a serious complication from developing. When to call the doctor between appointments should of course be clarified at the first visit.

☐ *When to Call the Doctor* The reason you have a private doctor is that you can get the personal care he offers, even during the times outside office hours when you may encounter difficulties that require his attention. Most doctors have telephone hours, or you can ask your doctor's nurse to pass on a message. Telephone conferences should not be abused. Don't call with trivial questions or questions that can wait until your next visit, but don't hesitate to call the doctor if you have an urgent question or symptom that disturbs you.

Never fail to get in touch with the doctor if you have a potentially severe problem such as bleeding—which could be a sign of miscarriage or ectopic pregnancy—or cramping—a symptom of premature labor or incompetent cervix—or a high fever or unexpected pain. Many serious problems can be prevented from harming a pregnancy if they are treated in the early stages. Premature labor, for instance, can often be halted if you see a doctor in time. If you are well informed, if you understand your pregnancy and know when to phone the doctor and what to ask when you call, you can not only save a question that does not require an urgent answer but you are more likely to be able to reach your doctor when there is a major emergency.

☐ *Education for All Pregnant Women* The only way we can achieve our goal of a better pregnancy outcome and fewer congenital malformations or miscarriages is by increasing the knowledge of every woman who intends to become pregnant. More than three and a half million children are being born every year in the United States. Some of these children are still unplanned, but it is to be hoped that one day every woman, whether she has finished high school or college, or whatever her job or family circumstances, will get enough education from her hospital or from her health educator or from other women, to understand the importance of proper nutrition and health care during pregnancy. We as obstetricians are trying to improve our hospitals by increasing the education of physicians and nurses and other health-care personnel and by increasing our educational services to patients. The only way we can achieve complete success and decrease our infant mortality rate to the low level of that in the Scandinavian countries is by caring for and educating everyone concerned in a birth—the pregnant woman, her husband, and the obstetrician. When this teamwork of understanding and caring is finally achieved, we will have reached our goal; we will be a nation of people who care about the unborn child as deeply as we care about ourselves.

8

The Birth Day

☐ *Calculating the Due Date* After a woman receives the news of a positive pregnancy test, her first question, almost inevitably, is, "When is the baby due?" Of course, the obstetrician would like to be able to satisfy a curious parent-to-be, but the due date, otherwise known as the estimated date of confinement (EDC), can be given only within a certain time frame unless you have a precise knowledge of the date of conception. For this reason it is important for any woman who is trying to conceive to record the dates of the beginning and end of her menstruation and to note on a calendar the days she and her partner have intercourse. The record will be a great help for you and your doctor when you try to estimate your delivery date.

The average human pregnancy lasts about 266 days from conception to full term. If a woman has a regular menstrual cycle of 28 days, her expected date of delivery would be 280 days from the first day of her last menstrual period. Two hundred and eighty days can also be thought of as 10 equal "months" of 28 days each.

☐ *How Accurate Is the Estimated Due Date?* In a recent analysis of 17,000 pregnancies that were carried past the seventh month of pregnancy, 54 percent of the women delivered before reaching 280 days from the last menstrual period. Only 4 percent delivered exactly on the due date—day 280, counting from the first day of the last menstrual period—and 42 percent delivered after the estimated date of confinement. To put it another way, 46 percent of the women delivered their children within a week before or a week after the estimated due date; and 74 percent of this group of 17,000 women delivered within a four-week span, beginning two weeks before and ending two weeks after the anticipated birth date.

Using these analyses, we can see that approximately one out of three women will deliver in the week around the estimated due date; one out of five women will deliver a week before the due date; and one out of five women will deliver after the due date. The delivery date, however, still varies a great deal, and a woman with a normal pregnancy may deliver anywhere between 240 and 300 days after the beginning of the last menstrual period. The estimated date of delivery follows a bell curve, with most patients delivering around the estimated date of delivery, but with other patients delivering at points ranging from 28 weeks gestation to 6 weeks after the date of confinement. These extreme points represent incidents of premature and overdue births.

☐ ***How to Calculate the Due Date***   In estimating the due date in single-term deliveries (twins tend to deliver early), the easiest way to calculate the approximate due date is to count back 3 months from the first day of the last menstrual period and add 7 days. For example: if your last period began on September 1, count back 3 months to June 1 and then add 7 days. The approximate due date will be June 8. You can make this simple calculation even easier by counting forward 9 months from the first day of the last menstrual period and adding 7 days. That should give a total of 280 days from the last menstrual period to the expected date of delivery of a full-term infant.

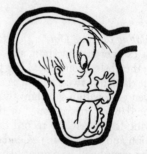

NEAR AS I CAN FIGURE... IT ALL STARTED AFTER THE RANDOLPH'S COCKTAIL PARTY.

Figure 14: Reproduced by permission from Lester Freidman, Monogram of California, San Francisco, California.

Your obstetrician will usually determine your due date by using a calculator wheel called the gestational calculator. One arrow is placed on the date when your last menstrual period began, then a second arrow indicates the estimated date of delivery. You can quickly determine your estimated delivery date by using Table I on the facing page.

☐ ***Why Is It Important to Know the Due Date?***   The approximate due date your obstetrician gives you at your first visit is an important calculation for several reasons. First, babies who deliver close to the due date usually have fewer problems in adjusting to their new environment outside the womb than babies who deliver prematurely. Now that various forms of treatment can be instituted in cases of premature labor, the obstetrician needs to know whether a woman's labor is premature or not. Second, almost half of all pregnancies deliver later than the expected due date. A birth occurring a few days after the estimated date of confinement usually has no negative effect on the baby, but if the birth is delayed

TABLE I

WHEN TO EXPECT THE BIRTH OF THE BABY

The calculation is made from the first day of the last menstruation, and is based on an average pregnancy period of 280 days

Month	1	2	3	4	5	6	7	8	9	10	11	12	13	14	15	16	17	18	19	20	21	22	23	24	25	26	27	28	29	30	31
January / October	8	9	10	11	12	13	14	15	16	17	18	19	20	21	22	23	24	25	26	27	28	29	30	31	1	2	3	4	5	6	7
February / November	8	9	10	11	12	13	14	15	16	17	18	19	20	21	22	23	24	25	26	27	28	29	30	1	2	3	4	5			
March / December	6	7	8	9	10	11	12	13	14	15	16	17	18	19	20	21	22	23	24	25	26	27	28	29	30	31	1	2	3	4	5
April / January	6	7	8	9	10	11	12	13	14	15	16	17	18	19	20	21	22	23	24	25	26	27	28	29	30	31	1	2	3	4	
May / February	5	6	7	8	9	10	11	12	13	14	15	16	17	18	19	20	21	22	23	24	25	26	27	28	1	2	3	4	5	6	7
June / March	8	9	10	11	12	13	14	15	16	17	18	19	20	21	22	23	24	25	26	27	28	29	30	31	1	2	3	4	5	6	
July / April	7	8	9	10	11	12	13	14	15	16	17	18	19	20	21	22	23	24	25	26	27	28	29	30	1	2	3	4	5	6	
August / May	8	9	10	11	12	13	14	15	16	17	18	19	20	21	22	23	24	25	26	27	28	29	30	31	1	2	3	4	5	6	
September / June	8	9	10	11	12	13	14	15	16	17	18	19	20	21	22	23	24	25	26	27	28	29	30	1	2	3	4	5	6	7	
October / July	8	9	10	11	12	13	14	15	16	17	18	19	20	21	22	23	24	25	26	27	28	29	30	31	1	2	3	4	5	6	7
November / August	8	9	10	11	12	13	14	15	16	17	18	19	20	21	22	23	24	25	26	27	28	29	30	31	1	2	3	4	5	6	
December / September	7	8	9	10	11	12	13	14	15	16	17	18	19	20	21	22	23	24	25	26	27	28	29	30	1	2	3	4	5	6	7

The light type in each column denotes the first day of the last menstrual period. The bold face type immediately beneath it indicates the estimated date of delivery.

more than two weeks after the estimated date, problems may arise. By that time the placenta may have begun to diminish in size. That in turn decreases the oxygen supply reaching the baby, with potentially serious consequences. An increased number of stillbirths and birth traumas occur in the group of women who deliver beyond the forty-second week after the onset of the last menstrual period. In a case of suspected postmaturity (an overdue birth) your physician wants to be sure that his estimated due date is accurate before he institutes various testing procedures or recommends artificial induction of labor. Sometimes in apparent cases of postmaturity the due date is off by two or three weeks because the patient is confused about her last menstruation or because her doctor didn't find out that she regularly ovulated late in her cycle.

Finally, your own planning during pregnancy will be much easier if you have a fairly accurate due date in mind. It will enable you to schedule visits to your obstetrician to give you the best care, especially at the end of the pregnancy; and you, your mate, and your immediate family need this information to make arrangements for the upcoming birth.

☐ *Are There Other Methods of Estimating the Due Date?*   Your doctor can use various methods to estimate the due date if you do not remember the date of your last menstrual period or if you tend to have very irregular periods. Some women become pregnant even though they have only two or three periods a year, and occasionally they conceive despite a history of amenorrhea. The first method is for the doctor to wait until he can hear the fetal heart rate through the fetoscope. Another method is to add eighteen to twenty weeks from the time the patient experiences quickening—the first noticeable movements of the fetus—

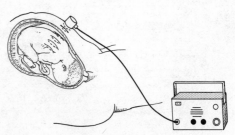

Figure 15: The Fetal Heartbeat:
The fetal heartbeat can usually be heard with a stethoscope (fetoscope) at approximately eighteen to twenty weeks from the first day of the last menstrual period. With the modern Doppler ultrasound machine, which many doctors now have in their offices, the heartbeat can be heard at twelve to thirteen weeks after the last menstrual period. The Doppler system utilizes ultrasound, which will change frequency as it is reflected against moving organs, such as the heart. The heartbeat can be picked up on the loudspeaker.

and arrive at a rough due date by this means. Neither of these methods is as precise as determining the due date from a woman's recollection of the date of her last menstrual period.

As pregnancy progresses, an estimation of the due date can be arrived at by palpating the uterus. The expanding uterus is usually still well hidden behind the pelvic bone at the end of the first trimester. Immediately after the three-month point, the fundus (the top of the uterus) can be felt right above the pelvic bone. Once the gestation of the pregnancy is at 20 weeks, the fundus is usually at the level of the umbilicus. Think of the umbilicus as an 0 and then place a 2 in front of it, denoting the 20th week of the pregnancy—a memorable point because 20 weeks marks halfway between conception and delivery. Then at 36 weeks' gestation the uterus is usually at its highest point and is pushing the rib cage up with it. After 36 weeks fetal engagement usually occurs and the fundus of the uterus begins to diminish.

☐ *The Use of Ultrasonography to Determine the Due Date*   Your obstetrician can determine an approximate due date by the use of ultrasound. An ultrasound device works pretty much like the sonar system of a submarine: it has the capability of transmitting sounds at such high frequencies that they cannot be heard by the human ear. These high-frequency acoustical waves are used to obtain an X-raylike picture of what is going on inside the uterus. The waves of sound are bounced off the fetus, and the returning sound waves produce the fetal image on a small screen that resembles a television set. It is rather like throwing a sound into the Grand Canyon and listening to the massive echoes bouncing off the canyon walls.

Once the baby's image is on the screen, the outline of the fetus can be studied to ascertain its stage of development and the head can be measured from one side to the other. The size of the fetal head follows a growth pattern linked to the weeks of gestation, and researchers have used ultrasonography to construct a curve of the average growth of the fetal head *in utero*. Once the so-called biparietal diameter—the distance between the temples of the fetal head—is measured, the results can be plugged into the natural curve, allowing the doctor to estimate, with some accuracy, how far along the pregnancy is. This will enable him to calculate the due date.

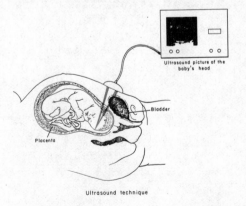

Figure 16: The Biparietal Diameter: One of the most precise ways to determine fetal size is the use of ultrasound. During an ultrasound examination, sound waves are directed against the baby's head and reflected from the head back to the Doppler transducer, which has the capacity to visualize the shape of the head on an ultrasound screen. By measuring the biparietal diameter, the doctor can estimate fetal age by comparing the results with the natural growth curve.

Ultrasound is an extremely powerful and impressive device, which, as far as we can tell, has no harmful effect on the child or the mother. Doctors now use it to examine the fetus for major structural abnormalities or to reassure themselves and the patient that the baby is developing normally. Some doctors suggest at least two ultrasonographies during a pregnancy to make sure that the baby's growth is following the natural curve of development.

☐ *Can X-Rays Be Used?*   X-rays cannot be used to estimate gestation age, because the X-ray picture is not capable of outlining the soft fetal tissues in detail. Furthermore, the potentially teratogenic effect of X-rays makes this an unacceptable method of determining the due date.

In the past, before doctors fully realized the damage ionizing radiation could do to the developing fetus, they frequently used X-rays later on in pregnancy to determine whether the epiphyseal lines (developmental lines in the bones) were developed or not. The epiphyseal lines are usually fully formed by the time the fetus is eight months old, and establishing their presence provided a rough guide to the baby's probable delivery date. Although the baby's limbs, brain, and vital organs are completely developed by the eighth month, it is possible for the fetal gonads to be damaged by ionizing radiation, and X-rays in pregnancy have also been tentatively linked to an increased incidence of childhood cancer. *Never* agree to such a procedure unless the doctor is looking for other parameters, such as the configuration of your pelvic bones, at the same time. This is *occasionally* necessary if there is a strong possibility of maternal/fetal disproportion during labor (see Chap. 30).

9

The Fetus

Conception and the development of the unborn child have always been great mysteries. Even after the past two centuries of research into conception there are still questions about the way the embryo develops to which we do not have the answer. Thousands of years ago primitive peoples realized that there was some link between menstruation and conception, since they observed that a pregnant woman ceased to bleed every month, but many tribal beliefs made no connection between sexual intercourse and pregnancy.

The ancient Hindus believed that there were three basic components needed for the creation of a baby: first, the father provided the white semen to form the child's bones; then the mother contributed the red semen to produce the skin, the hair, and the iris of the eyes. However, it was left to God to provide the expression of the face, and the child's sight, hearing, speech, and movements. But the ancient Hindus and Egyptians also thought that the ibis brought children, and young couples who wanted a child would offer up prayers to flocks of these sacred birds in the hope that the ibis would bless them. The myth that birds bring human children from some mysterious place persisted in folk culture through the Middle Ages in Europe and Asia, and up to a few years ago the stork was still used by parents to avoid embarrassing questions by children about their origin.

The ancient Hindu theory that both the man and the woman contribute somehow to the making of a child is to be found in other cultures as well, including those of the Greeks and the Jews. Hippocrates, who is acknowledged to be the founder of the modern profession of medicine, formed his own, more elaborate theory of conception in 400 B.C. He believed that conception was not only caused by the combination of male and female semen but that when conception occurred, the menstrual blood flowed daily into the uterus, and this accumulation of menstrual blood formed the flesh of a new child. Hippocrates believed that both the woman's ovaries and the man's testes produced semen, and the appearance of the conceptus was the result of the commingling of both the male and female semen.

This theory was hotly disputed by Aristotle, who felt that the woman was a purely passive partner in the act of conception and contributed nothing but the shelter of her body to the development of the unborn child. He based this belief on the observation that a woman could become pregnant while remaining completely passive during intercourse, while a man had to work to achieve conception. Therefore, he concluded, the man must be the only one to contribute the vital elements to the child, including the dynamic principles of thought, morality, and feelings. Aristotle's theory that the woman was merely an instrument in conception, whose only function was to nurture the young child, was not original with him. Many farming cultures likened the woman's body to the plot of ground in which the man sows his seeds. However, because of Aristotle's eminence in his own time and for many hundreds of years after, his idea of conception was widely taught and believed, right through the Middle Ages.

The Aristotelean thesis did not, however, prevent further speculation among the thinkers of medieval Europe. Later in the century the famous Italian doctor Fallopius examined the ovaries in an attempt to find semenlike elements. Because he failed to discover any trace of semen in the ovaries (at the same time, he quite accidentally found the tubes that are named after him), he agreed with the Aristotelean theory that women had no function in conception. This theory was challenged in 1621 when Fabricius arrived at a new theory of conception by dividing animals into two categories: those that produced eggs externally and those, including humans, that developed a fetus internally by a combination of an unknown substance from the mother and the semen fluid from the father.

In 1672 the ovarian follicle was discovered. This was overshadowed in the popular imagination by the discovery of sperm cells inside the semen, when a medical student examined the semen through the newly invented microscope, and Anton van Leeuwenhoek, the originator of the instrument, presented his sensational findings to the Royal Society in London. The society was in an uproar immediately. Some scientists firmly denied that sperm had anything to do with conception, while others described the appearance of homunculi, or miniature men, encased in the sperm cells, who, they declared, could be seen swimming around in the semen. This idea became immensely popular and found its way into most of the obstetrical textbooks of the time.

Then, approximately one hundred years later, an Italian biologist, Lazzaro Spallanzani, performed an experiment in which he fastened a tiny pair of "trousers" on a male frog. The frog, of course, failed to fertilize the female frog during the act of mating. He then collected the semen that the frog had spilled inside the "trousers" and mixed it with the eggs from a fertile female. The eggs became fertile. Even so Spallanzani failed to draw the logical conclusion from his experiment, and only as late as 1843 did Dr. Martin Barrie finally make the important discovery that a fetus originates from the union between the sperm and the egg. Since Dr. Barrie's pioneering experiments, scientists and medical researchers have agreed on the equal role of female eggs and male sperm in conception. However, only recently have we been able to identify clearly the process of conception and to photograph ovulation and conception as it occurs in the human being. This has given us a tremendous insight into conception and the incredible process of fetal development.

☐ *Does Life Begin at the Moment of Conception?* The theories as to when a conceptus can be considered a human being have varied greatly among different societies and countries and between different religious and legal authorities.

While we often say that life is created from the very moment of conception, many conceptuses never progress beyond the initial point of development. Many misfortunes can occur before the mass of cells goes beyond even the very earliest stage: there may be fetal wastage, resulting in a spontaneous abortion, because of uterine abnormality, or a hormonal imbalance, or a severe congenital abnormality incompatible with human life. Many scientists feel that we cannot realistically talk about life until a fetus is viable—that is, until it can exist, if only for a short time, outside the womb. Twenty-four weeks is presently held to be the point at which a fetus can be born alive and have some chance, however small, of surviving on its own. Consequently an abortion can be performed legally up to the twenty-fourth week. A miscarriage before the twenty-fourth week is considered a spontaneous abortion; after the twenty-fourth week we talk about a premature birth.

From legal and moral standpoints and perhaps in the future from a medical one as well, the concept of viability is constantly up for debate, but it is not within the framework of this book to tackle this difficult subject except as it touches on the development of the fetus through its gestational period. Twenty-four weeks marks a very significant point in the evolution of the fetus from a simple ball of cells to a vigorous and active baby, but there are other milestones that the fetus passes which are equally vital to a successful birth and a healthy child.

The first three months after conception are particularly important, because this is the time when the fetus is essentially formed, and the nervous system and the internal organs need the most advantageous environment to develop properly and avoid the possibility of congenital malformations. After these first three months the fetus is more or less formed, movement has begun, and the fetal heartbeat is evident. From the twelfth week on—with the important exception of the fetal brain, which is slower to develop than the other organs—the fetus merely grows in size, and the various organs subsequently reach full maturity.

☐ *How to Calculate Gestational Age* A woman is often puzzled by her doctor's interpretation of gestational age, since physicians and lay people often seem to speak different languages. While "everyone knows" that a pregnancy takes nine months, your doctor may confuse you by talking about the ten months of pregnancy.

It is important for you to understand why different people calculate gestational age differently, because it does affect your pregnancy. Your doctor or midwife is trained to calculate the gestational age from the first day of your last menstrual period. Professionals follow this rule, because a woman will usually remember when her last menstrual period began, and this makes it easier to determine a specific date of birth.

According to your doctor's calculation, a woman who has a regular menstrual period will deliver her baby at the end of 10 months of 28 days (a lunar month) each, calculated from the first day of the last menstrual period she experienced before she conceived. In other words, there are 10 lunar months from the last day of menstruation to the expected day of delivery. This means of determining gestation makes it much easier for the physician. However, in reality, a woman who has a regular menstrual cycle will usually conceive in the middle of the cycle, or two weeks after the onset of the last menstruation. This is the time that most lay people consider to be the beginning of pregnancy. By their interpretation, a woman can expect to give birth approximately 9 months later—full months of 30 to 31 days each, not lunar months.

Since your doctor uses the lunar calendar and calculates gestational age from the onset of the last menstrual period, I will be using that particular method in this book when I refer to gestational age. If you familiarize yourself with this calculation you will be able to communicate more easily with your doctor. For instance, when your doctor tells you that you are 20 weeks' pregnant, 20 weeks for him means that you conceived 18 weeks ago, and you have exactly 20 more weeks to go.

□ *Development of the Fetus*   Conception and fetal development are truly one of the world's greatest wonders. In this section we will travel through each stage of fetal development from conception to delivery to try to give you an idea of what is happening inside your womb. As the fetus is growing, it is attached to you by the umbilical cord. Approximately 25 percent of the pregnant woman's blood volume is directed to the uterus and the placenta. This is how the fetus is nourished during the months of pregnancy. The fetus derives food from its mother, but it can also take in deleterious substances, because anything you consume will be absorbed into your bloodstream. Since the placenta is unable to screen out poisons, traces of such substances as drugs, alcohol, and tobacco will be flushed right into the fetal circulation. Consequently what you eat, drink, and surround yourself with can influence and may even hamper the normal development of the fetus.

Intrauterine growth is largely governed by the placenta, which, at the beginning of fetal development, is almost the same size as the fetus. When a woman is five months pregnant, the placenta weighs one-quarter the fetal weight. At seven months the placenta weighs one-fifth as much as the fetus, and by the final month, once the fetal size has increased rapidly, the placenta weighs only one-seventh as much as the fetus. In other words, the fetus continues to grow in the last trimester while the placental growth slows down. This balance is naturally influenced by nutrition and other pregnancy conditions.

The fetus receives food and oxygen and gives off waste through the placental membranes. There are two layers in the early development of the placenta: the chorion, which surrounds the amniotic sac and the embryo, and the outer layer, containing the cells of the uterus. The tissues of the outer layer are filled with small blood-filled cavities and slender, branchlike extensions spread outward from the chorion into the cavities of the outer placental layer. This intricate pattern of blood vessels eventually forms three large blood vessels that pass through the body stalk and into the embryo. The body stalk is a piece of tissue connecting the embryo to the chorion. As pregnancy continues, the body stalk becomes more sophisticated and lengthens. It thus develops into the umbilical cord, which continues to nourish the fetus through the pregnancy and is severed

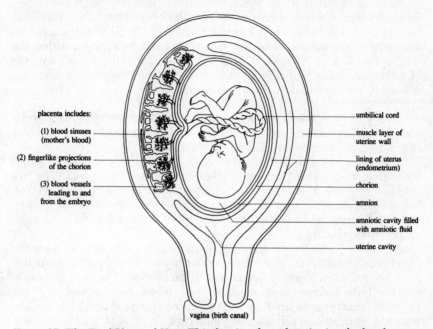

placenta includes:

(1) blood sinuses
(mother's blood)

(2) fingerlike projections
of the chorion

(3) blood vessels
leading to and
from the embryo

umbilical cord

muscle layer of
uterine wall

lining of uterus
(endometrium)

chorion

amnion

amniotic cavity filled
with amniotic fluid

uterine cavity

vagina (birth canal)

Figure 17: The Fetal-Placental Unit: This drawing shows how intricately the placenta is integrated into the uterus. Well-oxygenated blood is led through the blood vessels on the uterine side of the placenta to the umbilical cord and into the baby. Venous blood is led back in through the placenta to become oxygenated. The drawing also shows the fetal membrane, the chorion, and the amnion surrounding the amniotic sac.

only when birth is complete. This cord is the lifeline of the fetus, the only means by which the fetus is connected to the oxygen supply and life-giving nourishment of the placenta.

The fetus is surrounded by amniotic fluid throughout its development. This is fluid secreted from the fetus, mostly from the fetal urine. The protective amniotic fluid is essential, because it guards the growing fetus from shocks and rough jolts and allows enough space for the fetus to move during its development. It also has the vital function of protecting the umbilical cord from any obstruction or damage. Every hour, about 30 percent of the amniotic fluid is absorbed and resecreted back through the umbilical cord and the placenta. In this way wastes are returned to the mother's bloodstream, and new fluid is simultaneously secreted to protect the fetus. A portion of the amniotic fluid is swallowed by the fetus and then excreted as fetal urine. Analysis has shown that it contains protein and sugar.

At approximately three months' gestation about 12 ounces of amniotic fluid surround the fetus. At five months' gestation the volume of fluid is one pint, and at term it is usually slightly less than one quart, although, when a woman is suffering from hydramnios (an excess of amniotic fluid), enormous quantities of fluid have been found in a patient—as much as eight gallons have been recorded.

The amniotic fluid is a very effective sound conductor. The fetus can hear sounds from both outside and within the womb from a surprisingly early stage. By twenty-eight weeks fetal hearing is fully developed. Tests have shown that the fetus responds to vibrations and sounds produced by its mother's activities and those of the outside world (see Chap. 14). The environment within the mother herself is far from silent. The fetus hears its mother's heartbeat, the blood moving through her veins and the placenta itself, and a rhythmic whooshing sound created by the stomach rumbling.

☐ *The First Four Weeks of Life*   Since day one of your pregnancy is, by your doctor's calculation, the first day of your last menstrual period, you will not, in fact, be pregnant for another two weeks or so.

Conception occurs on day 14 or 15. On day 21 the fertilized egg enters into the uterine cavity, where the egg attaches itself to the uterine wall. The trophoblast—the cells around the outer surface of the fertilized egg—has by now formed little projections called *chorionic villae*, which catch onto the uterine lining and extract nutrients from the blood vessels in the endometrium to nourish the developing egg.

Once it has implanted itself, the egg starts to grow in the uterus, where the blood vessels from the endometrium continue to nourish and protect it. At this point the cell mass begins the process of differentiation. The outer cell layer, which will later become the placenta and supply blood, nutrition, and oxygen to the fetus, begins to grow rapidly, while the inner cell mass, the cells that will become the fetus, are also dividing and multiplying. With implantation, the next vital stage of human development has begun.

The hollow sphere of cells that implants into the uterus is called the blastocyst. It contains within it the potential development of the placenta, the umbilical cord, the amniotic fluid, and the fetus. Once the blastocyst is imbedded in the uterus, cell growth quickly continues. By the twenty-eighth day of pregnancy, just around the time menstruation would be due, the cell mass is just visi-

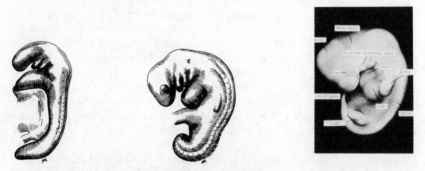

Figure 18: *The Fetus at Three Weeks' Gestation:* This drawing illustrates very early fetal gestation. Note that the nerve and cardiovascular systems are beginning to develop.   Figure 19: *The Fetus at Four Weeks' Gestation:* At four weeks' gestation the fetus has a more clearly developed head and body.   Figure 20: *The Fetus at Four to Five Weeks' Gestation:* After four to five weeks it is possible to see areas from which the various body parts will develop.

ble to the naked human eye—the conceptus is only one-hundredth of an inch in size.

☐ ***The Fourth to Eighth Week of Gestation*** Initially the uterus expands very slowly and the conceptus is very tiny. The fact that your pregnancy is not visible should not prevent you from thinking of yourself as pregnant. The minute conceptus goes through dramatic changes in these weeks. Within four weeks the blastocyst becomes an embryo, with a rudimentary skeleton, internal organs, a beating heart, a brain, and the beginning of recognizably human limb formations. This is a very critical time in the development of the fetus because the basic structure of human life, the nervous system, is being laid down.

☐ ***The Fifth Week of Gestation*** The fertilized egg is now sufficiently developed to move into the embryonic stage. The embryo at this point is a cell mass of undifferentiated tissue formation containing a small gray-white streak that will become the spine. The embryonic (or amniotic) sac is formed and surrounds and protects the embryo, which is now two-fifths of an inch in diameter. The embryo's spinal cord and rudimentary nervous system are also beginning to develop. By the end of the fifth week of gestation the brain, the spinal cord, and the beginning of the nervous system have been established. (The "head" at this phase is barely differentiated from the "body" of the embryo.) A primitive circulatory system is forming and the rudimentary heart begins to beat.

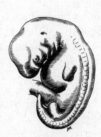

Figure 21: The Fetus at Five Weeks' Gestation: Note how the upper body develops before the lower body.

☐ ***The Sixth Week of Gestation*** First the head is formed; then follows the formation of the chest and abdominal cavities. The spinal cord has developed fully, but it still has a rudimentary tail, an early extension of the spinal cord, which will later disintegrate. The heartbeat is visible by the end of the sixth week and can be picked up by ultrasonography. The earliest parts of the stomach and intestines are forming inside the abdominal cavity.

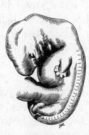

Figure 22: At the fifth week the head is formed, to be followed by formation of the chest and the abdominal cavity.

☐ ***The Seventh Week of Gestation*** By this time the chest and the abdomen are completely formed. The heart is sufficiently developed to allow cells to circulate through the blood vessels. The lungs still remain as solid organs on either side of the abdominal cavity. Other important internal organs—the liver and kidneys—are appearing, but their functions as yet remain dormant. The growth of the brain and spinal cord is now almost complete. The embryonic head is growing rapidly, and the outline of the head is starting to assume its final shape, although there are still some odd-looking lumps on the back and sides of the head. The location of the ears is quite visible now, and the inner parts of the ear are beginning to take shape. Depressions for the eyes are forming as well as the eyes themselves, although the eyelids are closed and the web of skin over the eyes is unbroken. The embryonic face is flatter and the openings of the nostrils are visible, although the nose itself will be formed at a later stage. The jaw and the mouth are continuing to develop, and the tiny embryo has clearly human features.

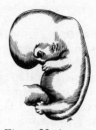

Figure 23: At seven weeks' gestation the chest and abdomen are completely formed and the fetus is taking on human characteristics.

The limb buds have grown to a point at which they can be distinguished as arms and legs, and the divisions of the fingers and toes can be seen at the ends of the buds. By the end of the seventh week the embryo has reached the stage at which it becomes a fetus; it is now about one-half inch long and weighs approximately one-thousandth of an ounce.

☐ *The Eighth Week of Gestation*   The internal organs are almost fully formed, and the heart and circulatory system are functioning strongly. The limb buds continue to grow, and lower joints at the shoulders, elbows, hips, and knees are becoming visible. The eyes and the inner ears are developing rapidly, the nostrils are well defined, and the general impression of a human face is increased by the fusion of the upper and lower jaws, which creates a recognizable mouth. The spine is now capable of the first, very tiny movements.

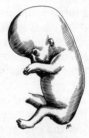

Figure 24: The Fetus at Eight Weeks' Gestation: At eight weeks the fetus is now almost completely formed. The internal organs are complete, though immature. The heart and the circulatory system are functioning strongly and the fetus looks almost human.

☐ *The Third Month of Gestation*   The fetus continues to grow rapidly and looks more and more like a human being. The head is completely formed by the end of the third month, although it is still a little larger in proportion to the limbs than it will be at birth. Arms, legs, hands, and feet are clearly formed. At this time an examination under a microscope (if that were possible) would determine whether the fetus is male or female, because the bud of tissue between the legs is now clearly a pair of labia or a penis.

By the end of the ninth week the fetus is about one and one-half inches long and weighs about one-fifteenth of an ounce (approximately 2 grams). The eyes are fully developed, although the eyelids are still tightly sealed. The nose and mouth are taking shape. Limb growth is proceeding rapidly and the beginnings of the hands and feet are quite obvious, with the ends of the limb buds clearly defined as fingers and toes.

At ten weeks the fetus can move its eyes, which are now fully developed and have grown considerably in size. The bumps on the back of the head have disappeared but the head remains overly large. The face looks more or less normal except for the jaws, which are still unformed. Inside the upper portion of the mouth the palate is taking shape. The outside part of the ears is now developing, and the inner ear is complete. Ankles and wrists are discernible, and differentiated fingers and toes are also visible, although they are still joined together by webbing. The liver, kidneys, intestines, and lungs continue to develop. By this time the fetal heart rate is well established and functions at approximately 120 to 140 beats a minute. The fetus is large enough at ten weeks for the fetal outline to be traceable by real-time ultrasonography.

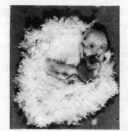

Figure 25: The Fetus at Eight to Nine Weeks' Gestation: Here the eight-week-old fetus is seen inside the amniotic sac and surrounded with white cloud-like placenta. The long, thick umbilical cord supplies the fetus with nutrition and oxygen.

During the eleventh week, limb growth continues rapidly, and by the end of this week the limbs have more or less their final appearance, although they are still rather short and thin, and the fingers and toes are still joined together. The face is almost fully formed, and the outer part of the ears is now discernible. The internal sexual organs—the ovaries or testes, depending on the chromosomal pattern at conception—are completely formed inside the body, and the external sexual organs are now developing fully. At this point the female clitoris appears much larger than it will later on.

By the end of the third month the tiny fetus is complete, with fingers and toes, developed ears and eyes, a functioning circulatory system, internal organs that are fully formed—although they need time to mature—and recognizably male or female sexual organs. The eyes are still closed, but the fetus

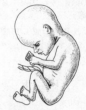

Figure 26: The Fetus at Fourteen Weeks' Gestation: At fourteen weeks' gestation the fetus is growing quickly, but the head and the upper body are still large in proportion to the lower body and the legs, which are the last to develop fully.

now opens and closes its mouth as it drinks the amniotic fluid. The mouth, the nose, and the ears are properly formed. Now that the neck is developed, the head moves freely, and the fetus is losing the "hunched" look of the early months.

At twelve weeks the fetus is sufficiently advanced to move freely within the amniotic sac, but because the brain is still undeveloped, fetal movements at this point are caused by reflexes from the spinal cord. These movements can be recorded by ultrasound equipment, and the fetus can be clearly seen turning inside the amniotic sac. Because the fetus is still so tiny—it is now about 3 inches long and weighs about 14 grams—the pregnant woman herself cannot feel it twisting and turning inside her uterine cavity.

The end of the third lunar month marks an important milestone in fetal development. The major organs are now fully formed, and the most sensitive pe-

riod of the fetus' development is passed. While it is still possible for the fetus
to sustain an injury that will have a lasting effect—especially to the brain, which
has barely begun to develop—the risk of a gross structural abnormality occurring in the last six months of pregnancy is very small. This was strikingly
demonstrated in the 1950s when women took thalidomide in the early
and later months of pregnancy. Limb reduction deformities appeared only in
the children of mothers who took the drug when they were four to twelve weeks'
pregnant, and after that sensitive time thalidomide had no noticeable effect on
pregnancy.

☐ *The Fourth Lunar Month (12 to 16 Weeks)*   A month can make a
crucial difference in the first four months of a pregnancy. After the third
month the main focus is on the growth of the fetus into a baby capable of surviving outside its mother's womb. In the last six months of pregnancy the baby's
weight multiplies seven or eight times over, and its lungs and other organs
mature sufficiently to allow it to survive without the protective environment
of the uterus. The amount the baby weighs at birth and the maturity of its vital
organs are the main indicators of its future success as an independent human
being.

The following chart is a simplified outline of the size and weight of the fetus
at various weeks of gestation.

FETAL SIZE THROUGHOUT THE WEEKS OF PREGNANCY

Weeks of Gestation	Average Weight		Average Length	
	POUNDS-OUNCES	GRAMS	INCHES	CM
8	0–0	1	1.6	3.1
10	0–0	4	2.6	6.5
12	0–0	14	3.0	9
14	0–1	25	4.9	12.5
16	0–3	100	6.3	16
18	0–7	190	8.1	20.5
20	0–10	300	9.8	25
22	0–15	430	10.8	27.5
24	1–5	600	11.8	30
26	1–12	800	12.8	32.5
28	2–4	1001	13.8	35
30	3–0	1350	14.8	37.5
32	3–11	1675	15.7	40
34	4–7	2001	16.7	42.5
36	5–2	2340	17.7	45
38	6–2	2775	18.7	47.5
40	7–3	3250	19.7	50
42	8–14	4001	20.7	52.5

☐ **The Fifth Lunar Month (*16 to 20 Weeks*)**   The fetus now looks almost completely "normal." The full development of the arms, legs, and head has been achieved, and the sexual organs are essentially formed. Fingers and toes are fully separated, and fingernails and toenails are present. Fetal movements at this time are vigorous but are still not apparent to the mother, although the fetus is growing fast—it is now approximately 8 inches long and weighs about 6 ounces (180 grams).

☐ **The Sixth Lunar Month (*20 to 24 Weeks*)**   At this point the pregnant woman will usually experience *quickening* when the fetus is particularly active. We know that the fetus has periods of activity and periods of rest; it will sleep for a while, wake up and move around, and then go back to sleep. This pattern of activity and rest is influenced by sensors in the fetus as well as by the activities of the mother herself, and it will be more and more noticeable as pregnancy progresses. The fetus generally becomes more active after a woman eats.

By the end of the sixth lunar month, in other words, by the twenty-fourth week of gestation, the fetus has grown rapidly and reached almost 12 inches in length and 1 pound 5 ounces in weight. The fetus' muscles enable it to move more strongly, and this is why quickening usually occurs during this period of development. The baby's body is now covered with a cheesy white protective material called the vernix caseosa, which keeps the baby's skin from becoming waterlogged by the amniotic fluid and will be an aid during the birth.

By this midpoint of pregnancy the baby's brain is entering an important growth spurt that will continue throughout pregnancy and postnatally for another four years. In studies on the brains of animals during gestation, a reduction in the total number of brain cells present at birth has been shown to occur when maternal nutrition has been seriously inadequate. The brain as well as the body of the growing fetus needs the nourishment of a good prenatal diet, especially in the last four or five months of pregnancy.

☐ **The Seventh Lunar Month (*24 to 28 Weeks*)**   The baby remains covered with the vernix caseosa. Hair is now beginning to grow on the head, and eyebrows and eyelashes are appearing. The eyes are capable of opening and shutting. Weight and length are both increasing steadily, and the fetus weighs about 2 pounds (906 grams) and is approximately 13 inches long. It still lacks the characteristic "baby fat" of the fully mature infant and looks more like a very tiny old man than an infant. The skin has a wrinkled appearance because of the absence of the layers of subcutaneous fat, and the skin texture is thin and brittle.

Sometimes a baby born prematurely during the seventh lunar month will be born alive and survive. Ten years ago such a tiny premature baby had only a 20 percent chance of survival, and most of those who did live were abnormal in some way. Now doctors are saving more and more premature children weighing between 1.6 pounds (750 grams) and 3.2 pounds (1500 grams), and many of the survivors will grow up normally. However, these very premature babies require intensive medical care and may, because of their immaturity, suffer from a variety of serious disorders, ranging from intestinal problems to brain hemorrhages.

☐ **The Eighth Lunar Month (*28 to 32 Weeks*)**   The fetus continues to grow rapidly. This is the point at which the testes in a male child descend to outside the abdominal cavity. Fetal movements are increasingly active, and at the end of this lunar month the fetus is approximately 16 inches long and weighs about 3 pounds 11 ounces (approximately 1700 grams). If premature birth occurs in the eighth lunar month, there is, thanks to recent advances in neonatal technology, a very good chance of survival at 28 or 29 weeks and an increased chance for each week after that. Some neonatal units report success rates of 80 percent among babies born early in the eighth lunar month, although a baby weighing under 1500 grams (3 pounds 2 ounces) is still at risk. The baby's lungs are immature, as are the other vital organs, and the skull is delicate and can be injured during labor.

☐ *The Ninth Lunar Month (32 to 36 Weeks)*   At this time the fetus is completely formed, and it is now only a question of the complete maturity of the vital organs and the achievement of a good birth weight. The pregnant woman herself can now feel how the baby's muscle development is progressing; the kicking and squirming is much stronger, and movements are visible on the outline of the abdomen. Sometimes a fist or foot will make a distinct bulge or sequence of bulges.

If this is your first baby, the ninth month is the time the baby will usually take up the birth position, normally with the head presenting first (cephalic presentation). During a second pregnancy there is more room in the uterus because of the stretching it experienced in the first pregnancy, and the baby can still turn itself around by kicking out with its feet. Once the baby stops shifting around, the mother will usually feel a distinct sense of kicking or some discomfort on one side.

At the end of 36 weeks' gestation the baby should weigh approximately 5 pounds (or about 2300 grams) and measure about 18 inches. If premature birth should occur during this month, the baby is estimated to have an 80–90 percent chance of survival.

☐ *The Tenth Lunar Month (36 to 40 Weeks)*   Increasing layers of fat are laid down at this time. Muscle tone continues to improve, and the lungs are fully developed. In a first pregnancy the baby usually descends into the pelvis at about the thirty-sixth week, and the fundus of the uterus becomes lower. "Lightening" may not happen until just before labor starts in a second or subsequent pregnancy, but the baby will have taken up the vertex position by the thirty-sixth week even in a second pregnancy, because it is too large to move around freely. Although a baby will usually survive if it is born during the thirty-seventh or thirty-eighth week of gestation, the liver and other vital organs may still be somewhat immature, and a successful pregnancy will go as close as possible to term, the full 40 weeks' gestation. By 40 weeks the baby will have achieved physical maturity and its full birth weight. Normally a baby will increase its weight considerably in the last four weeks of the pregnancy, being 2 or more pounds heavier at birth than it was at the end of the ninth lunar month.

☐ *Prematurity*   A baby is considered premature if it is born between the twenty-eighth and thirty-sixth week of gestation or if a full-term infant is less than 5½ pounds, or 2500 grams, at the time of delivery. Premature birth is a major concern in this country because it accounts for 90 percent of the present rate of perinatal mortality—the rate, that is, for babies who die just before, during, or after delivery. A baby who is very tiny is at grave risk because its body is not mature enough to adjust to living outside the protected environment of the womb. The lungs particularly function poorly until a baby is close to term, since the fetus inside the womb is breathing oxygen via the placental circulation. Furthermore, the skull of a premature baby is so fragile that the pressure during the birth process can cause intracranial hemorrhage. Such bleeding may result in nerve damage, which may manifest itself in later life as brain damage or cerebral palsy.

If a woman has a history of premature birth and recognizes the symptoms of prematurity at any time in her pregnancy, or she experiences cramping or spotting in the second or third trimesters, she should call her physician immediately. There are new medications and hormonal supports that can be helpful in delaying premature birth. If you feel your uterus is at all sensitive, it is very important to rest, stay off your feet, refrain from intercourse, try to avoid stress, and remember not to lift anything heavy. Although premature labor often occurs spontaneously, care and bed rest will sometimes prevent premature rupture of the membranes. These extra precautions in the last weeks of pregnancy are well worth the inconvenience they cause.

☐ **Term**   Term gestation is approximately 40 weeks from the beginning of the last menstrual period, although doctors usually count any time from 38 to 42 weeks as the term of the gestation. Once a pregnancy reaches this point, there are generally fewer problems associated with delivery—the baby is usually healthiest—and the closer the date of birth approximates to the 40-week term, the less likely it is for complications such as jaundice to occur in the postpartum period. This is because all the baby's organs are fully grown and developed.

☐ **Postmaturity**   A pregnancy that has gone beyond 42 weeks of gestation is considered to be postdate or postmature. This can be a dangerous time for the baby, because at this point the placenta sometimes starts to disintegrate. Eventually it will calcify and rot, decreasing the blood supply to the baby. This will also affect the volume of amniotic fluid, which surrounds the baby and prevents the kinking of the umbilical cord. As the fetal environment degenerates, dehydration will produce the characteristic appearance of the postmature baby with its shrunken, wrinkled skin. Labor and delivery may also be more difficult for women who have passed the forty-second week of gestation. In certain countries such as Great Britain, doctors try to bring a postdate patient into the hospital after the forty-second week and induce labor through the use of oxytocin, because they are so concerned about the possible complications of postmaturity.

☐ **You and Your Baby**   Now that you have traveled through the different stages of development, I hope it will be easier for you to imagine what your baby is like and why you sense his or her presence so strongly in the last few months. Most women feel very close to their children even before they actually see them physically. Indeed, the baby may seem to have a personality of his own long before he is born. Chapter 14 will explain more about what two writers (Thomas Verny, M.D., with John Kelly, Summit Books, New York, 1981) have called *The Secret Life of the Unborn Child.*

10

What to Expect During Pregnancy

Each pregnancy is different, and women who are pregnant for the second or third time still experience new events or emotions unique to that particular pregnancy. Even experienced women will say, "I don't remember that" or "I never felt that before" when they compare one pregnancy with another. If each pregnancy is different, a first pregnancy has a particular fascination for a woman, because everything about it is new, exciting, and unexpected. You have probably already noticed every minute change in your body.

The desire to experience pregnancy fully is usually associated with feelings of anticipation, happiness, and satisfaction—mingled with a sense of mild apprehension. This is understandable. There is always a natural uncertainty during pregnancy, because you can only guess at what is going to happen in the months to come. Reading about pregnancy and attending childbirth classes are valuable for just this reason—it is easier to cope with what lies ahead if you know what to anticipate and how to deal with difficulties.

Unavoidably, perhaps, many irrational fears about pregnancy and delivery surface in the early months, often triggered by old wives' tales and half truths that have little relation to reality. Millions of women give birth uneventfully every year, and the few problems you are likely to encounter can usually be overcome if you plan ahead, take good care of yourself, and don't get emotionally upset. If your immediate family is supportive, especially your partner, the months of pregnancy can be one of the greatest times of your life.

Your pregnancy should be a special experience. This is why it is important for you to feel positive about pregnancy. At the same time, plan ahead realistically and honestly and always keep in touch with your own feelings. All of us have different personalities, and our very different physical and emotional makeup means that every woman has a different experience of pregnancy. Some women are physically uncomfortable, some experience only a few uncomfortable days; some women are optimistic throughout the pregnancy, some have periods of doubts or indecision about whether they want to be mothers at all. These are all normal reactions, and no pregnant woman should be ashamed of mixed emotions or of physical discomfort.

Pregnancy is, however, a time in which certain rules must be observed if you want to stay healthy. See your doctor regularly, talk over your progress with him, and work out a realistic plan for your pregnancy. Most of the serious troubles that occur during pregnancy are the result of neglect or ignorance, and one of the purposes of prenatal care is to make sure that minor problems do not escalate into major ones. A woman who doesn't take proper care of herself during pregnancy often has a difficult pregnancy and an even more difficult labor and delivery. One of the best reasons for seeing your doctor at regular intervals is to let him screen your progress carefully and handle problems as they arise. With the medical advances of the last few years and our increased knowledge of nutrition and health, the margin of safety in pregnancy has increased considerably, and many problems that troubled women of an earlier generation can be detected and treated with our better knowledge of obstetrics and fetology.

It is quite natural for a pregnant woman to experience vague misgivings or physical discomforts from time to time. Don't be afraid to discuss them with your obstetrician, however trivial they may seem. Anxiety alone can lead to physical discomfort or can greatly intensify some existing discomfort. Talking over a problem or asking a question are excellent ways to demystify troublesome stories and encourage a positive attitude toward pregnancy.

☐ *The Earlier Months* It is not uncommon for a pregnant woman to feel miserable and depressed during the first three months. Many women find it takes time to adjust to the increased hormonal levels of the first trimester. The increased progesterone level has a similar effect in the two or three days before your period, when you may feel tired and depressed. Emotional concerns about what is going to happen before and after the baby is born are often difficult to cope with in the early weeks. You have probably asked yourself any one of the following questions: Do I really want this baby? Will I be a good mother? In addition, couples can experience some unexpectedly negative reactions from friends and family when they announce a first pregnancy. Mixed emotions at this stage of the pregnancy are normal, even though a majority of women today are better prepared for pregnancy than earlier generations were and seem to sail through the first trimester with a minimum of discomfort. Some women who have waited for years to become pregnant and have prepared themselves thoroughly still feel unwell or occasionally miserable during these early weeks.

Linked with this feeling of depression are the physical symptoms a woman often experiences in the early months, including nausea, occasional vomiting, and a bloated feeling. Constipation and flatulence are other common digestive problems that occur at this point of pregnancy. It is also normal to feel heavier than usual in the first trimester, because the increased progesterone and estrogen levels increase the body's tendency to retain water. This in turn leads to tenderness and enlargement of the breasts.

Most of these minor problems disappear spontaneously at the beginning of the second trimester; simple changes in diet and life-style usually take care of any remaining discomforts without the need for more complex treatment. A good way to overcome the problems of the first trimester is to adapt yourself mentally and physically to the idea of being pregnant and then learn to take care of yourself. Prevention is always better than treatment!

☐ *The Middle Months of Pregnancy*   The second trimester is usually the healthiest and most enjoyable period of pregnancy. To begin with, morning sickness almost abruptly disappears as soon as the majority of women enter their fourth month of pregnancy. The other side effects of the high progesterone and estrogen levels are also mitigated by this time, and the bloated, exhausted feeling usually gives way to a sense of renewed energy and a considerable increase in appetite.

About four and one-half months after the beginning of your last menstrual period you will usually experience fetal movements. Initially all you feel is the vague fluttering sensation called quickening, but as the weeks pass and the fetus becomes larger, movements are more definite and can't be mistaken for gas or some other normal disturbance. The confirmation that the fetus is alive is a turning point in pregnancy; once you detect fetal movements, doubts about the pregnancy usually give way to a new feeling of confidence.

There is a special contentment associated with the middle months of pregnancy. By now a woman has adjusted herself to the idea of being pregnant, and she feels better. Her increased appetite keeps her blood-sugar level stable and usually takes care of anemia and other diet-related complaints. Her skin is clear. By the fifth month the increased weight means that other people are aware of the pregnancy, and this often heightens a woman's sense of self-esteem. At this point you are not very large and can still move around easily, but you are certainly big enough for friends to take an interest in the pregnancy and enjoy your new physical appearance. (Most people, and this includes men, find pregnant women extraordinarily attractive.) Finally, the feeling that the fetus is alive and growing adds pleasure and happiness to the middle months, and any minor problems are usually overcome by the general sense of well-being.

☐ *The Third Trimester*   As her pregnancy enters the third trimester, a woman's abdomen grows more pronounced with each week, and by the end of the third trimester the baby is sometimes so large that the uterus presses against the stomach and right beneath the rib cage, making breathing and digestion difficult. This leads to indigestion and heartburn, because the stomach is unable to empty its contents properly. The discomfort is usually worse around the beginning of the eighth month when the uterus is most distended. Once the baby "drops"—in a first pregnancy, usually about four weeks before labor starts—this relieves some of the pressure on the stomach, and you will feel less burdened, although the new position of the baby can lead to other problems, such as pressure on and swelling of the legs.

Muscle cramps often cause discomfort in the last trimester, especially at night, and there may be an increased feeling of heaviness in other parts of the body besides the mid-section, because you are tending to retain more water. The heavy uterus is now resting on the large vein (the vena cava), and varicose veins and hemorrhoids often become worse in the final weeks. There are effective ways to take care of these problems through increased rest, a change in diet, or other minor adjustments.

By this point you may feel as if the baby is using you as a punching bag. Kicking becomes so strong as the baby grows larger that a very active baby can surprise you by the forcefulness of its movements. There are surprising differences, however, in the prenatal activity level of babies—which may, perhaps, indicate prenatal differences in personality. (This new idea is explored more fully in Chapter 14.) Kicking in general is a healthy activity, but if movements seem excessive, try to review your own activities to see if you are putting some unnecessary strain on the baby.

The last few weeks of pregnancy are often disturbed by mixed emotions about the delivery itself and the uncertainty caused by false labor contractions, which can start anywhere in the eighth month. Unfortunately the majority of Braxton-Hicks contractions seem to occur at night, and you may be awakened by false contractions several times before the onset of true labor. It is important to bear in mind that the great majority of first pregnancies normally go at least a week past the estimated date of delivery. A baby born at term or even a little after has a great advantage over an eight-month baby, because the birth weight is higher and the brain and the lungs are fully developed. You can look on the final, uncomfortable weeks as a time when your child is benefiting greatly from the uterine environment and should not be encouraged to leave it prematurely!

☐ *How Physical Changes Affect the Pregnant Woman* A woman's body undergoes a number of striking changes during the nine months of pregnancy. All the vital organs are affected. The heart rate increases to accommodate a 40–90 percent larger blood volume, the respiration rate quickens, and the kidneys work harder. And of course the hormonal levels alter to promote the successful continuance of pregnancy. These physical changes produce many of the classic symptoms we associate with a normal pregnancy. For instance, the increase in blood volume results in a significant retention of water in the blood vessels, and this in turn leads to the characteristic swelling that is otherwise known as edema of pregnancy. The higher lung capacity—a pregnant woman uses 15 percent more oxygen than a nonpregnant woman—increases the respiration rate and leads to quicker, shallower breathing. Since the kidneys work harder, the collection tract in the kidneys dilates and retains more urine, leading to an increased urge to urinate in early pregnancy, often accompanied by an urgent thirst.

The important hormonal changes of pregnancy are discussed elsewhere in this chapter and in other sections of the book. They are the direct cause of many of the minor discomforts of pregnancy, most of which disappear in time or can be controlled by special care. The most celebrated, of course, is morning sickness, which is discussed in Chapter 5, "The First Signs of Pregnancy."

☐ *Heartburn* Heartburn is a fiery, burning sensation in the chest, frequently associated with the taste of a small amount of bitter, sour fluid in the mouth. In spite of the popular name given to this annoying complaint, it has nothing to do with the heart but is simply the result of some of the acid content of the stomach overflowing back into the lower esophagus and producing an uncomfortable burning feeling in the stomach and the throat. This can happen at any time but is very common during the third trimester because of the upward displacement and compression of the stomach by the enlarged uterus. Susceptibility to heartburn is also increased by the sluggish action of the gastrointestinal tract. This results in a slower emptying of the stomach and enables the acid to stay in the stomach and irritate the stomach mucus. In other words, heartburn is simply an acute form of indigestion.

The best way to prevent heartburn is to avoid rich and greasy foods, such as mayonnaise, marbled steaks, cream, or fried foods, and to eat small portions at each meal. (Remember, you will probably be eating more meals a day than usual.) Plenty of fluids are valuable in combating heartburn, particularly milk, which has antacid properties, although some women are lactose-intolerant (see Chap. 17). Even so, you may still need to take an occasional antacid, such as Mylanta, Maalox, Riopan, or milk of magnesia, between meals to neutralize the extra acid in the stomach. Antacids in tablet form, such as Gelusil, Rolaids, Tums, and milk of magnesia are also useful. Avoid any products containing bicarbonate of soda (this includes Alka-Seltzer) and baking soda, because their high sodium content can bind water and lead to high blood pressure. Chewing gum after meals also seems to lessen heartburn for some people.

☐ *Excessive Salivation*   Pregnant women naturally produce more saliva, especially at the beginning of pregnancy. This complaint, called ptyalism, can be very annoying and often increases the tendency to nausea, because the extra saliva smells and tastes bitter. The increased secretion is sometimes so heavy that it floods the mouth, and you have to get rid of it by spitting it out. One of the best ways to deal with this embarrassing problem is to increase the number of times you brush your teeth. Rinsing out your mouth frequently and sucking on peppermints or chewing gum also helps control it. One theory about ptyalism is that foods containing high amounts of starch make the condition worse, so you might try cutting down on sugar and foods containing too much sugar to see if this makes any difference. In really severe cases women sometimes need medical attention, and, in a few instances, small doses of phenobarbital have been prescribed to prevent the constant flow of saliva. Ptyalism usually disappears, or at least diminishes, after the beginning of the second trimester.

☐ *Frequent Urination*   Early in pregnancy the urge to urinate becomes more frequent as the bladder muscles relax under the influence of the increased progesterone. At the same time the uterus begins to enlarge and exert pressure on the bladder, and you will feel the urge to urinate even when there is very little urine present. In the middle months of pregnancy the pressure is relieved temporarily because the uterus rises up into the abdominal cavity, and the need to urinate diminishes, only to increase once again in the eighth month, when the baby's head moves into the birth canal, pressing directly against the bladder. The problem is exacerbated because the body is making more urine than usual during pregnancy. When the greater blood flow from the heart reaches the vessels in the kidneys they in turn enlarge and produce more urine.

There are a few ways to lessen the discomfort: cut down on the amount you drink in the last hour or two before you go to bed, to avoid midnight trips to the bathroom; if the urge to urinate is high during the day, try to increase your bladder control by holding back and then voiding the bladder as thoroughly as possible.

Because of the distortion of the bladder and the urethra, it is much easier to develop bladder infections during pregnancy. See your doctor immediately if you feel even the slightest pain or discomfort in the bladder area; this may be a sign of cystitis or some other urinary-tract infection. Cystitis can be treated safely with antibiotics or other drugs. (See Chapter 19 on drug use in pregnancy.)

☐ *Constipation*   Some women suffer from constipation only during pregnancy, while other women find their natural tendency to constipation becomes worse. Still others discover that eating a proper diet and a larger amount of food than normal suddenly decreases their tendency to become constipated.

Pregnancy-related constipation occurs as the enlarged uterus presses down and back against the intestines and slows down the passage and elimination of the stool. During the early months constipation also increases because the high progesterone level relaxes smooth muscles, including the muscles of the intestinal wall. In both instances the stool moves more slowly through the intestines, and more water is absorbed through the bowel wall, increasing your chance of experiencing constipation. Occasionally a pregnant woman will notice a worsening of constipation as she increases her iron intake with a prenatal iron and vitamin medication. In this case try to change your brand of prenatal vitamins. Some prescription vitamins contain laxatives, and switching to one of these will generally take care of the problem.

Changes in diet are the best way to remedy constipation. Remember to eat more roughage to irritate the bowel and increase bowel function. Nutritious foods rich in fiber are whole grains, whole wheat bread, brown rice, dried peas and beans, and raw fruits and vegetables, including the skins. (Fruits and vegetables should always be washed thoroughly first to cut down on pesticide residues.) It is also helpful to eat yogurt with *live cultures* (read the label first because many commercial yogurts are pasteurized) to increase the natural flora in the stomach and intestinal tract. Remember to drink plenty of liquids—soup, seltzer, or water—at least eight glasses of fluid a day.

Regular exercise is valuable in controlling constipation as well as other pregnancy-related complaints. Walking increases muscle tone, strengthens the body, improves your emotional and physical well-being, and increases your desire for food.

If constipation cannot be controlled by natural means, it is safe to take an occasional over-the-counter remedy, such as Colace. Two Colace tablets daily will soften the bowel and aid proper bowel function. But always check with your doctor first before using this or any other medication when you are pregnant.

☐ *Flatulence*   The distention of the stomach and intestines by intestinal gas during pregnancy often results in a bloated feeling and frequent attacks of flatulence. The prevalence of this complaint in the first trimester is associated with the changes in the bowel, which can lead to constipation at the same time. Later on in pregnancy, as the uterus grows larger, it presses against the intestines and prevents the contents of the bowel from moving as rapidly as usual. The trapped bacteria in the stool consequently produce more gas. The tendency to flatulence is also more pronounced because the increased respiration rate of the lungs leads a woman to take more air into the stomach.

You can help overcome the discomfort of flatulence by eating slowly and chewing your food thoroughly. Avoid overlarge meals, fatty foods, and excessive amounts of protein—all of which tend to increase gas—and cut down on the notorious gas-producing foods: dried beans, corn, onions, cabbage, fried foods, and sugary desserts. Once again, regular exercise and plenty of liquids are helpful, and a mild antacid, such as milk of magnesia, can be taken occasionally to increase intestinal activity if you become really uncomfortable.

☐ *Hemorrhoids* Hemorrhoids are simply varicose veins in the rectum. You may notice them first when you are pregnant, although the tendency to hemorrhoids is partly genetic or may have been encouraged by previous episodes of constipation. When a woman is constipated, the veins around the rectum are improperly emptied, and the vein eventually blocks up, causing irritation and itching in a localized area because of the trapped blood. This means that proper bowel movements are important in preventing hemorrhoids, since they eliminate blockage (or stasis, as it is called) and bring the newly oxygenated blood into the affected area.

Hemorrhoids often become worse toward the end of the pregnancy and during labor, when the pressure of the baby prevents the venous blood from returning easily from the lower part of the body, including the bowels. During the last trimester you can reduce your susceptibility to hemorrhoids by lying on your side and elevating the foot of the bed. This enhances blood flow and helps eliminate pressure in the hips and legs.

One excellent way to prevent hemorrhoids is to prevent constipation from occurring. Another precaution is to avoid straining during bowel movements. If straining or pain occurs, a little petroleum jelly can be placed just inside the rectum to make elimination easier. With larger hemorrhoids, you can use an over-the-counter remedy or ask your doctor to prescribe Anusol suppositories to shrink them before they cause problems, such as skin irritation and bleeding. A small amount of bleeding is not uncommon with hemorrhoids, even though you should always report it to your doctor as a precautionary measure. One simple way to prevent bleeding is to apply petroleum jelly to the rectal area in the evening just before you go to bed.

Sometimes rather pronounced hemorrhoids cause a tender, swollen mass to protrude around the anus. In this case sit for several minutes in a tub of warm water, and then try to push the mass back with a well lubricated finger. If this is unsuccessful, lie on your back with your hips slightly elevated and apply a washcloth or a piece of cotton soaked in ice or witch hazel to the rectal region. An anesthetic ointment, such as Xylocaine or medicated Anusol suppositories, can be used if hemorrhoids do not shrink with this localized treatment.

Hemorrhoids that become very painful may indicate the presence of a thrombosed vein. The only means of relief is for your doctor to make an incision in the thrombosed hemorrhoid under local anesthesia and empty out the small blood clot from the hemorrhoid. In the unlikely event that you need major surgery, this should wait until after the baby is born.

☐ *Varicose Veins*   Varicose veins are so common during pregnancy that 10–20 percent of all pregnant women experience them, some more seriously than others. The condition is usually inherited, and a woman with a genetic tendency to varicose veins often develops them during a first pregnancy. The problem tends to become worse with each succeeding pregnancy. Since they can be very disfiguring, it is comforting to know that varicose veins usually disappear or improve after the baby is born if the condition is aided by some sensible precautions during pregnancy itself.

If you are aware of a family history of varicose veins, begin to use support hose *early* in pregnancy, and make a regular practice of sitting with your legs elevated to allow the venous blood to drain back from the veins in the legs. Although this is difficult when you have a job that involves standing, try to plan regular rest periods throughout the day when you can sit or lie with your feet up, and lie down with your feet up for at least half an hour after you reach home before you begin preparing dinner or doing any other chores. Walk as much as possible to keep the blood continually circulating through the legs, and if you are forced to stand at home or at work, flex your feet constantly to help the circulation in the legs. At night you can promote better circulation by elevating the foot of the bed.

Varicose veins sometimes appear as early as the second or third month, but they usually develop after the fourth month once the enlarged uterus puts pressure on the vena cava, the main vein in the body, preventing a free flow of blood back from the legs to the heart. Support hose are effective because they provide the extra pumping mechanism that pumps the venous blood back and helps avoid the development of blockages in the circulation of your legs. Always buy full panty hose support hose; knee-length support hose are useless during pregnancy. If the problem is serious, go to a surgical supply store and buy the firmest stockings you can find. (Jobst or Sivaris stockings are among the better brands.) Put the support hose on in the morning immediately after you wake up, and keep them on all day. Even with support hose on, elevate your legs several times during the day, and massage them from the foot up, to empty the excess blood from the veins.

Sometimes tiny red veins appear in clusters under the surface of the skin, usually on the thighs and calves. These are related to the much larger varicose veins that often bother pregnant women but usually disappear after delivery. If they do remain permanently, the more prominent spider veins can be minimized by injections or surgery.

A final word of caution: if you develop very large varicose veins, be sure to have your legs wrapped tightly with bandages during labor and delivery, otherwise there is the risk of a blood clot suddenly forming, which could have serious consequences. Continue to use support hose for a few weeks after the baby is born.

☐ *Headaches*   The commonest reason for a headache is emotional tension, and, unfortunately, anxiety or fear during pregnancy often results in headaches. An occasional Tylenol is usually helpful in relieving simple tension headaches. Headaches in pregnancy are also caused by the natural increase in the body's retention of sodium, brought on by the changes in hormonal levels. Increased estrogen causes sodium to bind water, and the resulting edema and water retention can result in a headache. In this case, cut out excess salt and try to rest more. Since headaches can also be the result of anemia, ask your doctor to take an extra blood count to determine your iron status. An increase in iron usually takes care of headaches as well as the other symptoms of anemia.

If you have persistent headaches or attacks of migraine, it is important to have them checked with your doctor. Headaches can be a sign of high blood pressure, which can develop quite suddenly when you are pregnant and can lead to toxemia. In fact, one of the classic signs of toxemia is a sudden headache, together with swelling and puffiness of the hands, feet, and face. If this occurs, *call your doctor immediately.*

☐ *Nosebleeding*   This is a very common side effect of pregnancy, particularly during the winter months. Nosebleeds rarely cause a serious problem, although I have seen one or two cases in which a nosebleed was so severe that the woman required hospitalization and a blood transfusion. A slight nosebleed is usually a result of the increased blood supply and dilatation of the blood vessels in the nasal mucosa. One is more likely to experience it in the winter, because the membranes that line the nasal cavity often become dried out as a result of central heating.

If you have a tendency to nosebleeds, be sure to lubricate the nasal cavity each night with a few drops of a 0.25 percent solution of menthol in white oil. Using a humidifier in the bedroom will also help. Remember, if a nosebleed does occur, rest and put your head forward immediately, put your thumb and forefinger on both sides of your nose and press them firmly from side to side to create a hemostasis (a blockage), or apply dry ice to the bridge of your nose. There are also vasoconstricting nose drops, such as Neosynephrine, which might be helpful if nosebleeds are a chronic problem. However, if the condition is really severe, you should consult your doctor.

Sometimes a woman is suddenly plagued by a runny nose or an allergylike condition. This is called pregnancy rhinitis (inflammation of the nasal passages). It will disappear in time, but decreasing the dryness of the mucous membranes helps control it temporarily. Keep the mucous membranes lubricated, and try to increase the humidity of your immediate environment.

☐ *Dizziness and Fainting*   Some women experience a feeling of dizziness, especially in the first half of pregnancy. The dizzy sensation occurs when you have been sitting or lying down for a long time and then get up rather suddenly. Although it can be unpleasant, there is a simple explanation for this characteristic symptom of pregnancy. Pregnancy-related changes in blood pressure result in dilation of the blood vessels, and if a woman moves too quickly from a lying to a standing position, her blood pressure suddenly drops and she feels dizzy or faint. If you find you suffer from hypotension (low blood pressure), try to prevent sudden changes of position and make sure to drink extra fluids and take in enough salt in the summertime, when the heat and humidity cause the blood vessels to dilate even more than usual. A higher sodium intake will increase your blood pressure and perhaps overcome some of the feelings of faintness.

One good way to combat dizziness is to breathe as deeply as possible in order to slowly introduce more oxygen to the brain. When you get out of bed in the morning, don't rush; sit on the edge of the bed for a while and breathe deeply before you start moving around. If you feel faint while you are out of the house, bend your head down and take several deep breaths; if you are still faint, press both your fingers firmly on both sides of the upper part of your nose at the same time. This will increase your blood pressure and help overcome the feeling of faintness. Carry smelling salts as a precautionary measure and use them if at any time you feel faint.

If the sensation of dizziness persists or you experience any blurring or disturbance of vision, talk to your doctor. Dizziness that occurs frequently is a sign of hypotension, and hypotension, if prolonged, can decrease the amount of oxygen reaching the baby. Very occasionally an obstetrician will see a patient who complains of bouts of dizziness for which he is unable to find a cause. A neurologist or a cardiologist should then be consulted. Tachycardia (fast heartbeat) and other heart conditions do occasionally appear without prior symptoms during pregnancy, and a cardiologist may elect to prescribe a digitalis drug to control the heart.

☐ *Leg Cramps*   Leg cramps are common in the middle and end of pregnancy, particularly when you lie for long periods on your back. The best way to deal with a sudden attack is to bend the foot upward and massage the cramped muscle, or ask your partner to elevate your leg and massage the muscles for you. These spasms in the foot or calf muscles can be very painful, especially as they tend to occur without any warning. Sometimes cramps are so violent that the calf muscles knot into an immovable, painful ball and the pain continues for some time after you have applied local massage or a heating pad to the affected area. Unfortunately this often happens at night, making sleep all but impossible.

Leg cramps can be such a nuisance during pregnancy that anything you do to prevent their occurrence is valuable. First of all, review your diet. You may not be getting enough calcium. Lack of calcium can lead to a calcium/phosphorus imbalance, and this in turn contributes to leg cramps. Unsuitable shoes may also be a contributory factor. Do you regularly walk around for long periods of time in high-heeled shoes, or have you recently bought shoes that don't fit correctly? If you change to a medium heel, which supports your increased weight better, you will be much more comfortable and less likely to suffer from foot or leg cramps.

There are some older remedies as well; one of the most popular is a small dose of Gelusil or Amphojel—two teaspoons or two tablets three times a day with meals. However, the best course is to talk to your doctor and have your calcium/phosphorus level checked with a blood count if the condition persists.

☐ *Fluid Retention*   A moderate amount of water retention and swelling are normal in the later months of pregnancy. About half of all pregnant women experience a slight puffiness of the hands, legs, and feet and a sensation of heaviness throughout the body. This edema of pregnancy is a normal condition. Approximately one-fourth to one-third of your weight gain during pregnancy is caused by increased water retention in the tissues, and this excess fluid tends to be concentrated in the parts of the body with soft tissues, such as the hands, feet, and ankles.

Edema of pregnancy used to be controlled by a completely salt-free diet. This is no longer considered advisable, since the body needs a certain amount of salt during pregnancy to function properly. Depriving a woman of salt completely led the body to conserve existing salt, and this in turn led to a rise in blood pressure and an *increased* amount of swelling. Instead of cutting out salt altogether, simply watch your salt intake and eliminate excessively salty foods. Eat nutritiously and drink plenty of fluids to wash out the waste products in the body.

Rest is important. Rest often, and when you sit or lie down, keep the legs elevated so the blood will circulate back from the legs to the heart and the pressure on the legs and ankles will be reduced. Most women find that the swelling disappears during the night, a fact that emphasizes the importance of rest in controlling edema. If you have poor circulation or varicose veins, remember to wear support hose at all times during the day; this will increase the blood supply and may eliminate swelling altogether. Since water retention is more pronounced in the summertime, take extra precautions during hot weather.

☐ *Breast Changes*   Changes in the appearance of the breasts are among the first signs of pregnancy. The breasts become much heavier, the surface veins become more prominent, and the pigmentation of the areola, the area around the nipples, deepens in color. These early changes are described in more detail in Chapter 5. As the breasts increase in size with the development of the baby in the second trimester, delicate veins appear just beneath the skin, and the nipples become larger, darker, and more erect. In about the fourth month of pregnancy a thick yellowish fluid called colostrum may be secreted or expressed from the nipple by gentle massage. At the same time the areola darkens and small elevations called Montgomery glands appear, scattered throughout the area.

During the later months of pregnancy, as the breasts become enlarged and the milk glands develop in preparation for breast-feeding, it is very important to buy a comfortable, well fitted bra to provide proper support. You can prevent any staining by slipping nursing pads or wads of tissue over the nipples. Excess colostrum can be removed from the nipple itself by a piece of cotton moistened in warm water, but make sure to dry the nipple area thoroughly to prevent dry or cracked nipples.

The breasts will remain enlarged for as long as you continue to breast-feed the baby. After weaning, they will return to approximately their former size.

☐ *Fatigue*   An increased sense of fatigue is a very common experience during pregnancy, especially in the first trimester. In these first few weeks the body is making new adjustments to pregnancy (see Chapter 5), and this increases the need for sleep and additional rest during the day. Then, at the beginning of the second trimester, the situation generally improves: the proper adjustments have usually been made, the hormonal levels stabilize, and the appetite increases. Eating properly has an immediate effect on your energy level, and proper amounts of protein, iron, and vitamins in your diet help eliminate any symptoms of anemia.

But even though the second trimester is often a time when you feel healthy and energetic, you still need more rest than the average woman. Whether you are at work or at home with a small child, you shouldn't automatically try to keep up your normal schedule. You need more sleep at night and, if possible, a rest period during the day. The hormonal and other physical changes of pregnancy mean that your body is working much harder, and the extra strain on the heart, lungs, and other vital organs has an effect on your fatigue level. Whatever her personal circumstances, a woman must try to get the extra rest she needs at all times during pregnancy. Don't be ashamed of being tired. It's a normal phenomenon, and the best way to overcome it is to rest as much as possible.

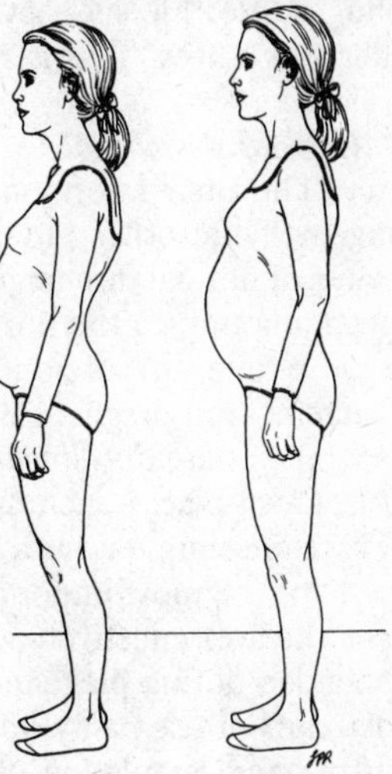

Figure 27: Posture During Pregnancy: As the pregnancy progresses a woman tends to lean backward to compensate for the extra weight in the front, increasing the tendency to lower-back pain. You can help overcome the problem by exercises. Straighten your body up several times daily by leaning with your back against the wall, your heels about six inches away, and iron out the hollow of your back by pressing your waist backward. Keep this up twenty times daily.

☐ *Backaches*   There is a traditional belief that aches and pains in the lower back, lower abdomen, and the legs are the result of the baby "lying on the nerve." In truth, almost all the backaches and leg aches women experience during pregnancy are caused by increased weight and alterations in posture. As the baby gets larger, a woman naturally tends to lean backward to compensate for the extra weight in front, and this puts increased pressure on the lower back, the most vulnerable part of the whole lumbar region.

Bending forward and lifting become difficult because of the size of the abdomen, and sudden, clumsy movements put additional strain on the lower back. This is why it is so important to bend your legs rather than your back when you lift anything. Back problems are often exaggerated because the joints in the pelvis tend to soften during pregnancy to allow for the expansion of the uterus, which leads to the characteristic waddling gait some women are forced to adopt just to get around. This temporary condition contributes to lower back pain and abdominal discomfort.

Backache can be prevented, or at least controlled, by regular exercises and by avoiding physical strain at work and at home. Some women find a light maternity girdle is helpful. Wearing low-heeled shoes that give your feet and legs proper support will reduce fatigue considerably and help distribute your weight correctly. Standing for long periods of time, of course, increases the pressure on your lower back a great deal. Try to walk around, even in a limited space, if your job requires a lot of standing; otherwise sit rather than stand, and, if possible, lie down rather than sit.

☐ **Shortness of Breath**　　Shortness of breath is a common complaint in the last few weeks before delivery because the baby is pressing against the rib cage and pushing up the diaphragm. This is particularly true of the eighth month, when the fundus (top of the uterus) is higher. In the last weeks before delivery the situation usually improves once the baby descends into the birth canal and the pressure is released.

Don't exert yourself physically in the last month of pregnancy, and lessen the feeling of breathlessness by resting on your side with a pillow or folded blanket under your knees. This is a comfortable way to sleep in the final weeks.

☐ *Vaginal Discharge*　　Vaginal discharge always increases during pregnancy. The altered hormonal levels in the body change the vaginal environment along with the other physical adjustments of early pregnancy, increasing the amount of normal discharge. This discharge will appear in every way similar, except in amount, to the normal white discharge of the nonpregnant woman. At the same time, the alterations in the vaginal environment make it less resistant to bacteria, and pregnant women often experience one of the common "yeast" infections, *Candida albicans*, or monilia. These annoying funguses thrive in warm, moist places, including the vagina.

There are simple ways to prevent or relieve monilia infections. Good hygiene is perhaps the most important. Sitting in a warm tub reduces the irritation and cleans the area effectively without the necessity for douching, which is *not* recommended during pregnancy. Avoid tight jeans and panty hose and use cotton underpants or use panty hose with a cotton crotch to encourage evaporation of moisture and circulation of air in the vagina. Wash everything that comes in contact with the discharge regularly to avoid reinfecting yourself. In the case of a persistent infection, your doctor will probably recommend suppositories or a medication such as Mycostatin or Monistat. Since the uterus is fully protected by the neck of the cervix, suppositories are unlikely to have an adverse effect on the fetus, and Mycostatin suppositories have a good record of safe use during pregnancy.

☐ *Stretch Marks*　　Stretch marks are the pink, slightly depressed streaks that appear on the skin of the abdomen, the breasts, and the thighs and buttocks during the later months of pregnancy. Why some women are affected by them and others escape remains a mystery. Blond women, women who are overweight, and women in their first pregnancy are apparently more susceptible. Interestingly, women who become pregnant later in life usually are less subject to stretch marks than very young women, perhaps because in a very young woman the skin has not completely grown, and the rapid weight gain during pregnancy causes breakages in immature skin areas. After the birth, stretch marks gradually fade away to an off-white color and may become all but invisible, although they will never disappear altogether. For this reason, anything you can do to minimize their occurrence is valuable.

Regardless of advertising hype, don't rely on oils or creams. They have no effect on stretch marks—although your skin will probably benefit from the increased moisture. Simply try to avoid gaining too much weight and keep your abdominal muscles in shape. (A controlled abdomen reduces the tension on your skin and the amount of stretch.) This is one excellent reason for following a routine of abdominal exercises conscientiously during the second and third trimesters (see Chap. 12).

☐ **Skin Changes**   The best known skin change is the appearance of darkened areas on the face, usually on either side of the nose. These darkish areas are called *chloasma,* or "mask of pregnancy." But the increase in pigmentation caused by the hormonal changes of pregnancy affect other areas of the body besides the face. A characteristic dark line called the *linea negra* develops in the center of the abdomen from the umbilicus to the region of the pubic hair, and the area around the nipples, the areola, also darkens, usually permanently.

These changes are the result of the body's increased production of melanin, the chemical substance that promotes suntan and freckles. Since the melanin level is higher during pregnancy, women with a tendency to moles will find that their size and number often increase during pregnancy. *Moles* are usually benign but can occasionally mutate into a deadly form of skin cancer called *melanoma.* The likelihood of this occurring is increased during and after pregnancy. Observe all moles closely. If one should begin to grow in size and change color, see your doctor immediately and have it biopsied.

11

Feelings During Pregnancy

At whatever point in your life you become pregnant for the first time, your life inevitably changes. This is usually a healthy and a happy change, but at the same time it is also a dramatic one. A first pregnancy is as important a turning point in a couple's life as their marriage. And for a woman it parallels the other great sexual passages: adolescence and menopause. Pregnancy is, like any other life crisis, a period of transition: as in adolescence you passed from childhood to adulthood, in pregnancy you move from manhood or womanhood into parenthood. Pregnancy, after all, is not simply a physical condition that ends abruptly after nine months when the baby is delivered. It is the beginning of a relationship with another human being who will be "your child" for the rest of your life.

Considering pregnancy as a life crisis does not mean that it is a state of continual tension or conflict. Most couples experience a wonderful sense of fulfillment when the woman is pregnant, heightened by moments of unusual tenderness and intimacy. Far from being destructive, pregnancy often strengthens a relationship, because the baby is created and nurtured in partnership. It is also a time of great personal satisfaction: we achieve a few things in our lifetime that we can be proud of, and one of them is having a child.

Nonetheless every pregnancy makes some unexpected demands as well as giving pleasure and fulfillment. This is not in the least surprising; any period of transition is bound to be difficult as well as rewarding. Because pregnancy changes your life, sometimes subtly and sometimes dramatically, it requires patience, understanding, flexibility, and toughness. Both partners in a successful first pregnancy should be prepared for the physical and emotional upheavals that occur in the nine months of the pregnancy and in the postpartum period as well.

Unfortunately, few women, and perhaps even fewer men, are aware of the potential for conflict or the inevitability of emotional crisis in an outwardly normal, happy, healthy pregnancy. Since most couples feel that this ought to be the happiest period of their lives, it makes it all the more difficult to admit to doubts or conflicting emotions. Until quite recently the best sources of information—the medical profession, books on childbirth, and prenatal classes—neglected to focus on the emotional aspects of pregnancy, leaving a couple without professional resources in a sometimes difficult situation. Happily this is changing as people begin to look on pregnancy as an emotional as well as a physical experience. Talking about conflicts or emotional crisis, however, does not mean that you are going to be miserable for nine months or that your relationship with your partner will suffer irreparably. I see women at all stages of their pregnancies, and I watch them and their partners making the transition successfully and enjoying the pregnancy. At those times I feel how fortunate I am to be an obstetrician because I can share at least a part of a couple's happiness.

☐ *How Are a Woman's Emotions Affected by Pregnancy?*   While personalities and personal circumstances differ greatly from one pregnancy to another, certain emotional states are almost universal in pregnant women. Perhaps the most common is a heightened sensitivity to a range of emotions. Pregnant women commonly experience sudden personality changes, they are more sensitive to joyful and upsetting emotions, and they tend to dream and fantasize more often during pregnancy than at other times. For the same reasons, emotions are often volatile: you might be euphoric at one moment and inexplicably depressed the next.

☐ *Mood Swings*   Many women are quite unprepared for the vehemence or the instability of their emotions during pregnancy. (In this respect pregnancy is akin to adolescence, another time in your life when emotions are both intense and rapidly changing.) Sometimes you feel radiant and serene or you wake up with a feeling of tremendous energy and self-confidence. Then the next day, for no explicable reason, you are depressed and anxious or you feel sure you will never get through the pregnancy or be able to cope with your life after the baby comes. Because emotions are so intense, trivial family arguments or minor tensions at work suddenly become difficult to deal with; you may also find yourself behaving irrationally—bursting into tears one moment and laughing the next. Many women experience moments during pregnancy when they feel more than a little crazy. Mood swings and similar psychological phenomena are so common during pregnancy that one obstetrician who surveyed a group of pregnant women found that over 80 percent of them experienced feelings of depression, while 70 percent of them reported inexplicable crying episodes, another manifestation of "pregnancy blues." In another study, 50 percent of the women who were surveyed said they experienced mood changes, anxiety spells, and insomnia during pregnancy. Other women report vivid dreams or fantasies or suffer from atypical obsessions or phobias when they are pregnant.

This heightened susceptibility to a variety of emotions is called emotional lability. It is characterized by a wide range of rapidly shifting moods and extreme reactions to apparently normal situations. It is not unique to pregnancy. Under certain types of stress many human beings respond more violently or experience mood swings of greater magnitude than usual. A pregnant woman who has crying fits or overreacts to a domestic argument is experiencing the tension that

146 /   *Childbirth with Love*

many of us feel during humid days in the summer when tempers are more on edge than at any other time of the year.

☐   *How Hormonal Activity Affects Mood Changes*   Although the emotional adjustment to pregnancy is the most important single cause of emotional lability, hormonal changes certainly play a part. Progesterone in particular seems to change the body's chemical balance, while progesterone and estrogen combined change the brain's metabolism to some degree. Consequently the pronounced hormonal changes of pregnancy appear to heighten the emotional tensions associated with early pregnancy. A high progesterone level has certain marked physical effects, including the relaxation of the uterus, food cravings, and the tired feeling associated with early pregnancy. Many of these changes are beneficial to the continuance of pregnancy. The decrease of the natural contractions of the uterus, for instance, helps prevent miscarriage. In addition, progesterone may well have a depressant effect on the mood centers in the brain in early pregnancy, just as it does when a woman uses injections of progesterone as a contraceptive means. Progesterone also seems to induce what are called regressive tendencies—immature and demanding behavior, which often shows itself in dreams, fantasies, and defense mechanisms of various kinds. This state is sometimes observable in the four to six days following ovulation, when the progesterone level is high. Finally, progesterone and estrogen changes during pregnancy are known to affect the action of the catecholamines, the chemical hormones believed to play a vital part in our emotions. There is some evidence that the corticosteroids, the hormones produced by the adrenal gland, are also altered during pregnancy and consequently heighten the moods of depression or elation.

In the past, doctors believed that hormonal changes were entirely responsible for the mood swings and the other emotional upheavals of pregnancy. To a certain extent this is true. As we have seen, higher levels of progesterone and estrogen, particularly at the beginning of pregnancy, affect a woman's physical and mental states in a number of different ways. However, this theory offers only a partial explanation for what is happening during pregnancy. While hormonal changes exacerbate mood swings in pregnancy just as they do during the menstrual cycle, they cannot be held responsible for the emotions you are experiencing. You feel alternately happy and unhappy or confident and confused because pregnancy *is* a time of uncertainty and difficulty as well as happiness. Don't worry; emotional lability is a normal part of pregnancy, and if you understand what is going on, it will be much easier to deal with.

The degree of emotional lability varies widely from woman to woman. To some extent it reflects your individual susceptibility to hormonal changes, but it is also influenced by your personality and the individual circumstances of your pregnancy. A woman who is under unusual stress or whose family is unsupportive is naturally more susceptible to violent mood swings or angry outbursts. In this respect it is not always the first pregnancy that is the stormy one: emotional lability is sometimes pronounced in a second or third pregnancy because of some new psychological or environmental factor. The same woman will experience quite different emotions in successive pregnancies even though she is carrying a child of the same sex. (There is some evidence that greater mood changes take place when the fetus is male, possibly because of the male hormone production.)

Although violent mood swings and extreme irrationality are experienced by only a minority of pregnant women, they are considered danger signals (see below) and may require professional counseling. A woman who is unremittingly hostile or chronically depressed, or feels that her life is out of control, is going through a severe emotional crisis and should get help. If she cannot do so herself, her family should contact her obstetrician and try to get professional counseling for her.

☐ *Dreams*   The dreams and fantasies experienced by pregnant women are often vivid, compelling, or frightening. The tendency to dream or fantasize is another aspect of the psychological "openness" of a woman during pregnancy, and both processes serve important functions in uncovering conflicting emotions or obsessions. The memory of a vivid or disturbing dream may recur over and over during the day. In the first trimester many women have powerful fantasies about the baby they can't feel or see but know is alive; or the embryo or fetus sometimes seems unimaginable, alien, or bizarre. Feelings about the baby can change from month to month. In the early months you may be more fascinated by the idea of being *pregnant* than the idea of having a *child*. This is a psychological defense that makes it easier to accept the baby, because it is not viewed as an individual whose separate life may threaten yours. Later on you may have dreams in which you lose or neglect the baby. Foreboding dreams about the baby are upsetting, but they don't mean that you are or are going to be a bad mother. You may be concerned about losing the baby through the separation process at birth or worried by the new responsibility of caring for a child.

☐ *Phobias and Superstitions*   Normally logical women often experience irrational moments when they are pregnant. Phobias are common, particularly those relating to physical vulnerability; dreams or superstitions may also become obsessive. Some women who cheerfully walk under ladders when they are not pregnant suddenly develop the oddest quirks or a firm belief in the supernatural. Occasionally a phobia or superstition appears or occurs because a woman has had a past experience that affected her profoundly. A woman who once had an abortion or had given her child up for adoption, for instance, might be afraid that her doctor or the hospital nurses are going to steal the baby. A phobia of this kind is extremely disturbing, but it does serve a useful purpose in expressing fears or guilt feelings that might otherwise be suppressed.

☐ *Will Mood Swings and Dreams Affect the Baby?*   There is no evidence of fetal distress from emotional lability, at least in a normal pregnancy. Nor is it likely to harm the baby, since the worst of it usually occurs in the early months when the fetus is relatively immature. The impact of severe stress, however, is a more serious matter. The final section of this chapter deals with the effect of different kinds of stress during pregnancy.

☐ *Conflicts, Doubts, and Other Uncomfortable Emotions*   Even though pregnancy is a time of great happiness, and a few women seem to remain serene and confident, most women experience periods of doubt, conflict, and anxiety when they are pregnant. Sometimes negative emotions surface together with joyful ones—at the beginning of pregnancy, for instance. One happily pregnant patient of mine recently came in for her second prenatal visit and broke into tears immediately when I asked her how she was feeling.

According to a recent informal survey many women experience a similar feeling of ambivalence: over 60 percent of the women interviewed in this survey said there were times during their pregnancies when they didn't want the baby. I suspect a survey of expectant fathers would yield much the same result.

Ambivalent feelings about becoming pregnant can sometimes surface in an odd or troublesome way. A few women stubbornly deny the very existence of their babies by ignoring the cessation of menstruation or the onset of nausea and vomiting. When a woman is really troubled by the pregnancy, she may go so far as to disbelieve the obstetricians' diagnosis or a positive pregnancy test. Some psychiatrists believe this indicates a conflict about sexual behavior, since conception is proof of the couple's sexual relationship, but anxiety about the pregnancy is the more likely explanation. When a woman cannot face up to the reality of her pregnancy, her partner's reaction is often crucial. If he wants the baby, this is often sufficient to resolve her ambivalence, but if the man is anxious about this turning point in his life or worried about the economic implications of having a child, the partners can drag each other down into deeper and deeper emotional difficulties. At this point a couple should seek professional help.

Ambivalence is usually worse at the beginning of pregnancy when your body is making the initial adjustments to its new state. Physically the first trimester is not always a comfortable or rewarding period, and you may find yourself becoming unexpectedly resentful about the pregnancy, especially if your partner is outwardly healthy and energetic while you are queasy and depressed. (However, many men do experience the *couvade syndrome*—physical changes that parallel the physical symptoms of their mates during pregnancy.) This ambivalence is part of an important psychological process, the process of accepting the pregnancy, which begins in the early weeks and may continue for several months. Even after you have accepted the pregnancy, you can expect ambivalent feelings to return when you are feeling unwell or under emotional stress.

Fear is often part of the initial conflict. What happens if you lose your job or your marriage breaks up? Is the baby all right? Suppose you can't cope with the delivery or learn to look after the baby? These and other frightening questions can surface quite unexpectedly. You may be afraid to discuss them with your partner, and he is probably experiencing anxieties of his own that he is afraid to discuss with you. Sometimes women try to hide their feelings because they seem "unnatural" or they think they will harm the baby. However, fears are far more dangerous if they are suppressed, and only a very tense or fearful woman will adversely affect the development of the fetus. Anxieties also have a useful function because they prepare new parents for the birth and care of the baby. The best way to deal with your fears is to talk to your partner and make some plans for the future instead of allowing yourself to become more and more depressed. Once fears are openly expressed, you can at least begin to deal with them.

It is important to realize that doubts and conflicts are a normal part of the experience of pregnancy. Pregnancy is a time of rapid change when you are making choices that affect your own life and the lives of your partner and your baby. Although becoming a parent is exciting and challenging, it is such a momentous process that you are bound to feel uncertain, depressed, or overwrought at times. The anxieties women commonly feel during pregnancy are not unreasonable. In most cases they are based on some concern that is more than relevant—the well-being of the baby, for instance. A woman is faced with unfamiliar choices just because she is pregnant—a situation that naturally leads to uncertainty and anxiety.

Anxieties also help you work through what is, after all, a major transition in your life, the process of becoming a parent. It has been said that a woman who does not express certain fears in pregnancy or who doesn't feel occasionally depressed is indeed reacting abnormally to a major turning point in her life. Psychiatrists who deal with cases of postpartum depression in women regard the absence of anxieties in pregnancy as a warning signal. Women who say they are *always* happy appear to suffer far more severely from postpartum depression than women who face up honestly to the problems of parenthood before the baby's birth.

However, it is valuable to learn how to deal with stress, because it can be damaging. Pregnancy is often a stressful time and common anxieties can become disproportionally magnified. One good way to cope with stress is to learn relaxation techniques. Deep breathing and other measures conducive to relaxation (see pp. 177–182) have a calming effect physically and mentally and also circulate more oxygen through the placenta, reducing the effects of stress on the baby. It is, of course, important to talk over any problems or anxieties with your partner, your family, close friends, and the professionals with whom you are in close contact.

☐ *The Stages of Pregnancy*   Psychologically, a pregnancy can be divided into two stages. In the first stage a woman comes to terms with the knowledge that she will be a mother; she learns to accept her pregnancy. The second stage is the perception of the fetus as a separate individual, a phase that often begins with quickening. For most pregnant women the early months are the time when they accomplish the first psychological task—acceptance of the pregnancy. In this first trimester a woman is physically and emotionally adjusting to pregnancy, a stage that is characterized by certain physical symptoms and, very often, conflicting emotions such as those described in the previous section.

Physically, the early months are often a confusing time. Although you know you are pregnant, it is hard sometimes to believe that you really are. This is why it is important for a woman to recognize the early symptoms of pregnancy—enlarged breasts, a different appetite level, or fatigue. (Indeed, if a woman is unaware of physical changes, it may indicate an abnormal pregnancy or a denial of pregnancy itself.) At the same time, your pregnancy is usually invisible to the outside world. Many women enjoy the secrecy that surrounds the first trimester, but the lack of visibility can be frustrating. You are pregnant, but you don't look or perhaps even feel pregnant. You may find yourself compulsively reviewing your symptoms over and over again to make sure you are really pregnant, or eating twice the usual amount of food to put on weight quickly. This frustration often persists into the fourth or fifth month, when the sudden weight gain makes the pregnancy visible to the outside world.

In early pregnancy a woman's thoughts usually turn inward. Often she is more concerned about being pregnant than about having a child. Sometimes the lack of a visible pregnancy leads a woman to treat the pregnancy as an illness rather than the beginning of a new phase in her life; she may complain bitterly of nausea, bloated breasts, exhaustion, and the other side effects of early pregnancy. Usually this passes, but a few women continue to complain of severe physical symptoms into the second or even the third trimester. Undue nausea or an obsession with food that persists beyond the fourth or fifth month may be signs that a woman is having trouble accepting the fetus as a part of herself (see "Danger Signals," below). In general the first trimester is the time of greatest tension in any pregnancy, when a woman undergoes the rewarding but difficult process of learning to accept the pregnancy.

A reawakened identification with the pregnant woman's mother is another crucial stage in the adjustment to pregnancy. Sometimes close contact is resumed between mother and daughter after several years of separation. Often the unexpected closeness of this mother-daughter relationship leads a woman to reexamine the feelings she had toward her mother when she was a child. Although uncomfortable as well as pleasurable memories can surface at this time, a woman who is about to become a parent herself must look at the way she was brought up if she is to define the qualities that will determine her relationship with her child. By examining her past a woman begins to take on the nurturant role herself instead of remaining the child of her parents. Thoughts about one's relationship toward one's mother may persist throughout the pregnancy, but they are generally less obsessive by the second trimester.

Some women come to accept their pregnancies at an earlier point than others. Accepting the pregnancy does not mean that you have resolved all your doubts, only that you have dealt with your conflicts sufficiently to go on to the next turning point—the perception of the fetus as an individual with a life separate from yours. Before you can accomplish this important step it is necessary to "make room" for your child by accepting your role as a parent. Unfortunately some women delay completing this essential stage until very late in the pregnancy or even until after the baby is born. Such a late acceptance of pregnancy can have serious consequences; it may indeed be a factor in the onset of postpartum depression (see Chap. 33).

☐   *The Second Trimester*   Physically and emotionally this is generally the most rewarding period of pregnancy. Many women who find the first trimester disappointing begin to enjoy their pregnancies in the second trimester. First of all, there is the physical confirmation of the baby's existence, which comes with the first discernible fetal movements. Once you experience quickening, you will find that many fears disappear, including a conscious or unconscious fear of miscarriage. Women who find it difficult to think of themselves as pregnant up to the fourth or fifth month often find that quickening changes their perception of the pregnancy completely. At the same time, the more unpleasant side effects of pregnancy tend to disappear, and most women have a renewed sense of energy and well-being.

Once she knows the fetus is alive, a pregnant woman may pass on to the next important stage of pregnancy: conceptualizing her baby as an individual with a life separate from hers. One no longer asks oneself: "Does this child exist?" Instead one might ask oneself: "Who is this baby? What does it look like? What can I do to care for it?" After quickening, fantasies about the unborn child increase, especially guesses as to the baby's sex. A woman may also be suddenly afraid of injuring the fetus accidentally (although the fetus is well protected by the amniotic fluid and the muscle layers of the uterus). Dreams about injury to oneself change to dreams about "someone else." Surprisingly, husbands are often more nervous about fetal well-being than their wives, even if they enjoy watching the belly grow rounder as pregnancy proceeds. In one informal survey of expectant couples, many of the men interviewed spoke about anxieties that they had been afraid to share with their wives, particularly anxieties about the health or the normalcy of the fetus. Such apprehensions often surface in a couple's sexual relationship when a man may be reluctant to have intercourse for fear that he might injure the baby.

In the second trimester the baby nonetheless brings his parents together as he kicks and turns within the uterus. First fetal movements are too fleeting for a man to detect, but by the end of the trimester the baby has become large and vigorous enough for the outline of a fist or foot to appear on the outside of the abdomen. As he realizes that he is really a father, a man may become involved in the pregnancy for the first time. Generally too a woman finds that she moves closer to her partner in the second trimester as she learns to think of the fetus as *their* baby rather than *her* baby. Partners who have had a difficult time in the early months of pregnancy often find that the middle months are ones of greater tranquillity, not to say happiness. Sexuality changes too in the second trimester. (See Chapter 13 for a full discussion of sexual changes during pregnancy.) Most women find they are more easily aroused because of physical changes that take place in the area of the pelvis. The new emotional involvement with the partner may also have a good effect on the couple's sex life. Much will depend, however, on the physical changes during the second and third trimesters. Reaction to the pregnant body often depends on negative or positive body image before pregnancy.

A woman who is at ease with herself physically is usually excited by the change, although there are always moments when the pregnant body seems burdensome or clumsy. A woman who is ambivalent about her physical appearance in the nonpregnant state may find the adjustment more difficult. Occasionally a woman has such unremittingly negative feelings about her body that she, in effect, rejects her pregnancy. This is a danger signal, a sign that a woman is in trouble and needs professional help. Her partner's attitude too will have a great effect on a woman's feelings as her body begins to alter radically. A man can do much to help his wife adjust to her pregnancy by reassuring her that he still finds her desirable. This is easier for some men than for others. A man may be delighted by the visible growth of his child. He may equally find it difficult to accept the momentous change in his partner, out of fear or out of jealousy. When one group of expectant couples were asked to draw a picture of the wives during pregnancy, the women pictured themselves with shapeless bodies and beatific facial expressions. Many of their husbands, on the other hand, created images that were either ambiguous or hostile: one showed the pregnant wife with a pointed devil's tail and bared teeth; another pictured a blimp with a woman's head. Both men confessed they had hidden their feelings from their wives because they were afraid to hurt them. A husband's reaction may depend in part on his own adjustment to the new demands of the pregnancy: a man who is not sure how good a father he will be will naturally be more disturbed by his wife's pregnant body than a man who has successfully come to terms with becoming a father.

The second trimester is a good time for a couple to go over plans for the later months of pregnancy and the delivery. Anxieties often disappear once you think ahead and deal with questions of work, living arrangements, and practical help after the birth. Because couples usually feel very close to each other in the middle months of pregnancy, the conflicts associated with the early months are generally resolved in the second trimester, and you can begin to look forward to the future. It is important to use this opportunity well because the last months of pregnancy, like the first, are often a time of emotional upheaval, although for different reasons.

☐ **The Third Trimester**   As you pass into the third trimester the baby's movements are more and more insistent as each week passes. The pregnancy has become an inescapable reality for both expectant parents. By now most couples will have solved the conflicts of the early months and will be looking forward to the birth. The baby is also clearly perceived as having a life of its own. In fact at this point of pregnancy it may begin to disrupt its mother's life as the uterus swells to accommodate the rapid growth of the last trimester.

Physical changes in the last trimester are momentous. As the abdomen becomes larger it pushes up the rib cage and pushes down on the bladder, causing such side effects as breathlessness, insomnia, and loss of bladder control. It is more difficult to move around. Even finding a comfortable sitting position can be a problem for a woman in the final weeks. By the end of the pregnancy a woman may be exhausted and impatient; she may find herself looking forward to the delivery just to be rid of the discomfort. By the eighth or ninth month frequency of sexual intercourse tends to decrease because the woman is too tired or too clumsy to enjoy making love or the man finds her pregnant abdomen to be visually as well as physically obstrusive. Again, this is an individual matter, since some women say they feel more sexually attractive during the last weeks of pregnancy than at any other time in the pregnancy.

One especially pleasing aspect of later pregnancy is the attention you can expect to receive from friends, family, and even strangers. One writer has described the special position a very pregnant woman occupies as a "biologically based dominance," an identity that transcends the individual. So compelling is the sight of a visibly pregnant woman that friends will pat you on the belly or strangers will stop on the street to ask you when the baby is due. The special privileges of the last weeks of pregnancy may be looked back on later with nostalgia.

Now that you know the pregnancy is coming to an end, physical preparations for the baby become a priority. Almost every pregnant woman experiences what is known as the "nesting instinct," an urgent need to make the physical environment ready for the baby's arrival. The onset of the nesting instinct is a sign that the separation stage of the pregnancy is almost complete. Some women begin buying baby clothes or equipment in the second trimester, others wait until later, sometimes as late as a few weeks before the due date. This depends on the circumstances of the individual pregnancy. If a woman is ordered to bed in the second trimester because of the threat of premature labor, she will naturally wait for two or three months before ordering anything for the baby. Similarly, a woman whose pregnancy has been unusually troubled emotionally may not be ready to make practical preparations until the third trimester. Sometimes a woman will wait until after the birth to complete her plans for the baby. Do not be concerned about an apparent lack of interest in practical matters early on. An absence of the nesting instinct in the third trimester could, however, be a sign that a woman is rejecting her pregnancy.

As the abdomen continues to grow, a woman who welcomed the first fetal movements may find herself unexpectedly alarmed or even angered by the extraordinary changes she is being forced to undergo. It is natural to be afraid of losing control over your body as the baby insistently kicks at the walls of the uterus, disturbing what rest you can manage to take at night or during the day. Some women manage to regard the changes humorously, others become frightened by the loss of control.

Violent fetal movements are of course a reminder of the imminence of the baby's birth. Most expectant parents make initial plans for labor and delivery in the first or second trimester and then turn to more immediate practical concerns. By the last trimester the birth is usually a couple's most urgent concern. You may find yourself looking for the first symptoms of labor several weeks before your due date. Some women pass through the last month of pregnancy in a state of perpetual anticipation. Not surprisingly, you may find yourself experiencing dreams in which you are trapped or in which you lose or misplace the baby. Such dreams express a natural apprehension of labor and delivery, a state that is normal even though you will have acquired a theoretical knowledge of labor from books and childbirth classes. It is good to remember that anxieties do have a useful function in preparing a woman mentally and physically for the stresses of labor. Women who are fearful but are unable to express their anxieties are often those who find labor most difficult. It will help to discuss your feelings in your childbirth class, where you will have the support of the prenatal instructor and the other members of the class. Open discussion is important for your partner as well. Men are often worried that they will not be able to support their wives successfully through labor and delivery.

By the ninth month the baby has almost reached its full birth weight and is vigorous enough to keep its mother awake at night. You can still only speculate as to your child's sex and appearance, but the guessing games become more fascinating as the due date approaches. Naming is another activity that makes the unborn child real in the eyes of its parents. Sometimes a woman becomes regretful as she contemplates the end of her pregnancy; she may want to hold on a little longer to her full belly and the other physical satisfactions of pregnancy. At the same time, a woman in her last month typically experiences a final burst of energy in which she cleans the house, finishes the baby's room, or exhibits some other compulsive behavior that recognizes the reality of the birth. Time may seem to move slowly in the final two or three weeks, especially if you pass the due date without going into labor, which many women do in a first birth. An unexpected delay can be irritating and will become more irritating as time goes on without any sign of labor. Even if they are nervous about what will happen during the birth, most women feel a tremendous relief and excitement as they recognize the first symptoms of progressive labor. It is, after all, the culmination of nine extraordinary months and the beginning of a new life for themselves and the people closest to them.

☐ *Ellen's Story*   There were so many difficult decisions in the early years of my life. Then I met Jeff, and my life began to change for the better. When I was 26 and Jeff was 29, we had been together for 4 years and had been married for one year. Many things had changed in the year we had been married. Our relationship had had its difficult times but we had begun to develop a constant trust, an endurance, and we felt so much of a unity that we wanted to combine our lives and start a family. We were beginning to believe in ourselves, to love each other and trust each other. If someone believes in you, this trust will make you stronger and give you confidence. We thought we had reached a point where we trusted each other enough to start a family. We felt great about that moment— that we were now doing and building something together. We knew we were going to have our baby.

I felt immediately that something had happened to me. I was sure I was pregnant, but we realized it would take time before we knew for sure. In the meantime we began to ask ourselves, "Do we know what we are doing?" We began to have doubts. "Are we really ready for this? What about our financial responsibility? Do we really want to have a baby? What's going to happen to us?" The ups and downs continued. Of course we knew it was too early [to confirm that I was pregnant] and we would have to wait for at least another week.

Deep down I knew my menstruation would not occur. Even though we both felt uncertain, even scared at times, we continued to talk, to feel, and to reach out to each other. Now that we needed each other, it was so important that we be honest with each other. Finally, I missed my period and awaited the date of my examination and the pregnancy test. I felt beautiful in the doctor's office but somehow disappointed by Jeff's lack of excitement. I realized later how much more there is to think about after a pregnancy test is confirmed. I thought to myself, I hope I am pregnant, I want to tell everyone. But the doctor told me the test wouldn't be ready until the evening. I wanted life to begin to grow inside me. I wanted it much more than I had ever wanted anything in my life. It was a long day and a long evening before I got the answer about the pregnancy test. I received a call at my office and the test result was positive. Hurrah! We celebrated!

Almost 2 months have passed. The initial shock is over and the pregnancy is becoming more of a reality. Morning sickness reminds me of how real all this is.

Figure 28: "I wanted so much to have a healthy child! During the doctor's visit, I was both excited, ecstatic, and nervous. Will my blood pressure be okay? Will they discover anything wrong with my baby? The doctor's visits always turned out to be reassuring and my thousands of questions and the calming answers from the nurse and doctor helped give me confidence until the next visit."

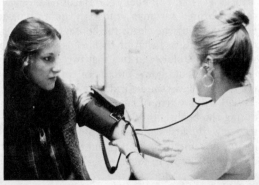

I look at myself in the mirror; I don't look different, though my waistline is expanding and I don't feel like eating a thing. I wonder if there really is life—a tiny little person growing inside me. It seems so unbelievable. We had a positive feeling about this baby, even before we got the test result. Now the high is slowing down and new thoughts and feelings cross my mind. I am pleased but worried about this new experience, childbearing. It is sometimes frightening to be innocent; fear of the unknown can be very difficult. I want to know and prepare myself as much as possible. Most of all, I want to be healthy so that my unborn "little one" will be healthy too.

I experience many ups and downs, not realizing yet that this is a temporary state of mind and that a pregnant woman is much more sensitive and emotional than she would be in the nonpregnant state. I decide I must find a healthy balance, mentally, physically, and spiritually, to be able to channel these feelings in a positive way, realizing as I do that so much affects the unborn. I am more aware and in touch with myself than I ever have been before in my life. I try to have a positive attitude, to be happy, to read and educate myself as much as possible, keeping physically fit, eating food that has natural nutrition and vitamins. I have become a nutrition expert through my pregnancy experience. It is good to know the way the unborn baby develops and the need it has for proper nutrition. Feeling good about myself is the most important responsibility I have, because my unborn is my responsibility. It is my responsibility to feel good.

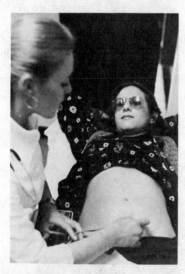

Figure 29: The Fetal Heart Rate: "Donna [the nurse] and I listened to the baby's heart rate with a Doptone, a special machine that can pick up the heartbeat early on. It was then that I realized I was pregnant; that I was really carrying a life inside me. I felt so good afterward."

Still, there are days where I feel terrible, unable to deal with my increasing size and the body changes that are absolutely incredible to me. I have become a little more withdrawn, yet I still want comfort and affection from my family and friends—especially Jeff.

I am sure it is terribly difficult for a man to understand these emotional changes in an exciting, though extremely difficult time. Changes in my body weight contribute to irritability at times, but educating myself helps me deal with the anxieties that we are going through. Ours is a total involvement, com-

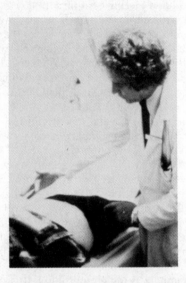

Figure 30: The Antenatal Visit:
"I always brought a long list of
questions with me for each visit.
It was important to me that I was
not rushed through the visit, but
had sufficient time to get everything explained: what was happening to me, and what I could
anticipate."

mitment, and responsibility. It is also a great feeling to know that the baby is
growing inside you. Everything is so important. I had trouble in the beginning
coping with these changes. I found myself always getting upset, feeling bloated,
nauseated until the third month. I often felt guilty when I felt I should be
happy. I'm pregnant and I should be radiant, but I often felt down, depressed,
sweaty and unattractive. There are days, however, when I look in the mirror and
feel good about myself—an inexplicable moment when everything is wonderful.

Now at the end of the fourth month I am experiencing the feeling of becom-

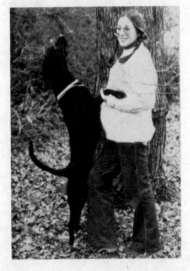

Figure 31: "When I felt alone or
sad, the best therapy was usually
long walks with Friday. Friday
seemed to know that something
was going on and I was naturally
worried that one day he would be
jealous of the baby. However, he
was such a great friend and gave
me so much comfort and happiness during the pregnancy."

ing heavier and slower. Having been so physically active up to now, playing paddle ball almost every day, I find myself hardly being able to go for a ball. Instead I take long walks in the forest or in the park with my dog Friday. We walk together and enjoy each other's company. It is almost as if Friday knows that something is happening. The dog knows that I am weak and need protection. He also seems to know there is something growing inside me that needs to be protected too. As I begin to grow bigger, I have to learn to rechannel my energy to fit my limited activity. Exercising is a good start to my day, but after a short period of exercise I am usually exhausted. I come back to the house tired. Then, after breakfast I feel the baby move. This new feeling of life inside me usually gives me energy. I began to plan, plan ahead for the baby. Many times I feel a special spurt of energy, the so-called nesting instinct. I feel I have so much energy that I can prepare the baby's room, clean everything, play with the dog and walk for miles. I feel I am able to do everything. Then, later that day or the next day it suddenly feels as if I have lost all my energy. The "high" disappears, I feel weak and tired. Sometimes I even experience crying spells. This up-and-down mood continues; however, as time goes on, I feel stronger as I feel the baby getting bigger.

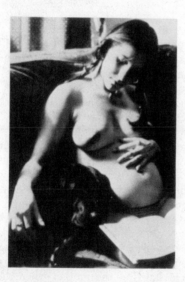

Figure 32: "I felt my abdomen growing. Some of the most wonderful moments were when I was relaxing with my hands on my abdomen and I could feel the baby move. Then I knew that the baby was really alive. Friday always understood my moods."

I really enjoy my body, looking at it changing. As I gain weight I watch my abdomen move sometimes as if my belly is like an ocean wave. I sometimes have to stop and catch myself smiling as I feel the baby's continuous movements inside me.

These last few weeks of the pregnancy are harder because the baby is large and is pressing against my stomach. I don't feel as well as I have before, but my doctor always brings back my confidence. I look forward to seeing him in the office. Each time I hear the baby's heartbeat I feel a new sense of strength—and this, together with the support of Jeff and my family, makes me feel as if I am sailing through this last part of the pregnancy.

When I finally went into labor, I was all ready. We had taken classes, so we were well prepared. It was a most wonderful experience—Jeff and I together in the hardest and most serious thing we have ever done. And we did it! We managed to have a beautiful natural birth. And when I look at my daughter Sara, I think back many times to what a wonderful pregnancy it was, although how difficult, how frustrating, and how frightening some moments were. Sara is so wonderful. She has such a pretty little face, she is so sweet, she hardly ever cries. But when I watch her I wonder, Will I really be a good mother? Will I be able to give her what she needs? But then Jeff comes to my support with his love and with his understanding and with his help. We feel we need to know that we all love one another and need one another—Sara, Jeff, and I.

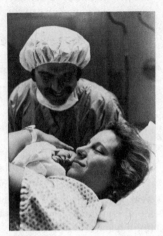

Figure 33

Ellen sent me this letter a week after the baby was born. It was a great pregnancy and the experience certainly changed her and Jeff's lives. Ellen's story, however, is no different from many other people's as they go through the conflicting emotions of pregnancy and learn to support one another.

☐ **Stress and Pregnancy**   There are differing theories about stress. One eminent psychiatrist, Helene Deutsch, believed that anxiety during pregnancy was desirable because it prepared a woman emotionally for the stresses of labor. In fact, she felt that childbirth classes that attempted to take away the fear of labor interfered with a woman's "important work of worrying." A celebrated contemporary authority on stress, Dr. Hans Selye, is another psychiatrist who believes that certain kinds of stress are beneficial. He points out that the complete avoidance of stress would destroy life itself by taking away the means by which humans pursue happiness and express their talents and energies. On the other hand, excessive stress at any time causes exhaustion, nervous breakdowns, and illness, and in pregnancy it can have a serious effect on the mother and the baby.

The deleterious effects of prenatal stress on infants is believed to come about through changes in the hormonal status of the mother when the hormones usually produced by stress, epinephrine and cortisone from the adrenal glands, and hormones produced by the pituitary gland, are released on signal from the brain. Studies on laboratory animals have discovered that pregnant animals exposed to excessive stress experience a decreased heart rate and a decrease in fetal blood pressure, since less oxygen is carried to the fetal brain.

When a pregnant woman is exposed to stress, her heart rate increases and the uterus begins to contract. This, of course, is also a trigger mechanism caused by the epinephrine and cortisone produced by the woman's adrenal glands. (Since the uterus is made up of muscles, it is directly responsive to hormonal changes.) Sometimes contractions of the uterus are so severe that a woman actually experiences pain. Since prolonged uterine contractions can deprive the baby of oxygen and affect the baby's growth, children exposed to severe prenatal stress are often smaller and have lower birth weights than normal children, and they may be psychologically disturbed in childhood. Stress may also affect sexuality: a link has been made between prenatal stress and menstrual irregularities in young women, and some researchers think there may be a connection between homosexuality and maternal stress (see Chap. 14). (Once again, we are talking about severe or prolonged stress of women who are chronically anxious.) And according to a recent study, women who are under excessive stress because they resent their pregnancies seem to experience a higher rate of miscarriage, accidents, and infections.

☐ *How Emotion Can Affect Pregnancy*   After studying eight thousand pregnant women in California, a group of researchers came to an important conclusion: a woman's emotional state does indeed affect her pregnancy. They found that women who dislike being pregnant have a significantly higher rate of serious problems, including a higher risk of miscarriage and a higher death rate among newborns than women who welcome their pregnancies. In the group under study the death rate of fetuses among women who resented their pregnancy was twice as high as the rate among women who looked forward to having a child. Furthermore, the babies of women with negative attitudes toward pregnancy had about one and a half times more congenital abnormalities than the children of the control group. The California researchers felt that stress-related changes in the mothers' hormonal levels may have caused the congenital malformations and miscarriages among the fetuses of the unwanted pregnancies. It is to be hoped that fewer children are being born now under such difficult circumstances since the pregnancies took place between 1959 and 1967, before therapeutic abortions were widely available in the United States.

☐ *Danger Signals*   Certain physical and emotional danger signals are considered signs that a woman is rejecting her pregnancy and needs professional help. They are:

Excessive nausea and vomiting or nausea that persists beyond the fourth month.
Vague feelings of discomfort, especially in the stomach or genital area, that are medically inexplicable.
Lack of response to fetal movement.
Excessive fears, including an overwhelming feeling of physical vulnerability and fears about the baby.
Lack of the so-called nesting instinct during pregnancy: no attempt to prepare the baby's room or clothes or make arrangements for the homecoming of the newborn.
Prolonged periods of depression or unusually violent mood swings that are without rational explanation.
Excessive preoccupation with physical changes or a complete distaste for the pregnant body.
Obsession with food or unwillingness to put on weight.

☐ *If Professional Help Is Needed*   Do not hesitate to seek professional help if you feel you are under unusual stress. There are therapists or crisis groups that work regularly with pregnant women. Ask your obstetrician or the staff at the hospital to refer you to a source of help.

After investigating a number of causes of prenatal stress, researchers now believe that extreme or prolonged stress affects the mother's ability to carry the pregnancy successfully, and they link certain behavioral and physical abnormalities in children with the stress their mothers experienced before they were born. While psychologists also point out that many problems of infancy are reversible in later life, the new findings should encourage the medical profession to give the relief of stress as high a priority as the relief of the physical symptoms of pregnancy.

☐ *The Emotional Aspects of High-Risk Pregnancies*   A woman in a high-risk pregnancy is under unusual emotional as well as physical strain. Stress and fear, as well as resentment toward the baby, are commonly experienced in high-risk pregnancies, more so than in a physiologically normal pregnancy. This is hardly surprising. Emotions are more intense because there is a fear of losing the baby and because a high-risk pregnancy usually requires more medical care and therefore loss of working time, which may cause economical burdens as well. Very often a woman's activities are restricted or she is on a strict diet, and the resulting frustration is difficult to bear.

Sometimes parents have unnecessary fears. The normal fear of loss or a birth defect is magnified in a high-risk situation since couples are aware that "high-risk" implies abnormalities. Parents may firmly believe that their baby will be abnormal when the doctor has talked about only *possible* risks, and this of course leads to even more anxieties. Genetic counseling and testing are important in this situation because they provide a realistic assessment of the baby's health, and both the husband and wife should be in close touch with their obstetrician.

Many parents in these difficult months may feel resentment toward the baby and may be afraid to express their emotions out loud. Once again: It is important not to keep your emotions to yourself because this can lead to serious problems later on. Here a sympathetic obstetrician can be invaluable. Today, when many more doctors are specialists in high-risk pregnancies, there is far more professional understanding of the emotional factors involved.

☐ *Partnership and Pregnancy*   There is always the possibility of marital conflict during pregnancy. It is, after all, a time of dramatic change when both partners are naturally apprehensive about the future, and unexpected tensions can surface even in an otherwise tranquil marriage. One common problem is a breakdown in communication as one or the other partner becomes withdrawn and uncommunicative in the face of difficulties. This lack of contact just at the time that both partners need love and reassurance can lead to further tension, and tension in turn may lead to open conflict.

A difficulty faced by many expectant couples is that a man and a woman tend to adjust to pregnancy at different rates. In the first trimester the man is usually a few weeks behind his wife in coming to grips with the pregnancy, and he may find her mood swings mystifying or upsetting, especially if she is difficult to live with because she is not feeling well or is ambivalent about the pregnancy. Later on, the man must make his own adjustment to parenthood, when he in turn needs the support of his wife. As each month passes, different adjustments have to be made, and this can be hard.

Becoming a parent may indeed be more difficult for a man than a woman, because outside of his role as labor coach the expectant father still does not have a well defined role in a pregnancy. Once the initial excitement is over, many men don't know what to do or how they fit into the new family situation, even though a successful transition to fatherhood is just as important as the woman's transition to motherhood.

☐ *Emotional Conflicts of Fathers*   During the first few months a man often experiences conflicting emotions that he may be afraid to share with his partner because they make him seem less than a man. He may be nervous about taking on the added responsibilities that fatherhood implies. He may be afraid of losing his independence or be concerned about the additional financial pressure involved in raising a family. The prospect of becoming a father may make him very proud and at the same time bring back conflicting memories of his own childhood. Many men look back on their relationships with their fathers and are determined to be better fathers to *their* children. But sometimes it is difficult to feel like a father when the fetus is still a tiny, invisible organism, and many men feel irrelevant early on in a pregnancy because there is nothing for them to do. Since a woman is often moody or self-absorbed in the first trimester, she can contribute to her partner's feeling of rejection. Unfortunately this feeling of exclusion sometimes grows rather than lessens as pregnancy goes on. Sometimes his resentment at being excluded results in the man's running away from the pregnancy by taking on extra work, a compulsive hobby, unnecessary business trips, or, occasionally, an extramarital affair. A man can end up feeling unwanted and superfluous even if he began the pregnancy determined to involve himself fully along with his wife.

Financial worries can be another source of stress. The need for extra income to meet the expenses of the pregnancy sometimes forces the man to take on additional work, even though more women do plan on going back to their jobs after the birth. Consequently he has less time at home and the couple have less time together. Sometimes a man takes on this extra financial burden because he feels it is his duty to take care of his wife rather than review the financial situation with his partner's help. At the same time, worries about money can increase both partners' fear of being trapped by pregnancy. Loss of independence is a powerful fear, one that increases resentment toward the other partner.

☐ *The Couvade Syndrome*   Some men go through bizarre physical changes during their partners' pregnancies. As many as 60–70 percent of the men interviewed in one study complained of common pregnancy symptoms such as nausea, fatigue, backache, vomiting, and weight gain—symptoms that disappeared promptly once the baby was born. These physical responses to the emotional conflict of pregnancy are known as the *couvade syndrome,* from the French verb *couver,* which means "to brood or hatch." In certain other cultures men go through elaborate formalized rituals during pregnancy and childbirth. Men of the Kurtatchi tribe in the Pacific Islands go into complete seclusion when their wives are delivering children, and the Chaorati males of South America are expected to take to their hammocks and rest until several days after the delivery, waited on by their families. These are primitive but psychologically satisfying methods of including the male in the female process of labor and delivery. The unpleasant symptoms that males experience in our culture might be allayed if men had more acceptable ways of participating in their wives' pregnancies.

12

The Pregnancy and Your Daily Life

Being pregnant for the first time can be a somewhat daunting experience since everyone you talk to seems to have a different idea about what a pregnant woman should or should not do. The shrewdest course of action is not to listen to too many people's advice, although this can be difficult, because you are probably uncertain yourself about the safety of your normal activities. During pregnancy even the simplest decisions suddenly seem open to question, from a visit to the dentist to choosing a brand of toilet soap.

There are two things to bear in mind. First of all, pregnancy is a time to feel good, and second, it is a time to take proper care of yourself. The second consideration does not mean you can't live an active life. In most pregnancies women can expect to enjoy normal activities. It is important, though, to appreciate what is happening to your body and to watch for any signals that indicate something should be changed.

Pregnancy in Victorian times was often regarded as an illness. It is not, of course; quite the contrary, it may be the healthiest time of your life, because you are eating well and taking care of yourself. But there are still some precautions you should take, even though most pregnant women go to work, continue their routines at home, and enjoy themselves. It is, after all, a time in your life when you are making decisions that not only affect you and perhaps your partner but your unborn baby as well. You might be willing to take risks for yourself, but not for the baby.

I hope this chapter will give you some guidelines as to what is and what is not healthy during pregnancy and what you can or cannot do. Since women have so many questions about health care and their normal activities during pregnancy, the material here may not be sufficiently comprehensive for your particular needs. If you are ever in doubt about your activities, consult your doctor before going ahead with any plans, and if something goes wrong, see him immediately. Be a partner in your own health care at all times and especially during pregnancy.

☐ *Is a Holiday or a Business Trip Advisable During Pregnancy?*   You can certainly take a holiday or a business trip while you are pregnant, but traveling during pregnancy is not quite as easy as traveling at other times. To begin with, your tolerance of such normal travel hazards as motion sickness and cramped seating arrangements is different during pregnancy. Any long trips, especially abroad, need careful planning and the approval of your obstetrician. A woman whose pregnancy is abnormal in any way will not be safe or comfortable on an extended trip, especially in countries where the medical facilities are unfamiliar or inadequate.

The second trimester is usually considered the best time to take a holiday during pregnancy. In the first trimester you are adjusting to pregnancy and there is a slightly higher risk of miscarriage; in the third trimester the additional weight is a deterrent to sightseeing and there is the possibility of premature labor. If you must take a business trip, you can travel at any time during pregnancy up to the ninth month, providing your doctor feels it is safe for you to do so.

A few pregnant women should not travel at all. If you have a history of miscarriage, if you are expecting twins, if you have a serious complication, or if you are older, you need to be close to your obstetrician and hospital at all times. Another contraindication is a sudden attack of vaginal bleeding, however slight. Although vaginal bleeding does not necessarily indicate the onset of miscarriage, it does require a period of comparative rest.

There are certain precautions you should take whether you travel by road or by air. Try to plan your journey so you are not subjected to long, uncomfortable trips without a period of relaxation. Sitting in one position for a long period will impede the circulation in the legs and may result in the formation of blood clots. As a rough guide, plan a break of at least half an hour every two hours during a lengthy road trip, and take even more frequent breaks if the roads are rough. As far as any car or bus travel is concerned, the length of time you are forced to sit in a cramped position is a more important consideration than the number of miles you cover. On a plane, ask for an aisle seat, and get up at regular intervals and walk around. Move your feet up and down to increase the circulation in your feet and legs while you are in your seat.

Motion sickness can be a problem. Some women find they are more susceptible than usual, and the problem is increased because Dramamine and other motion-sickness drugs are not considered safe for use during pregnancy. If you are a very poor traveler, this may deter you from traveling altogether. However, pregnant women's tolerances vary greatly, and some women who normally suffer from motion sickness travel without discomfort when they are pregnant.

If you are traveling abroad you may need to take extra supplies, such as powdered milk and, of course, an adequate supply of prenatal vitamins. Pack any over-the-counter drugs and products, such as sun creams, from your own medicine cabinet—making sure to get the approval of your obstetrician. Don't buy any over-the-counter drugs abroad. Even in English-speaking countries, drug labeling can be inadequate or misleading. Food and drink are more of a problem than usual. Be particularly careful about following sanitary regulations in countries where the water supply is suspect; in the case of intestinal illness it may be difficult to get a doctor—and, of course, drug use should be avoided if possible.

Getting medical help in a foreign country can sometimes be difficult, especially if you do not understand the language. For a small fee you can obtain names of foreign doctors trained in English-speaking countries through an organization called the International Association for Medical Assistance to Travelers. Their address is: Suite 5620, Empire State Building, 350 Fifth Avenue, New York, N.Y. 10001. Your doctor can give you a letter stating your due date and any special considerations in case you do need medical assistance. It would also be a wise precaution to take out a special traveler's health-insurance policy if the country you are visiting does not have free medical services. If you are traveling inside the country and are planning to be away for several weeks, ask your obstetrician to supply you with a reference to a local doctor or hospital. This is particularly important if you are traveling during the last trimester.

In general, don't restrict yourself, but don't overdo things either. Many women travel during pregnancy and travel successfully, but there is always an added element of risk for a pregnant woman, and this has to be taken into consideration whenever you plan a holiday or schedule a business trip. You can protect yourself by taking intelligent precautions, but an unexpected emergency might still occur, although fortunately this is rare. Don't overtire yourself, don't expect to have the same energy as usual, and be sensible about exposing yourself to unnecessary hazards.

☐ *Airline Regulations*   Most international and domestic airlines permit a pregnant woman to fly without restriction up to the sixth month of pregnancy. After that point regulations differ according to the airline. Some airlines place no restrictions until the eighth month, when they require a letter from your obstetrician giving your due date and declaring your fitness for travel; and a few carriers will not allow a pregnant woman on board under any circumstances in the ninth month. Although pregnant women often go on board unchallenged, it is sensible to contact the airline in advance, because you may be turned away at the ticket counter without the proper clearance.

☐ *Is the Body Scanner at Airports Safe?*   Most people think flying is hazardous only when you actually leave the ground. However, aircraft personnel are being subjected daily to quite significant doses of radiation within the airport. Anyone who operates one of the electronic scanners used in routine body checks is receiving up to 50 millirems of radiation a month, or 500–600 millirems a year—approximately three times the normal amount received from background radiation. This could pose a decided hazard to the fetus, which is much more sensitive to radiation than the adult. The radiation hazard is of primary concern to people who work in close proximity to the machines. There should not be any particular danger in passing through the machine once or twice during a pregnancy; but if you are a frequent air traveler or an airline attendant, don't pass through the scanner. Any pregnant woman can ask for a body search instead of going automatically through the machine.

☐ *How Long Can I Go on Driving the Car?*   You can continue driving as long as your abdomen fits comfortably behind the wheel and you feel confident about driving. Driving requires extra care during pregnancy. You will probably find that your reflexes are slower and less accurate than usual. I would advise against driving once you become very large, because you don't have complete control over your body and if you have to brake rapidly, you might throw yourself and the baby against the steering wheel, with possibly fatal results.

Always break up a long car journey with frequent rest periods. A back pillow is useful in preventing fatigue. If you are a passenger, the best place to sit is in the back seat where you can have more room and the risk of injury is lessened. In the last half of pregnancy try lying halfway on your side during the car trip so the baby is in a comfortable position and is receiving enough oxygen during the trip.

Most roads in the United States are smooth enough to make driving safe for a pregnant woman. Do not plan a trip in which you are likely to be jostled or banged around. Excessively bumpy roads can result in the onset of premature labor through the displacement of the uterus, or in premature separation of the placenta, which often will lead to fetal death.

☐ *Seat Belts*   A pregnant woman should always wear a safety belt. The American Medical Association recommends the use of a seat belt as long as it is fastened under the abdomen and across the pelvis—not across the top of the abdomen. Use the shoulder harness as well. Correct placement is important, because in an accident or an emergency stop the belt may jar the abdomen so severely that the baby is injured or killed. The safest way to ride is in a back seat equipped with the shoulder type of safety belt.

A final warning: carbon monoxide exposure can be dangerous to you and the fetus. Carbon monoxide concentrations in large cities with a heavy volume of traffic now often reach as high as fifty parts per million, at which point there are alterations in mental, visual, and other functions for the mother and adverse effects to the fetus similar to those incurred by cigarette smoking (see Chap. 17). There have been several cases of acute carbon monoxide poisoning in the Los Angeles area involving people exposed to the fumes of nearby cars idling in a gas station.

☐ *Can I Play Tennis or Any Other Sport?*   Once again the answer is yes— and no. Many women who play tennis, jog, or swim as part of their normal routines find they don't need to give up sports immediately after they become pregnant. In fact, a sensible sports program is often valuable during pregnancy; exercise improves the cardiovascular system, encourages proper circulation and increased respiration, and builds muscle tone and physical stamina, which are great assets during pregnancy and in labor and delivery. Exercise also has psychological benefits—perhaps the most important to a pregnant woman is its ability to relieve tension. On the other hand, each woman is different and each pregnancy is different. Some women go on jogging or bicycling up until the seventh or eighth month, while in some pregnancies unavoidable or unexpected complications occur that make a sports program inadvisable. Advanced age, high blood pressure, severe back pain, episodes of bleeding, history of miscarriage, or cervical incompetence are some of the more common reasons for abstaining from sports at any time during pregnancy. In addition, "sports" does not mean contact sports. Contact sports in which you are jostled or pushed around involve unnecessary hazards to you and the baby and must be avoided.

The demands of each sport are different, and some are more suited to the pregnant woman than others. In general, sports that require tremendous speed and mobility (squash, for instance) are almost impossible to play beyond the first trimester, and some sports are hazardous, especially for the inexperienced. I would not advise even an experienced horseback rider or skier to continue once the reflexes slow down and increased weight shifts the balance of the body. A few sports are absolutely contraindicated during pregnancy. Water-skiing is inadvisable at any point because water could penetrate the cervix during a fall. For the same reason, avoid diving from a height of more than three feet throughout pregnancy. Sports you can enjoy safely include swimming, bicycle riding, bowling, tennis, and jogging in the first half of pregnancy. (The strain on your ligaments can become severe once you carry more weight.) But in every case consult your doctor before planning any active sports program. There may be some health problem you are not aware of.

Whenever you exercise during pregnancy you should always observe some simple precautions. "Exercise" does not mean a full training program. Even international athletes stop competing during pregnancy. While reasonable exercise is beneficial, really strenuous exercise can severely restrict the amount of oxygen reaching the fetus and result in impaired growth. At the same time, unless you are in superb physical condition to begin with, a full training program during pregnancy will put an unnecessary strain on your own body. The physical functions are already working harder to keep up with the extra demands of pregnancy itself, and eventually the extra weight will slow you down and reduce your stamina and agility. You would be wise to slow down gradually as pregnancy advances, and give up exercise altogether if you begin to feel uncomfortable. Whenever you exercise during pregnancy you must always be aware of your body and slow down when your body tells you. Many women who are avid joggers or tennis players find walking, swimming, or a simple exercise routine more beneficial in the last trimester than a four-mile run or a full game of tennis.

Pregnancy is a time to have fun rather than win competitions. Don't be unrealistic about your body's capacity to take strain or stress successfully. Whatever you play or do to keep fit, take regular "time outs," don't exercise when weather conditions are hazardous, especially during excessive heat, and *stop* immediately if you become tired or stressed. The latter is particularly important, because it will take you longer than usual to recover from any form of strenuous exercise. Whatever you play or do, do only to the extent of your physical capacity, even if it means limiting your overhead strokes in tennis or your golf swing; and reduce the risk of falls by avoiding overcompetitive situations in which you may lose your coordination. Remember, your reflexes are not as swift and your balance not as sure as usual. During pregnancy the health and well-being of the baby outweigh the value and enjoyment of sports.

☐ *What Should I Do if I Don't Go in for Sports?* With the current emphasis on a healthy, active pregnancy, many pregnant women feel they should do something to keep fit. Sometimes this can lead to problems. If you don't normally play tennis or jog two miles a day, pregnancy is not the time to start. You will only strain your muscles or become overtired or simply frustrated, because any kind of physical exercise during pregnancy requires more effort and skill than at any other time. Concentrate instead on a daily routine of simple physical exercises designed to increase your strength and flexibility, and walk as much as possible. Walking is healthy exercise; it does not overtax the body unless you set unrealistic goals for yourself, and brisk walking promotes good circulation and deep breathing. Be sure to walk in comfortable clothes and sturdy, low-heeled shoes. Remember, even a modest exercise program may be difficult to achieve in the last trimester. Some women find the joints in the pelvic region become so loose that it is difficult to walk at all in the last month or two.

Moving around the house or the yard is exercise in itself. Correct standing, walking, reaching up, and bending down are all exercises, or what Elisabeth Bing, the famous Lamaze teacher, calls "nonexercises." In her book *Moving Through Pregnancy** Dr. Bing describes a number of these nonexercises—normal activities such as walking upstairs, carrying home groceries, watering the plants, and lifting a small child out of the bathtub. For instance, she suggests the following way to strengthen the abdominal muscles. Standing at the kitchen sink, round the lower back slightly, straighten it, and tuck in the buttocks at the same time, to hold the baby with the abdominal muscles, then relax the abdominal muscles and go through the same sequence again. Dr. Bing points out the advantages of moving around the house normally during pregnancy because reaching up, squatting down, and walking are all valuable forms of exercise that can be done without setting aside a special period for exercise routines.

Of course there is a right and a wrong way to perform any normal activity or household chore during pregnancy. Changes in balance and weight affect sitting, standing, walking, and lifting, especially in the last trimester. A later section in this chapter will teach you how to achieve proper posture, relaxation, and breathing.

☐ **Is It Safe to Go to the Dentist?**   Yes, it is, as long as you don't undertake dental work that requires full anesthetic or multiple X-rays. It is, in fact, important to keep your teeth in good condition during pregnancy because the sensitivity of the mouth changes under the influence of progesterone. Changes in the soft tissue of the mouth can lead to a gum condition called *pregnancy gingivitis*, which is so common that it affects at least half of all pregnant women.

In general, though, pregnancy is a favorable time for your teeth because you are eating well and taking extra calcium. Furthermore, pregnancy is a time a woman becomes seriously interested in taking care of herself, and this includes attention to dental as well as medical care. It is also time to retire some persistent myths. In the past, people believed a pregnant woman's teeth became brittle because the unborn child absorbed calcium directly from his mother. This is the origin of the old saying "Every child costs a tooth." But we now know that tooth loss occurs only when a woman's store of calcium is seriously depleted by a subsistence diet or repeated pregnancies.

See your dentist in the first trimester and ask him to clean your teeth and inspect your gums. After that he may require a repeat visit or visits if gum problems persist or grow worse. Cavities can also be attended to during pregnancy, but, ideally, treatment should be undertaken after the first trimester if you re-

---

* Elisabeth Bing. *Moving Through Pregnancy*. New York: Bantam Books, 1980.

quire a local anesthetic. And at whatever point you see your dentist, first be sure to tell him you are pregnant before he begins any dental work or takes routine X-rays. Drugs and X-rays can harm the fetus at several stages of development. Finally, try to put off any elective dental work until after delivery. Even minor dental procedures can put you under extra stress at this time, and major work usually involves prolonged anesthetics, X-rays, and pain-killing drugs, all of which are undesirable during pregnancy.

☐ *Pregnancy Gingivitis and Other Gum Conditions*   Pregnancy gingivitis is an inflammation of the gums surrounding the teeth and is characterized by swollen, bleeding gums. When oral hygiene is poor, the condition can become aggravated, and you may require more frequent checkups and plaque removal than usual during pregnancy. Since gingivitis can begin as early as the second month, try to arrange for a checkup and cleaning as soon as you know you are pregnant. Once your teeth and gums are thoroughly cleaned, use dental floss as well as regular brushings to keep the mouth as free of plaque as possible. If you notice bleeding or swollen gums after your initial treatment, go back to your dentist and have the affected areas cleaned out. The condition usually grows worse as pregnancy progresses and may linger on for a few months after the baby is born. Fortunately it is not permanent, and gingivitis disappears promptly once hormone activity returns to the nonpregnant level.

Occasionally a rare gum disorder called pregnancy tumor affects a localized area of the mouth, usually the gum area between the upper front teeth, or on the tongue, cheek, lip, or roof of the mouth. Despite its alarming name, a pregnancy tumor is nonmalignant and more of a nuisance than a danger. If the growth is large or annoying, it can be surgically removed; otherwise it usually disappears spontaneously in the postpartum period.

Sometimes the teeth become increasingly mobile during pregnancy. This is normal. Even if you do not have gingivitis, the soft tissues of the mouth respond to the altered hormonal levels of pregnancy, and the color and texture of the gums change slightly. The changes in the gums are temporary, and your teeth will become firm again after your pregnancy is over.

☐ *Dental X-Rays and Drugs*   Although the amount of X-ray exposure in a dentist's office is rather small, *don't* permit dental X-rays to be taken routinely. Particularly during the first trimester, X-rays should be restricted to localized areas of the mouth. If an X-ray is required, the dentist or dental assistant must safeguard you and the fetus by limiting the beam size, using an electric timer, and *shielding your abdomen with a lead apron* to prevent secondary radiation hitting this sensitive area.

Treatment involving local anesthetics should ideally be carried out in the second trimester. Although the safety of novocaine has not been seriously questioned, it seems sensible to avoid its use in the first trimester, unless dental work is urgently needed. Even small amounts of lidocaine, a local anesthetic commonly used by dentists, are known to cross the placenta and could, theoretically, affect the fetus. In the last trimester any dental work involving drugs should be kept to a minimum because of the (very small) chance of a dental procedure irritating the uterus and precipitating premature labor. Do not permit your dentist to give you nitrous oxide at any point during pregnancy. Although some dentists will tell you it is safe as long as it is administered with oxygen, it has been frequently linked to an increased rate of miscarriage.

The risks of a general anesthetic during pregnancy are discussed later in this book (see Chap. 27). In the case of a dental emergency, you should discuss the pros and cons of anesthetics with both your dentist and your obstetrician.

If you need pain relief before or after dental treatment, an occasional Tylenol is considered safe. Prescription pain-relief products pose a problem because they have not been adequately tested on pregnant women. A consultation with your obstetrician as well as your dentist is advisable before you take a pain-killer of any kind. Since antibiotics are frequently prescribed to control oral infections during pregnancy, be sure to read the section on antibiotics in the chapter on drugs in pregnancy. Avoid the use of tetracycline, which can lead to permanent staining of the baby's teeth, and streptomycin, which can result in deafness in the newborn.

☐ *Can You Be Vaccinated?*   Vaccination with live vaccines, such as those for rubella, measles, mumps, and tropical diseases such as smallpox and yellow fever, should not be given during pregnancy. All vaccinations of this type should be given *at least three months before conception.* (See Chapter 2 for more information on vaccinations before conception.)

Certain other vaccinations can be given with comparative safety if their use is indicated. The flu vaccine (inactivated type A and type B virus vaccine) is often recommended for pregnant women who have heart disease, bronchial problems, diabetes, or some other chronic complaint that puts them in a high-risk category. Doctors do not like to give a flu shot routinely during pregnancy, and your need for vaccination should be discussed individually with your obstetrician.

Certain other vaccines are given under special circumstances, including epidemics, unavoidable foreign travel, and household exposures. If you have been exposed to hepatitis A strain, for example, you should ask your doctor for the immune serum globulin shot to protect you and the fetus. A polio shot would be given to an unprotected woman in the case of an epidemic or personal exposure to the disease even though a routine shot is normally considered inadvisable.

Note: Most adults have received a diphtheria/tetanus immunization at some point but may not have had a booster shot for some years. If you have not received a combined tetanus/diphtheria booster within the previous ten years, your doctor may advise you to get one before pregnancy. You should not receive a shot during pregnancy except if it is really needed. Tetanus in particular is fatal in at least 60 percent of all reported cases.

☐ *What to Do in Case of a Fall or Accident*   First, try to find out whether you have sustained any injury yourself. Are you in pain? Are you bleeding? Are your movements restricted? If you can answer these three questions in the negative, you are probably uninjured, but if there is any doubt, see a doctor at once. Next, turn your attention to the pregnancy. If there is no vaginal bleeding and the fetus continues to move, you can presume that the pregnancy is unaffected. If you are too early on in pregnancy to have experienced fetal movements, the only criterion is vaginal bleeding. Fortunately the fetus is so perfectly protected by the amniotic fluid and the natural shock absorbers built into the uterus that it is very rare for even a direct blow to the uterus to disturb the fetus or the position of the placenta. If there is vaginal bleeding, you should, of course, get in touch with your physician at once. If you can't detect fetal movements, don't panic; wait an hour or two, and if they have not resumed, call your doctor.

If you have a serious car accident or a fall, you could do some damage to the placenta that will not show itself immediately. In some cases there can be internal bleeding or bleeding into the amniotic fluid, which won't produce severe symptoms immediately but can within a day or two result in fatal injury to the fetus. After any serious accident, call your doctor and arrange for an immediate ultrasonography. If you have to go to the emergency room, insist on seeing an obstetrician as well as the regular emergency room personnel. Be checked carefully before you leave the hospital, and be sure the doctor listens to the fetus' heartbeat. You should not consent to any X-ray unless the doctor feels it is absolutely necessary. You could even check with your obstetrician before you permit the X-rays to be taken.

☐ *What About Any X-Rays in Pregnancy?*   X-rays should not be taken routinely during pregnancy *unless* the mother requires the X-ray to safeguard her own health. Even at the comparatively low level used in diagnostic procedures, there are unacceptable risks to the fetus. The most dangerous X-rays are abdominal, pelvic, and lumbar X-rays, which expose the fetus to the direct beam of the X-ray unit. The amount of radiation is increased when the procedure involves continuing exposure through the use of a fluoroscope. (The fluoroscope shows the interior of the body in continuous motion rather than in one single exposure.) X-rays that fall into this category should *never* be taken during pregnancy unless there is a life-threatening emergency for the mother. Direct exposure of the fetus has been linked to growth retardation and possibly intelligence loss, a higher incidence of childhood leukemia, and menstrual and reproductive disorders among young women. Even though the amount of radiation in the average pelvic X-ray is small—about 2 rads—it is still believed to increase a child's chance of developing leukemia by one to one and a half times.

The most sensitive period is the first six weeks, when embryonic development is proceeding swiftly. At this point radiation above 10 rads (well above that used in the normal X-ray) can cause a miscarriage; or a chromosomal aberration can result, even at a lower rad dosage. This makes it very important to follow the American Association of Radiologists "ten-day rule": *If you are trying to conceive or suspect you have conceived, do not schedule any X-ray of the pelvic, lumbar, or abdominal area any later than during the ten days immediately following the onset of your last menstrual period.* (Chapter 2 includes a fuller discussion of the effects of X-rays before conception.)

Other X-ray procedures, those that do not expose the fetus to a direct beam, are reasonably safe as long as the abdomen is fully shielded from any scattering of radiation, the technician is properly trained, and up-to-date equipment is used to minimize the exposure. The head, limbs, chest, and neck can all be X-rayed without exposing the fetus directly. But your doctor or dentist would be exposing you and the baby to unacceptable risks if he insisted on any X-ray without proper indication. Don't hesitate to question his judgment if a situation arises in which an X-ray of any kind is involved. If you need to visit an emergency room at any point during pregnancy, tell the nurse you are pregnant, and refuse any

X-ray that seems unnecessary. Emergency rooms often take X-rays "just in case."

X-ray pelvimetry, which involves the irradiation of the fetus, is another area of dilemma. This procedure will be discussed further in the chapter on labor and delivery.

☐ *Is It All Right to Move to a New Home During Pregnancy?*   Try, if possible, to avoid moving to another home when you are pregnant. Moving is physically strenuous and also causes anxiety. What so often happens is that a couple suddenly decides their home is too small or the neighborhood is unsuitable for a young child, and they begin looking frantically for another house. House- or apartment-hunting is in itself a strenuous and time-consuming activity. Once you find a place, there is the pressure of the move itself and the organization of your home. All of this may be too much strain for both of you. I would advise you to stay in your present place—unless it is completely unsuitable—at least until the baby is born. When the baby is a few months old, you can weigh your need for space and other factors more calmly.

If you must move, the second trimester is usually the best time for the move itself. By the third trimester you will be too heavy to manage successfully. Don't try to do too much yourself, and get someone else to lift heavy furniture or boxes. Too much lifting and moving around can lead to high blood pressure, swelling of the ankles, and possibly protein in the urine. For the same reason, avoid heavy housework until after the baby is born.

☐ *Can You Redecorate or Have the House Painted?*   During pregnancy you will find you are more susceptible than usual to paint fumes because your respiration rate is greater and your lungs take in more oxygen. Toxic fumes may also cross the placenta and affect fetal development or the fetal circulatory and respiratory systems. This applies not only to paints, especially lead-based paints, but to other chemicals used in redecorating, including polyurethane, turpentine, and paint strippers. Redecorating involving chemical substances should ideally be done several months before you conceive—or after delivery, providing that the baby is adequately protected from any toxic fumes. If your partner or a professional crew is painting or using chemicals, make sure the house is well ventilated, and avoid areas of the house where work is going on.

☐ *Personal Hygiene*

Bathing Many women, especially when they are pregnant, prefer bathing to showering. They feel it relaxes and cleanses them better. If you observe a few precautions, you can go on taking a daily bath at least until the end of the second trimester, and possibly right up to delivery.

One reason women feel nervous about taking baths is the fear of water penetrating the cervix and entering the uterine cavity. This is very unlikely to happen in the first two trimesters unless water is literally forced up the vagina by some extraordinary means such as douching. Contrary to popular belief, the vagina is a space that is collapsed and closed rather than an open hole, and for the first two trimesters it is usually impenetrable to fluid. Until the third trimester you can take a bath safely as long as the bath water is fairly cool and you do not use harsh detergent soap. If an irritant enters the vagina, there is a slight chance that it could irritate the cervix. In the last three months it is safer to switch to a daily shower, since the cervix may begin to open and bathwater might penetrate the vagina, possibly leading to irritation and premature rupture of the fetal membranes. In a normal pregnancy the risk is small, but it should be taken into consideration.

Be careful as pregnancy advances. As the baby grows larger, your balance is affected. Put a nonslip mat in the bath or the shower *and* on the bathroom floor to prevent falls as you get in or out of the tub or shower. A fall at this point could be serious. Once you become very heavy it may be easier to take a shower rather than clamber awkwardly in and out of a tub, unless a member of your family is available to steady you.

An Important Note: Never take a bath once the membranes have ruptured. At this point the amniotic fluid has ceased to protect the baby and the vagina could become a source of serious infection.

☐ *Hot Tubs or Jacuzzis*   Normally the fetus is surrounded by the amniotic fluid, which acts as a natural buffer and keeps the fetus' body at the correct temperature. Experiments with monkeys and observations of human pregnancies have confirmed that when the temperature of the amniotic fluid rises beyond a certain level, the heat can trigger labor. This sometimes occurs when a woman suddenly develops a high fever as the result of a urinary-tract infection during pregnancy. The unusually high temperature of the water in a hot tub can also result in the same syndrome. Moreover, according to a new California study, a temperature of over 102 degrees Fahrenheit in the first trimester may cause congenital defects in the fetus. Among the group of women in the study who either suffered from a virus infection or used a hot tub in the first trimester, a significant number gave birth to babies with congenital defects.

☐ *Douching and Pregnancy*   Avoid douching during pregnancy. Douching with any solution, even lukewarm water or a vinegar-and-water solution, can be dangerous, because if the cervix is open, the force of the water may penetrate through the cervix and enter the fetal membranes. Any irritation of the thin fetal membranes can disrupt their normal protective mechanism and perhaps lead to an irritation that triggers labor; or the fetal membranes may be ruptured and a miscarriage or premature labor may result. Instead of douching, you can keep the vaginal area clean by inserting one or two fingers to rinse the outer portion of the vagina. Don't use a soap or detergent, to avoid irritating the vagina.

Warning: Douching with a chemical solution during pregnancy is particularly dangerous. There is a possibility that the douching solution may enter into the circulatory system, pass over the placenta, and cause a congenital defect. Some douching solutions contain phenylmercuric acetate (PMA), a mercury compound. Prenatal exposure to mercury can result in severe fetal abnormalities. While not all douches contain mercury, few chemical douche solutions have been tested for safe use during pregnancy, and none of them can be considered advisable. Therefore, *don't douche!*

☐ *Skin Care*   When you are pregnant, your body temperature is one degree higher than normal, and you will find yourself perspiring more than usual. Increased perspiration is one of the ways in which the body copes with the disposal of waste materials. Take a daily bath or shower to remove perspiration and relieve the skin of the excess wastes that may tend to clog the enlarged pores. Since the skin is particularly sensitive during pregnancy, use a mild toilet soap, and make sure to dry the skin thoroughly after you have bathed, finishing off, if you like, with a dusting powder or lotion to prevent dryness, possibly mixed with vitamin E cream to avoid stretch marks.

As your weight increases, the skin on the body is more susceptible to cracking, friction, and heat rashes. You can relieve dryness effectively by using a lotion or oil on the abdomen, thighs, and other affected areas. If a rash appears, it is usually the result of chafing from clothes or from the lower abdomen rubbing against the pubic area and can be treated by frequent baths or a change of clothing. Do not use special skin creams without consulting your doctor first. Some over-the-counter skin products contain cortisone, and steroids such as cortisone are not considered safe for use during pregnancy.

Skin coloring changes as pregnancy progresses. In the beginning many women, especially brunettes, notice a distinct facial pallor, and sometimes dark circles appear under the eyes. Later on in pregnancy the increased circulation of the blood brings more color than usual to the face, and you may have a distinctly flushed look. Facial skin texture also changes. Usually it becomes drier, but occasionally the overactivity of the sebaceous glands produces a skin condition resembling acne. You can help control any blackheads or pimples by washing your face regularly and applying a mild astringent lotion to the affected areas.

☐ *Breast Care*   The breasts require special care. In the second and third trimesters the skin is overstretched and sensitive, and as the breasts grow larger, there is a natural leakage of colostrum from the nipples. Sponge the nipple area daily with cotton wool dipped in water and soap suds, and dry the nipples thoroughly. This will prevent the excess colostrum from drying and irritating the delicate tissues surrounding the nipples. If the tissues do become cracked, you can use ointment or vitamin E lotion to keep them moist.

☐ *Hair*   Hormonal changes affect the hair as well as the skin. Some women find that their hair becomes oilier, some notice that pregnancy has a drying effect. In either case you can safely alter your normal routine to accommodate the changes in your hair. Shampoos and most other hair products are safe to use during pregnancy; the one notable exception is hair dyes. Many hair dyes contain substances that are suspected carcinogens, and since they are absorbed through the skin, they could, theoretically, cross the placenta and adversely affect the fetus. Although a link has not been proven between childhood cancer and hair dyes, their use is not recommended for pregnant women.

☐ *Clothes*   The clothes you wear during pregnancy will reflect your individual taste, finances, and way of life. From a doctor's point of view, it doesn't matter what you wear as long as you are comfortable, although there are psychological benefits to looking attractive. The way a woman dresses often reflects her general attitude to health care. A woman who can't be bothered to dress decently and take care of her appearance is usually careless about far more important things than clothes, and this includes her own health and the health of the baby.

Clothes to avoid are tight dresses and pants, girdles, panties, and brassieres that inhibit the proper circulation of the blood and make you feel hot and uncomfortable. Remember, you are not only larger, your temperature is higher during pregnancy, and you are more susceptible to heat rashes and other irritations caused by tight clothing. The increase in your temperature should also be borne in mind when you look at summer- and winter-weight clothing, since you will feel warmer and perspire more, especially in the last few months.

Loose dresses are probably more comfortable than suits or pants, although you may not feel like wearing dresses if you have to use heavy support hose throughout pregnancy. The best maternity dresses and shirts fit closely on the shoulder and hang loosely around the abdomen. Slimmer women can usually continue to wear pants, but remember to buy proper maternity slacks that have a stretch panel in the front to avoid pressure against the abdomen. Don't wear a belt beyond the fourth month. It will restrict the blood supply to the baby and put an uncomfortable strain on your abdomen.

What you wear underneath your dress or slacks should be as comfortable as the dress itself. For a first baby you shouldn't need to wear a girdle unless your doctor recommends one. If you are experiencing backaches you may find a maternity girdle useful in giving additional support, but this is not usually necessary until a second or third pregnancy. Don't try to wear a normal girdle. It will not give sufficient support and will constrict your abdomen.

A good supporting bra is important for appearance and posture as your breasts grow heavier. Make sure that the cup is large enough and the underarm is cut high enough to cover all the breast tissues. Wide shoulder straps will give you the most comfort and support. If you are planning to breast-feed, you can buy a nursing bra before delivery. These usually have a front clasp to facilitate nursing, and adjustable eyes in the back, making it easier to achieve a proper fit as your breasts grow larger. If at all possible, have an experienced salesperson help you choose your bra and girdle; you should have the best possible fit and support.

Many pregnant women find normal underpants uncomfortable during pregnancy because the elastic around the waist is constricting. In this case buy the bikini-type panties in which the elastic fits under your abdomen.

Even doctors appreciate how much maternity clothes have changed in the last few years. Now that it is once again fashionable to be pregnant, there seems to be a variety of light, comfortable, and colorful maternity clothes that women enjoy wearing. They need not be expensive. There are all kinds of discount maternity stores, resale shops, and mail-order catalogs. And friends are usually generous about lending maternity clothes.

□ *What Kind of Shoes Should I Wear?* Shoes that fit you properly are a great asset during pregnancy. Once you grow heavier, it is harder to keep your posture and your normal balance, because the back tends to compensate for the extra weight in front by tipping backward. Well fitting shoes will help balance your weight and may prevent leg pain, backache, and fatigue. By the second trimester, change to low- or medium-heeled shoes and choose those that offer proper support (moccasins and sneakers are not recommended, because they don't support the feet sufficiently). You can test the suitability of a pair of shoes by placing the shoe on a firm surface, such as a table or the floor, and pressing your thumb down on the part of the shoe that comes under your arch. A shoe that gives under pressure is not worth buying.

Don't wear high heels routinely, especially toward the end of pregnancy. Very high or very slender heels can be dangerous in the last trimester, because they may cause you to lose your balance or slip and fall. For the same reasons, buy or use a pair of boots with nonslip heels and soles for protection in wet weather or snow. Inside the house it is better to go without shoes altogether if you have comfortable rugs and nonslip floors. Walking without shoes reduces tension in your feet and helps eliminate foot and leg cramps. Try to change your shoes several times during the day. Your feet tend to perspire more during pregnancy, and you are more likely to develop a fungal infection as a result.

□   *Posture*   When you are pregnant, the normal balance between the muscles of your abdomen and lower back is altered. Instead of counterbalancing each other, the increased weight of the abdomen tilts the pelvis forward, and the back is suddenly arched into a larger, hollow curve (see Fig. 27). This places unaccustomed strain on the back muscles, particularly those in the lower back, and produces the backaches so many women experience during the later months of pregnancy. Although some strain is unavoidable, attention to the way you stand and walk—even to the way you relax—will help ease the worst of the discomfort.

□   *Sitting*   Sit evenly on both buttocks and make sure your back is supported fully by the back of the chair or sofa. Wherever possible, sit with your feet and legs elevated to promote proper circulation and retard the development of varicose veins. *Do not cross your legs* when sitting. It could obstruct the circulation, cause blood clots, and promote varicose veins.

□   *Standing*   Standing correctly will ease the strain on your back and legs. Keep your feet parallel and be sure to place an equal amount of weight on both feet. Keep the knees straight and the legs spread slightly apart. Then tighten the abdominal wall, pull it in and up, and tuck in your buttocks. Let your arms hang naturally down your sides and be sure your head is kept erect on your shoulders. When you walk during pregnancy, move your left leg forward if you are right-handed and vice versa if you are left-handed. This will enable you to shift the weight from foot to foot and turn your body without difficulty.

□   *Lifting*   The best way to lift an object is to keep your back straight and bend down slowly with your knees bent. Then put your hands underneath the object and lift it up as you gradually straighten your back. Never bend down from the waist; this will put a tremendous strain on your back and abdomen and may lead to problems later on. An alternative method is to lower yourself to the floor, put one foot forward, and lower yourself to the other knee. Then draw the object toward you and lift it by using the front foot as a lifting device and the rear foot as a balance. As you get up, try using the thigh muscles to avoid straining the lower back.

Note: Heavy lifting should be avoided during pregnancy.

☐ *Reaching*   Opening a lower desk drawer or file cabinet can be difficult in the last trimester. Again, never bend from the waist. Lower yourself to a squatting position, and keep the knees and feet well apart to balance yourself and reduce tension on the abdomen. Rise carefully, using the thigh rather than the back muscles.

☐ *Sleeping*   Lying on your back is the most comfortable position in early pregnancy. This position is also safe. You may, however, find it helpful to have a pillow or folded blanket under your legs to keep the knees flexed. Let your legs and arms relax and roll outward. This will prevent tension from building in the legs, hands, and feet.

As pregnancy advances, the sleeping position changes. At this point it is important for you to lie on your side rather than on your back, to take the weight of the uterus off the large abdominal aorta and the vena cava. When the uterus rests against the vena cava, insufficient blood is returned to your heart, and the fetal circulation will decrease, resulting in a drop in blood pressure, which in turn will decrease blood and oxygen to the baby. This could be dangerous. The syndrome, which is called supine hypotension, can be prevented by simply lying on your side, preferably on your left side. Place one pillow under your head, one under your shoulder, and one between your legs, with your right arm and leg behind you, and your left arm and leg in front.

When you are getting out of bed, roll to one side, draw up your knees, and turn your shoulder and hip at the same time. Follow this procedure whenever you change positions. Before standing up, sit on the edge of the bed for a short while to allow your blood pressure to adjust itself before you start to move around.

☐ *Relaxation Position*   Learning to relax completely is important during pregnancy and especially during delivery. You can practice relaxation when you come home from work or after an exercise period. The normal sleeping position can be used for relaxation in early pregnancy, or you may prefer to lie flat on the floor in the classic yoga *suvasana* position, with arms and legs apart and relaxed. Later on, move into the side-lying position described above.

If you are in the office, there is a way to rest without lying down. Sit back in your chair, relax your back, let the head fall slightly forward, allow the knees and arms to relax completely, with the feet spread apart, and breathe deeply. This is an effective way to counteract lunchtime fatigue.

☐ *To Relieve Muscle Tension at Home or at Work*   Change positions frequently. Sitting in one position or standing still for long periods of time places unnecessary strain on the body and promotes problems such as varicose veins and leg cramps. Always shift the weight from one foot to the other if you are forced to stand, and move the feet in a circular motion when you are sitting down, to increase the circulation. If you are working around the house, don't involve yourself in any one physical activity for too long. Moving from a squatting to an upright position or stretching up occasionally will help reduce fatigue and relieve muscle tension.

☐ *To Relieve Backache*   Sit on a hard chair with your buttocks firmly placed on the front of the chair and lean back, with your hands placed at the back of the seat. Hollow your back slightly and then round your back as much as you can. This can be done standing up and lying down as well. Another effective way to relieve back tension is to practice the *pelvic rock*, the prenatal exercise designed to strengthen the abdominal muscles in preparation for the second stage of labor (see below). Carol Dilfer, a fitness expert and author of *Your Baby, Your Body** suggests an exercise she calls the "lower back stretch." Lie on your back, bend your knees, and put your feet flat on the floor. Then clasp the fingers of both hands around your right (or left) knee and gently pull your knee toward your chest. Hold this for a slow count of five and release. Do the lower back stretch with alternating legs and both legs together. In each case let the buttocks and lower back come off the floor as you pull your knees toward you.

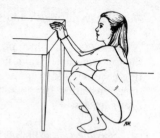

Figure 34: *The Squat Exercise:* This is an excellent exercise to strengthen the legs and to learn correct lifting. Stand next to a table with your heels flat on the floor and feet slightly apart. Slowly lower yourself to a squatting position as you exhale through the lips. Remain in the squatting position for a few seconds; breathe in through the nose, and slowly resume the upright position with your back remaining straight. Repeat this ten to twenty times daily. Remember: use the leg muscles for lifting rather than the back muscles to mitigate the stress on the back and abdomen.

☐ *Exercise Routines for the Pregnant Woman* ▬ Pregnancy tests certain areas of a woman's body more stringently than at any other time of her life. The muscles in the pelvic-floor area, the abdomen, and the backbone are all required to lift and support the unusual weight of the baby and the other contents of the abdominal cavity. If the muscles in these areas are poorly toned, stress will result, and you will experience backache, abdominal discomfort, and possibly hemorrhoidal and urinary problems as well. Toning of the abdominal and pelvic-floor muscles is also important because these are muscles you will be relying on to help you push the baby out in the second stage of labor.

Any one of the different prenatal exercise programs you may encounter will involve the strengthening of the back, abdomen, and pelvis. A good exercise program will also help you relax and increase your flexibility and fitness. Because there are so many different programs in different parts of the country, it is impossible to advise you specifically on any particular regimen. However, I would suggest at least an exploratory visit to a prenatal exercise class even if you exercise regularly in some other way. Regular sports activities do not necessarily strengthen the muscles required in pregnancy and delivery. You should, of

---

* Crown Publishers, 1977.

CAT STRETCH

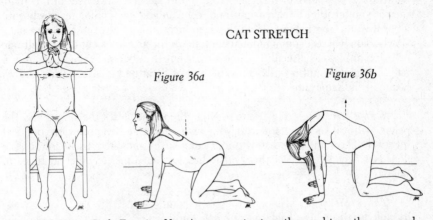

Figure 36a

Figure 36b

Figure 35: Upper Body Exercise: Here is one way to strengthen and tone the arms and alleviate tension. Sit on a chair with your legs together. Extend both elbows out to the side and keep the palms together. Press the palms tightly together. This exercise is good for strengthening the arms, especially the hard-to-firm upper muscles in the upper arms near the armpits, and the upper chest muscles. It also alleviates tension in the back and the upper arms. This exercise should be repeated several times daily. It could easily be performed at work.   *Figure 36: Cat Stretch: 36a:* Kneel with your knees and your palms flat on the floor. Your legs and arms should be comfortably apart, and your body weight equally distributed between your hands and knees. Make sure your arms and legs are like posts forming right angles at the shoulders and hip joints and supporting your body at the four corners. Begin the exercise by inhaling. Curve your back. Then raise your head and allow your back to relax into a hollow.   *Figure 36b:* Exhale as you drop your head between your arms and push your back up toward the ceiling. As you tighten the abdominal muscles you should continue to exhale deeply through the mouth. Then inhale again as you relax your abdominal muscles and lift your head. Repeat this exercise ten to twenty times daily. This exercise is called the *Cat Stretch* because an angry cat often puts itself in this position.

course, inform your doctor first before you plan to take a course of prenatal exercises.

An Important Note: Don't try to work beyond your capacity in a class or while exercising on your own. Exercises should not be carried out to the point of muscle tension or fatigue. Begin with a simple warm-up before going on to the more demanding exercises, and don't expect to perform every exercise perfectly or for an extended period the first time you try it. Take a few minutes' rest at the end of each class or exercise period to practice deep relaxation and prevent fatigue. Finally, if any unexpected complication such as severe abdominal pain or bleeding should occur, stop exercising immediately and call your doctor.

☐ *Deep Breathing*   Learning to relax through deep breathing is valuable at any time of your life. It increases your lung capacity and strengthens the abdominal area. This deep breathing exercise should be practiced throughout pregnancy until it becomes the natural way for you to breathe at all times. Lie down on your back and bend your knees, keeping the feet flat on the floor. Put your hands on your stomach (this will enable you to feel the movement of the abdomen as you breathe). Inhale deeply and feel your abdomen filling up slowly with air as if you were a balloon. Hold the deep breath for a few counts. Then exhale slowly. You will feel your abdomen contract as the air passes out of it. Continue exhaling until you sense all the stale air has left the abdomen, the chest, and finally the mouth and nostrils. This method of breathing is invigorating and relaxing at the same time.

☐ *Tailor Stretch*   This exercise strengthens and flexes the thighs and the pelvic area. Sit on the floor with your knees apart and the soles of your feet together. Then put your hands under your knees and press them toward the floor (see Fig. 37). Repeat this *gently* three or four times at different times of the day.

☐ *Tailor Sitting*   Tailor sitting is a comfortable way to relieve back pressure and limber the pelvic area. Sit on the floor and bring your left foot toward you. Then bring the right foot back toward the left foot, without crossing the ankles. Round your back and bend forward slowly until your knees touch the floor. Slowly sit up straight. You can sit in the tailor position whenever your schedule permits—another good example of a nonexercise.

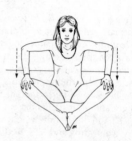

☐ *Pelvic Rock*   Lie on the floor with your knees bent and your feet apart. Your feet should be as close to your body as you can comfortably get them. Keeping buttocks and shoulders pressed to the floor, breathe deeply and arch the back slightly so it is lifted from the floor. Then exhale slowly and press the back against the floor, pulling in the muscles of the abdomen at the same time. Repeat several times. This exercises the pelvic region and helps eliminate the

Figure 37: The Tailor Stretch: Sit on the floor in the tailor position with your knees apart and the soles of your feet together. Put your hands on your knees. As you lift your legs upward, push your arms downward to help tighten your pelvic muscles. Repeat this exercise several times daily.

extra strain on the back muscles. Once again, you can do this exercise safely at different times during the day (see *Figure 38*).

☐ *Stretch Exercises*   The arms, shoulders, and upper torso are all areas where you tend to become tense, especially if you sit at a desk for long periods. Relax and strengthen your arms and upper body by the following exercises:
  1. *Tailor reach:* Use the tailor sitting position and reach both arms above the head. Using first one arm and then the other, stretch up as far as you can from the shoulder and waist to relieve tension on each side of the upper body.
  2. *Side stretching:* Still using the tailor position, place one hand on your abdomen or knee and raise the other arm above your head. Stretch down gently toward the opposite side and hold the position, bouncing gently, for a few seconds. Repeat several times, using each arm. A similar exercise can also be done

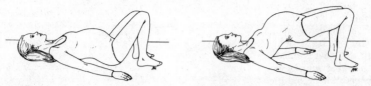

Figure 38a: Lie on the floor with your knees bent and your feet slightly apart. Breathe in and out slowly. As you exhale, press your back against the floor, pulling in the muscles of the abdomen.   *Figure 38b:* Inhale deeply as you raise your buttocks as high as possible and arch your back until it leaves the floor, still keeping your arms and neck flat on the floor. When you feel the full stretch of this position, exhale again as you lower your body and resume the first position with your back pressed against the floor. Repeat this exercise ten to twenty times daily.

standing up, with both arms following the alignment of the body. This is a useful way to firm the muscles of the waistline and upper arms.

□ *Leg Lifting*   Lie flat on your back with your arms by your sides. Stretch one leg, point the toe upward, and slowly lift the leg into the air as you inhale through the nose and mouth. (Lift the leg only as far as you can without straining.) Then flex the foot and slowly lower the leg. Repeat, using the other leg (see *Figure 42*).

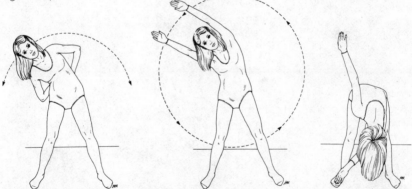

Figure 39: Side Stretching: Place your feet parallel, slightly more than hip distance apart. Put your hands on your back and continue to face forward. Keep your feet firmly in one position. Then lean as far as you can to the left and then to the right. Repeat ten to twenty times.   *Figure 40: Side Stretching:* Remain in the same position as in Figure 39, with your feet apart, but raising your arms above your body. Then rotate your arms and hands in a circular movement, bending at the waist and moving your arms out in front of your body. Repeat this circular arm swinging ten to twenty times.   *Figure 41: Side Stretching:* Stand on the floor and place your feet parallel and somewhat more than hip distance apart. Stand erect with your arms extended to the side. Keep your knees straight, then touch your left toe with your right hand. Return to the original position with your arms apart, then bend down and touch your right toe with your left hand, and return to the original position. Repeat this side-stretching exercise ten to twenty times.

Figure 42: Leg Lifting: Lie flat on the floor or on a mattress on your back with your arms by your side. As you inhale through your nose, raise one leg straight up with your toes pointed. Make sure that your leg is completely straight and the toes are pointed upward. Then slowly flex the foot and lower the leg. Perform the same exercise with the other leg. Repeat the exercise ten to twenty times.

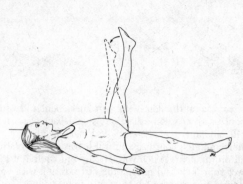

☐ **Feeling Fine**   Try to find a proper balance during pregnancy. Don't overtax yourself. When you are pregnant it is very important to be aware of your body and not exercise beyond your capacity to do so. If something doesn't feel right or seems troublesome, stop the exercise and rest.

13

Sex During Pregnancy

Pregnancy is a time when the special relationship between a couple is very important, a time when there is a new emotional closeness, and for some a sense of heightened sexuality. A couple no longer fears an unwanted pregnancy nor is there pressure to become pregnant. This means that pregnancy is potentially a time when a woman is free to enjoy a good sexual relationship with her mate. I would like to be able to say that sexual relations during pregnancy are always this satisfying. Unfortunately there are emotional and other factors that sometimes make the sexual relationship less than perfect. This chapter will discuss the pros and cons of sex during pregnancy, obviously not to cause fear and worry but to give the expectant couple enough information to make decisions and communicate knowledgeably with their obstetrician.

Possibly no issue is more controversial than the safety and advisability of sexual relations throughout a pregnancy. Nothing would please an obstetrician more than to report that sexual intercourse is always perfectly safe for the expectant couple. Unfortunately some research has suggested that this might not be so (although other researchers have shown no contraindication to normal sexual relationships in a low-risk pregnancy). These conflicting findings often confuse and worry expectant couples. I hope my discussion of sexuality during a normal pregnancy will reassure you and your sexual partner.

☐ *Sexual Response During Pregnancy*   According to Masters and Johnson, the pregnant woman experiences the basic sexual response cycle commonly known to the nonpregnant woman, although with certain notable differences. The female sexual response cycle, as defined by Masters and Johnson, begins with an excitement phase, moves on into a second, or plateau, phase, reaches a brief orgasmic phase, in which the vasocongestion accumulated in the previous two phases is released, and resolves itself in the last, or resolution, phase. There is a difference between the pregnant and nonpregnant experience in each of the four different stages of sexual response. When the nonpregnant woman enters the excitement phase, a rush of blood reaches the sexual organs, the vagina expands to make way for the erect penis, and the breasts enlarge slightly and the nipples become erect. But in the pregnant woman there is natural congestion in the pelvic area at all times, and an increased lubrication from the end of the first trimester is not unusual even without external sexual arousal. (This is more pronounced in multiparous women—those who have given birth at least once.) By the third trimester the whole genital area is often so swollen that any added swelling or lubrication from sexual excitement is almost undetectable by the woman or her sexual partner. This is the reason that a pregnant woman, although she is easily aroused, may have difficulty reaching orgasm.

Breast response, which is a normal part of the arousal stage, may not be as pleasurable as usual during the first trimester of pregnancy, because the breasts are enlarged and tender, and a rush of blood during sexual arousal often causes increased tenderness or even pain, particularly in the nipples and the areolar area. Breast sensitivity gradually decreases as pregnancy progresses. The change is more obvious in the nulliparous woman (one who is bearing her first baby) than in the multiparous woman.

In the second phase of sexual response, the plateau phase, the external sexual organs become completely engorged and the vagina lengthens and narrows. Vasocongestion develops in the outer third of the vagina as localized blood in the walls of the vagina increases tension and enables the vaginal walls to close and tighten around the penis, creating what is known as the orgasmic platform. Once a woman is pregnant the blood supply reaching the vagina increases to such an extent that the vaginal walls meet at the midline, a phenomenon that is more pronounced as pregnancy advances. Vaginal engorgement causes the vagina sometimes to feel too constricted to contain the penis comfortably, but this may also increase the sexual pleasure of both partners.

In the final resolution phase the body gradually returns to its preorgasmic condition as the blood leaves the external sexual organs and the pelvic area. Here the pregnant woman may well experience an unusually prolonged state of sexual tension, since it can take as long as fifteen to thirty minutes for the blood to drain from the pelvic organs. A heightened state of physical tension in the sexual organs persists despite the achievement of a satisfactory orgasm. This is the phenomenon that is probably responsible for the unusual and enjoyable level of sexual tension experienced by many pregnant women, who may become multiorgasmic in the second and third trimesters. Continued sexual tension can also be frustrating, since full release often takes so long to achieve, and is the reason that certain women feel unsatisfied even if they have actually reached orgasm. Again, this is an experience unique to pregnancy.

☐ *Does Sexual Desire Increase or Decrease During Pregnancy?*   Patterns of sexual responsiveness during pregnancy are often said to follow a well defined timetable: (1) *first trimester*, a decreased desire for sexual relations; (2) *second trimester*, a considerable rise in sexual interest; and (3) *third trimester*, a gradual but decided decline, which continues up until the time of delivery. This in general was the pattern observed by Masters and Johnson under laboratory conditions.

They found considerable fluctuation from woman to woman in the first trimester, when some women rejected all forms of sexual activity and a few reported a significant increase in libido.

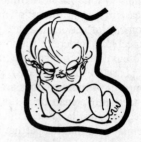

AW, LAY OFF, MOM...IT'S SUNDAY!

Figure 43: Reproduced by permission from Lester Freidman, Monogram of California, San Francisco, California.

Other researchers have made contradictory findings or discovered variations on the Masters and Johnson pattern. According to the majority of these research findings, a large number of women seem to experience a steady decline in sexual interest from the time pregnancy is confirmed up to the time of delivery, although certain women do report higher levels of sexual enjoyment in the second trimester and the beginning of the third, which in a few instances continue until term. The decline in sexual interest is most obvious in the last two months of pregnancy, when couples who normally have frequent sexual relations stop having sex or have intercourse only infrequently. The woman's interest in sex seems to decline as her partner's interest declines, a pattern that contradicts the notion that a man is always ready for sex, whatever the circumstances (see below).

Unusual elevations and depressions in sexual response are entirely normal during pregnancy, and no woman should be surprised or concerned if her responses fall well below or well above her normal levels. Decreased desire is natural, especially during the first trimester, when nausea and fatigue often interfere with sexual pleasure. You may also be afraid of injuring the fetus or be deterred by a previous first trimester miscarriage. Other women simply find their enjoyment decreases naturally as they become heavy and uncomfortable from the beginning of the third trimester on. On the other hand, many pregnant women notice a heightened state of arousal, more noticeably perhaps in the second trimester but not infrequently in the first and third trimesters as well. This can be attributed to the changes in the body that heighten sexual tension and increase orgasmic capacity, as well as to the general feeling of pleasure that many women feel in pregnancy, especially in the middle months. Women who have been nonorgasmic before pregnancy may well experience a first orgasm during pregnancy, while others become multiorgasmic for the first time.

These findings would suggest that a pattern of sexual behavior can be established, but that individual experience varies more than has been believed. Your own responsiveness would obviously depend greatly on your physical health, your relationship prior to pregnancy, even the hormonal variations you experience from week to week. How you feel at any one time is usually less important than sharing your feelings with your partner and continuing the sexual behavior you still find enjoyable.

☐ *Do Men's Sexual Feelings Change During Pregnancy?*   The pregnant woman is not the only sexual partner who experiences considerable changes in sexual response. A man can expect to go through a number of transitions—periods when he is far more anxious than usual to have sex with his wife, followed by times when he too experiences a diminished sex drive. None of these variations

186/   Childbirth with Love

seems to follow a neat trimester-by-trimester pattern, although the general decrease in sexual interest at the end of pregnancy is reported by men as well as
women, for reasons that are probably complementary. A man's feelings can be
expected to undergo variations that he should not be surprised by or ashamed of.
His emotions are inevitably influenced by his adjustments to the pregnancy, his
response to his partner's physical condition, and his partner's feelings about
him. All of these feelings are highly individual.

Certainly a man need not be afraid of losing his sex drive when his wife is
pregnant, just because some men do report a loss of libido. Quite the contrary,
he may find that his partner's heightened responsiveness makes sexual relations
more pleasurable during her pregnancy than at any other time.

□ *Do Husbands Have Affairs When Their Wives Are Pregnant?*   Most
couples report some decrease in sexual relations during pregnancy, particularly
toward the end of pregnancy. This has given rise to countless stories about a
husband's extramarital affairs when his wife is pregnant. In reality, a man is
more likely to fantasize about approaching other women than actually start an
affair, although Masters and Johnson did report some extramarital affairs among
their research population.

□ *Sexual Positions During Pregnancy*   In the first trimester the uterus is
small and well protected and intercourse can take place in any position that gives
pleasure to the couple. Then in the second trimester the uterus expands up
within the pelvic bones and moves freely beneath the abdomen, where it can be
felt above the pelvic bones. At this point the missionary position, with the man
resting on the uterus with his full weight, usually becomes uncomfortable, and
sexual intercourse is more pleasurable with the couple lying on their sides in a
face-to-face or face-to-back position. The side-lying position has another advantage: the man cannot penetrate as deeply, and there is less risk therefore of the
penis injuring or stimulating the sensitive cervix. A rear-entry position also
allows the man to be close to his partner and fondle her breasts at the same time.
(As she becomes heavier, the woman might be more comfortable with a pillow
under her thighs.) Standing and kneeling positions are favored for the same reasons, since the man's weight during these forms of lovemaking does not rest
directly against the baby.

Some women prefer the superior position, because they have more freedom to
move and they feel in control of the sexual friction needed to achieve an orgasm.
This is not a position for women with short vaginas, since there is a greater
chance of the man's penis hurting or overstimulating the uterus, particularly if
the woman is moving vigorously.

Whatever position is used, it should be one best suited to the couple, a position in which both partners feel pleasure without causing harm to the developing fetus. With care and gentleness, there is no reason that sexual intercourse
could not continue enjoyably until close to term. In the eighth or ninth month,
couples often find intercourse cumbersome and turn to other forms of sexual expression until after the birth. This does not mean the end of the sexual relationship, which can, after all, take many satisfying forms among sympathetic
couples.

☐ *Touching*   A loving relationship between expectant couples can be greatly enhanced by touching and stroking. This is pleasurable for the couple and of positive benefit to the unborn child, since touching rids both partners of tension and stress, loosens the woman's abdominal muscles, and increases the flow of blood to the uterus.

Physical closeness and sensuous touching can be as important as sexual intercourse in cementing a relationship, and they can replace intercourse at those times during pregnancy when the woman is not feeling well or is not allowed to have intercourse. Such intimacy can be important to a couple during the changes their lives undergo in a pregnancy, when the normal sexual relationship is inevitably altered, physically and emotionally.

☐ *Vaginal Discharge*   The amount of normal vaginal discharge increases during pregnancy because the cervix is protected by continuous mucus secretions that help form a barrier against infection. This, together with the other changes in the internal balance of the body, increases the likelihood of vaginal infection. While a simple vaginal infection is not harmful, it may well decrease your sexual pleasure if you and your partner normally enjoy oral genital sex. This increased vaginal discharge is, of course, only temporary and will not continue to influence sexual relations in the postpartum period. If you experience any annoying discharge, report it to your doctor. He can evaluate and treat the condition appropriately.

☐ *Why Is Intercourse During Pregnancy Sometimes Uncomfortable?*   Some women who normally experience no discomfort during intercourse complain of unexpected discomfort when they are pregnant. The cervix is sensitive, and deep penetration can lead to pain or even occasional spotting. A simple change in position or more gentle intercourse will usually solve the problem. If it does not, you should talk to your obstetrician. On the other hand, there are women who find that the increased lubrication in the vagina makes intercourse easier and more pleasurable than usual.

☐ *Will Sex Harm the Baby?*   Men who find it difficult to have normal sexual relations with their pregnant wives are often consciously or unconsciously afraid of harming the baby. These fears are usually groundless in the normal pregnancy. The baby is well protected by the amniotic sac and the mucus plug—at least up until the eighth month of pregnancy, when extra caution may be in order. Understandably, it is not always easy for each partner to comprehend all the changes that occur during a pregnancy, but it is important for a man to know that he will not harm the baby or the pregnant woman by making love to her.

But it is not only men who are afraid that intercourse will injure the fetus. Although women are generally more confident than their partners, a number of women whose pregnancies are not in any way high-risk stop having intercourse either in the first trimester or once the pregnancy becomes visible, because of the fear of trauma. Often this fear is based on nothing more substantial than conversations with friends or a cultural tradition. If you are aware of fears of this kind, even though your pregnancy is low-risk, try to discuss them with your partner, and make sure to talk to your obstetrician. All you may need is reassurance. It is important for each partner to deal with his or her fears rationally, because a long period without normal sexual relations can affect a marriage long beyond the duration of the pregnancy itself, and some marriages are permanently damaged. If you jointly decide to forgo intercourse for a few months, then at least you will have made the decision together, and you can look forward to normal relations after the birth.

☐ *Are There Times When a Couple Should Not Have Intercourse?* Intercourse is not advisable if a woman is experiencing bleeding or shows signs of premature labor or has a previous history of these conditions. It is definitely contraindicated when the fetal membranes have been ruptured. This occasionally happens when a couple is having intercourse and the cervix is ripe for labor. If you experience a sudden gush of water from the vagina during intercourse, or at any other time, call your doctor immediately and refrain from any further intercourse. Penetration could theoretically introduce an infection into the unprotected cervix. Otherwise, you can continue to enjoy normal sexual relations up to the last month before delivery as long as there is no complicating high-risk factor. Shallow penetration is advisable toward the end of pregnancy, because the vagina becomes more sensitive and the ripened cervix is softer and more susceptible to pressure from the penis.

An Important Note: Air blown into the vagina during oral sexual relationships may be pleasurable for some women, but it is exceedingly dangerous. The pressure can form an airtight seal, trapping the air and causing a fatal air embolism. The practice is potentially fatal for any woman, pregnant or not, but the venous channels are open wider during pregnancy, making it a greater hazard then than usual.

☐ *What About the High-Risk Pregnancy?* Any woman with a high-risk pregnancy or any woman who has had previous difficulties with bleeding and other problems at the beginning of pregnancy, or who has lost several babies in the past, should refrain from sex for at least a part of the current pregnancy. A woman with a history of prolonged infertility who has finally conceived must also have a different outlook on sexual intercourse from that of a low-risk woman, because in her case too sexual intercourse might indeed stimulate the uterus to contract more, leading to miscarriage or premature birth. Even if there is no bleeding or other abnormality in the current pregnancy, a pregnancy complicated by a past history of problems is more fragile than others. With this or any other high-risk pregnancy, sexual intercourse should be continued only with the permission of the couple's obstetrician. This includes pregnancies complicated by incompetent cervix, uterine abnormalities, fibroid tumors, previous preterm births, placenta previa, or multiple births.

☐ *Safety of Intercourse During Pregnancy Questioned* Most couples continue to have intercourse without any apparent influence on the pregnancy, and most stories about the harmful effects of sexual relations on pregnancy are wildly exaggerated or unfounded. Unfortunately, however, the safety of intercourse throughout a low-risk pregnancy is still a controversial issue. The following information is provided not to give rise to fear or hesitancy about sexual relations during pregnancy but rather to encourage enlightened decision-making and intelligent communication between partners.

In one influential study of more than 26,000 women who gave birth in Philadelphia, intercourse during pregnancy was described as less safe than doctors once presumed. The study concluded that infections of the amniotic fluid were more common among women who had intercourse one or more times a week in the month before delivery than among women who abstained from intercourse during that time. In addition, the researchers found that newborns whose mothers had had intercourse in the month before delivery were far more likely to die as the result of an amniotic-fluid infection than other babies with similar infections whose mothers had not had sexual relations in that time. According to the study, the problem was even more serious when intercourse occurred in the month before a premature birth, probably because infection-fighting substances in the fluid become more potent as pregnancy progresses. If bacteria enter the sac comparatively early in the pregnancy, an infection is more likely to develop at this early stage than it would at term. At the same time, the fetus is more vulnerable to infection because of its immaturity.

Additionally, the study found a sharp increase in amniotic-fluid infections after the thirty-eighth week, when the cervix starts to efface and dilate, exposing the fetal membranes to semen and the bacterial flora of the vagina and cervix. This would suggest that the normal decrease in sexual relations at the end of a pregnancy is nature's way of protecting the infant.

The new idea that intercourse in late pregnancy is harmful has been challenged by a number of researchers, including one group from Israel who found no data to connect a higher risk of prematurity with intercourse. In their hospital, preterm delivery was no more frequent among those having intercourse than among those abstaining, and newborns whose mothers had had intercourse in the month before birth had the same rate of infection as other babies. The second group of findings clearly adds to the confusion, since two well conducted research studies have drawn exactly contrary conclusions. (This is one of the reasons why doctors and childbirth educators often give different advice.) To resolve this dilemma yourself, you must understand that each pregnancy is different and each couple needs to listen to advice from health professionals, but in the end each couple must make their own decision.

My recommendation in a low-risk pregnancy is that a woman without difficulties can enjoy sensitive, gentle lovemaking up through the eighth month of pregnancy. Beyond that point intercourse is not always advisable, since the fetal membranes might be exposed and an infection or premature labor could be spread or triggered by the penile thrusts. Women with bleeding or other disturbing signs should discuss their situations individually with their obstetrician.

☐ *Is Orgasm Harmful to the Fetus?*   As pregnancy progresses, pronounced uterine contractions often accompany orgasm. These differ from the normal uterine contractions observed in nonpregnant women during orgasm, because the gravid uterus is highly sensitive in the last trimester, and a series of contractions will cause it to harden and tighten into a prolonged muscle spasm. Occasionally these spasms are prolonged enough to cause pain or alarm.

How these contractions affect the pregnancy is a matter of dispute. Some researchers believe the uterine contractions produced by orgasm are strong enough to gradually efface and dilate the cervix and bring on labor at term or prematurely. Others feel a link between premature labor and orgasm is unproven, at least in the low-risk pregnancy.

Women who might be asked to refrain from orgasm, particularly after the twentieth week of pregnancy, are those whose previous pregnancy ended in premature labor or whose current pregnancy is complicated by spotting, threatened prematurity, or placenta previa. Strong contractions induced by intercourse might be sufficient to irritate the sensitive uterus into premature labor. Self-stimulated orgasm achieved by masturbation is more powerful than that achieved through vaginal intercourse, so masturbation should also be eliminated in the high-risk pregnancy.

Fear of miscarriage in the first trimester is often enough to deter a woman from achieving orgasm. If abstinence is based only on old wives' tales, a couple can be reassured and a normal sexual relationship encouraged. Among couples with a past history of early first trimester miscarriage, it may be desirable to refrain from orgasm for a few weeks until the sensitive period is over.

☐ *Prostaglandins and Premature Labor*   The semen contains prostaglandin, first discovered during artificial insemination and so called because it was thought to be secreted by the prostate gland. This is one of the hormones that both triggers the onset of menstruation and induces labor. The prostaglandins are definitely known to have uterus-contracting effects, although a full understanding of the relationship between intercourse and the onset of labor is only theorized. One belief is that intercourse induces labor because the prostaglandin content in the sperm signals the uterus to begin labor. Another, less creditable, belief is that labor results when semen is swallowed by a pregnant woman close to term. Neither of these observations has been scientifically proven, but certainly prostaglandin hormones, either in pills or in suppositories, are used successfully to induce labor and abortion, confirming some relationship between prostaglandins and the inception of labor.

☐ *Does Sexual Intercourse Stimulate Labor?*   A connection has been posited between intercourse and the beginning of labor. Penile stimulation of the uterus is thought to release prostaglandins and cause labor contractions. The sperm also contain prostaglandins, which could possibly stimulate contractions of the uterus, leading subsequently to labor. Finally, there is the risk I have already cited of the penis introducing an infection into the vagina, which could damage the fetal membranes and stimulate the reflex mechanism that causes labor to begin. There is, therefore, a possible link between intercourse and premature labor even in the low-risk pregnancy, but intercourse is more likely to stimulate labor in a postterm pregnancy, in which the labor mechanism is already ripe.

☐ *Can You Talk to Your Obstetrician About Sex?*   In the past, many pregnant women never discussed the subject of sex during pregnancy with their obstetricians. It was something that simply wasn't done. The only mention of the subject was likely to be the obstetrician's automatic prohibition of intercourse for two six-week periods, one before and one after the birth, for reasons that were not discussed with the patient or her husband. There was no attempt to recognize the nature of a woman's sexuality during pregnancy or to prepare a woman for the changes in feeling she and her partner were likely to experience.

In certain respects the current attitude among obstetricians is not very much different from what it was twenty years ago. There is a natural embarrassment associated with the subject even now that makes it a difficult topic for discussion in the obstetrician's office. But at least the modern obstetrician is less likely to lay down rigid rules for his patients and more likely to treat each pregnancy individually. Increased openness about sexual matters and recent research on the role of sex in pregnancy have also had their effect, and more obstetricians are prepared to answer questions, even though it may be the couple's responsibility to initiate the discussion. It is still true, though, that the topic of sexual relations is usually confined to the aspect of safety.

With the contradictory evidence on the safety of sexual relations in a normal pregnancy, it may be difficult for the obstetrician to advise his patients with confidence. But he can still share his up-to-date information on the safety of intercourse with you and encourage you to discuss your feelings with him. Today obstetricians generally feel that sexual activity can continue safely through eight months of a healthy pregnancy, although whether or not it can continue safely in the ninth month is still questionable. Most doctors appreciate the importance of continued sexual activity to a couple's relationship and are reluctant to discourage intercourse unless its safety is clearly doubtful.

☐ *Caring—The Most Important Sexual Expression*   There is probably no time in a woman's life when she is more in need of emotional support than during pregnancy. Physically, and therefore sexually, a pregnant woman often feels vulnerable and not particularly attractive, even though there are times in pregnancy when the sexual relationship is unusually satisfying. Preconceived ideas of sexual attractiveness sometimes make it difficult for a woman and her partner to accept the physical changes of pregnancy easily. A few women feel more sensual during pregnancy than at other times, but most women seem to vacillate between increased sexual enjoyment at certain moments and a lack of desire at others. A man can do much to reassure his partner in difficult times by kissing, touching, and other affectionate behavior. Caring is such an important part of a couple's relationship during pregnancy that, whether a couple has intercourse or not, I cannot encourage a husband enough to share the enjoyment of pregnancy with her and to do everything he can to make her feel happy, desired, and loved.

14

The Emotional Life of the Unborn Child

Some fascinating research has begun to expand our understanding of prenatal life and the prenatal development of personality. This is a new area of developmental research, one that received very little attention in the United States until a few years ago, even though Europeans have been investigating the prenatal development of personality for several decades.

Although most of the research is new, the idea that a child's personality is shaped in the womb is a very old one. The Chinese, for instance, believe a child has already passed through nine months of existence by the time it emerges at birth. Ancient peoples were certain a catastrophic event during pregnancy marked the unborn child for life and tried to protect the mother from painful prenatal experiences.

The idea that the mother's impressions affect the child persisted right up to Victorian times, when conscientious mothers-to-be went to concerts or visited art exhibitions to encourage their children's appreciation of "finer things." (This is not so fanciful as it might seem; a number of eminent musicians have attributed their musical tastes to the compositions they heard prenatally.) These traditional beliefs were ignored by scientists and psychiatrists, who assumed that the human newborn was a helpless, malleable being whose unformed personality was shaped solely by the environment after birth. In fact, Freud thought a child's personality did not begin to develop until he was two or three years old.

Slowly this view of personality development has begun to change, in part because we have a better appreciation of the newborn's amazing physical capabilities. Far from being helpless, the newborn has well developed sight, hearing, and sucking reflexes. Immediately after birth a baby will respond to his parents' voices and faces. In the first few hours the baby also reveals distinct behavioral characteristics that are quite individual; two newborns side by side in a nursery rarely display similar levels of activity or go through the same sleeping/waking cycle. Sometimes a child's temperament is distinctive from the moment of birth. I have delivered babies who remain calm and quiet despite the activity and bright lights in the delivery room, while others cry and squirm around so furiously that the slippery vernix makes it difficult to hold on to them.

What produces these distinct personality differences in newborns? How does the prenatal environment shape our personalities? What is our relationship with our parents before birth? These are fascinating questions, which the new studies of prenatal development are attempting to answer or at least explore. By focusing on the prenatal as well as the natal period, such research is gradually altering our perception of the unborn child and his relationship with his environment in the womb. One important result of the research—of particular concern to parents—is evidence that a stressful or neglectful pregnancy can affect the baby's emotional as well as physical development and perhaps jeopardize a child's growth and behavior later in life.

These new studies of fetal behavior, which include research on the interaction of the mother and her baby before birth, have led to the foundation of several new disciplines, including fetal psychology, behavioral embryology, and a research area called behavioral teratology, which deals with behavioral abnormalities caused by an adverse prenatal environment. In most cases the pioneering studies were done in Europe (including the USSR), Australia, and Canada. The interest in this subject is now so great that an increasing amount of research will probably be carried out in the next decade. Continued research, both on animals and humans, will further help us appreciate the importance of viewing the unborn as needing the same love and emotional support we give the newborn baby.

☐ **Life in the Womb**   Babies can hear, respond to sounds, and discriminate between light and darkness several months before they are born. Although the womb is a dark, warm place that protects the baby from temperature fluctuations or bright light, it is not completely shut off from the outside world. Vibrations and sounds reach the unborn baby through the few inches of skin and amniotic fluid that keeps the baby safe inside the mother's abdomen. The unborn child responds with increased movement or a quickening of the fetal heart rate. As the mother's pregnancy advances, the baby is increasingly aware of external stimuli and responds to them more vigorously.

Spontaneous movements of the limbs and head begin early in pregnancy. By the twentieth week of gestation a sophisticated brain and nervous system exist that continue to mature as the time of delivery grows closer. A five-month-old

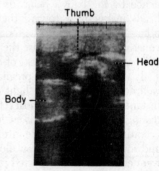

Figure 44: Ultrasonography of a fetus inside the uterus. Note the head at the right upper corner of the picture and the baby's body to the left. The fetus is sucking its thumb in a relaxed fashion, apparently enjoying its intrauterine environment.

fetus is already highly active; it can turn its whole body, kick its legs, move its arms, squint and display other facial expressions, suck its thumb, occasionally even hiccup. From the sixth month on there is evidence that the unborn child not only senses but responds to external sensations in a remarkably discriminating way.

Hearing is probably the most developed of the unborn baby's senses—which is not surprising when we consider the amount of noise going on within the womb itself, including the sound of the mother's heartbeat and the constant rumbling of her stomach. A baby in the last trimester also hears loud external noises and perhaps softer ones as well. Mothers have been aware of this for centuries, because a sudden loud noise will startle the baby into a spasm of violent kicking and body movements. (The fetal heartbeat also increases when the baby is startled or excited.) In the 1920s one German doctor who had several concert-going patients was fascinated by their inability to sit through a concert because their babies' increased activity was so painful. At the time this was a mystery. Fifty years later a New Zealand researcher, Dr. Albert Liley, discovered exactly why these music lovers had been made uncomfortable. According to his experiments, a twenty-five-week-old fetus becomes so excited by the beat of a drum that it literally jumps up and down inside the womb.

Unborn babies not only respond to music, they respond differently to different kinds of music. In one experiment in which researchers played the works of several composers, the babies became extremely agitated when they heard works by Brahms and Beethoven. Vivaldi or Mozart, on the other hand, had a delightfully soothing effect, while rock music excited the babies to the point of frenzy.

Voices appear to reach the baby too, particularly its parents' voices. One prenatal researcher believes that the unborn baby not only hears the mother's voice quite clearly from the twenty-fourth week on but responds to it by moving in rhythm. The idea that the baby recognizes its parents prenatally is given credence by the baby's behavior after birth. Newborns are known to turn their heads instinctively toward their mothers' voice, even when there are several other people talking in the room. Sometimes a baby can distinguish the father's voice as well. In either case the familiar voice appears to soothe and reassure the newborn, even to the point of causing it to cease crying.

By the sixth month of pregnancy other fetal senses, including sight, are fairly well developed. A bright light directed at the mother's abdomen will cause an instantaneous reaction; most fetuses move away as if startled by it. The ability to distinguish tastes, which is evident in the newborn, is also established prenatally according to Dr. Liley. He introduced sugar into the amniotic fluid of one child and found that the fetal swallowing rate increased considerably, as if the baby were enjoying an unexpected piece of candy.

Many of the baby's responses inside the womb are caused by interaction with the mother. At times, you can sense this for yourself. You may find, for instance, that increased blood sugar makes the baby's movements more noticeable after a meal. Sometimes babies are more active when their mothers are in a hurry, and settle down once the mother herself sits down and rests. This continuous interaction between mother and child happens daily in many different ways.

It is important to recognize why such interaction occurs. Almost everything the mother ingests also crosses the placenta and enters the fetal bloodstream; in this way the mother's tastes and personal habits have a direct influence on the fetal environment, even to the point of changing it in undesirable ways. Researchers have measured fetal responses to a number of such situations, including cigarette smoking. By using sonography they have observed how the fetal heart rate speeds up when the mother smokes a cigarette (an increased heart rate is often a sign of stress or discomfort). But in one study the fetal response was so sophisticated that the heart rate increased tremendously *before* the mother lit her cigarette. Somehow her desire to have a cigarette conveyed itself to the baby, who became agitated. This is a good example of the way maternal emotions as well as physical actions affect the baby *in utero.*

Some researchers believe that communication between the mother and child before birth is so finely tuned that the unborn baby responds to subtle emotional states such as contentment or pleasure in the pregnancy. In this way, they feel, the mother helps to shape her baby's personality prenatally by increasing confidence in the unborn child and trust in other human beings. Some research has already been done on the emotional effects of stress during pregnancy, certainly enough to indicate that the mother's emotions reach the unborn baby through her hormonal activity and affect prenatal behavior.

Fetal movements and consciousness increase considerably in the final weeks as the baby becomes more mature. A sign of this maturity is the establishment of spontaneous breathing movements, which take place even though the lungs will not be fully inflated until the baby is outside the womb. Some women say they are aware of the baby's breathing, and the movements are occasionally visible. This is particularly true of very slender women, whose abdomens sometimes visibly rise and fall with the rapid rhythmic movements of the baby's chest wall. (When I saw a clear example of this recently and asked the mother what she thought it was, she replied without any hesitation, "That's my baby breathing.")

Another important sign of the baby's maturity is the increased capacity of the brain, especially once the cerebral cortex (the section of the brain that permits consciousness and full response to stimuli) is developed, in the thirty-second week. After this point the baby is capable of dreaming, or something very like dreaming, because brain-wave tests on babies older than thirty-two weeks have detected REM (rapid eye movement) during periods of sleep. During the final month of pregnancy the increased sophistication of the baby's brain fosters the unique sleeping/waking cycle, the individual pattern of sleeping and waking that we follow throughout our lives.

☐ *Is the Baby's Personality Shaped Prenatally?*   This is, of course, one of the crucial questions raised by the new research on prenatal life. As I have already pointed out, the very idea of personality development in young children is relatively recent, and the idea of prenatal personality development is even more so. Since the fetus cannot be tested or observed by conventional techniques, the whole idea of tracing prenatal personality development may seem absurd to some people. But there are some clues, and, once again, pregnant women themselves are sometimes the most observant judges of the way babies develop before birth.

There are distinct and measurable differences between the activity levels of individual children before they are born. These differences are observable not only when the baby of one woman is compared to that of another but when mothers themselves recall the activity level of previous children. Most women notice distinct differences in prenatal activity from pregnancy to pregnancy, differences that enable them to make confident judgments about the personality of the baby.

Even if this is your first baby, you can often tell how active it will be after birth by the amount of movement you feel in the last few weeks of pregnancy. If you sense that the baby enjoys long periods of sleep, the likelihood is that he or she will settle down into a comfortable pattern of sleeping and waking soon after birth. A more lively baby will probably sleep less and demand more attention. In many babies these differences in sleeping and activity levels persist for several months after birth.

One group of researchers was so fascinated by the distinct prenatal differences between babies and the implications of this in terms of personality development in infancy that they ran two sets of tests on a group of children, one measuring activity levels before birth and the second at six months. The results were hardly unexpected: at six months the children who were active prenatally were still more active—and physically more advanced—than the children whose activity level was lower during pregnancy. Unfortunately these children were not tested beyond the sixth month, which makes it impossible to tell how accurately these tests foreshadowed their development as they grew up.

At the same time, these researchers did not speculate on the origin of prenatal and postnatal behavior—in other words, whether the active children were genetically so or whether the environment in the womb had something to do with their higher level of activity. The latter is important, because some prenatal researchers feel that a higher level of activity may be an indication of discomfort experienced within the womb itself. They point out that flurries of prenatal activity sometimes indicate nervous disorders such as colic, which seem to have a prenatal origin and make the baby difficult to handle in the weeks immediately after birth.

The fetal heartbeat may be another clue to the baby's personality. Each human being possesses a characteristic heartbeat, which remains more or less consistent from birth to old age and differs noticeably from person to person. Personality tests have led psychiatrists to believe that a highly variable heartbeat is associated with a distinct personality type (especially in males), the so-called cardiac labiles, who are said to be impulsive, indecisive, and introspective. Researchers at the Fels Research Institute in Yellow Springs, Ohio, who were interested in the marked differences between fetal heartbeats, followed this up by interviewing and testing a small group of adults whose fetal heart rates were on record. Although the group was too small to make any definite conclusions possible, the results suggested that individuals maintain the same heartbeats throughout their lives, which also suggests that certain personality traits can be predicted from physical characteristics measured prenatally.

Another difference that can be measured prenatally is the degree to which individuals respond to stress. Some children, for instance, start to kick violently when they hear a sudden loud noise, and at the same time the fetal heart rate increases considerably, indicating the extent of their agitation. Other children appear relatively undisturbed. Researchers have tried to find out whether these differences in response are significant and have come up with some interesting answers. In one study in particular, the researchers interviewed a group of adolescents whose responses had been tested *in utero* and found that there were quite different ways of thinking and perceiving events between adolescents who had shown strong responses and those who had remained calm when exposed to stress. The "strong reactors" apparently exhibited a more imaginative approach when they were presented with a picture test than the "low reactors" and projected feelings and emotions into the picture that the low reactors did not seem capable of. On the other hand, the low reactors had a greater degree of emotional and behavioral control in all kinds of situations. In other words, both sets of children exhibited desirable characteristics, and in many cases these personality traits could have been predicted prenatally with some accuracy.

Since we still know comparatively little about prenatal personality development, it is impossible to tell how much the environment in the womb and the baby's relationship with his mother shape his personality before birth. Some of the differences between children may simply be inborn. But sensitive parents who provide a good prenatal atmosphere are doing all they can to foster healthy physical and emotional development for their baby. What happens after birth is equally important. Children are very flexible and can change in quite surprising ways as they grow up. A good relationship between parents and child after birth may compensate for a less than ideal pregnancy.

☐ *Bonding Before Birth*   The discovery that the newborn baby is capable of complex responses to his environment and, in particular, to his parents has fostered our appreciation of the crucial period called bonding. During bonding the new parents hold, stroke, and speak gently to their newborn, and the newborn in turn responds in his own way to his parents. By this reciprocal interaction an unshakable attachment is formed between the new baby and his parents. According to Marshall H. Klaus and John H. Kennell, the doctors who pioneered the study of bonding, "this attachment is crucial to the survival and development of the infant. . . . The power of this attachment is so great, it enables the mother or father to make the unusual sacrifices necessary for the care of their infant day after day, night after night—changing dirty diapers, attending to his cry, protecting him from danger."

But, as we have seen, attachment begins prenatally, and parents and child form a unique relationship long before the birth itself. This means that bonding can and should take place in the prenatal period as well as immediately after birth. In addition, prenatal care is as crucial to the survival of the baby as postnatal care, making bonding before birth (known to fetologists as intrauterine bonding) a vital part of healthy fetal development. If you think of the sacrifices you make in the months of pregnancy to ensure your baby's future, you will realize that this bonds you and your child just as surely as the physical closeness you experience after birth. And as each week of your pregnancy goes by, the prenatal bond between you and your baby grows stronger, because the baby is more and more able to respond to your care and love.

☐ *Talk to Your Baby*   Although you cannot see your baby, you still have ways to communicate and reassure him or her of your love and caring. To start with, don't be afraid to touch your abdomen. Pregnant women instinctively put their hand to their abdomen when they feel the baby move. Touch it often. There is only a fraction of an inch between your skin and the baby, and the baby is so close to your hand that you can stroke the head or leg gently when movement occurs. Your husband will enjoy this contact with the baby too, and he can put his head to your abdomen and listen to the baby's movements.

Occasionally you may sense that the baby is kicking too much. This can happen in the evening after you have just eaten dinner, or the baby may be awake because you are watching television. Many babies seem restless in the evenings and continue to move around even when you are trying to sleep. Sudden bursts of movement also occur when there is a loud or unexpected noise in the room. If this happens and the baby seems startled or upset or you sense there is too much movement, put your hand to your abdomen and rub it gently. Talk soothingly to the baby at the same time. He or she already recognizes the sound of your voice and will be reassured by your presence.

Talking to your baby before birth increases the closeness of your relationship and fosters communication after birth. In fact, hearing your voice is believed to be an important part of your child's language development, another example of the way the fetus experiences and learns prenatally. In experiments performed in Sweden a professor of pediatrics at the University of Miami, Dr. Henry Truby, determined that babies can hear external noises during the entire last half of the pregnancy. He believes that when a child overhears his mother's conversations from inside the womb, a subtle "imprinting" goes on that affects his speech patterns when he begins to talk. In this way we begin learning our native language from our parents long before we can master words ourselves.

Encourage your mate to talk to the baby at the same time you do. Newborns recognize their father as well as their mother and are attracted or consoled equally by the voices of both partners. This is one way for a father to begin bonding with his child before the birth itself, and it seems to hasten bonding between father and child in the first weeks home. Sometimes the absence of the father for long periods during pregnancy seems to affect bonding, at least temporarily.

I have in mind one couple I know. The husband was constantly away on business during the last trimester, and both parents noticed that the baby girl was slow in adjusting to her father's presence, even though he was very proud of his daughter and enjoyed being with her.

☐ **Stress and the Unborn Child**   While it is impossible to come to definitive conclusions about human behavior from animal studies, we know that certain kinds of intrauterine stress have a similarly harmful effect on the unborn baby. The mother's heavy smoking, for instance, cuts down fetal oxygenation and results in a smaller, lighter baby. Too much alcohol has a stressful effect that results in growth retardation or more subtle behavioral abnormalities in the newborn. Lack of nourishment from the mother can produce such severe stress that it results in premature delivery. These are well documented instances of the way physical stress changes the baby's environment for the worse.

Another, perhaps surprising, example of the influence of physical stress is the aftereffects of strenuous exercise during the last two trimesters of pregnancy. Strenuous exercise will cause the muscles to utilize all the available oxygen and the blood to be shunted away from the uterus, leaving less oxygen for the baby and compromising fetal growth. A certain amount of exercise is valuable, because it strengthens your muscles and keeps your body flexible, but a strenuous athletic program in the second and third trimesters is not good for the baby, however invigorated you may feel as a result.

When you are pregnant, think before taking any action that directly or indirectly affects your baby. Parents who want to encourage bonding before birth can start by evaluating their baby's physical environment and eliminating the hazardous conditions that increase fetal stress. A happy, healthy pregnancy with proper care is undoubtedly one of the best ways you can relate to your child before birth.

What happens if the stress is emotional rather than physical? This is an important question, because a certain amount of stress naturally occurs during pregnancy, when so many changes are taking place in the lives of both parents. And if this is your first pregnancy, the stress is usually increased, because everything happening is unfamiliar.

Emotional stress produces certain observable physical reactions in both mother and child. When a pregnant woman is upset or fearful, hormones called catecholamines are released from the hypothalamus gland in the brain and enter her bloodstream, producing the physical changes in the body that we associate with stress: a rapid heartbeat, sweating, and a rise in blood pressure. These hormones cross the placenta and enter the fetal bloodstream, which results in a pronounced increase in the activity level of the baby. In women who are under sudden and severe stress the phenomenon is so marked that fetal movements have been known to increase as much as ten times over.

Two cases in particular were cited by the Fels Institute, where researchers used a group of mothers to measure normal fetal responses. One woman in the group suddenly lost her husband in a car accident, the other came to the institute one night to seek refuge after her husband had suffered a psychotic breakdown and threatened to kill her. In both instances the baby's kicking was so violent that it was actually painful. I myself have known cases in which an emotional crisis was so overwhelming that the mother's oxygen level decreased profoundly, triggering premature labor. Although the causes of premature labor are too complex to attribute solely to emotional factors, premature births often occur after a sudden separation or a fight between husband and wife. Pregnant women who are under profound stress need particular care and reassurance if prematurity is to be avoided.

Prenatal stress may affect the baby in less dramatic ways than prematurity. The babies of the two women in the Fels Institute study were born at term, but both of them were irritable, hyperactive, and suffered from colic—nervous traits that the staff of the institute attributed to the babies' experiences *in utero*. Sometimes pediatricians see a restless, fretful baby with a feeding problem whose symptoms cannot be explained by illness. In this case too prenatal stress may be the reason for the baby's difficulties. I must emphasize that this is only a theory, although observations indicate it's a well founded one.

Before you become concerned about your own baby and the effect of your emotions on his or her development, you should understand that most researchers are talking about situations of extreme or prolonged stress, not the normal anxieties women experience during pregnancy. Although at times the baby may sense your concern or minor anxieties, he or she is likely to be unaffected unless great difficulties occur during pregnancy and stress becomes chronic. Even then, some writers on prenatal development believe that if a woman really loves her baby, the baby will sense her attachment and will be spared the more serious side effects of maternal stress. Remember too that children change as they grow older, and a good environment after birth can make up for a great deal. Nevertheless, if it is at all possible, try to moderate the effects of stress when you are pregnant. If conditions in the home are emotionally upsetting, talk to your mate. A loving partner is your best support during any difficult times.

☐ ***Does Prenatal Stress Lead to Homosexuality?***   Researchers have conducted animal studies that seem to suggest that a stressful environment *in utero* alters the baby's behavior to such a degree that abnormal sexual preferences appear later in life, at least in males. In the early 1970s groups of young male rats were exposed to stress prenatally and postnatally in experiments conducted at Villanova University in Pennsylvania, and some fascinating results were obtained. The prenatal group whose mothers had been subjected to bright light for long periods of time in the final week of gestation appeared at puberty to be demasculinized and actually feminized. Put in a cage with young female rats and normal males, they made no attempt to mate. When other male rats approached, many of them assumed the crouching position the female rat usually assumes before being mounted by the male. Other male rats, who were exposed to stress postnatally and kept separate from females, and females subjected to prenatal stress showed normal sexual behavior. Researchers theorized that the first group of males were deprived prenatally of the male hormone testosterone, which their mothers lost as a result of stress. The female brain and hormonal system does not need testosterone to promote female sexual behavior, and this difference explains why the female rats were unaffected. It is important to add that the researchers made no assumptions about the origins of human homosexuality from this study.

A second study by the same researchers is particularly fascinating for anybody interested in pre- and postnatal behavior in animals and humans. Instead of separating the males and females after they were born, researchers put male rats exposed prenatally to stress in a cage with female rats of their own age, and, surprisingly, the males were found to have normal sexual development in spite of their prenatal experience. This suggests that the harmful effects of the environment before birth can be reversed by a favorable environment after birth.

☐ ***Love Your Child Before It Is Born***   Research is expanding rapidly into the area of fetal psychology, including behavioral abnormalities that may be caused by the maternal environment during pregnancy. The present studies clearly indicate that, in animals at least, changing the fetal environment for the worse can have a sometimes permanent effect on the young. It is difficult as yet to translate these studies in terms of human beings, and some psychologists feel it may take a long time before we can completely verify the effects of prenatal influences on children. We know enough, however, to encourage every couple who are expecting a child to take care of their unborn baby from the moment of conception.

Loving your baby before birth means more than showing your child affection, although, as we have seen, this is very important. Loving your child means changing your life as well. Think of pregnancy as a time invested in yourself and your unborn baby, a time in which you give generously of your own life to make sure that your baby gets the best possible start in his or her life. This means a lot to you, but it also means a lot to the child you deliver. If you can avoid stress, if your pregnancy is healthy, you will find it easier to take care of yourself and your baby, and the delivery and postpartum period will be more rewarding as well. You will probably find your child will be much better adjusted, much easier to take care of, will probably sleep longer, and will have less tendency toward colic than a child of a more stressful pregnancy.

Of course much of the research into prenatal life remains to be done, and we may never find out everything we would like to know about life inside the womb and its effect on our postnatal existence. At the same time, I believe that it doesn't matter if our knowledge is incomplete. We don't need research paper after research paper to appreciate the importance of caring for and communicating with the unborn child. This is something parents have known intuitively for centuries, and it is knowledge that the mothers and fathers of our generation will in turn pass on to their children.

15

Weight Gain in Pregnancy: Then and Now

□ *Why Were Our Mothers Not Allowed to Gain Weight?*   The dietary habits of pregnant women have received close scrutiny throughout history. Certain African tribes, for instance, prepared a girl for pregnancy long before she was married. A girl who reached puberty was kept inside the house and fed rich and fattening foods to make sure that when she married, she would have plenty of body fat to draw on. Each culture has developed its own approach to prenatal nutrition, according to its own prejudices, observations, and religious, social, and scientific beliefs.

In the Middle Ages the pregnant woman was advised to keep up her health and spirits by eating and drinking well. In the sixteenth and seventeenth centuries the new practitioners of medicine who were becoming fashionable based their advice on the old Greek authorities—Hippocrates, Aristotle, and Galen—and combined this with their scientific observations of the course of pregnancy. The obstetrics of the time faced two great problems—miscarriages and premature deliveries—and special diets were recommended to combat these tragedies. A good diet was believed to prevent an abortion by feeding the fetus sufficiently so that it did not come out of the womb before its time to seek nourishment. The pregnant woman was encouraged to eat more food as the child inside her grew larger, and not to be afraid of overeating. Midwives and doctors appreciated the connection between a large, healthy child and a good maternal diet.

Unfortunately this approach changed in the late eighteenth century, when obstetricians became the fashionable birth attendants and childbirth began to be seen as an illness instead of a normal event. The obstetricians of the time were much concerned with what we now call fetal/maternal disproportion—an overlarge head passing through a too small pelvis. In 1788 Dr. James Lucas, a surgeon at Leeds General Infirmary, recommended a special diet for pregnant women to overcome the difficulty of labor in such cases. He advised a restricting diet and other treatments to diminish the size of the child and make the delivery easier. The distinguished doctor's suggestions were as follows: "Temperance in diet, a diminution in the usual quantity and a change in the quality of the food, and increase in exercise, the occasional loss of a few ounces of blood, and the moderate use of cooling asperients." Dr. Lucas' theory on diet found enthusiastic acceptance among contemporary doctors and was commonly practiced in the nineteenth century. Although we know now how harmful such advice must have been, it is easier to understand the popularity of this approach at the time, when the fear of Cesarean section was so great and doctors believed that smaller children were easier to deliver vaginally.

In 1889 a German physician, Dr. Ludwig Prochownick, published a diet plan, which was to become the standard for the obstetrical profession. In order to reduce the necessity of Cesarean section among women with small pelvises, he recommended a diet in the last six weeks of pregnancy that was low in liquids and carbohydrates and rich in protein. This considerably reduced infant size and was similar to the diet adopted by diabetic patients. The medical profession in the United States enthusiastically adopted Prochownick's ideas because the conventional medical wisdom of the time held that infant size and nutritional status were two quite different entities. Despite an attempt by an English physician, C. F. G. Smith, whose study, published in 1916, concluded that poor nutrition during pregnancy led to infant mortality and illness, doctors in the United States and western Europe continued to recommend a modern version of the Victorian "lowering" diet well into the twentieth century. Women who dutifully obeyed their doctors and kept their weight gain at or below the recommended 15 pounds, undoubtedly suffered from anemia and physical exhaustion in the final weeks of pregnancy, at the very time when the physical demands of pregnancy are highest.

It took a long time, particularly for American doctors, to comprehend the relationship between prenatal care, prenatal nutrition, and a successful pregnancy and delivery. Fortunately in the 1960s the situation changed radically. In a famous study in 1968 two doctors at the Johns Hopkins Hospital in Baltimore found that a greater weight gain was related to a decrease in low-birth-weight children and concluded that a weight gain of less than fifteen pounds depleted the mother's body of mineral and protein stores and should not be recommended. Another study in the same year for the Cerebral Palsy Association linked a greater weight gain to superior health, growth, and intelligence in the first year of life. These pioneering studies heralded a return to the old emphasis on good nutrition in pregnancy and a proper weight gain. A mother's nutrition is extraordinarily important to the child she carries. If all women in the United States ate better, before and during pregnancy, we would have healthier children, less perinatal mortality and fewer childhood diseases, and our children would get a far better start in life.

☐ *How Much Weight Should You Gain?*   Pregnant women are now being advised to gain more weight than was fashionable twenty years ago, because recent studies indicate that a good weight gain reduces the chance of premature birth, intrauterine growth retardation (low birth weight even though the baby is delivered at term), and poor health after birth. If you talk to your mother about her pregnancies she will probably tell you how strictly her doctor watched her weight because he believed she would be healthier and the baby would be smaller and easier to deliver. Unfortunately there are still obstetricians who try to enforce weight restrictions. This is quite unjustified. Don't listen to a doctor who tries to put you on a diet during pregnancy. In fact, this is a very good reason to change doctors and find one more in line with modern thinking, since all the recent studies would support your stand against an obstetrician with an outdated attitude advocating weight restriction.

Most obstetricians now recommend a weight gain of 24 to 27 pounds: 7 to 8 pounds in the first half of the pregnancy, and about 1 pound a week in the second half. This is based on studies showing that a pregnant woman who is allowed to gain weight naturally will, on average, gain about 27 pounds. When, for instance, a group of women in Aberdeen, Scotland, were taken off a restricting diet, the average weight gain of these women proved to be about 27 pounds. These mothers were compared to another group of women, who were restricted during pregnancy, and the nonrestricted women were found to have fewer complications and fewer low-birth-weight infants. Furthermore, this study linked a weight gain of about 20 pounds in the last twenty weeks of pregnancy to a lower incidence of toxemia and a lower infant death rate during labor and delivery and postpartum. However, 27 pounds is only a number. Many healthy women show weight gains that vary greatly. Young women, for instance, tend to gain slightly more weight than older women. A woman in her first pregnancy usually gains more than in a subsequent pregnancy. Thin women put on more weight than obese women. Weight gains also vary from area to area as well as from race to race.

You certainly do not need to be as weight-conscious in pregnancy as women a few years back so often were. In fact, many doctors worry more about a woman gaining too little weight rather than too much, although a very large amount of weight or a rapid weight gain may indicate a serious problem, such as diabetes or toxemia of pregnancy (see Chap. 25). Finally, don't be concerned about putting on too much weight during pregnancy because you think it will be difficult to lose it afterward. Much of the weight is lost almost immediately, and the rest usually disappears within a few months if you go back to your prepregnancy diet. Most doctors no longer have a strict upper limit for weight gain, but, ideally, a healthy woman should not gain in excess of 35 pounds. If you gain too much, your doctor will ask you to cut out superfluous calories.

Nutritional needs change as pregnancy develops. During the beginning of pregnancy good nutrition is important. Even so, what you eat at this time is probably more significant than how much you eat. With the early development of the placenta and the fetus, an increased blood supply flows into the uterus, changing the maternal environment and removing waste from the placenta. This increased blood flow increases your need for iron and vitamins and other nutrients that are used for the finer development of the fetal nervous system. The main body weight of the baby is gained in the final twenty weeks of pregnancy. During this period the mother's body further adapts to ensure proper fetal nutrition, and her metabolism changes so that enough fat will be deposited to provide for the baby's growth, for the breasts to enlarge, and for milk to be produced.

Actually, a series of changes occur in pregnancy. A woman may not be particularly hungry at the beginning of pregnancy, but the need for food is higher toward the middle months and even higher toward the end of pregnancy, when she will have a considerably increased appetite and eat far more than she would normally. Furthermore, nature has provided for other changes to accommodate the needs of the fetus. The absorption rate in the intestines alters, resulting in a more efficient utilization of important nutriments such as calcium in the latter part of pregnancy. Of course, if there is not enough food at this point, the baby's growth will be limited, even so.

Some women become so alarmed by the changes in their body during pregnancy, and so fearful of losing their figure, that they cut back on calories, believing that dieting will protect them from obesity in the future. This belief is based on an old wives' tale. It has been proven that the weight gain in pregnancy has no relationship to your future weight and the way your body will look several years hence. Remember, you need to gain at least 25 pounds to insure a desirable birth weight of no less than 7½ pounds for your baby. Both of you will benefit, because a baby who is smaller is often more fretful and more prone to disease than a heavier baby.

Your weight gain should be achieved through the right kind of nutrition. If your weight gain comes only from junk food, your body may not get the right balance of vitamins, calcium, and iron. During pregnancy your need for vitamins, minerals, and protein increases considerably. For example, you need more calcium-rich foods such as milk to help your baby form strong bones and teeth. You need vitamins and minerals to give the right balance to the baby's growth: the minerals and vitamins in vegetables and fruit aid the development of the eyes, skin, hair, and the heart and the other internal organs; the B vitamins in cereals and bread enhance blood and nerve functions. You need increased protein to build the baby's body cells and contribute to brain development. A proper balance of foods will give the right impetus to the baby's growth and assure the birth of a healthy and strong child. *as well as giving you the energy to be active in physical exercise.*

☐ *Why Is It So Important for the Baby to Have a Good Birth Weight?* Statistically an infant has a better chance of surviving and developing normally after birth if its birth weight is not too low. In most industrialized countries, 5½ pounds (2½ kilos) is considered to be the lowest adequate birth weight. Below 5½ pounds a child is said to be premature, whether it is a full-term baby or not. But a desirable birth weight is much higher than 5½ pounds; doctors now feel that 7½ pounds is probably an optimum birth weight for babies born in the United States. Unfortunately many babies in this country are premature or underweight for their gestational age, and these are the babies who account for our high infant-mortality rates. In this respect the United States is notably behind other countries—in fact, we rank eighteenth in the world, which is not a good record for a rich country. This means that a child born in Sweden, Denmark, Japan, Australia, Germany, France, or Great Britain has a better chance to survive than if it were born in the United States—not a situation to be proud of!

The highest rate of infant mortality is found in the poorest sections of the American population. In some of these groups infant mortality is two or three times higher than it is among middle-class Americans. Also, babies from these disadvantaged mothers weigh on the average one-half pound less than a child born to a middle-class family. Some health professionals feel that this difference in the birth weight between different sections of the population almost entirely explains the higher infant-mortality rates among poorer women. Thus, they reason, if we could educate all women and give practical help during pregnancy where it is needed, we could eliminate poor maternal nutrition and have far healthier babies, and the United States would have birth records to equal or better the Scandinavian countries.

□ *How Much Should an Underweight Woman Gain During Pregnancy?* Most doctors, backed up by considerable research, now agree that being seriously underweight before you become pregnant is a potentially dangerous situation unless you put on enough weight during pregnancy. Even so, if you are underweight, your body's storage system is probably deprived of the vitamins and minerals that are so important for the development of the fetal nervous system in the first few months of pregnancy. Since many women have morning sickness in the first trimester and are unable to eat properly until the second trimester, an underweight woman, whose body is already depleted, will be weakening herself even further and possibly endangering her baby.

In the second half of pregnancy, when an adequate weight gain is so important, a woman who starts her pregnancy underweight should ideally gain as much weight as a normal woman *plus* the number of pounds she lacked in her prepregnancy weight according to average standards. If a woman is very thin or undernourished, she may therefore need to gain more than the 35 pounds usually recommended.

Recent research has shown how important it is for an underweight woman to have a good weight gain during pregnancy. An insufficient weight gain in a woman who is underweight may have very serious consequences. Miscarriages and prematurity are much higher among this group of mothers. (Premature delivery is responsible for 75 percent of infant deaths during labor and delivery and in the first few months of life.) Toxemia, preeclampsia, and eclampsia (seizures caused by toxemia) are also more prevalent among underweight women who fail to gain sufficiently during pregnancy. The incidence of low-birth-weight babies has been shown to be approximately twice as high in this group of women as in normal pregnancies. A baby born with a low birth weight because of prematurity or poor nutrition is not only smaller in size but has a smaller brain size and smaller organ weight than a normal baby. The risk with these children, if they survive, is that they may never catch up in later life either in body weight or in brain function. Remember, your baby is not a parasite—it can get only so much from your body without your help. If you are really undernourished and do not put on weight properly, the baby's birth weight and general health will be adversely affected.

□ *The Overweight Pregnant Woman*   Too little and too much have always caused problems. Very overweight women, just like underweight women, suffer from problems during pregnancy that can be serious. Obese women have a higher incidence of stillbirth, an increased chance of prolonged labor, and a greater incidence of Cesarean section. It is often standard practice for extremely obese women to be delivered by Cesarean section if it is estimated that the baby is very large. When a woman is obese, her blood sugar increases, which may result in gestational diabetes (diabetes caused by weight gain during pregnancy in a nondiabetic woman). The increased blood sugar will in turn cause the baby to gain too much, often leading to a difficult birth. Obese women suffer far more frequently from hypertension than do women of normal weight. Furthermore, there is a far higher incidence of toxemia (seven times greater, according to one study) in women who are overweight.

Dieting should be undertaken before pregnancy begins. It is important not to try dieting during pregnancy, because a body deprived of food begins to burn up its own storage system. Under these circumstances the body rapidly becomes acidotic, and this can damage or even kill the fetus.

Although an obese woman should gain weight during pregnancy, her increased stores of fat make a high weight gain unnecessary, because her calorie reserves give her a greater natural supply from which the fetus can draw. However, some nutritionists feel that the quality of the nutrition from this source is not as high as that derived directly from food. They therefore recommend that overweight women should gain about 16 to 17 pounds and should watch their nutrition carefully. Unnecessary and useless calories should be avoided, but plenty of protein should be encouraged. Prenatal vitamins are particularly important, because many obese women have a lifelong history of poor eating habits.

Most of these recommendations are based on studies of very overweight women. Before you follow them, find out what is appropriate for you by discussing your plans carefully with your doctor. You may think of yourself as overweight although you are only a few pounds over standard weight for your height and build. Don't curb your calorie intake in pregnancy without consulting your doctor first.

If you really are obese (that is, 20 percent heavier than normal for your height and body type), remember that pregnancy is not the time to go on a diet but it is a time to carefully observe what you eat.

☐ *Does the Mother's Height Affect Birth Weight?*   Yes, it does, to some extent. Shorter women usually have babies who are smaller and lighter, and taller women have larger and heavier babies. These differences between women are quite normal, and a baby in either case can be perfectly healthy. Height is important in one respect. Obstetricians feel that populations in which women are normally over 5 feet in height have much better pregnancy records than populations in which women are small, because height is often an indication of a woman's lifetime history of nutrition. In the United States most girls eat adequately as children, and height is not a very large factor. It is more important to have the proper weight for your height and a good weight gain through proper nutrition.

☐ *Is It Important When You Gain the Weight?*   If you are of average height and build, you can expect to gain about 24 to 28 pounds. However, the exact weight you gain may not be as important as the way you gain the weight. In the first three months of pregnancy the fetus is still very small, and you may only gain 2 to 4 pounds. During the next six months you should probably average about 1 pound a week. When your doctor weighs you at each visit he is looking for a regular weight gain, which will indicate that the baby's development is progressing well. If the baby stops growing, he may suggest an ultrasound examination of the baby to evaluate the problem and then place you on a protein-rich diet with proper vitamins and minerals.

If you suddenly begin to gain weight very rapidly, it could be the first sign of toxemia or preeclampsia (early form of toxemia before occurrence of seizures), and this is a warning signal that you should point out to your doctor. Preeclampsia, if uncontrolled, can lead to eclampsia, which depletes the fetus of oxygen and may be fatal both for the baby and the mother (see Chap. 25). One common symptom of toxemia is the sudden swelling of the face, hands, and fingers, and you may find it difficult to remove your rings. If this occurs, call your doctor immediately.

☐ *How the Weight Gain Breaks Down*   An average weight gain of 28 pounds might break down in the following way, according to the number of weeks of gestation:

At 10 weeks you would expect to gain 1½–2 pounds;
at 20 weeks, approximately 8 pounds;
at 30 weeks, approximately 18 pounds;
at 40 weeks, (in other words, at term), approximately 28 pounds.

However, you don't need to follow this pattern slavishly. Your weight gain will vary, depending on your height, your prepregnancy weight, what you eat during pregnancy, and your obstetrical history.

☐ *How the Weight Is Distributed*   If your weight gain is about 24–28 pounds, the various elements will break down in the following way:

The baby will be about 7½ pounds at the time of delivery.
Fat and water in the maternal tissues weigh about 6–10 pounds.
The placenta, 1½ pounds; the amniotic fluid, 2 pounds; the increase of the uterus, 2 pounds; increase in breast size, 1 pound: all equaling another 6½ pounds.
Increase in blood volume, 4 pounds.

Within a week or two after the baby is born you will have lost 18 to 20 pounds. Within three or four months you will have lost everything you gained during pregnancy if you are not breast-feeding. If you are breast-feeding, it is not advisable to lose weight too fast. Stop breast-feeding if you plan to go on a diet. Eating well during breast-feeding is just as important as eating well during pregnancy (see Chap. 32).

protein. Vegetable sources: ¾ cup of cooked legumes, one ounce of nuts, or ¼ cup of peanut butter are the equivalent of a serving.

Calcium: The best source is *milk*, whole or dry, and *milk products*—hard cheese or cottage cheese, ice cream, and yogurt. Milk and milk products are also a good source of protein.

Calcium requirements are met by 3 cups of milk in the first three months and 4 cups in the second and third trimester. One ounce of a hard cheese such as cheddar is the equivalent of 1 cup of milk.

Grain Products: Grain products—preferably whole grain—provide vitamins and minerals and some protein. These include bread, cereals, pasta, wheat germ, and rice.

You need *at least three servings.* One serving is: 1 slice of bread, ¾ cup of granola, ½ cup of cooked rice, 1 whole-wheat pancake, 1 muffin or biscuit, ¼ cup of wheat germ. Whole-wheat breads and cereals are nutritionally far superior to so-called enriched products.

Vitamins: From vegetables and fruits. *Leafy green vegetables*—broccoli, Brussels sprouts, cabbage, watercress, Boston lettuce, kale, and collard greens supply B vitamins and iron.

You need two servings of leafy green vegetables (one cup raw or ¾ cup cooked).

Vitamin C is provided by oranges and other citrus fruits, strawberries, tomatoes, broccoli, pineapple, green peppers, and cabbage.

You need at least one orange or one serving of a vitamin C-rich vegetable or fruit.

Other vegetables and fruits that are useful sources of vitamins are: potatoes, squash, carrots, peas, apples, bananas, apricots, plums, pears, dates, prunes, raisins, grapes, watermelon.

You need at least one daily serving, more if possible.

Fluid Intake: Plenty of fluids are important at any time. During pregnancy drink at least 8 to 10 cups of fluid a day. Avoid drinking too much tea, coffee, or soft drinks that contain cola, especially during the first trimester, because caffeine is now suspected of causing birth defects (this is discussed fully at the end of the chapter).

☐ *How Closely Do You Need to Follow a Diet Plan?* The food plan included here is only a guide to the *basic* requirements during pregnancy. Once you have enough calcium and protein-rich foods, and a minimum of vegetables and fruits, you can go on to eat whatever you want. Don't feel you can't eat 4 pieces of bread if you want to just because the diet plan says 3. A thin woman, after all, needs to eat more than a woman who is overweight, and a woman who is 6 foot 2 needs more calories than a woman who is 4 foot 11.

☐ *Calories in Pregnancy* An adult nonpregnant woman needs at least 2000 calories a day to function properly if she is of average weight and build. A very active woman needs more. The most important recommendation during pregnancy is to increase your food intake so the number of calories you eat is increased by at least 300, and possibly 500 if you remain active. This should be sufficient to provide a good healthy growth for the baby. Calorie intake strongly influences the course and outcome of the pregnancy as well as the baby's weight by supplying you with more energy at a crucial time, and giving your body a proper balance.

Calories are the way your body builds and stores energy. Much of your body energy during pregnancy is channeled into forming and developing the placenta and the fetal tissues. If you restrict your calorie intake the baby will be small and poorly nourished, you will become exhausted, and both of you will be deprived of essential nutriments because of your limited food supply.

Many doctors recommend that your increased calories come from protein foods. Some nutritionists, however, believe that the source of the extra calories is not important to the fetus because the mother's body converts so-called useless calories into protein when a woman is pregnant. A few years ago women in a Guatemalan village, whose babies were generally growth-retarded because of their poor diets, were given 20,000 extra calories throughout their pregnancies and the babies' birth weights increased by an average of one pound. It seemed to make no difference to the babies whether their mothers received extra protein or carbohydrates. However, when a woman's diet is lacking in protein but is high in carbohydrates, maternal muscle tissue is broken down to supply the necessary amino acids. This is eventually detrimental to the health of the pregnant woman.

If you have been used to counting calories to prevent yourself from eating too much you may suddenly find old habits reversing themselves. Now you should count calories to make sure you are getting enough.

☐ *"Useless" Calories?*   It is easy to exceed the minimum requirement of 2500 calories daily if you eat three meals a day and four pieces of chocolate cake for dessert. Eating a tremendous amount of food will only make you overlarge and uncomfortable. The best advice is to eliminate junk foods—foods that are loaded with refined sugars and are very heavy in calories—and concentrate on foods that provide calories *and* nutrition. But there is nothing wrong with the occasional piece of chocolate cake or some ice cream.

☐ *Protein and Pregnancy*   A pregnant woman needs to increase her intake of protein quite considerably. Protein is vital in the development of the fetus because it supports the new growth of the fetal tissues. At the same time protein enables the pregnant woman to maintain her own tissue growth, which is considerably increased during pregnancy.

Protein is digested by the body into amino acids, the essential substances in growth and development. While the body manufactures many amino acids by itself, eight of the twenty amino acids can be supplied only through the food we eat. These are called "essential amino acids." The function of protein during pregnancy and at any other time is to enable the body to produce these essential amino acids.

A pregnant woman is generally advised to increase her daily pure protein intake by 30 grams (1-1/10 ounces). Since a nonpregnant woman should consume about 45 grams of pure protein daily (in more familiar terms, the protein found in about 6 ounces of lean meat) a pregnant woman needs about 75 to 80 grams (7½ ounces) daily.

Animal foods such as meat, fish, and poultry are by far the best source of complete protein. A 3-ounce serving of lean meat or fish provides 20 to 25 grams of protein. Dairy products and eggs are good sources, but contain somewhat less protein than lean meat. One egg has a protein content of 5 to 8 grams; so does one glass of milk, and one ounce of hard cheese. A woman who eats meat or fish regularly and drinks milk in the quantities recommended during pregnancy should easily meet her protein requirements. Protein is also available from vegetable sources. Soybeans are an outstanding source of protein; one cup of soybeans has 25 grams of protein, the equivalent of a lean piece of beef. Nuts, peanut butter, bread, cereals, dark green vegetables and potatoes also contain some protein, although not in amounts large enough to meet the daily requirement.

A woman who follows a vegetarian diet is probably already aware of the need to combine vegetable sources with milk or cheese, or with each other if she is a strict vegetarian, to form complete amino acids. If you are not a vegetarian but you eat very little meat, this is also an important rule to follow. Kasha, for example, which is an incredibly good source of protein and vitamins, is always combined with an egg to complete its full complement of protein.

☐   *Fat and Pregnancy*   Fat is an essential and integral part of all our body tissues. It is a necessary vehicle for getting the fat-soluble vitamins into the cell tissues. Fat provides energy for the body functions and is necessary for a proper diet, although too much fat intake is unhealthy and unwise.

Fats are widely distributed in foods, so you do not need to be concerned with getting enough. A majority of people in America, as a matter of fact, eat too much fat. Foods that contain fats and are highly nutritious are milk and milk products, egg yolks, nuts, and peanut butter. Since red meat contains too much fat, you should cut down on the red meat you eat. Additional fat in the form of butter, margarine, and oil are added to food during preparation and serving. If you are gaining too much weight during pregnancy you must immediately cut down on the fat content and amount in your diet.

Fat comes from animal sources (saturated fat) and plant sources (unsaturated fat), such as soybeans, cottonseeds, and plant oils. No more than 35 percent of a pregnant woman's total daily calorie intake should come from fat, and only half of these fat calories should come from saturated fat. Although many people should be more careful about the amount of fat they consume, a certain amount of fat is necessary for energy and some essential nutriments.

☐   *Carbohydrates and Pregnancy*   Carbohydrates are the natural starches and sugars in foods from which calories are produced. A low-carbohydrate diet is definitely to be avoided during pregnancy because your body will be deprived of body heat energy and some very important vitamins—in fact, a diet of this kind is best avoided at any time. Good advice during pregnancy is to eat cereals, breads, vegetables, and fruits that are high in carbohydrates and will give you plenty of calories. Adding starches and roughage to your diet will also help your digestive system.

☐   *Minerals and Pregnancy*   A healthy diet is composed of several important nutrients that help to nourish your body and keep it strong. Your diet
should contain adequate amounts of calcium, iron, and the so-called trace minerals: zinc, phosphate, and magnesium. Another mineral, salt, is also needed to
achieve a proper balance of fluids in the body.

Minerals are just as important as vitamins in assuring the maintenance of a
healthy body during pregnancy, even though we tend to think of vitamins as the
key to good health. Unfortunately mineral requirements are sometimes difficult
to achieve through the normal diet because the overrefining of foodstuffs removes so many trace minerals, and because women lose iron every month when
they menstruate. Now that you are pregnant, this is a good moment to evaluate
the mineral content of your normal diet. This does not mean carefully watching
and weighing every ounce of food, but you should survey your diet and try to get
a basic idea of the minerals it contains. If you find out you do not get enough,
increase your intake. Information on some important minerals is included in this
section to help you increase your intake through regular meals or through supplements. At the same time, there is no need to be a slave to nutrition. If you eat
a variety of foods you will usually meet most of the mineral requirements—with
the important exception of iron, which is always given supplementally during
pregnancy. For instance, a simple change to whole-wheat breads and cereals will
add more trace minerals as well as vitamins to your diet. Adding extra cheese or
yogurt will increase your calcium intake. By making some simple adjustments it
is very possible for you, and your partner, to enjoy life and eat well during your
pregnancy, which is, after all, one of the few times in your life when no one
minds if you gain weight.

☐   *How Much Calcium Do You Need?*   Calcium is needed during pregnancy to form the bones and teeth of the developing baby. It also helps the normal clotting action of the blood; it assists the normal reaction of the muscle
fibers; and it helps tired muscles relax. The need for calcium is not so great in
the first trimester because most of the growth of the skeleton takes place later on
in pregnancy. This means that if you are suffering from morning sickness or you
don't feel well enough to eat properly in the first trimester, don't worry too
much about drinking enough milk. Even before pregnancy begins, your body is
storing calcium to help its absorption in the first few months. However, as soon
as the first trimester is past, you should begin increasing your calcium intake.

The intestines change during pregnancy to absorb calcium from food more
efficiently. This does not eliminate your need for extra calcium. The recommended daily amount (the RDA) in the second and third trimesters is 1200
milligrams (1 cup of milk supplies 300 milligrams of calcium) and a woman may
need even more than that to assure the body of an adequate supply. In addition,
teenagers need more calcium than adult pregnant women do. Any excess calcium is simply excreted from the body, so you can afford to take in more calcium
than you in fact need.

During pregnancy your body absorbs and stores calcium very efficiently.
About 30 grams (1-1/10 ounces) of calcium are deposited in the mother's body
before the baby is born. Almost all of that is used for the building of the baby's
bones and teeth; an estimated 300 milligrams of calcium is deposited in the fetal
skeleton in the last three months of pregnancy. But the mother also stores cal-

cium in her body as a reservoir, which can be used if necessary during pregnancy or after delivery to assure adequate calcium for breast-feeding.

In many cultures people do not keep milk-producing animals, the best natural producers of calcium. Babies in these cultures do not universally suffer from calcium deficiency, probably because the mother's body compensates to some extent. Consequently, some nutritionists feel we overemphasize calcium intake. However, if a woman does not take in enough calcium, the body will eventually compensate by removing calcium from the mother's bones and teeth. After several pregnancies the ill effects of calcium deficiency can be serious. Many women in the past who didn't eat properly and had one child after another and breast-fed them all finally suffered spontaneous fractures and lost teeth because their calcium stores were so depleted. Children born to these women often had poor bone formation as well, and developed rickets in early childhood.

Calcium is closely related to phosphorus—the two build together in the body and keep one another in balance. This calcium-phosphorus balance is important for the bones as well as for the nerve and muscle functions; for example, if you suffer from leg cramps during pregnancy, which many women do, it may be because you are not getting enough calcium. Phosphorus is found in foods such as milk and cheese, which also have a high calcium content.

☐ *How to Get Enough Calcium*   Calcium is unevenly distributed in food. The highest amount is found in milk and milk products. For instance, 1 cup of milk has about 300 milligrams of calcium, and 1 ounce of hard cheese, such as cheddar, has 225 milligrams. Soybeans are quite high in calcium. Dark green leafy vegetables also contain a substantial amount. The best way to assure a sufficient amount of calcium is to drink approximately 4 cups of milk a day. This doesn't necessarily mean drinking 4 *glasses* of milk, something many adults have not done since they were small children. There are plenty of substitutes. The calcium in 1 cup of milk is found in 8 ounces of yogurt, 1 ounce of hard cheese, 12 ounces of cottage cheese, 6 ounces of ice cream, and 1½ ounces of processed cheese. Cheese is particularly good because it is very high in protein as well as calcium. Milk and cheese can also be used in cooking—in soups, casseroles, pasta dishes, and puddings. Liquid milk or dry milk powder are both useful in preparing calcium-rich foods; dry milk is very economical—1 cup of powdered milk is the equivalent of 3 cups of regular milk. Whole milk, however, is better than low-fat or skimmed dry or fresh milk because it supplies more protein.

☐ *Lactose Intolerance*   Some women find it very difficult to drink milk because it is high in lactose. Lactose intolerance is commonly found among people whose cultural background does not include dairy products—in the United States it often affects women who are black or Chinese. Milk drinking can, in fact, be quite harmful to a woman with lactose intolerance because it can cause severe intestinal cramps and diarrhea. The best alternative is hard cheese, which is low in lactose and high in calcium. Cottage cheese is also low in lactose. Sometimes a woman who is very uncomfortable after drinking a glass of milk can eat ice cream without any trouble because it is well chilled. For the same reason, yogurt also seems to be better tolerated than whole milk. Occasionally a calcium supplement is recommended, but only if a woman can't or won't eat enough cheese to supply her calcium requirement.

☐ **Phosphorus Intake**   Phosphorus is essential to a good diet. A balance of calcium and phosphorus is necessary for a good bone structure in the fetus as well as for muscle and nerve development. Phosphorus is present in milk and cheese, and in seafood, eggs, meat, and onions as well. A satisfactory level of phosphorus intake is, therefore, easier to achieve in the normal diet. If you eat cheese or drink 4 glasses of milk a day you will get plenty of phosphorus. Phosphorus is usually added to calcium supplements, so if you think you need extra calcium and phosphorus because you are not eating milk products, you might ask your doctor to prescribe calcium and phosphorus tablets.

☐ **Iron Requirements in Pregnancy**   Most women do not get enough iron in their ordinary diet, and a pregnant woman becomes a prime candidate for anemia because her need for iron is substantially increased. Iron is a vital substance in achieving a high blood count and in the development of the red blood cells. These cells are needed to carry oxygen to the body tissue of the growing fetus.

The body is remarkable in its ability to regulate the absorption of iron. When it needs more iron, the intestines are usually able to take in iron and as the need diminishes, the rate of absorption also slows down. This prevents the absorption of too much iron, either from your diet or from an iron supplement. Before pregnancy an average woman absorbs about 10 percent of the available iron in her diet; but halfway through pregnancy, almost three times the usual amount of iron can be taken in by the body. However, at the same time the fetus is demanding iron from the mother to form its own red blood cells and build up its own storage. If enough iron is not available through the placental blood flow, the baby will take what it needs from the mother's body.

The fetus, the placenta, and the expanded maternal blood volume increase a woman's need for iron considerably, so much so that an iron supplement is always recommended during pregnancy. The RDA for a nonpregnant woman is set at 20 milligrams; the amount a pregnant woman needs is 5 to 6 milligrams more. About half of this goes to the fetus and the placenta; the remainder contributes to the expanded blood volume in the woman herself. Women who are anemic prior to pregnancy may need a higher amount of iron to fill the storage. This increased need is usually impossible to supply through changes in diet alone, although you should try to include iron-rich foods in your diet as well as taking a supplement. Your doctor will usually recommend iron tablets in the form of ferrous gluconate, ferrous sulphate or ferrous fumarate tablets—at least 30 to 60 milligrams daily, to assure an adequate supply, since the iron in supplements is less efficiently absorbed than iron from food sources.

Iron absorption will be considerably increased if you eat foods that are high in vitamin C, folic acid, and vitamin B_{12}. These are important substances in aiding the body's efficient storage of iron. For instance, a meal in which meat is served with a watercress or tomato salad will supply you with far more available iron than meat served with a cooked vegetable. At least 7 milligrams of vitamin C should be taken for each milligram of iron to increase absorption. In some cases, combinations of foods seem actually to decrease iron absorption. Tea, for instance, seems to decrease iron absorption by binding iron to form an insoluble compound. These are important considerations when you think about your everyday diet during pregnancy.

Iron deficiency can be a serious matter, especially if you lack sufficient iron stores before you become pregnant. The best way to avoid anemia in pregnancy is to see your doctor as early as possible and have him prescribe an iron supplement for you. Regular prenatal vitamins usually contain sufficient amounts of iron for the normal woman. However, your doctor will usually take a blood count at the first visit and give you an extra iron supplement if he finds you are somewhat anemic. In more serious cases, he will take a battery of blood tests to find the source of the anemia (see Chap. 7) and adjust his treatment accordingly to enhance your iron intake. If you find yourself becoming overtired during your pregnancy, you should have your iron status checked a second time. You might need either additional iron tablets or two prenatal vitamins.

Although women are particularly vulnerable to iron deficiency during pregnancy, in most cases iron supplements will eliminate the problem. If a woman is still tired and anemic despite iron supplements, a different approach may be needed. Signs of anemia should not go untreated. Serious anemia during pregnancy has been linked to a higher rate of premature delivery and an increased likelihood of stillbirth. There is also a greater chance of toxemia and other complications for the mother.

The best way to make sure of your iron intake is to check your iron status before pregnancy and take a supplement. This will prevent anemia in the first three months of pregnancy when your iron needs are very high.

☐ **Which Foods Contain Iron?**   Meat, eggs, leafy green vegetables, dried fruits, soybeans, peanut butter, potatoes and bread all contain some iron, although organ meats such as liver are by far the best source. But however well you eat, it is still advisable to take an iron supplement. A hamburger, for instance, has an iron content of only 3 milligrams. A half cup of leafy cooked green vegetables has only 2 milligrams. This will give you some idea of how difficult it is to meet iron requirements through the diet alone.

☐ **Should You Use Salt in Pregnancy?**   During pregnancy the increased estrogen binds sodium in the body tissues just as it does before menstruation begins. The sodium in turn binds salt, sometimes causing the body to swell. You will notice puffiness in the limbs, hands, and feet, and the development of what doctors call edema, which is caused by increased sodium in the extravascular space. Some slight degree of edema is quite normal during pregnancy, although a few years ago doctors routinely advised women to adopt a salt-free diet and take diuretics (pills that increase urination) if any swelling appeared. This is no longer considered acceptable practice. We now know that a pregnant woman needs more rather than less sodium to maintain a normal fluid balance in the body, and that diuretics can damage a woman's kidneys and harm the fetus.

Edema can sometimes be the first symptom of a marked increase in the body's water retention, a condition known as toxemia of pregnancy (see Chap. 25). Toxemia used to be linked to a high-sodium diet. However, doctors no longer believe this is so. Toxemia is most common among women who have poor diets or are under eighteen or over thirty-five and does not seem to be related only to sodium intake. The best advice during pregnancy is to use a normal amount of table salt without oversalting your food.

Don't eat salty processed foods such as potato chips or salted nuts. A regular diet of these foods is not advisable for anyone, and will definitely cause you to retain extra water. Foods that are especially high in sodium are ham, pastrami, sausage, bacon, sardines, anchovies, frankfurters, and tuna packed in oil. Seasonings such as mustard, chili, ketchup, and soy sauce also have a high salt content. If you feel too heavy, cut out excess salt and drink extra water to flush out your system.

☐ *How Much Iodine Do You Need?*   A small amount of iodine is necessary during pregnancy. Iodine is needed to create and metabolize the thyroid hormones, which are extremely important for the normal growth of the baby, and a serious iodine deficiency may lead to fetal brain damage or cretinism. The use of iodized table salt is the best way to make sure you have enough iodine. Shellfish and commerical dough products also contain iodine.

☐ *Do You Need Chromium?*   A pregnant woman needs a small amount of chromium; the exact amount, however, is unknown. Chromium deficiency has been tentatively linked to gestational diabetes, a condition in which diabetes appears during pregnancy as a woman gains weight (see Chap. 24). Many people in modern industrialized countries do not get enough chromium because the traditional source was unrefined whole grains. However, a simple solution during pregnancy is to switch from refined foods to whole-grain cereals and bread. Brewer's yeast also provides a significant source of chromium.

☐ *Zinc—A Very Important Mineral*   Zinc is a very important mineral at any time. It forms part of most of the enzymes in the body and is involved in nearly all aspects of cellular metabolism. If there is not enough zinc in the body, hypogonadism and dwarfism can result.

Recent studies have shown that many women have marginal zinc deficiency during pregnancy. The plasma concentration of zinc naturally decreases at this time because some of the zinc is taken up by the fetus. It has been estimated that a pregnant woman must retain approximately 750 mcg (micrograms) of zinc daily for the normal growth of the baby in the last two trimesters. There are some good sources of zinc in our diet (see below), although the refining of staple foods such as bread has reduced the zinc content of the normal American diet. A severe zinc deficiency in pregnant animals has been shown to produce abnormalities of the skeleton and nervous system, and a few such cases have also been reported in humans. Recent studies have also shown that women with complications of pregnancy, including those with malformed babies, sometimes have a lower level of blood zinc than normally pregnant women, while an abnormal zinc level in the newborn can cause behavioral abnormalities due to biochemical effects on the brain. Zinc deficiency has been recently linked to an increased infection rate after delivery, and the role of zinc in wound healing is well known. Poorly nourished women will, therefore, have more infections after delivery and a slower healing and recovery.

☐ *Where to Find Zinc in Foods*   Beef, liver, eggs, nuts, and seafood—particularly oysters and herrings—are very good sources of zinc. Milk and whole-grain products contain moderate amounts, and so do carrots, potatoes, and turnips. Deficiencies in zinc are more prevalent in people whose diet is lacking in sea and animal foods.

☐ *Copper Requirements During Pregnancy*   Copper is involved in the storage of iron and its transformation into hemoglobin. Copper deficiency, therefore, can lead to anemia, and to defects in the connecting tissue.

The need for copper is particularly important in the early months of life. Copper deficiency has recently been reported in premature infants. It also appears that if a pregnant woman does not have sufficient copper in her diet, the baby will be born with an inadequate copper storage. Copper deficiency is also seen in stress situations.

The estimated human daily requirement for copper is 2 milligrams, although recent data indicate that the average diet supplies closer to 1 milligram. One good solution to this problem is to go back to natural foods that have not been refined. These will supply copper and other trace minerals, which are often deficient in a diet of refined cereals and flour.

☐ *Vitamins and Pregnancy*   During pregnancy, a woman makes new tissues at a faster rate than at any other time in her life. At this time you need not only extra calories but more minerals as well. Equally important is the extra intake of vitamins demanded by pregnancy—particularly vitamins A, B_1, B_2, B_6, B_{12}, C, D, and folic acid. In fact, vitamin and mineral needs increase by a greater percentage than the number of calories do.

Vitamins are extremely important substances, which in many cases cannot be synthesized by the body. This means that your diet every day should include a wide variety of vitamins. When the food you eat is lacking in vitamins, the body will operate inefficiently. During pregnancy this can lead to an adverse effect on the fetus. The dangers of vitamin "starvation" have been well understood for a long time and most pregnant women are aware of the importance of vitamins even though they may still not be getting all they need.

If you are unsure about your vitamin intake, the first step is to look at what you eat, and plan a sensible diet for yourself. The second is to use a prenatal vitamin supplement. During pregnancy, the need for certain vitamins increases quite considerably. The most important of these is folic acid, which is needed during pregnancy as a protection against anemia. Folic acid is found in some foodstuffs but not generally in large enough quantities to prevent a deficit, and most doctors now recommend prenatal vitamin supplements containing folic acid and other important vitamins.

☐ *Is It Possible to Consume Too Many Vitamins?*   In general, if you eat too many vitamins, the body will not absorb more than it needs, and will simply excrete the excess. However, this is true only with what are called water-soluble vitamins. A few vitamins such as A, D, and E are not water-soluble and will be stored up in the body fat. Vitamins that are readily stored in the body may have a dangerous effect during pregnancy when they are taken in excessive amounts. Structural changes, including deformities, can result in the fetus.

Here is a guide to the water-soluble and fat-soluble vitamins and a recommended daily amount (RDA) for each one during pregnancy:

VITAMIN	RDA	EXCESSIVE DOSE
Vitamin A	5000 IU	greater than 50,000 IU
Vitamin B₁ (thiamine)	1.3 mg	no level known
Vitamin B₂ (riboflavin)	1.5 mg	no level known
Vitamin B₃ (niacin)	15 mg	greater than 3 grams
Vitamin B₆ (pyridoxine)	2.5 mg	no level known
Vitamin B₁₂	4 mcg	no level known
Folic acid	800 mcg	no level known
Vitamin C	60 mg	greater than 2000–3000 mg
Vitamin D	400 IU	greater than 2000 IU
Vitamin E	25 IU	greater than 800 IU

Vitamin A: This is important in maintaining the skin and the mucous membranes. It prevents night blindness and aids in normal eye function. This makes it a valuable aid against eye and skin abnormalities. It also helps to form the baby's tooth enamel and hair, and assists the growth and functioning of the thyroid gland. Vitamin A is found in high amounts in carotene, the red or orange coloring of such plants as carrots, and in deep-green leafy vegetables. It is also found in fortified whole milk (vitamin A is normally present in the fat portion of white milk), butter, margarine, egg yolks, and in some other fresh fruits such as peaches and watermelon. Dried skim milk may also be fortified with vitamin A.

Excess vitamin A is not excreted by the body and an excess of it can be very dangerous. Several recent research papers have shown that excessive doses of vitamin A during pregnancy can be teratogenic. Specifically, hypervitaminosis A in humans may cause a variety of congenital malformations in the fetus, including abnormalities of the urinary tract. The Committee on Drugs and Nutrition of the American Academy of Pediatrics now recommends no more than 5000 to 6000 international units (IU) of vitamin A daily.

☐ *The B Vitamins*

Vitamin B₁: Called also thiamine. This is an essential vitamin in the maintenance of the digestive function; it encourages the bacterial breakdown of food by the intestines and assures a good appetite. During pregnancy it aids the baby's growth and contributes to successful breast-feeding. Thiamine is not fat-soluble, so you need a regular intake during pregnancy. The best sources are pork, beef, oysters, soybeans, peas and beans, and whole-wheat breads and cereals. Wheat germ is an excellent source. Asparagus, cauliflower, broccoli, and milk also provide some vitamin B₁. Acute B₁ deficiency produces a disease called beriberi, which is characterized by abnormal muscle tone. While beriberi is still common in some parts of the world, a severe lack of B₁ is rarely seen in the United States, except among acute alcoholics. A valuable source of B₁ is lost when the outer layer of grain seeds is removed during milling. The regular use of wheat germ in cooking or cereals is a good way to compensate for this loss. About 1.3 milligrams is recommended daily during pregnancy.

Vitamin B$_2$: Called also riboflavin. This is involved in energy metabolism, helping the body utilize food to produce energy. It is a very important part of the fetus' proper growth and development from conception on. Vitamin B$_2$ is widely available in food, particularly in milk; however, riboflavin is damaged by exposure to light, although it is pretty stable during cooking and food preparation. It is best to keep all milk in a plastic coated container to preserve its vitamin B$_2$ content. Other good sources of riboflavin are beef, liver, cheese, eggs, and various vegetables and beans.

The daily requirement is at least 1.5 milligrams during pregnancy. B$_2$ is water-soluble and is easily absorbed by the body. There are no toxic side effects of megadoses of vitamin B$_2$.

Vitamin B$_3$: Called also niacin. This is a coenzyme playing a vital part in the chemical reactions that produce energy in the human body. In pregnancy it helps to build brain cells and transfer energy for the developing fetus. Vitamin B$_3$ can be synthesized by bacteria in the intestines and can also be formed from the amino acid tryptophan. In a case of severe deficiency of niacin a condition called pellagra can result. "Pellagra" is an Italian word meaning "rough skin" because pellagra sufferers develop a red skin rash on their face, hands and feet as soon as they are exposed to sunlight. This condition was once common among poor people whose diets were lacking in lean meat and whole-wheat foodstuffs, which are good sources of niacin. Beef liver, peanuts, and butter are other foods with high amounts of vitamin B$_3$.

The estimated daily requirement during pregnancy is about 15 milligrams. The amount of niacin in your food is not affected by the way it is cooked. Niacin is not recommended in the excess of 3 grams daily.

Vitamin B$_6$: Called also pyridoxine. This is extremely important in successful fetal development and should be taken in sufficient amounts prior to conception (see Chap. 2). B$_6$ must be an essential part of your vitamin intake during pregnancy, both to aid the proper development of a healthy fetus and to ease depression, nausea, and vomiting in the early months. Pyridoxine is found in high amounts in liver, muscle meats, and wheat germ. It is found naturally in whole grains, but if you eat refined breads you may not be getting enough vitamin B$_6$ because the refining process removes it from the outside of the grain through the husking process.

The daily requirement of B$_6$ varies from person to person. A woman under stress needs a higher amount. The RDA for vitamin B$_6$ is 2.5 milligrams, but you will need more if you are very active or stressed during pregnancy. Vitamin B$_6$ is water-soluble, and there are, therefore, no known effects from too much of this vitamin.

Vitamin B$_{12}$: This vitamin is essential in the development of the red blood cells and will prevent a specific form of anemia called pernicious anemia. If a pregnant woman does not have enough vitamin B$_{12}$, red blood cells will not develop, and the fetus may be deprived of oxygen, resulting in congenital malformations. Vitamin B$_{12}$ is developed in the body from bacteria and fungi in the intestinal tract.

Dietary sources of B$_{12}$ are liver, meat, fish, eggs, shellfish, whole grains, and some dairy products. Most women get enough B_{12} from their diets, but if you are a true vegetarian you may be suffering from a deficiency. In this case you may need a B_{12} supplement. B_{12} can be found in pill form, but is often given by injection since this vitamin is not absorbed very successfully through the stomach.

The daily recommended amount of B_{12} is 4 micrograms. There is no known side effect from too much B_{12}.

Folic Acid: This is the one vitamin whose increased requirement in pregnancy cannot be satisfied by a balanced intake of foods. Folic acid is vitally necessary in the process of cell division and blood formation. During pregnancy, when both the placenta and the mother herself are manufacturing so many new cells, a folic acid supplement is definitely advisable to assure healthy fetal development. In the absence of this vitamin, some rather serious complications such as premature separation of the placenta and toxemia of pregnancy have been known to occur. It is also important in the synthesis of fetal tissue.

There are a few good sources of folic acid: yeast, liver, dark green vegetables, legumes, and whole-wheat products. However, the folic acid content of food is easily destroyed by cooking at high temperatures. Furthermore, the storage of vegetables for more than three days also destroys this vitamin. This is why folic acid deficiency is among the most common of all vitamin deficiencies. Because it is so difficult to get enough folic acid in your diet, however carefully you eat, be sure to get extra folic acid either in your prenatal vitamins or in a special folic acid supplement which your doctor should prescribe for you.

The RDA for folic acid is 800 micrograms daily. Excess amounts are harmlessly excreted from the body.

Vitamin C: This is very important in pregnancy since it is involved in the formation of collagen, a protein found in the skin, tendons, and bones of the fetus. If a woman suffers from a vitamin C deficiency there will be abnormalities of the fetal bones, teeth, and gums. Furthermore, vitamin C is valuable in aiding the absorption of iron and it helps fight infections. We also know that wounds heal slowly when there is not enough vitamin C. This can adversely affect the postpartum period. A severe deficiency of vitamin C produces scurvy, which used to be common during the long European winters, or on sea voyages. Fruits and vegetables are primary sources of vitamin C; however, they should be left uncooked because the vitamin C is easily destroyed when they are overcooked or placed in too much hot water. Vitamin C is also affected by exposure to air. It might be wise to take extra vitamin C tablets if you don't get enough fresh orange juice, cantaloupe, strawberries or other fresh fruits, tomatoes, or broccoli—otherwise enough vitamin C is easily supplied by the diet.

The recommended intake of vitamin C is 60 milligrams daily. The requirement is higher during stress. A pregnant woman should not take more than 3000 milligrams daily. Vitamin C is active metabolically and very large doses are potentially dangerous to the fetus.

Vitamin D: This vitamin helps the body make proper use of calcium by absorbing it and building the calcium into the bones and tooth buds of the developing fetus. Vitamin D is made naturally by the body from the exposure of your skin to ultraviolet light (a component of sunlight). People in northern climates, especially those who live in cities where the sun's rays are weakened by city air, need extra vitamin D because they do not get enough sunlight to manufacture their own vitamin D. Because so many people live under these conditions, homogenized milk is regularly fortified with vitamin D to prevent childhood bone disorders. The amount of vitamin D should be clearly listed on the outside of the milk container. Pregnant women who drink milk will get plenty of vitamin D regardless of their skin type (dark-complexioned women need more sunshine to manufacture vitamin D) or their regular exposure to sunlight. Vitamin D is also found in other dairy products and in tuna, sardines, and herrings. A few women may need to supplement their daily intake by vitamin D capsules if, for instance, they are lactose-intolerant.

The daily requirement of vitamin D is approximately 400 IU. This is the amount of vitamin D in a quart of fortified whole milk. Excessive doses can be toxic—it would be wise to restrict your intake to 2000 IU daily.

Vitamin E: Called also tocopherol. E is a somewhat controversial vitamin. There have been studies showing that vitamin E taken in the amount of 800 IU daily can help improve red-cell survival, at least in the face of some blood abnormalities. It is believed that vitamin E can help the body fight infection, and act as a vasodilator and an anticoagulant. It also seems to accelerate the healing of burns in severe cases. Vitamin E is believed to have an important role in reproduction, although at this time studies have been done only on pregnant animals to determine the specific reproductive functions of vitamin E. In experiments on pregnant rats researchers found that a serious lack of vitamin E led to reproductive disorders; the rats suffered destruction of the red blood cells, muscle degeneration, and very high fetal loss. It has been impossible so far to establish a similar pattern in humans. However, vitamin E does have a therapeutic effect on newborn babies—it can be used to correct various forms of anemia associated with low birth weight where abnormalities of platelets are present; and vitamin E in large doses has been given to premature infants to lessen lung damage due to prematurity. In some cases, vitamin E given to the mother seems to protect the baby from neonatal jaundice.

☐ ***What Are the Best Natural Sources?***   The best natural sources are wheat germ, soybeans, vegetable oils, broccoli, Brussels sprouts, leafy greens, spinach, whole wheat and whole-grain cereals and eggs. The daily recommended intake of vitamin E is approximately 400 IU in a normal adult. Pregnant and lactating women or women on the pill or on other hormones need to increase their intake of this vitamin. Vitamin E in large amounts appears to be well tolerated although symptoms of fatigue, headaches, and nausea are occasionally seen.

Vitamin K: This helps the body form the proper blood-clotting mechanism. It is not produced directly from food—instead, the bacteria in the human intestines manufacture it in the digestive process. Normal adult women do not need vitamin K supplementation because it is produced naturally. However, a newborn baby's bowel is sterile, which means that there are not enough bacteria present in the first few days of life to produce the necessary vitamin K, and babies have been known to hemorrhage. This is why newborns are routinely given an injection of vitamin K to hold them over for a few days until they develop enough bacteria by themselves.

☐ *How Much in the Way of Vitamins and Minerals Do the Prenatal Vitamins Contain?*   There are a variety of commercially available prenatal vitamins. Each brand usually has various strengths and concentrations of vitamins and minerals. For comparison, a few of the more commonly prescribed prenatal vitamins are listed below. For further information regarding other brands, please refer to the PDR (*Physician's Desk Reference*), which is available in any public library.

VITAMIN AND MINERAL CONTENT OF PRENATAL VITAMINS

	FILIBON F.A.	MATERNA 1.60	NATABEC RX	NATALINS RX	STUART PRENATAL
Vitamin A	8000 IU	8000 IU	4000 IU	8000 IU	8000 IU
Vitamin D_2	400 IU	400 IU	400 IU	400 IU	400 IU
Vitamin E	30 IU	30 IU	—	30 IU	30 IU
Vitamin C	60 mg	120 mg	50 mg	90 mg	60 mg
Folic Acid	1 mg	1 mg	1 mg	1 mg	0.8 mg
Vitamin B_1	1.7 mg	3 mg	3 mg	2.55 mg	1.7 mg
Vitamin B_2	2 mg	3.4 mg	2 mg	3 mg	2 mg
Niacinamide	20 mg	20 mg	10 mg	20 mg	20 mg
Vitamin B_6	4 mg	4 mg	3 mg	10 mg	4 mg
Vitamin B_{12}	8 mcg	12 mcg	5 mcg	8 mcg	8 mcg
Calcium	250 mg	350 mg	600 mg	200 mg	200 mg
Iodine	150 mcg	0.3 mg	—	150 mcg	150 mcg
Iron	45 mg	60 mg	150 mg	60 mg	60 mg
Magnesium	100 mg	100 mg	—	100 mg	100 mg
Copper	—	2 mg	—	2 mg	—
Zinc	—	15 mg	—	15 mg	—
Docusate Sodium	—	50 mg	—	—	—

☐ *Food Additives and Pregnancy*   It seems wise to cut down on food additives and other substances during pregnancy, even though many of these substances have not specifically been linked to birth defects. Because of the link between nitrosamines and cancer, women at all times should be careful about eating smoked meats and fish and lunch meats.

Processed foods that are high in additives, are, once again, not to be recommended at any time. No one knows at this point how detrimental additives such as BHA and BHT are, but it is a good idea to be cautious. *At all times* it is important to wash fruits and vegetables thoroughly. Unless produce comes from your own or a neighbor's organic garden, you can be sure that the produce has been sprayed. Peeling fruit is another sensible precaution.

☐ *Caffeine and Pregnancy*   Recently the Food and Drug Administration advised pregnant women to cut down or eliminate caffeine-containing products because of some new studies linking the heavy use of caffeine to birth defects. The FDA reached this conclusion after a study was conducted in which pregnant rats were fed very large amounts of caffeine—the equivalent of 12 to 24 cups of coffee a day. This caused serious skeletal defects, limb reduction, missing toes and other abnormalities in their offspring. A lower level of caffeine also had a definite effect: Rats that were fed the equivalent of 2 to 4 cups daily had a significant reduction in weight and size in their offspring. Although there is no a direct link at this time between birth defects and caffeine in humans, the FDA feels that pregnant women should be cautious about their use of caffeine.

Caffeine is one of the substances that freely crosses the placenta and enters the fetal tissues. Experiments on newborns have shown that it is metabolized very slowly. It is also a substance that adult women and men consume with incredible regularity. Caffeine is not found in only tea and coffee—it appears in a wide variety of soft drinks and over-the-counter remedies. A cola soft drink, for instance, contains 50 milligrams of caffeine; one Excedrin tablet contains 60 milligrams; over-the-counter stimulants contain 100 milligrams. By comparison, a cup of tea has about 40 milligrams; instant coffee has about 90; and freshly brewed coffee has about 125 milligrams. Milk chocolate also contains a very small amount of caffeine.

CAFFEINE CONTENT IN OUR FOOD

	CAFFEINE CONTENT
A cup of coffee	75–155 mg
A cup of tea	28–44 mg
A cup of instant coffee (not freeze-dried)	90 mg
A cup of freeze-dried coffee	66 mg
A cola drink	50 mg
An Excedrin tablet	60 mg
Over-the-counter stimulants	100 mg
Milk chocolate—1 square	6 mg
A cup of decaffeinated coffee	3 mg

At the present moment, until the FDA conducts further studies to assess the effects of a "normal" consumption of caffeine in humans, pregnant women are being advised to watch their caffeine consumption, especially in the first three months of pregnancy. Interestingly, this is a time when many women "go off" caffeine naturally because they cannot tolerate it, so abstinence may not be so difficult as you think even if you are a confirmed coffee drinker. If you must drink coffee, use decaffeinated.

17

Smoking and Pregnancy

The incidence of smoking among American women of childbearing years is now higher than it has ever been—just as the incidence of smoking in men is going down. Forty percent of working women over the age of twenty smoke; and teenage girls smoke even more heavily than teenage boys do. More than 26,000 women now die of lung cancer each year—4,000 more women than die of gynecological cancers of all types. This marks a great change, because women, up until a few years ago, smoked far less than men. It also means that we are only just beginning to see the effects of large numbers of women smoking during pregnancy.

Recent figures on women smokers estimate that 30 percent of women continue to smoke while they are pregnant, and a majority resume smoking after childbearing. Unfortunately, when a pregnant woman smokes, it means she is damaging two lives—her own and her baby's! Whatever you inhale—and it is impossible *not* to inhale—is absorbed into your bloodstream and transferred with the blood into the placenta and the umbilical cord. In this way it inevitably reaches the baby, and subtle or dramatic changes can result, depending on the amount you smoke and other factors having to do with your health and pregnancy.

☐ *What Happens if You Smoke During Pregnancy?* Briefly, smoking during pregnancy stunts the baby's growth and possibly diminishes its IQ; it increases the risk of miscarriage; it can cause serious complications in pregnancy and delivery, such as placental separation, which can be fatal; and it increases the chances of a child's dying just before or just after birth. These are the disturbing reports from two decades of studies conducted in many countries throughout the world. One of the largest and most thorough investigations, the

United States Collaborative Perinatal Project, examined more than five thousand pregnancies at twelve major hospital centers in the United States and concluded that smoking during pregnancy produces a long list of risks to the unborn and newborn child. Researchers in this study noted an increased risk of fetal death or damage, a delay in fetal growth, and an increased likelihood of pregnancy-related complications for the mother.

Cigarette smoking involves repetitive exposure to a mixture of potentially harmful teratogenic compounds, such as nicotine, carbon monoxide, hydrogen cyanide, tar, and resins, and potential carcinogens (cancer-causing agents), such as diazobencoptyrene, which can cause mutations. A pregnant woman who smokes twenty cigarettes a day inhales this lethal mixture approximately 11,000 times during the nine months of pregnancy and spends perhaps 10 percent of her day smoking.

☐ *What Causes the Damage from Smoking?*　Extensive research has shown that two major components of smoking play the most significant part in injuring the developing fetus: *nicotine* and *carbon monoxide*.

Smoking produces a large increase of nicotine in the arterial blood supply, which in turn causes constriction of the arteries and veins in the blood-circulation system. The effect of nicotine is not direct but is mediated by a release of the hormones called catecholamines. Studies on animals have shown that nicotine injections cause a drop in blood flow to the uterus and the placenta and a decline in the oxygen supply to the fetus. Furthermore, smoking produces a 25 percent greater decrease in the oxygen supply to the fetus. Several studies in humans have shown a decrease in the placental blood supply as well as in fetal breathing and movements during smoking.

Carbon monoxide is a major component of smoking. The carbon monoxide is absorbed by the pregnant woman and bound to the hemoglobin (red blood cells) to form a relatively stable compound. The carbon monoxide crosses the placenta easily and reduces the oxygen-carrying capability of the fetus, which results in decreased fetal size.

Other potentially harmful components involved in tobacco smoking are: oil, tars, hydrogen cyanide, resin, and diazobenzopyrene, which work in combination with the carbon monoxide.

☐ *Growth Retardation and Smoking*　As early as 1957 there were reports that the children of smoking mothers were an average of 200 grams (7 ounces) lighter and were shorter than those of nonsmokers. However, other contemporary reports disputed this finding, and *no* public emphasis was placed on the danger of smoking during pregnancy until several years later. By the 1970s the situation had entirely changed. No longer could there by any doubt about the connection between lower birth weight and smoking. In study after study it has been found that mothers who smoke are more likely to give birth to underweight babies who are either premature or growth-retarded. The effects of smoking have been found to be directly dose-related. In one study researchers calculated that light smokers (women who smoked under one pack a day) were 30 to 170 percent more likely to give birth to a smaller than average baby, while the children of heavy smokers (over one pack a day) had a 90 to 340 percent higher chance of being growth-retarded! The wide range of percentages is caused by variations in cigarette smoking from woman to woman and other variable factors such as a woman's health.

The most vulnerable women seem to be older women who smoke heavily, have a poor diet, are anemic, and already have several children. A woman in her early twenties who is pregnant for the first time and who enjoys good health and is only a light smoker has, perhaps, a 10–20 percent chance of having a baby who is slightly underweight. These differences explain why some women who still smoke in pregnancy seem to have healthy children. However, a 10–20 percent chance of harming your baby is not worth the risk of continuing to smoke.

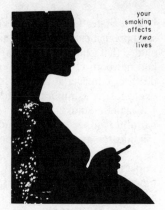

your smoking affects *two* lives

Figure 45: Courtesy of the National Institute of Health and Child Development.

☐ *Why Are Smokers' Babies Smaller?*
Nicotine absorbed into the mother's lungs and from there into the maternal blood flow is passed freely across the placenta and reaches the fetus. By constricting the blood vessels in the baby's developing body, the nicotine diminishes nutrition to the growing fetus and impairs the heart rate, the blood pressure, and the oxygen supply, resulting in a retardation of fetal growth.

The carbon monoxide inhaled during cigarette smoking is even more damaging to the baby's growth. Carbon monoxide reduces the oxygen-carrying capacity of the mother's blood at a time when this capacity would normally increase considerably. To protect itself, as it were, from this deprivation of oxygen, the fetus grows at a slower rate. The more the woman smokes, the greater is the growth retardation. At the same time, curiously, the placental weight remains higher than normal in smokers' pregnancies, presumably to allow more oxygen to reach the fetus. The result of this oxygen starvation is a child who is lighter, shorter, has a smaller head circumference, and may have slight learning disabilities that will become evident later. In many cases these children do not seem to catch up in growth and development as they go through infancy and childhood, and one can presume that they will be shorter and lighter as adults as well.

☐ *The Effect of Smoking on the Baby's Lung Development*   In the months of growth inside the mother's womb the fetus constantly exercises not only its limbs but its immature lungs in preparation for the task of breathing on its own after birth. By 40 weeks, fetal breathing averages about 60 breaths a minute. However, among women who smoke, this breathing pattern is greatly diminished. Specific monitoring of the fetal breathing, using ultrasonography, has shown that the smoking of even one cigarette temporarily depresses fetal breathing because of the powerful effects of the nicotine on the fetal nervous system. A significant reduction in fetal breathing seems to occur within five minutes after the mother starts her first cigarette, and this state appears to last for about an hour. Using this information, we can assume that the consumption of a whole pack of cigarettes would depress fetal breathing movements for a full 18 to 24 hours. Reduced fetal breathing normally indicates fetal distress; extreme stress can result in the death of the baby before birth.

☐ *The Baby's IQ and Smoking*   In several recent studies, including a very extensive one in Britain, groups of children born to mothers who smoked during pregnancy were tested at regular intervals in the years after birth. In general these children were found to have slightly lower IQ scores and lower reading levels than comparable groups of children whose mothers were nonsmokers. The British study concluded that children of mothers who smoked ten or more cigarettes a day during pregnancy were slightly shorter on the average and between three to five months behind in reading, mathematics, and general ability when they were compared with children of nonsmokers. Most of the other studies have shown similar patterns of development. It is only fair to say that one study in the United States does not seem to bear out these differences in intelligence but instead attributes the lower IQs to other factors. In the U.S. study the growth retardation among babies of smoking mothers was still significant.

One new study appears to find a decided and alarming link between smoking and the brain abnormalities we see in hyperkinetic (hyperactive) children. In a study of a group of twenty hyperkinetic children, researchers found that only four of the mothers did not smoke during pregnancy; these women had suffered traumatic deliveries. The rest of the mothers were all heavy smokers. The conclusion of the study strongly suggested that smoking was a decided factor in the appearance of hyperkineticism in children.

These findings, however tentative, should be so alarming to any woman who smokes that she will immediately quit once she becomes pregnant. Even if fetal brain damage is so minimal that it isn't really noticeable in later life, careful observation may still reveal that one child is just a little slower than his or her friends. If smoking causes minimal brain damage, this is one retardation factor that is totally preventable.

Stop smoking, or at least cut down to one or two cigarettes a day during pregnancy. This will assure your child of better health and full intellectual development.

☐ *Behavioral Abnormalities in Newborn Babies of Smoking Mothers*   Recently a group of newborn babies was tested in a hospital nursery in Britain. They were normal newborns whose mothers had smoked more than fifteen cigarettes a day during their pregnancies. Although in many respects the infants showed the responses expected of young babies, as a group their hearing ability was less developed than that of other infants. At the same time, they showed a higher level of irritability and a general lack of interest in their surroundings. The researchers concluded that the behavioral patterns and the hearing ability of infants might indeed be affected by a concentration of carbon monoxide in the prenatal environment.

☐ *Smoking and Birth Defects*   The most widespread aspect of maternal smoking is its adverse effect on the baby's weight gain and general development. There does not seem to be a large increase in congenital malformations among the children of smoking mothers, with one notable exception, namely, damage to the central nervous system. A correlation has been found between smoking and certain *neurotubal defects* such as *spina bifida* and *anencephaly* among the offspring of very heavy smokers. There seemed to be *no* correlation between the mothers' smoking habits and skeletal, gastrointestinal, or genitourinary defects but there does seem to be a higher incidence of *cleft lip* or *cleft palate* in babies of moderate to heavy smokers. Major structural defects seem to appear in those few cases of unusually heavy smokers in which carboxyhemoglobin levels are so concentrated that they exceed those normally found in women who smoke.

The likelihood of structural defects has concerned doctors far less than the threat of miscarriage or growth retardation. However, the later health of the child may be affected by prenatal smoking in ways that we are only just beginning to guess at. A recent investigation has theorized that smoking may damage the major blood vessels and contribute to heart and arterial disease later on in life. Other studies in animals have raised the possibility that exposure to tobacco smoke in the womb may increase the adult's susceptibility to cancer. Cigarette smoke contains several substances that are transplacental carcinogens in animals, including diazobenzopyrene, anthracenes, nitrosamines, hydrazines, and urethane. Although there is no conclusive evidence that human infants are equally susceptible to these substances, it is possible that exposure to transplacental carcinogens may heighten a person's vulnerability to cancer in later life. The risks may be increased if a child is exposed prenatally and postnatally to cigarette smoke. Until a large group of people born to smoking mothers reach middle age—which will not be for a few more years—these questions on the long-term effects of prenatal exposure will probably remain unanswered.

☐ *Pregnancy-Related Complications and Smoking*   Since smoking reduces the blood flow to the placenta, it weakens its structure and may result in its premature separation from the uterine wall. This condition is called abruptio placentae. Abruptio placentae may occur without warning during labor and often results in the death of the fetus or in serious brain damage. This life-threatening emergency is seen far more frequently among women who smoke heavily, and it is possible that 20–25 percent of the cases of abruptio placentae can be directly attributed to smoking. The condition occurs because smoking constricts the arteries in the uterine wall that lead blood into the placenta. Significant decrease in the blood supply may then result in a spasm reaction, and the placenta is shed prematurely.

Another abnormality of the placenta, placenta previa, also appears more frequently in women who smoke. In this case the placenta is attached abnormally low in the womb, leading to complications in labor and birth or to premature labor. Placenta previa is of particular concern because its incidence seems to be directly related to the number of years a woman smoked *before* she became pregnant. An unusual amount of dead tissue also seems to appear on the placenta of women who smoke or used to smoke. These are among the factors that make it very important for a woman to avoid smoking entirely or at least stop smoking years before she plans to have a baby.

Smoking increases the risk of spontaneous abortion, premature birth, and stillbirth. The perinatal death rate—that is, the death of children just before, during, or just after they are born, is 35 percent higher for women who smoke heavily than for women who smoke less than one pack a day. This mortality rate includes spontaneous abortions after the fifth month and deaths among full-term babies.

☐ *Spontaneous Abortion* Smoking may increase the likelihood of spontaneous abortion. One recent study in New York estimated that the risk of spontaneous abortion was 70 percent higher among heavy smokers than among nonsmokers. Again, the risk appeared to be dose-related. Women who smoke also have an increased incidence of irregular bleeding and spotting during pregnancy. Often this is the first sign of an impending miscarriage or of problems during labor.

Many of the deaths associated with maternal smoking are avoidable. They occur in otherwise normal children. Sometimes babies are born prematurely and have related respiratory problems, but there is usually no congenital malformation present. The immediate cause of most smoking-related deaths is placental complications and bleeding. In other cases the oxygen supply simply seems to fail from reduced carrying capacity because of the presence of carbon monoxide in maternal and fetal blood. Since there is usually nothing congenitally wrong with these babies, their deaths would, presumably, be averted if women did not smoke during pregnancy.

☐ *Are SIDS and Smoking Connected?* Recently the Collaborative Perinatal Project found a direct relation between *sudden infant death syndrome* (SIDS) and maternal smoking, although smoking does not seem to be the most significant factor in SIDS. Smoking appears to contribute to amniotic-fluid bacterial infection and to anemia in the mother, both of which appear to place the infant at risk. Researchers have also noted the effects of cigarette smoke on infants, especially when children already have respiratory problems, as so many SIDS babies do. Two doctors researching the causes of SIDS deaths began to investigate parental smoking habits when they noticed the amount of cigarette smoke at meetings of parents who had lost children to SIDS and found that a significant number of SIDS parents were heavy smokers. Whether prenatal or postnatal exposure to smoking is more important cannot be determined, although, as I have said, these are believed to be only contributory factors in the incidence of SIDS deaths. Even so, SIDS is one of the saddest events that can happen in a couple's life, and the evidence should encourage every pregnant woman to stop smoking immediately.

☐ *Passive Smoking—The Effect of Tobacco Even if You Don't Smoke* Your friends, family, and coworkers who smoke should be aware that you are inhaling carbon monoxide from their cigarettes even if you are not smoking yourself. The effects of passive smoking can be very damaging if a pregnant woman is constantly exposed to cigarettes. In one case study a group of women who were not smoking themselves were so heavily exposed to cigarette smoke at home that their children exhibited the classic growth-retardation pattern of the children of smoking mothers. If someone in your family feels he or she must smoke, ask that person to confine smoking to one particular area, so you will have at least one or two smoke-free rooms in your house or apartment.

After the baby is born try to establish the same carbon monoxide-free atmosphere for your child. A child inhales smoke passively when you or another family member smokes. A new study in Boston testing children aged five to nine whose parents smoked found that these children had definitely impaired breathing abilities. Breathing motions and gas exchange were affected. This condition was worsened if both parents smoked. Other studies have linked heavy parental smoking to a higher incidence of childhood lung diseases, including bronchitis and pneumonia. Children thus affected were found to spend more time in hospitals and had a higher death rate from diseases such as pneumonia than children whose parents did not smoke.

☐ *Alcohol and Smoking*   There is strong evidence that smoking and alcohol each have a detrimental effect on the growing baby. However, when both cigarettes and alcohol are combined, the chance of congenital malformations, miscarriages, or other damage is accentuated. The combination of alcohol and tobacco also adds to the probability that a woman is not eating properly, increasing the risks to the baby even further. In cases in which babies are born after a double exposure to nicotine and alcohol, growth retardation or birth defects seem even more pronounced than in instances in which alcohol or tobacco appear alone. Try not to mix alcohol and tobacco, even at a low level, especially in the first trimester.

☐ *Smoking and Breast-Feeding*   Women who smoke should know that the nicotine in their bloodstream is excreted in the maternal milk. The nicotine is passed to the baby through the milk. If the concentration is heavy enough the nicotine constricts the vascular system, and the baby may experience slower growth than a normal child. Furthermore, the nicotine may have a stimulating effect on the baby, diminishing its appetite. Eventually this will restrict growth considerably. It has been theorized that a nicotine infusion of this kind can lead to neonatal death or sudden infant death syndrome (SIDS) if the baby is not fed frequently enough to keep the nicotine level at a steady state.

Significantly lower levels of vitamin C have been found in the milk of women who smoke. This lack of vitamin C may damage the fetus prenatally and cannot be corrected by supplementing the mother. Women who are heavy smokers and cannot give up smoking should, perhaps, consider the option of not breast-feeding, since this may do more harm than good to the baby.

☐ *Why Smoke During Pregnancy?*   Remember, when a woman smokes, so does her baby! Why pregnant women still continue to smoke is a complex question and involves physiological and pharmacological factors. Many women, pregnant or not, are dependent on smoking for stimulation. Other women smoke only because they can't break a bad habit. Recent evidence indicates that nicotine dependence may be a very important factor in a woman's inability to give up smoking. In a series of experiments nicotine was infused into adult men, and the number of cigarettes consumed fell as the nicotine infusion increased. People who chew nicotine-infused chewing gum also find they reduce their cigarette smoking. This recent confirmation of the dependence factor in smoking makes it easier to understand why so many women who are genuinely alarmed by the harmful effects of smoking in pregnancy still find it so difficult to stop.

Pregnancy is a time when a woman is both highly motivated to quit smoking and emotionally vulnerable to the old reassurance of cigarettes. She can find herself in the middle of a battleground in which she is pulled two ways—one way by her conscience and the pressure of her family and friends, who keep telling her to give up smoking, and the other by the tension induced by the tremendous physical and emotional changes and the new concerns about managing her life after the baby is born. One dictates that she give up smoking, the other increases her dependence on it.

Help should come from people at work, from friends, husbands, other family members, and also from doctors and other health professionals. Many doctors, unfortunately, don't warn women in time about the dangers of smoking, because they feel unable to effect any useful change in their patients' habits. I hope in this chapter to compensate in part for such neglect by helping you understand the dangers to which you and your baby are exposed if you continue smoking.

Many women do give up smoking—at least during the time they are pregnant. It has been estimated that about 75 percent of smokers stop smoking during pregnancy, although the majority of them resume after the baby is born.

□ *Quitting During Pregnancy*   When a woman who smokes heavily gives up smoking or cuts down considerably by the beginning of the second trimester, she avoids the most common complication of smoking in pregnancy—the low-birth-weight child. The main stages of a child's growth, physically and mentally, take place after the fourth month, and so this growth is not affected if the mother has given up smoking. Other complications, unfortunately, are not necessarily avoided. The risk of placenta previa is directly related to the number of years a woman has smoked; it is not reversible as soon as she quits. However, the chance of a premature delivery or late miscarriage is considerably reduced, because without nicotine and carbon monoxide, the baby's environment in the womb is far more favorable to the continuance of pregnancy. If you are pregnant now and are still smoking, it is not too late to stop. I would urge you to do so!

□ *Talk to Your Obstetrician*   Your obstetrician should ask you about your smoking habits when you make your first prenatal visit. You may be reluctant to discuss the whole subject with him because you are ashamed of your dependency on tobacco and nervous about its effects on the baby. It is, however, important to talk with him frankly; a good obstetrician, a man or woman who cares for his or her patients, will undoubtedly try to help you. This help should go beyond pointing out the adverse effects of smoking and using scare tactics to get you to stop smoking. You already know some of the horror stories. What you need is his advice and encouragement. Many smokers have said they would quit smoking if only their doctors encouraged them to do so. It is the responsibility of every doctor to help his patients conquer habits that are destructive to themselves or others.

18

Alcohol—The Most Dangerous Drug?

Alcohol acts as a powerful depressant on the central nervous system and will adversely affect almost every organ in the body if drunk in large quantities. Besides damaging the liver and poisoning the brain, alcohol addiction leads to emotional and psychological disasters that have ruined family life for many people. But there is also increasing evidence that alcohol can cause other life-threatening problems. A recent study has shown that the risk of a major stroke is increased three times for men under forty who are alcoholics and three to four times for women alcoholics. Acute alcohol intoxication has not been previously recognized as a risk factor for stroke in young adults.

Unfortunately a very large group of people in the United States are seriously addicted to alcohol, including more than one million women of childbearing age, and their number seems to be increasing.

☐ *Alcohol and Pregnancy*   Until a few years ago the effect of heavy alcohol consumption on the fetus was only guessed at, because most doctors still believed that the placenta had the ability to screen out toxins from the mother's bloodstream before they reached the baby. Now we know that any alcohol a pregnant woman consumes reaches the baby in the same concentration that is found in her own bloodstream. In other words, every time she has a beer or a glass of wine, the baby is drinking too. With heavy alcohol use, the fetus can be very seriously affected, both mentally and physically.

In the late 1970s pregnant women were suddenly alerted to the danger of alcohol consumption in pregnancy when the media reported new findings on the fetal alcohol syndrome (FAS). FAS is a distinctive group of birth defects that affects the children of alcoholic mothers. Some major studies in the United States confirmed the dangerous effects of alcohol on the developing fetus and questioned the wisdom of drinking at all during pregnancy.

"Can I drink?" is a question that patients now commonly ask their obstetricians. Because this is a matter of much concern, a full understanding of the implications of drinking during pregnancy is essential for any woman who is pregnant or is about to become pregnant. Pregnancy is an important time for a woman to evaluate—and perhaps change—her drinking habits, even if she drinks only occasionally.

□ **What Happened in the Past? Was Drinking in Pregnancy Always a Problem?** Two thousand years ago people already understood that there was some link between heavy drinking and the birth of malformed children, even though the precise reason for it was unknown. In the biblical story of Samson, the angel commands his mother, "Behold, thou shalt conceive, and bear a son; and now drink no wine nor strong drink . . ." (Judges 13:7). An ancient Greek custom forebade the bride and groom to drink wine at the wedding feast to prevent the conception of a child when the parents were intoxicated, and Aristotle observed that "drunken women bring forth children like unto themselves." The same observation was made periodically during the next two thousand years. At the height of the gin fever in London in the 1720s, when poor Londoners, including thousands of women, became addicted to cheap gin, the London College of Physicians cited it as a "cause of weak, feeble, and distempered children," and a contemporary writer described children who "often looked shrivel'd and old as though they had numbered many years."

But the first scientific observation on alcohol-related growth and developmental abnormalities did not appear until 1849, when Dr. William Carpenter of London was awarded a prize for his essay, "The Use and Abuse of Alcoholic Liquor in Health and Disease." In this study he described instances of mental disability in the offspring of alcoholic parents and quoted a contemporary authority, W. A. F. Brown, the resident physician of a lunatic asylum, who had this to say about the habitual drunkard: "His daughters are nervous and hysterical. His sons are weak, wayward, eccentric, and sink insane under the pressure of excitement of some unforeseen exigency in the ordinary call of duty." (Interestingly, researchers now suspect there may be a link between alcoholic fathers and birth defects in their children.)

Aldous Huxley made ingenious use of the connection between brain damage and alcohol. If you have read his *Brave New World*, you may remember Bernard Marx, the Alpha Plus who is a misfit in the ordered and happy world of assembly line humans. The rumor in his conditioning center is that Bernard's "strangeness," he is small and ugly and likes to spend time by himself, was the result of an unfortunate error when a careless laboratory technician dropped alcohol into his test tube before he was decanted (the new method of birth), thinking he was a lower class Gamma.

Huxley wrote *Brave New World* in 1930, long before any of the modern studies on alcohol and the fetus were published.

Contemporary research on the effects of alcohol was encouraged by a German study published in 1957. This clinical report by a group of scientists found behavioral abnormalities and structural deformities in the infants of mothers who were heavy drinkers. A research paper was subsequently published by Dr. Lemoine in France, who observed in 1968 that newborns of mothers who were alcoholics had signs of behavioral abnormalities and were congenitally malformed in the more severe cases. Lemoine reported that these children had delayed physical and mental development, language abnormalities, and an IQ that was below normal.

Although these first reports on alcohol's impact on pregnancy were released from Europe, American researchers were the first to use the phrase "fetal alcohol syndrome" and clearly describe this syndrome, which was popularized in the United States by Drs. Ulleland and Jones. In 1972 Dr. Ulleland reported on his findings: newborns whose mothers were alcoholics had a smaller head circumference, were smaller on the average in weight, and had delayed growth after birth. This work was followed by a five-year study of women in the Boston City Hospital. By the end of the 1970s there was no doubt that the fetal alcohol syndrome existed, and the harmful relationship of pregnancy and alcohol was widely publicized in the American press.

☐ **The Fetal Alcohol Syndrome (FAS)**   This is termed a syndrome because certain characteristics have been found to appear in a large number of cases. The baby is born with a small head size (microcephaly), low birth weight, distinct facial characteristics—a short, upturned nose with a flat surface across its bridge, small eye openings, and a receding jaw. There is damage to the central nervous system. Many of the babies are mentally retarded, some mildly, some severely. The physical and mental retardation persists after birth, and these babies often fail to thrive and remain physically smaller and more backward than other children. There are often abnormalities in the internal organs, with discernible damage to the heart and the kidneys. Cleft palate is another common defect associated with FAS. Often the effects of very high levels of alcohol are so threatening that a pregnancy ends in miscarriage: 70 percent of the alcoholic mothers in the Boston City Hospital study were found to have a history of spontaneous abortions. Many of these women drank from 8 to 16 ounces of absolute alcohol a day, or, to put it in more familiar terms, about a quart of vodka a day.

Babies may be born with a full spectrum of FAS-related defects. In most cases, however, only some of the characteristic symptoms of FAS are present. The children of severely alcoholic mothers—not surprisingly—are most likely to exhibit the full syndrome. Sometimes a child has only a slight neurological impairment or seems jittery or hyperactive. Because no major birth defect exists, it does not preclude abnormalities in growth and development or "just" a small but discernible lowering of the IQ level.

Researchers feel that as a pregnancy progresses, heavy drinking will have different effects on the fetus. In the first trimester, alcohol attacks the cell membranes and the fetal organ system. This is the most likely time for congenital abnormalities to occur, because the nervous system and the major organs are being formed. Drinking heavily in the prepregnancy period is particularly dangerous. In one group of women, 11 percent of mothers who drank heavily in the month before they realized they were pregnant had babies with FAS symptoms. Heavy drinking in the later months is linked with growth deficiencies, impairment of brain functioning, and behavioral development. Women who stop drinking altogether or at least cut down considerably in the last trimester have a good chance of giving birth to a child with normal growth and brain development.

Several animal studies have shown that the blood level of alcohol is the best indicator of the damage to the fetus. When the alcohol concentration is at a very high level the risk of congenital abnormalities is also high. With a lower level the effects on the fetus are lessened.

☐ *How Common Is the Fetal Alcohol Syndrome?*   Unfortunately it is quite common. Estimates in the United States range from one case in 600 births to one in 1500. It is certainly one of the nation's leading causes of mental retardation, together with Down's syndrome and neural-tube defects.

☐ *FDA Warning*   Recently the Food and Drug Administration asked the Treasury Department to place a warning label on liquor bottles advising women of the risks of heavy alcohol consumption during pregnancy. A final decision has not yet been made. At present the Treasury Department and the FDA have begun a campaign to educate the public on this issue and are waiting to see the results of the campaign before proceeding with a warning label.

☐ *Has the Type of Alcohol Something to Do with FAS?*   It appears from the studies that there is no distinction to be drawn between beer, wine, or spirits. The type of alcohol ingested by the mother is immaterial; the total amount of alcohol consumed is the crucial factor. Researchers working with laboratory animals have found that they can produce a fetal alcohol syndrome in baby rats which is strikingly similar to the syndrome in humans simply by dosing the mothers with pure alcohol. When the dose is increased the symptoms become more severe.

☐ *What About Nutrition and the Fetal Alcohol Syndrome?*   Because women who drink heavily tend to have poor diets, it has been suggested that specific nutritional deficiencies in association with alcohol consumption are a contributing factor in fetal alcohol syndrome. Some investigators have suggested that the effect on the fetus would be modified if a woman's nutrition was improved. However, the children of poorly nourished mothers who do not drink do not show the characteristic birth defects of FAS children, even though both groups are underweight for their age. In Denmark during World War II, for instance, pregnant women were severely malnourished, and their babies were born underweight, but there was no recognizable increase in the frequency of birth defects during that time. The same observation has been made in other countries in which the food supply is inadequate. The fetal effect of malnutrition is clearly different from that of alcohol.

☐ *Smoking and FAS*   Many of the alcoholic mothers in the Boston City Hospital study also smoked up to two packs of cigarettes a day. This is not unusual among women who drink heavily. Some researchers into FAS believe that other substances frequently ingested during pregnancy, such as nicotine, may contribute to the appearance of the syndrome in babies. FAS, they feel, may be the result of interacting factors, because similar birth defects have been seen in the children of women who took certain drugs during pregnancy but did not use alcohol. Other researchers dispute this, and studies are still continuing.

☐   **What Does "Heavy Drinking" Mean?**   The FDA has concluded from the recent evidence on FAS that six drinks a day constitute a major risk to the developing fetus. A "drink" is defined as one 5-ounce glass of wine, one 12-ounce can of beer, one mixed drink, or 1 ounce of rye, Scotch, bourbon, rum, or gin. Two drinks can also be thought of as 1 ounce of absolute alcohol. This means that a woman who drinks 3 ounces of absolute alcohol a day, or *sometimes* has as many as six drinks at one time, is endangering her baby.

☐   **What Can We Do to Prevent FAS?**   The saddest aspect of FAS is that it severely cripples babies although it is totally preventable. When a woman has a drinking problem, she should be encouraged to get help from her doctor or from a counseling center before she becomes pregnant. If she doesn't have the resources or the strength to do this initially, therapy during pregnancy can still be very helpful. Pioneering alcoholism programs in prenatal clinics have already enabled women to control or cut out alcohol completely through sympathetic counseling. Women who conquer their alcohol habit before their third trimester usually have larger and healthier babies than those born to women who continue to drink heavily.

If someone in your family or among your friends is planning to have a child or is already pregnant and is drinking too much, try to help her find counseling. Encourage her to talk with her doctor. Sometimes, unfortunately, a doctor neglects to ask a patient whether she needs special help even if he suspects that something is wrong, or he may not be alerted to a drinking problem in time. It is encouraging that doctors, therapists, and counselors often have good results with women who are pregnant because they are highly motivated to change their lives for the sake of their unborn children.

☐   **Would One Drink Harm My Baby?**
This is a difficult question to answer at this time because researchers are only beginning to collect data on women who are not heavy drinkers. However, based on the current findings, the FDA feels that even *moderate* drinking may carry an increased risk for growth and developmental abnormalities.

In one recent study investigators from the University of Washington observed newborn babies in a hospital in Seattle. These were normal newborns whose mothers' drinking patterns had been recorded by the hospital during their pregnancies. According to their observations, the babies of mothers whose consumption averaged at least 1 ounce of pure alcohol a day seemed to be more wakeful but less alert than other babies. They appeared more nervous and jittery and

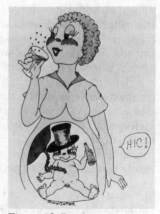

Figure 46: *Drinking During Pregnancy:* When you drink, your baby drinks too.

tended to turn their heads to the left instead of the right, which is unusual in newborns. This may indicate some neurological damage. The researchers also found that the babies scored lower on tests measuring their reflexes and their responses to sounds or visual stimuli. An earlier study found that 19 percent of infants born to a group of mothers who had more than four drinks a day showed abnormalities in growth and development. Ten percent of the babies in the same study whose mothers took two to four drinks daily during *early pregnancy* showed a pattern of abnormalities similar to those found in FAS children, although somewhat milder.

Since the present evidence is definitely disturbing, a woman who is pregnant should be cautious about how much she drinks, particularly in the first three months. Consequently I would advise you not to drink or to drink only occasionally during the time you are trying to conceive and for the rest of the first trimester. This will eliminate the risk of alcohol's affecting the developing fetus. After that an occasional drink or two is unlikely to do any harm when a pregnant woman has a good diet. Don't exceed a limit of two mixed drinks or two 5-ounce glasses of wine or two 12-ounce cans of beer a day, and don't "save up" drinks and then drink five or six at a time. "Binge drinking" is even more suspect than steady drinking because the peak blood-alcohol concentration is probably the most crucial factor in producing congenital malformations, especially in the first trimester.

Many women find they stop drinking alcohol naturally in the first trimester. This may be another example of the body setting up its own defenses against harmful substances in the early weeks, since women who smoke often experience this too.

So far the FDA has not established a safe level for alcohol consumption in pregnancy, although it would not absolutely advise against alcohol, based on the available evidence. A pregnant woman who is uneasy about the risks involved would be well advised to give up drinking altogether.

☐ ***Don't Mix Alcohol and Other Drugs*** Whether you are pregnant or not, *never* combine alcohol and other drugs, including aspirin. It can be dangerous. The enzyme in the liver that breaks down alcohol also breaks down other drugs. They then compete for the enzyme, neither is broken down with normal speed, and their combined dangerous effects are heightened. This phenomenon is called *synergism*. This interaction of alcohol and other substances can cause far more serious symptoms than either the amount of alcohol alone or the drugs alone would. Drinking also lowers the safe limits of many medications. Sleeping pills, sedatives, pain-killers, and cold medications all depress the central nervous system just as alcohol does, so their combination means a double depressant. Particularly dangerous drugs from this point of view are narcotics, barbiturates, sleeping pills, and major tranquilizers such as Valium. Antihistamines, cold-relieving drugs, and motion-sickness drugs can also produce serious side effects when they are combined with alcohol.

☐ ***How to Get Help*** When drinking is out of control, it affects the basic realities of life, health, physical safety, emotional well-being, family and personal relationships, work, and a family's financial situation. Alcoholism is an illness that is suffered by 10 million Americans of all ages and professions. But it is a treatable condition. A woman can get help from women's centers, mental health agencies, her own doctor (doctors are a neglected but often good source of counseling), and from Alcoholics Anonymous (AA), which has done an excellent job in forming groups throughout the country to help people with their drinking problems. You can write to the National Clearing House for Alcohol Information, Box 2345, Rockville, Maryland, 20852, for information on self-help and counseling groups in specific locations. Relevant names and addresses can also be found in the local telephone directory.

☐ *What About an Alcohol Infusion to Delay Labor?*   Alcohol blocks the release of oxytocin from the brain and relaxes the uterus. Alcohol drips have been used for many years to prevent premature labor and enable a woman to carry her pregnancy until the fetus is viable. Many of the babies have been followed up later in life, and the studies have shown no significant difference between the babies of women who were given an alcohol drip for a short time and those who were not. This is probably because alcohol given in premature labor cases is administered for only one or two days during the second and third trimesters, and the women are usually well nourished.

☐ *Can You Take a Drink to Check If You Are in Labor?*   Many doctors and Lamaze instructors recommend a glass of wine or a mixed drink once patients think they are in labor. This is because in a case of false labor the alcohol will stop the contractions, but once labor has really begun, a drink will have no effect. Elisabeth Bing, the most noted of the Lamaze practitioners in the United States, also recommends a glass of wine or spirits to relax the pregnant woman in early labor. The test to detect the status of labor is still a recommended one. A drink or two this late in pregnancy should not affect the baby in any significant way.

☐ *Nursing and Alcohol Consumption: Be Careful!*   A large intake of alcohol in association with breast-feeding is not a good combination. When you drink alcohol, it goes right to the baby via your milk. However, there is no problem with an occasional drink—a cocktail, a glass of wine, or a beer—when you are nursing. It may actually relax you and help to bring the milk down.

A heavy, steady consumption of alcohol in any form can be detrimental to the breast-fed child. One case was recently reported in which a mother who drank seven cans of beer daily and a large amount of hard liquor was breast-feeding a little girl. The baby developed some bizarre symptoms, including a moon-shaped facial appearance, a high level of blood glucose, and extra body fat. The woman's milk was tested, and her doctors found that the baby was, in effect, being alcohol-fed. Once the woman stopped drinking, the baby's facial appearance gradually returned to normal and the other symptoms also disappeared.

Occasionally an otherwise conscientious nursing mother goes to a party, has a great time, and forgets that the alcohol is going straight to her milk. I know of one case in which a baby was completely knocked out by the aftereffects of a New Year's Eve party and slept for nine hours without waking. Fortunately no harm was done, but the mother was terribly frightened. Always stay away from large amounts of alcohol if you are breast-feeding.

By all means, have an occasional drink when you are nursing, but remember that the same rules of moderation apply to the weeks or months of breast-feeding as to the months of pregnancy.

19

Drugs and Pregnancy

Pregnancy is usually a memorable and joyful time for a woman and her family, a time when a couple feels happy, confident, secure, and proud—proud of being able to conceive and happy about creating a new human being and sharing the development of a new life. In spite of all the pleasures and happy moments parents experience during pregnancy, they still worry at times about the health and well-being of their unborn child. Once their baby is safely delivered, fathers and mothers often look back with amusement at the sudden moments of anxiety they experienced during pregnancy when they felt sure something was "wrong," even though they had no apparent reason to suspect an abnormality. And there is no doubt that natural parental anxieties have been fueled by the recent alarm over a woman's exposure to drugs and other toxic agents during pregnancy.

The seemingly endless reports on one or another medical or environmental hazard are often so troubling that many patients ask me anxiously about some medication taken early in pregnancy, even if the drug in question is only aspirin. Other patients want to know whether medications their husbands took around the time of conception could possibly cause harm to the baby. These are not irrelevant questions. People are right to be alarmed about drug use during pregnancy, especially because fetal tolerance is so different from that of a child or an adult. This makes it very difficult to estimate the effect of any drug on an unborn child. In fact, much of the necessary research still remains to be done, although our knowledge is increasing.

☐ *Is There Any Safe Drug?*   In a sense there is no such substance as a safe drug during pregnancy, although in many cases no adverse effects have been noted from drug use. Nevertheless this does not mean to say a safe drug does not exist; it simply means that evidence either way is lacking. What happens when a woman is pregnant and apparently needs a particular drug? The rule of thumb among medical professionals is that *no drug should be given to a pregnant woman unless it is necessary for her health or for the well-being of the fetus.* This means that each time a doctor writes a prescription during pregnancy he must weigh the drug's benefit to the mother against its known or suspected effects on the fetus. This sounds more frightening than it often is in practice, because drugs can be used that do not seem to pose a significant risk to the baby. Usually a doctor likes to prescribe a drug that has been around for many years and has proven to be reasonably safe for use during pregnancy. A drug that has just been put on the market is always questionable inasmuch as it has not been tested on a large number of unborn children. The thalidomide case in particular confirmed the wisdom of this unwritten rule. There were plenty of alternative tranquilizers on the market which had been used for years. Although no tranquilizer can be prescribed safely, none of the alternative drugs had the incredible teratogenic potential of thalidomide.

☐ *Are Drugs Responsible for Most Birth Defects?*   The answer, at this point, seems to be no. Genetic factors are probably responsible for more birth defects than environmental or drug-related factors, even when we include tobacco and alcohol in the drug category. Chromosomal abnormalities appear to account for approximately 20 percent of all major malformations, and disorders of multifactorial inheritance (caused by several genetic factors) are said to cause another 30 percent. Estimates of the effects of environmental factors are as low as 8 percent and as high as 40 percent. Many researchers believe that birth defects are often due to a combination of causes—the result, perhaps, of a defective gene and exposure from a toxic substance or substances—which makes it very difficult in many cases to pinpoint the exact cause of a birth defect.

Since other factors are more likely to produce birth defects, you should not overreact to the issue of drugs in pregnancy. Instead of simply alarming yourself over your past or present use of drugs, take some positive steps. Try to inform yourself about the safety of different drugs. Do not be afraid to question your doctor if he prescribes a drug for you. Never prescribe a drug for yourself. And never take any drug that has been found to be unsafe.

☐ *What Is the Patient's Responsibility?*   As soon as you realize you are pregnant, or better still, even before you become pregnant (see Chap. 2), carefully evaluate your environment and your regular drug therapy. Your present drugs, and any alternative drugs, should be carefully evaluated and a decision made as to the therapy best for you during pregnancy. If your doctor is not an expert on the effects of drugs on the fetus, he or she can usually get the required information through professional resources.

Immediately after you become pregnant, or even before you become pregnant, change your life-style to eliminate the obvious hazards of smoking and drinking. If you are in the habit of using hashish or cannabis or any other social drugs, don't do so while you are pregnant. The effects of social drugs on the fetus are as yet unknown, but we must assume that they could be harmful to the baby, especially if you use them often. Never take any medication from a friend unless you know it's a safe over-the-counter drug.

This cautious approach to drugs applies to minor health problems as well as major ones. Here is an example. At the beginning of pregnancy you might find yourself with a cold or sore throat you can't get rid of and feel you would like some medication because the cold is making you so miserable. But even if you only suspect you are pregnant, be very explicit when you call your doctor to get a prescription. *Always inform him you are pregnant or think you may be pregnant.* Don't simply ask for your usual prescription and don't allow your doctor to pre-scribe your normal medication for you automatically. If you are still in doubt after you receive a prescription because you know that somewhere—in a newspa-per story perhaps—you have seen the safety of the drug questioned, do not hesi-tate to bring this up with your doctor.

Remember, if you can possibly do without a drug during pregnancy, do so. The best course is to take no medications at all and to avoid social drugs. If you do need medication, and if you have been assured by your doctor that a drug is safe *and* you have verified its safety yourself, you are reasonably sure in assuming that the benefits to you probably outweigh the risks to the baby. Many, many drugs have been used for years without, apparently, harming the unborn child. Just be sure that the decision is an honest and informed one.

☐ *How to Look Up the Safety of a Drug*   Later on in this chapter you will find an updated review of the known hazards of various commonly used drugs, both prescription and nonprescription. This list is not, however, comprehensive, simply because of reasons of space. If you want to check the side effects of a drug yourself, go to your local public library and consult a copy of the *Physicians' Desk Reference.* This lists generic and brand-name drugs and gives their known effects on the fetus and the pregnant woman. Entries include references to re-cent studies on the safety of drugs during pregnancy and explicit warnings wher-ever drug use appears to be questionable or dangerous.

☐ *Nonprescription Drugs*   Never take a nonprescription drug without checking with your doctor first. Self-medication is absolutely contraindicated in pregnancy. Many nonprescription drugs have not been clinically tested for use in pregnancy, and a few are known to be harmful, especially when taken in large doses. Who would have thought, a few years back, that common aspirin would be suspected of causing bleeding disorders in labor?

☐ *The Doctor's Role*   There is evidence that drug use in pregnancy is far greater than most people suppose, even after the adverse publicity of the last few years. When a group of patients was recently asked about their drug use in preg-nancy, almost 95 percent of them reported receiving seven to ten different drugs during the prenatal period, including the drugs used in labor and delivery. One patient in this group told researchers she took thirty-two different drug products, nonprescription as well as prescription, while she was pregnant. A woman who takes such an enormous variety of drugs is guilty of self-medication as well as abusing prescription drugs, but obstetricians themselves don't have a good record in this area. The majority of obstetrical patients appear to receive at least three to five drug prescriptions during pregnancy, including prenatal vitamins, an average that suggests that their doctors are not using the proper restraint in many instances.

However, some doctors have reacted so strongly to the evidence that drugs cross the placenta and may damage the fetus that they have become almost too conservative about drug use in pregnancy. Concern about malpractice suits as well as the health of the fetus means they may refuse to prescribe any drugs at all for the pregnant woman, even vitamins. This is an understandable but possibly damaging overreaction and may cause harm in cases in which medication really is indicated. Instead of outlawing drug use altogether, I believe a doctor must try to have a balanced attitude.

One important way a doctor can protect his patients and himself is to discuss the pros and cons of different drugs with his patients and make sure that the patient and her partner are completely informed of the risks they run in using a particular drug. If a woman feels that her doctor's advice is endangering her child or the doctor seems completely insensitive to the issue of teratology, it is her right to find another physician immediately.

☐ **The Legal Position**   Physicians may be liable for failure to inform pregnant patients of the possible risks to the fetus. Legislation in New York State now requires physicians and nurse midwives to inform the expectant mother of the drugs they intend to administer during pregnancy and childbirth and explain their possible effects. This law was passed in 1978 after one woman brought suit against her obstetrician for inducing labor with oxytocin, which, according to her and her lawyers, resulted in significant brain damage to her son. As a result of this legislation we can expect physicians who take care of pregnant women to give them full information on drug use during pregnancy and delivery.

☐ **FDA Labeling on Drugs**   Because of the increased publicity regarding the safety of drugs taken during pregnancy, the Food and Drug Administration now requires that all available information on teratogenicity and other adverse effects appear on an insert with prescription drugs that may be used during pregnancy. Drugs with a recognized use during labor and delivery must also list their effects on the mother and child. The FDA has established five categories indicating a drug's potential for causing birth defects. Category X lists drugs that are absolutely contraindicated in pregnancy because they are associated with fetal abnormalities and their risks clearly outweigh their benefits.

☐ **Men Should Be Warned as Well**   Men should also be warned against drug use near the time of conception. There is a growing body of evidence to suggest that paternal drug absorption can affect the outcome of the pregnancy. For example, there is evidence that babies born to fathers who take antiseizure drugs for epilepsy have an increased incidence of malformation. The same adverse effects have been found in male animals exposed to morphine and other narcotics before pregnancy, and LSD use has been linked to alterations in the chromosomal arrangement of the male sperm, leading to miscarriages and, perhaps, an increased likelihood of anencephaly in the offspring of its users.

A man should review his prescription-drug use with his doctor to discover any known mutagenic side effects of his medication several months before he and his wife plan to conceive. In exactly the same way, he too may be able to modify or change his therapy to make a healthy conception possible. Remember, changes in medications should be made at least three months before conception, because traces of drugs can be found in the sperm for a long time. Social drugs should also be used with great moderation during this period. (See Chapter 2 on the effects of various substances on male fertility and more advice on male drug use during conception.)

In any instance in which a couple use a potentially dangerous drug at the time of conception, they should not be afraid to discuss the whole matter thoroughly with their doctor. Your doctor can usually give you information on the teratogenic effects of a drug or refer you to an expert for genetic counseling. In all probability your doctor will be able to reassure you about the side effects of your drug use, although in a very few cases he might want to discuss the advisability of continuing the pregnancy.

☐ *Commonly Used, and Abused, Drugs*   At some point your doctor may prescribe a drug for you or you may wonder about the safety of drugs you already have in your medicine cabinet. The following list is not comprehensive, but it does include drugs that are widely prescribed or used during pregnancy. By consulting this reference guide you can check the safety of some common drugs for yourself.

☐ *Alcohol*   See Chapter 18 for a full discussion of alcohol use during pregnancy. Alcohol is a drug and as such should be treated with caution by the pregnant woman.

☐ *Allergy Drugs*   There are a large number of allergy drugs, which are also referred to as antihistamines. They include: *Actifed, Benadryl, Chlor-Trimeton* (12 mg), *Dimetapp Extentabs, Optimine,* and *Sudafed.*

Actifed is a widely prescribed antihistamine, but its effect on the fetus has not been established, and its use cannot be recommended during pregnancy. *Benadryl* is safe to use in the second and third trimesters but should not be prescribed in the first trimester because one study has indicated a connection between Benadryl use and an increased incidence of cleft palate. No studies are available on the effects of *Chlor-Trimeton* on the fetus; this drug has not been linked to the appearance of congenital malformations. The absence of the proper studies means that Chlor-Trimeton should be used with caution during pregnancy. *Dimetapp Extentabs* contain *brompheniramine,* which presents an increased risk of malformations in the fetus and should not be used by a pregnant woman. *Optimine* and *Sudafed* are two other drugs whose safety in pregnancy has not been established, and Optimine's atropinelike action makes it inadvisable for use in patients with hypertension.

Caution: All allergy drugs should be avoided during breast-feeding because they enter the breast milk and may prevent lactation.

☐ *Amphetamines*   Benzedrine, Biphetamine, Dexedrine: Appetite-suppressant drugs should not be used during pregnancy. At a time when nutrition is so important there is no reason to control your appetite by taking drugs. In addition, amphetamines can have serious side effects during pregnancy. Animal studies show that amphetamines may cause cleft palate and heart defects in the fetus when taken in the first trimester. Amphetamines have been extensively abused, and this has resulted in drug dependence and intoxication. Control of narcolepsy is perhaps the only reason for using amphetamines during pregnancy.

☐ *Analgesics*   Prescription drugs (*codeine, Darvon, Demerol*): The safety of *codeine* use during pregnancy has not been established, and there may be adverse effects on fetal development. Codeine compounds should, therefore, not be used except with great care and under special circumstances. Caution is also recommended with *Darvon* and other prescription pain-killers. Always consult with your doctor first before using any prescription pain-killers already in your medicine cabinet.

Prescription analgesics, particularly *Demerol*, are widely used in labor and delivery. For a full discussion of this important subject, see Chapter 27.

Nonprescription pain-killers: The most widely used are the salicylates (aspirin). *Aspirin* use may be potentially harmful during pregnancy under certain conditions, especially if consumption is very heavy (more than 25 aspirins a week). Aspirin appears to alter the clotting action of both the mother's and the fetus' blood by interfering with the platelets, the cellular bodies that normally repair any tears in the body's blood vessels. This can result in prolonged bleeding during delivery and neonatal blood loss if aspirin is taken in large doses just before delivery. Heavy consumption of aspirin also appears to prolong the length of pregnancy and the duration of labor through its adverse effect on the prostaglandins, the hormones that regulate gestation and labor. For these reasons women are now being advised to use aspirin only *very* occasionally in the last trimester and to be careful about aspirin use at any time during pregnancy. According to an Australian study, very heavy aspirin use may, in addition, be responsible for the closing up of the ductus arteriosus (the blood vessel that shunts the blood from the right to the left side of the heart) in the fetus, resulting in an increased risk of stillbirth. Although aspirin is still a useful pain-killer, less dangerous than a prescription drug under many circumstances, pregnancy is not a time to use aspirin routinely. This caution also applies to aspirin compounds such as phenacetin and aspirin.

Acetaminophen (Dandril, Nebs, Tempra, Tylenol): Acetaminophen compounds appear to be safe for use during pregnancy as long as you do not exceed normal dosage. Although they do appear to cross the placenta, no ill effects to the fetus have been reported. Used sensibly, *Tylenol* and related products are good alternatives to aspirin if you need an occasional mild analgesic during pregnancy.

☐ *Antacids*   Prescription drugs (*Tagamet, Pro-Banthine*): *Tagamet* inhibits acid secretions and is used in the treatment of ulcers and preulcerous conditions. Little is known about its side effects in pregnancy. While it does cross the placenta, studies on animals have not shown it to have a teratogenic effect. Since it is secreted in human milk, Tagamet use is not advisable during nursing. *Pro-Banthine* tablets are also used to decrease gastric-acid secretion. Since there are no studies on Pro-Banthine's effect on either animals or humans, this drug should be used only when its benefits to the mother appear to outweigh a possible risk to the fetus. It does not appear in significant quantities in breast milk. Discuss their use with your doctor before you take either of these drugs.

Nonprescription antacids include products that contain aluminum hydroxide, calcium carbonate, sodium bicarbonate, and magnesium compounds. Of these over-the-counter compounds, the one to avoid at all times during pregnancy is *sodium bicarbonate,* which can cause edema and weight gain and may lead to systemic alkalosis. Other antacids are generally considered safe for use in the second and third trimesters as long as you do not exceed the recommended doses. Try to avoid antacids in the first three months of pregnancy, because one inconclusive study has suggested an association between major and minor congenital malformations and antacid use in the first trimester. Chronic use of any antacid product is to be avoided, since both the mother and the fetus may experience adverse reactions, including drowsiness and respiratory distress in newborns, and constipation and other side effects for the mother. Use of aluminum hydroxide also slightly affects the proper absorption of vitamin C, vitamin A, and proteins, and may increase calcium absorption to an undesirable level. Over-the-counter antacids should always be treated with caution.

☐ *Antibiotics* There is a wide spectrum of antibiotics, which are divided into groups according to the bacteria they fight. These include the aminoglycosides, the cephalosporins, penicillins, and the tetracyclines.

Aminoglycosides (Streptomycin, Garamycin, Kantrex, Nebcin): The aminoglycosides are used to treat serious gram-negative infections such as tuberculosis, streptococcus, peritonitis, and serious skin infections. Your doctor will always keep you under close observation if you have a serious infection of this type, because both in the pregnant and nonpregnant woman the aminoglycosides carry the risk of rash, fever, itching, and renal damage. *Streptomycin* and *kanamycin* (*Kantrex*) have been associated with deafness in the newborn and are not recommended for use during the first trimester or in doses exceeding a total of 20 grams in the last half of pregnancy. Beyond this, the effect of this group of drugs on the fetus is not known at this time. The benefits to the mother seem to outweigh the possible risk to the fetus when a very severe infection can only be controlled with aminoglycosides.

Cephalosporins (Duricef, Ancef, Mefoxin, Keflex, Keflin): This group of drugs is often used during pregnancy to combat staph infections, salmonella, and infections caused by streptococcal bacteria. Side effects are less serious than those of other antibacterial drugs, although gastrointestinal disturbances and allergic reactions may occur. While the cephalosporins cross the placenta, they do not appear to have a toxic effect on the fetus, and tests on pregnant laboratory animals have, so far, indicated no teratogenic effect. They can, therefore, be prescribed during pregnancy and are often used when women are allergic to penicillin. However, your doctor should still be cautious about prescribing these drugs until more data about their safety has been accumulated.

Penicillins (ampicillin, Penicillin G, Penicillin V): Penicillin compounds are the safest antibiotics for use during pregnancy. Although they cross the placenta, they do not, as far as we know, have any teratogenic effect.

If you are allergic to any form of penicillin or normally suffer side effects from penicillin use, pregnancy will not usually alter your penicillin tolerance. Always inform your doctor of your reaction to penicillin and make sure it is noted on your medical chart.

Tetracyclines (Declomycin, Terramycin, Sumycin): Tetracyclines should not be used during pregnancy because they are deposited in the baby's bones and teeth. Tetracyclines can retard normal bone growth and permanently stain a child's second teeth when administered to the mother in the second and third trimesters. However, these antibiotics do not appear to be teratogenic, and an inadvertent use of tetracycline early in pregnancy is unlikely to impair the growth of the fetus (see also "Urine Tract Infections" below).

☐ *Anticoagulants (Blood-Thinning Drugs)*   (*Warfarin, Heparin*): Anticoagulants are used in the treatment of thrombosis and pulmonary embolism. *Warfarin*, an oral anticoagulant and one of the commonest of the anticoagulant drugs, is associated with a syndrome of severe congenital malformations in the fetus and an increased incidence of spontaneous abortion. A woman who needs an anticoagulant is usually given *Heparin* instead during pregnancy, beginning in the preconception period. Heparin does not have a teratogenic effect, even though there is still an increased risk of miscarriage and stillbirth—which may, however, be a side effect of the woman's health rather than her drug therapy.

☐ *Anticonvulsants (Antiseizures)*   (*phenobarbital, Dilantin, Mysoline*): These drugs are used in the treatment of epilepsy. Phenobarbital can also be prescribed as a sedative during pregnancy. No woman should receive anticonvulsant medications unnecessarily during pregnancy, but the seizures themselves may be more dangerous to the fetus than the effects of the drugs. Anticonvulsant medications are known to cross the placenta and may increase the risk of congenital malformations such as cleft palate or heart defects, which are more common among the children of epileptic mothers. However, a woman with epilepsy still has a 90 percent chance of giving birth to a normal child. Most physicians favor using phenobarbital when a woman becomes pregnant because this is a drug that has been around for many years, and thousands of women have been treated with it, apparently with relative safety.

☐ *Antidepressants*   (*Elavil, Desipramine, Dosepin, Vivactil*): In a few known instances the children of women who took any of these antidepressant drugs just prior to delivery suffered heart failure and respiratory distress. Their use during pregnancy is not recommended (except in a few cases involving bouts of severe depression), since withdrawal symptoms have been noted in newborns, and a connection between this group of drugs and congenital malformations is suspected.

☐ *Antihistamines* (see also Allergy Drugs)   *Nonprescription antihistamines:* This large group of over-the-counter medications includes any drug used to control the side effects of motion sickness and the relief of allergy symptoms, and certain over-the-counter sedatives. Although, with one exception, these drugs appear to be relatively safe when used during pregnancy, they should still be treated with caution. During pregnancy it is far better to stay away from substances to which you are allergic or to avoid situations that could lead you to take drug relief than to rely on over-the-counter remedies.

Caution: Never use antihistamine compounds that include *brompheniramine*. Brompheniramine may, according to one large-scale study, pose an increased risk of congenital malformation for the fetus.

☐ **Antihypertensive Drugs** (*Aldomet, Apresoline, Inderal,* compounds with *reserpine*): Hypertension is a fairly common problem among pregnant women. Most doctors prefer to use *Aldomet* to treat cases of hypertension because it has been fully tested and is generally presumed to be safe during pregnancy. In one test the birth weight and maturity of a group of babies whose mothers had been treated with Aldomet were assessed and pronounced normal. There were no signs of congenital abnormality that could be attributed to the use of the drug. However, there may be adverse side effects for the mother when Aldomet is used for more than six months.

Animal studies indicate that *Apresoline* is teratogenic in mice. Although a similar effect has not been proven in humans, it should not be used during pregnancy except under special circumstances.

The use of *Inderal* should be limited in pregnancy. Frequent use of this drug by pregnant women has been linked to growth retardation in the fetus and hypoglycemia (low blood sugar) in the newborn. It has been used intravenously during labor, but this use is controversial, since it severely distresses fetal breathing (see Chap. 24).

The compound *reserpine,* which appears in several drugs used to treat hypertension, including Sandril, Serpasil, and Raurine, causes fetal distress by depressing fetal breathing and can have adverse and possibly long-term effects on the pregnant woman. There is a possible association between it and breast cancer, and it also appears in breast milk. For these reasons it is not usually recommended for the treatment of hypertension during pregnancy.

☐ **Antinausea Drugs** (*Bendectin, Compazine, Tigan*): *Tigan,* a compound of trimethobenzamine, is commonly used to prevent nausea and vomiting during pregnancy. Several large studies have failed to show an increased risk of damage to the fetus with the use of Tigan. Tigan is usually effective in controlling nausea symptoms.

Compazine is a widely prescribed antinausea drug that should, however, be used with caution because adequate studies have not been performed. Use it in suppository form if you are suffering from severe nausea or vomiting.

Bendectin, a commonly used antinausea drug, has been removed from the market (see Chap. 5).

☐ **Asthma Drugs** *Ephedrine* and *Isuprel:* The use of these drugs is not usually recommended for the relief of asthma during pregnancy. *Ephedrine* is used extensively during labor (see Chap. 27) after the administration of a spinal or epidural anesthetic.

Potassium Iodide: Never use potassium iodide during pregnancy. When iodide enters the fetal bloodstream, it may bind to result in the formation of fetal goiter.

Brethine: The safety of Brethine in pregnancy has never been established; animal studies, however, have not shown any adverse effects from Brethine use prenatally. When your doctor prescribes Brethine for you during pregnancy, he should weigh its therapeutic benefits against the possible hazards to you and the baby.

Vanceril: The effects of Vanceril on the fetus are presently unknown, but studies in animals indicate that Vanceril may cause birth defects in humans and may enter human milk. Its use during pregnancy and breast-feeding requires very careful consideration by your doctor.

☐   *Barbiturates (Nembutal, Seconal, Tuinal, and Quāāludes)*   (see *Sedatives*)

☐   *Caffeine*   Caffeine is perhaps the most commonly used of all drugs. It may have a deleterious effect on the fetus if taken in large enough quantities (see Chap. 16).

☐   *Cardiovascular Drugs (Digoxin, Amyl Nitrite)*   Digoxin is widely used to treat congestive heart failure, and it is the most frequently prescribed of the digitalis drugs. Although it crosses the placenta, digoxin does not appear to produce malformations or signs of distress in the fetus. *Nitrites*, such as amyl nitrite and nitroglycerin, are often used to treat cases of angina, which is, fortunately, rare among young women. *Amyl nitrite* increases the heart rate, and deaths have occurred when it has been used as a social drug in large amounts. It crosses the placenta and could, if inhaled in large quantities, result in fetal death by speeding up the fetus' heart rate.

☐   *Cocaine*   Cocaine is a powerful central-nervous-system stimulant and a vasoconstrictor. Taken as a social drug, it produces a state of high excitement, nervousness, and wakefulness. Its effects on the fetus are unknown, but it is such a powerful stimulant in adults that we can only conclude that the effect on the fetus must be disturbing.

☐   *Diabetic Drugs*   Insulin: A woman who is diabetic usually needs to continue taking insulin, although insulin requirements tend to drop in the first trimester and increase in the second half of pregnancy. At this point, insulin itself is not suspected of causing malformations or other serious side effects in the fetus. Most of the problems associated with diabetic pregnancies are the result of erratic high maternal blood-sugar levels, and control of blood sugar by insulin or diet is generally the first concern of a doctor in a diabetic pregnancy. Congenital malformation in the fetus of a diabetic mother is usually connected with abnormally high blood-sugar levels in women out of insulin control (see Chap. 24).
Oral diabetic drugs (Diabinese, Orinase): Both of these drugs are contraindicated during pregnancy. You should discontinue your regular diabetic medication and be controlled by insulin prior to conception. If you become pregnant while you are still using either of these drugs, call your doctor immediately and arrange to be switched to insulin for the rest of the pregnancy.

☐   *Diet Pills* (see also *Amphetamines*)   *Nonprescription appetite suppressants (Dexatrim capsules)*: Do not use over-the-counter appetite suppressants while you are pregnant or nursing. You have no reason to take them during pregnancy, and their effects on the fetus or the newborn have not been established.

☐   *Diuretics (Thiazide, Diuril, Hydrodiuril)*   Thiazide diuretics were once used extensively during pregnancy in the treatment of edema. It was believed that the control of maternal edema through a salt-free diet and the use of diuretics prevented the onset of toxemia and preeclampsia (see Chap. 25). Diuretics are no longer used except in a few, very specific situations, since it has been proven that diuretics do not prevent the onset of preeclampsia and, in fact, can do great harm to the mother and the fetus. The thiazides, the most commonly prescribed group of diuretics, have been associated with severe maternal complications leading to fetal death. Fetal complications are low birth weight, salt and water depletion of the fetus, low blood sugar, and neonatal depression with decreased blood platelets at birth; fetal nutrition and oxygenation may also be affected adversely. Antihypertensive drugs, some with a diuretic effect, are still used during pregnancy (see above), but they should be prescribed with caution.

☐ *Fungal Infection Drugs* (*Fulvicin-U/F, Grifulvin V, Grisactin, Micatin, Monistat, Monistat 7, Mycostatin, Milstat, Candeptin*)
Products containing *griseofulvin* (*Fulvicin-U/F, Grifulvin V, Grisactin*) are *not* recommended during pregnancy. Griseofulvin crosses the placenta freely and has been shown to be teratogenic in laboratory animals. Topical products containing *miconazole* (*Micatin, Monistat, Monistat 7*) can be safely used for the relief of vaginitis as long as the membranes are not ruptured. Ask your doctor *not* to prescribe the new intravenous preparation; its safety has not been established, and heavy use may possibly result in miscarriage. *Mycostatin* and *Milstat* are safe to use in treating fungal skin and mucous membrane infections. Once again, they should not be applied vaginally once the membranes are ruptured. *Candeptin*, which is available in ointment and tablet form, is also safe to use if the same precaution is observed.

☐ *Headache Medications* (see *Analgesics* and *Migraine Drugs*)

☐ *Heart Drugs* (see *Cardiovascular Drugs*)

☐ *Hemorrhoid Medications* Prescription drugs (*Anugesic, Anusol-HC, Anusol suppositories* or *ointment*): Do not use *Anusol-HC* or *Anugesic*; they contain steroids and are, therefore, not recommended during pregnancy. *Anusol suppositories* or *ointment* are preparations that can be used safely in the relief of hemorrhoids, a common and sometimes annoying side effect of pregnancy.
Nonprescription drugs (*Pazo, Preparation H*): These are probably the most common of the over-the-counter remedies for hemorrhoids. No studies have been done on these drugs to establish their safety in pregnancy, but occasional use, especially in the second or third trimester, is unlikely to cause any harm.

☐ *Hormones* (*oral contraceptives, estrogens, progestins*) This is an important and notorious group of drugs, including as it does the now discredited synthetic hormone, *DES*.
Oral contraceptives: Estrogen-progesterone oral contraceptives may be teratogenic when taken inadvertently in early pregnancy. The principal birth defects that may result from oral contraceptive use are cardiac malformations and

lymph-reduction malformations. Fortunately, both of these abnormalities occur infrequently, affecting only one out of every 5000 live births.

Estrogens: Estrogen use during pregnancy can result in congenital malformations in the fetus. The discovery of a connection between estrogen use and cancer and birth defects means that steroidal and nonsteroidal estrogens are now contraindicated during pregnancy—a ban which, unfortunately, came too late to save many DES daughters and sons from a lifetime of concern and reproductive problems. The only estrogen use still permitted during pregnancy is the "morning after" contraceptive pill. This very large dose of estrogen is designed to prevent the implantation of a fertile egg, but at the same time it can cause severe birth defects if implantation still takes place. In such cases, an abortion is usually recommended.

DES (diethylstilbestrol) is a potent synthetic hormone still used widely in cattle feed to fatten livestock, as a "morning after" pill, and as a medication to dry up breast milk after childbirth. In the 1950s, thousands of doctors prescribed DES as a "pregnancy support" to prevent miscarriage, inspired by the example of two influential doctors in Boston who claimed great success with DES among their diabetic patients and women with a history of reproductive problems. Infants born to these mothers apparently not only survived pregnancy more successfully, but, according to the first reports on DES babies, were bigger and healthier and "more rugged" than normal children. Despite the fact that proper studies were not performed and in the face of stilbestrol's known carcinogenicity in animals, obstetricians all over the United States continued to prescribe DES with confidence for the next twenty years. So convinced were the medical profession and the general public of the efficacy of DES and other hormone supports that a University of Chicago study that found no difference between the outcome of DES pregnancies and that of a control group was almost completely ignored (the DES women in this study were not informed of the nature of the experiment—an oversight which the university has subsequently paid for by several million dollars' worth of legal settlements).

The immediate maternal side effects of DES were nausea, vomiting, skin changes, and pulmonary embolism, as well as potential jaundice, but it took a number of years before the serious side effects of DES use were seen in the children of DES mothers. In 1966 and 1967, three cases of an extremely rare cancer, *clear-cell adenocarcinoma,* were reported by Massachusetts General Hospital. The only link in these unusual cases was the use of DES by the mothers of the young women during pregnancy. By 1971, the number of cases had risen to eight, and an article that year in the *New England Journal of Medicine* alerted the medical profession and the public to the magnitude of the problem. The era of "pregnancy supports" had come to a hasty and inglorious end.

Fortunately, the incidence of clear-cell adenocarcinoma has turned out to be low—affecting perhaps only one in every 10,000 DES daughters. Fortunately, too, this type of cancer rarely appears once these young women are past their teens. After twenty, doctors are far more concerned about the development of a second type of cancer—squamous-cell cancer which affects the cervix. As a routine precaution, women who were prenatally exposed to DES are advised to have a Pap smear twice a year. Then, if any abnormality appears, a colposcopy can be performed and a biopsy obtained.

Perhaps the most common side effects of DES exposure are menstrual and reproductive problems. Stillbirths and miscarriages appear more frequently among DES daughters than among other young women, apparently because of cervical incompetence and unusual changes in the shape and appearance of the uterus. Although most DES daughters will ultimately bear children successfully, they face perhaps a 60 percent greater chance of encountering serious problems during pregnancy. For further information, you can call this toll-free number: 1-800-462-1884.

☐ *Does DES Affect Men?*   Some young men who were exposed to DES *in utero* have also been found to have serious abnormalities of the genital organs. There is a high incidence of cysts in the testicular tissue of these young men, and low sperm counts are common. At this time, it is still too early to tell just how much this will alter the fertility levels of this large group of men, although the present evidence suggests that some DES sons are unlikely to father children. Fortunately, so far there have been no abnormalities suggesting cancerous or precancerous conditions in men exposed prenatally to DES.

A woman or man exposed to DES *in utero* has no reason not to attempt pregnancy, although they may have a higher chance of infertility or an increased chance of pregnancy-related problems. Careful observation by an obstetrical specialist is recommended.

☐ *Progesterone: The Second Female Hormone*   *Progesterone* is a hormone that occurs naturally during pregnancy and has been used in both synthetic and natural form to prevent the onset of miscarriage due to the inadequate production of progesterone from the placenta, or from a so-called inadequate luteal phase, when the corpus luteum is not producing enough progesterone to maintain the pregnancy. In its synthetic form, progesterone was given to thousands of women in the 1950s and 1960s as a "hormonal support" to prevent miscarriage. However, certain birth defects, including cardiac and main-vessel malformations, limb-reduction defects, and the masculinization of the female sexual organs became associated with its use. Health professionals also increasingly questioned its efficacy. Finally, in 1977, the FDA inserted new labeling on progestinal drugs warning doctors and consumers of the possible teratogenicity of progesterone taken in early pregnancy. The use of *synthetic* progesterone is now contraindicated in pregnancy. However, government regulations regarding natural progesterone are still unclear, and the whole subject remains controversial.

Natural progesterone works at the intercellular level and relaxes the uterine wall. When the production of progesterone from the corpus luteum, the body's source of progesterone, seems inadequate, natural progesterone suppositories (25 mg daily) have been used to increase the chance of conception. Instead of suppositories, some doctors prefer to use injections of 17-hydroxy-progesterone to stimulate the corpus luteum to produce increased progesterone; the usual dose is 250 milligrams once a week intramuscularly until at least the twelfth week. Side effects for the mother include weight gain and occasional episodes of depression, but the side effects to the fetus are apparently not harmful, although progesterone use remains controversial. Of course, it should be restricted to those very specific cases in which there is an inadequate luteal phase with a low progesterone level. If a woman experiences spotting or staining at the beginning of pregnancy or has a history of repeated miscarriages, her doctor will take a blood test first, and only in cases in which the progesterone level is low should natural progesterone in either form be used.

☐ ***Does Progesterone Increase a Child's Intelligence?***   According to one Rutgers University study, conducted on a group of children exposed prenatally to synthetic estrogens and progesterones, distinct personality differences are evident after progesterone and estrogen exposure. In this study, the "progesterone" children were observed to be more independent, more individualistic, and more self-assured; and the "estrogen" children were apparently less independent and more highly socialized. According to the researchers, the findings were equally true of both boys and girls. This study does not stand alone. One British study went even further and linked intelligence as well as a more assertive personality to prenatal progesterone exposure. On the other hand, a group of California researchers investigated the IQ scores of hormone-exposed children and their untreated siblings and found no significant difference between them. This led them to conclude that synthetic hormones were neither detrimental nor beneficial to later mental development, at least as far as it was measured by a standard IQ test. Perhaps, they suggested in conclusion, those children who were exposed to a large prenatal dose are the ones who show the most marked increase in intelligence. This might explain the high IQs of a group of little girls investigated by the Johns Hopkins University in Baltimore, who were born with rudimentary penises as well as female genital organs as a result of intensive hormone therapy. Such unlooked-for side effects make attempts to produce more intelligent human beings through prenatal hormone exposure hardly worth the risk.

☐ ***Hypertension***   (see *Antihypertensive Drugs*)

☐ ***Laxatives***   The occasional use of an over-the-counter laxative is not harmful during pregnancy, but one of the best ways to prevent constipation without using drugs at all is to increase the amount of roughage in your diet. Do not use laxatives routinely; consult your doctor if there is a persistent problem. Stool softeners, such as *Colace tablets*, are frequently used during pregnancy, and no adverse effects have been reported.

☐ ***Marijuana***   The active ingredient of marijuana, tetrahydrocannabinal, is known to cross the placenta and depress the fetal heart rate and change fetal brain-wave patterns. In experiments with mice who were exposed to dosages of marijuana smoke comparable to the amounts inhaled by heavy smokers, fetal death increased considerably. Although there is no proof that marijuana has a teratogenic or life-threatening effect in human pregnancy, marijuana is a drug, and no drug should be used that directly affects the fetus unless you need it for medical reasons. There is another factor: a woman smoking marijuana usually inhales the drug so deeply that the carbon monoxide level in her blood is higher than if she smoked a cigarette. With heavy or even moderate marijuana use, the carbon monoxide concentration might well retard fetal growth and intellectual development just as seriously as in heavy cigarette smoking. Did you know that one rolled cigarette of marijuana is the equivalent of seven tobacco cigarettes?

☐ *Migraine Drugs*   Prescription drugs (*Cafergot* with caffeine): do not use drugs such as *Cafergot*, which contain ergotamine tartrate. *Ergotamine tartrate is known to cause uterine contractions and may result in an increase in maternal blood pressure.* When this drug was fed to pregnant rats, growth retardation in the fetus and miscarriages resulted.

☐ *Motion Sickness Drugs (Antivert, Dramamine)*   *Antivert* is an effective drug in the prevention of nausea and vomiting caused by motion sickness. At the same time, it should be used with caution during pregnancy, especially in the first trimester. In one study, rats fed high doses of Antivert prenatally developed cleft palate.

Dramamine should *not* be prescribed during pregnancy even though it is a popular drug among nonpregnant women. A tentative link has been made between Dramamine use and an increased incidence of premature labor.

☐ *Nausea Drugs*   (see *Antinausea Drugs*)

☐ *Pain-Killers*   (see *Analgesics*)

☐ *Prostaglandin Inhibitors (Motrin, Naprosyn, and Ponstel)*   Prostaglandin inhibitors are used increasingly in the management of menstrual cramps and for arthritis. Some women might, therefore, find themselves pregnant while taking these drugs. Reproductive studies on *Motrin* and *Naprosyn* have been performed on rats, rabbits, and mice at doses much higher than the human dose, and no evidence of fetal abnormality has been found. However, no human data has been obtained. It is not expected that any fetal harm from these drugs will occur when taken during the first two trimesters. Since Motrin and Naprosyn might postpone delivery and prolong labor, they are not recommended during the third trimester of pregnancy. Reproductive studies with *Ponstel* in animals have shown decreased rate of fetal survival. Ponstal is, therefore, not recommended during pregnancy.

☐ *Saccharin*   *Saccharin* products now carry a warning label advising consumers of animal studies which have found saccharin to be carcinogenic in very large amounts. Saccharin has also been tested on pregnant rats and monkeys, and the results are not altogether reassuring. While saccharin does not enter the fetal nervous system, it does persist in fetal tissue, and experiments involving two generations of rats reveal a higher incidence of bladder cancer in the second generation. This suggests that a pregnant woman would be well advised to watch her consumption of saccharin carefully.

☐ *Sedatives*   Barbiturates (Mebaral, Nembutal, Seconal, and Tuinal): *The safe use of Mebaral, Nembutal, Seconal, and Tuinal during pregnancy has not been established.* The use of any sedative during pregnancy should be avoided if possible, since sedatives are known to cross the placenta and induce sedation and withdrawal symptoms in the newbo. baby. Your doctor should prescribe a sedative only when he feels the benefits to you clearly outweigh the risks to your baby.

Nonbarbiturates (Noctec, Quāālude): Animal studies have not been done to establish the safety of Noctec in pregnancy, and the active ingredient in Noctec, chloral hydrate, is known to cross the placenta and induce withdrawal symptoms in the fetus. It also enters human milk. For these reasons it should be used only in cases of special need.

Quāālude use during pregnancy is *contraindicated.* Skeletal abnormalities may occur after Quāālude use even in small quantities. This makes it very important to stay away from this potent teratogenic social drug if you are pregnant.

Placidyl: This sedative is used in the treatment of insomnia. Adequate animal studies have not been done to establish the safety of Placidyl, and the same precautions apply to it as to any other insomnia drug.

☐ *Over-the-Counter Sedatives or Sleeping Aids (Cope, Quiet World, Sleep-Eze, and Sominex)*   Over-the-counter sedatives and sleeping aids are heavily advertised, and many pregnant women may be tempted to use them.

Cope, Quiet World, Sleep-Eze, and *Sominex* are among the most familiar. Most of these over-the-counter sedatives contain one main ingredient, the antihistamine pyrilamine. Do not take any sleeping aids of this kind without consulting your doctor first. No known ill effects have been reported from their use, but the FDA still recommends that it is better not to use any over-the-counter sleeping aids during pregnancy. Since they are classified as antihistaminics, you should also take a look at the more detailed cautions described under *Allergy Drugs* and *Antihistamines* in this chapter.

☐ *Social Drugs*   (see *Alcohol, Caffeine, Cocaine, Marijuana, Tobacco,* and *Quāālude*)

☐ *Tobacco*   Smoking during pregnancy is not advisable under any circumstances. Its use has been linked to low birth weight, prematurity, and other pregnancy-related complications. Chapter 17 presents a full discussion of tobacco use during pregnancy.

☐ *Toxemia Drugs (magnesium sulfate, phenobarbital, diuretics)*   *Magnesium sulfate* is used in the treatment of severe cases of preeclamptic toxemia. In these severe cases, the baby is usually delivered immediately after the stabilizing effect of the drug has taken place. The administration of magnesium sulfate can cause weakness and respiratory difficulties in the newborn, but this is an instance in which the benefit to the mother usually outweighs the risks to the fetus. Magnesium sulfate also causes a calcium decrease in the mother and baby. *Phenobarbital* is widely prescribed in cases of mild to moderate preeclampsia often in combination with bed rest. Phenobarbital is an "old" drug which has been used for years, and its adverse effects are believed to be negligible. Phenobarbital may be given to nursing mothers, but drowsiness can be expected in the baby.

Diuretics, which used to be widely prescribed in cases of toxemia, are now no longer used except in very special cases (see *Diuretics*).

☐ *Tranquilizers*   Prescription tranquilizers: These drugs will be dealt with in three representative groups:

Valium: Valium is one of the most frequently prescribed drugs in the United

States, and the great majority of these prescriptions are written for women. One in every ten Americans used this tranquilizer in 1980. In a recent laboratory test Valium appeared to halt muscle growth and to interfere with protein synthesis in the cells of fetal laboratory animals. It is possible, too, that Valium and other tranquilizers may have subtle but long-term effects on fetal nervous-system development. Regular use of Valium is not recommended during pregnancy or breast-feeding. Valium readily crosses the placenta, entering the fetal circulatory system. During breast-feeding, the drug is excreted into the mother's milk and may cause lethargy and weight loss in the baby. Heavy use during pregnancy may result in fetal withdrawal symptoms, which are similar to those experienced by the children of mothers addicted to narcotics.

Thorazine, Compazine, Phenergan, Stelazine: This group of tranquilizers does not appear to cause malformations, but may induce neonatal jaundice followed by hyperactivity and depression. Since the safety of these drugs during pregnancy has not been established, they should not be used by a pregnant woman except in very rare instances.

Eskalith, Lithane: These are potent tranquilizers that should only be used during pregnancy to control severe symptoms of manic depression. The use of *lithium* (Lithane) has been shown to increase the risk of congenital malformations, and the newborn's respiratory system and sucking instincts may be adversely affected.

☐ **Urinary-Tract Infections (*Thiosulfil Forte, Gantanol, Gantrisin, Macrodantin, and NegGram*)**   Urinary-tract infections are fairly common during pregnancy. Such infections are often treated by a group of antibiotics called sulfonamides, which include sulfa forte, *Gantanol* and *Gantrisin*. Sulfonamides should be used with caution at any time, and your doctor will monitor your blood count carefully if he prescribes one of these antibiotics. Sulfonamides can be used in the first six months of pregnancy, although there are insufficient studies to establish their safety. In the last trimester, they may lead to the development of severe jaundice in the newborn. For the same reason, they should not be used in the nursing period. *Macrodantin* is widely used to treat pregnant women, but its safety in pregnancy and lactation has not been established, and cases of anemia have been reported in newborns after its use just before delivery. In this case, your doctor will have to weigh the benefits to you against the possible risks to the baby. *NegGram* has been used in the second and third trimesters without any noticeable ill effects to mother or baby, although its safe use in the first trimester has not been established. *Penicillin* is also used frequently in urinary-tract infections and has been found safe for use in all trimesters.

☐ **Drugs Used in Labor and Delivery**   This is an important group of drugs and one whose use you will want to discuss with your obstetrician well before your due date. Although certain drugs may be necessary during labor, the routine use of some common drugs in labor and delivery is now highly controversial. This subject is dealt with fully in Chapter 27. Drugs used to arrest premature labor are described in Chapter 25.

☐ **Addictive Drugs and Pregnancy**   Although the numbers of women addicted to heroin and methadone are comparatively few, most of them are young.

The average age of women addicts in the mid-1970s was twenty-two years, which means that many addicted women are able to have children and do so. (While addiction to heroin affects pregnancy outcome, it does not seem to affect a woman's fertility.) The obstetrical histories of addicted women make very depressing reading. Many of them take so little care of themselves that they do not see a doctor until just before they give birth, by which time their poor eating habits and susceptibility to diseases have already taken their toll on the mother and child. And it is then, of course, much too late to try detoxification procedures and reduce the fetus' as well as the woman's dependence on hard drugs. It is not surprising that children of addicts are usually underweight, are often delivered prematurely, and may have congenital syphilis or other serious infections. Sometimes they are stillborn or die soon after birth. Addicted babies who survive are restless, overactive, appear to be in considerable pain, do not want to be held or cuddled, and show very little interest in sucking. When these babies are not given intensive care immediately after birth, they can die from the severe convulsions brought on by their sudden withdrawal.

Heroin and *methadone* cross the placenta and enter the fetal bloodstream. Both of them are teratogenic in laboratory animals, but the effect on fetal health and growth is usually more serious than the threat of congenital malformations. This means that the most devastating effects of addiction can be mitigated if a woman is treated while she is pregnant. With special care and counseling, addicted women have been known to give birth successfully to full-grown and nonaddicted babies.

Any woman who is addicted to drugs should try to get help immediately after she becomes pregnant.

20

The Rhesus Disease: It Could Affect Your Baby

Twenty years ago almost 20,000 children in the United States alone died soon after birth or were permanently brain-damaged by a disease they had contracted prenatally. This is Rhesus disease, or Rh blood disease, an immunological condition that develops through a simple incompatibility between the blood types of a mother and her unborn baby.

The Rh disease was such a serious threat to newborns that researchers tried for years to evolve new methods of treatment—an effort that was finally successful. In the last decade, thanks to better detection of the disease prenatally and effective means of prevention, the incidence of Rh disease has declined precipitately. Fewer than 6000 American children are now born with Rh disease each year, and even fewer die or are seriously crippled. In fact, so many babies have been saved in the last few years that Rh disease is no longer considered a major public health problem. This is unfortunate, because the number of babies suffering from it is still far higher than it need be, given the effective means of prevention we already have. Because of the present discrepancy between the number of babies born with the disease and the tiny number one would expect to be affected, this is yet another area of health care in which parents themselves can act to protect their unborn babies.

If every woman in the United States knew her blood type, and knew how and when she needed protection, and made sure that she got it, it would take only another decade for Rh disease to be effectively eradicated. This is not to say that doctors don't bear the primary responsibility for their patients' well-being, but doctors can't be held responsible if women don't come to them when they need care. If you are one of the large group of women whose pregnancies could be affected by Rh disease, you too need to learn how to protect yourself and your children. The aim of this chapter is to show you how.

DEVELOPMENT OF Rh DISEASE

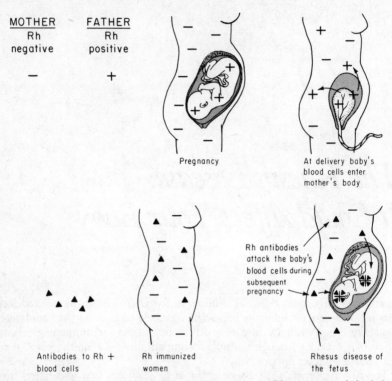

MOTHER	FATHER
Rh	Rh
negative	positive
−	+

Pregnancy

At delivery baby's
blood cells enter
mother's body

Antibodies to Rh +
blood cells

Rh immunized
women

Rh antibodies
attack the baby's
blood cells during
subsequent
pregnancy

Rhesus disease of
the fetus

Figure 47: Development of Rhesus Disease: If a mother is Rh negative and the baby is Rh positive, the baby's red blood cells could enter into the maternal bloodstream during delivery and sensitize the mother so that she will have antibodies to Rh positive blood in her body. These rhesus antibodies will attack the fetus of a subsequent pregnancy if the fetus has Rh positive blood. Consequently, the fetus will run the risk of developing Rhesus disease with severe complications and possibly fetal death.

☐ *The Rh Factor*   The Rhesus, or Rh factor is a substance found on the surface of the blood cells. The word "Rhesus" is derived from the rhesus monkey, the laboratory animal used in the basic studies of the working of the red blood cells. The Rhesus factor is commonly found in human beings, so commonly in fact that 85 percent of the white population of the United States and 95 percent of the black population are described as "Rh positive," because they have Rh antibodies in their blood. Those who do not possess the Rh factor are said to be "Rh negative." Lack of the Rh factor has no effect on the individual's health and is significant only when a blood transfusion is required or when a woman is pregnant.

☐ *What Is Rhesus Disease?*   The existence of the Rhesus blood group system was determined in 1940. One year later a group of doctors established a connection between the Rh factor and an often fatal disease called *erythroblas-*

tosis fetalis, or *Rh hemolytic disease.* This disease, which can kill the fetus or cause severe birth defects, is the result of an immunological incompatibility between a mother with Rh negative blood and a fetus that has inherited its father's Rh positive blood type. This simple incompatibility can have tragic results if fetal blood enters the bloodstream of a mother who has already developed antibodies to the fetus' RH positive blood. Antibodies develop when sufficient numbers of Rh positive blood cells from the baby cross over into the mother's circulatory system. Her body then chemically perceives them as "foreign" substances and fights them off by producing antibodies, anti-Rh substances, which in turn will attempt to destroy the baby's Rh positive blood when it once again enters the mother's bloodstream. While this rarely has a serious effect in a first pregnancy, because the mother usually develops antibodies after the first baby is born, the maternal antibodies remain in the bloodstream and there is the risk of damage in a second or subsequent pregnancy. Once the mother's antibodies attack an Rh positive fetus, the baby's red blood cells begin to break down, and the fetus can die, become seriously anemic, or develop a condition called *erythroblastosis fetalis,* a form of edema that often leads to serious and irreversible brain damage because of the serious decrease in oxygen caused by severe anemia.

Because of the large number of Rh negative women in the population, the results of Rh disease were only too evident at the time the factor was discovered. Fortunately, in 1945 an eminent pediatrician introduced the technique of blood-exchange transfusions immediately after birth, and the perinatal mortality rate from Rh disease was halved. This new method of treatment also reduced the deaths and brain damage caused by high levels of bilirubin (the waste product produced in the liver when blood is destroyed) in the newborn, a condition called *kernicterus.* Then, twenty years later, the discovery of a special vaccine revolutionized the treatment of Rh disease by preventing its occurrence prenatally.

☐ *How Is the Disease Now Prevented?*   The need for heroic measures at birth has been greatly diminished in the last decade because of the invention and widespread use of the vaccine called *Rhogam,* a specially prepared gamma globulin that contains a small but concentrated group of Rh positive antibodies. Antibodies are substances commonly found in the blood which form the basis of our natural defense system against toxic agents. A normal individual's blood contains hundreds of different antibodies capable of destroying bacteria, viruses, and other entities that attack the human body at all stages of its existence. The concentration of Rh antibodies in the Rhogam vaccine binds the Rh positive blood cells in the mother's circulatory system. These Rh antibodies provide a protection against any foreign Rh positive blood cells that leak from the fetal circulation during the delivery of a Rhesus positive infant, or through a miscarriage, ectopic pregnancy, amniocentesis test, or abortion. One injection of Rhogam provides virtually complete protection in any future pregnancy by preventing a woman from producing her own permanent antibodies.

The invention of the Rh vaccine by a pioneering British research team in Liverpool, England, and two American doctors working in a clinic in New York was one of the great medical breakthroughs of the late 1960s. One of the American doctors, Dr. Vincent Freda, was drawn into work on the vaccine after

PREVENTION OF Rh DISEASE BY RHOGAM INJECTION

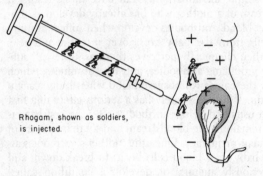

Rhogam, shown as soldiers, is injected.

Rhogam (soldiers) are attacking and destroying the Rh + blood cells so no antibodies develop.

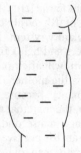

Rhogam was given within 72 hrs of delivery and the mother is completely normal with no Rh antibodies.

Figure 48: Prevention of Rhesus Disease by Rhogam Injection: In order to prevent Rhesus disease, any woman who is Rh negative should receive an injection of Rhogam, an anti-Rh positive substance, after a miscarriage, a pregnancy interruption or the delivery of an Rh positive baby. If a Rhogam injection is given within twenty-two hours of miscarriage or delivery, the Rhogam will act like soldiers that will attack and destroy any positive blood cells which might enter a woman's bloodstream. Any subsequent pregnancy will then proceed without the danger of sensitization.

his experience as a young obstetrician delivering babies who were seriously ill or brain-damaged from Rh incompatibility. He established the first specialized clinic for Rh negative mothers at Columbia Presbyterian Hospital in New York, where he and another doctor, Dr. John Gorman, tested the vaccine by giving Rh antibodies to Rh negative mothers at the time of delivery. Their faith in the Rh antigen, which persisted in the face of great skepticism, helped to establish its widespread use in the United States.

☐ *How Does the Vaccine Work?*   Since the vaccine contains antibodies to Rhesus positive blood, these antibodies trap the Rh positive cells that enter into the mother's bloodstream from the fetus during delivery and form a new complex that is completely different from the original fetal blood cells. This complex then circulates harmlessly in the mother's bloodstream and traps any Rh positive blood cells that attempt to enter it. In this respect it acts rather like a group of soldiers in battle formation who move out to repel the enemy before it can stage an attack.

A standard dose of Rhogam contains 300 mcg of the Rh immune globulin. If the injection is given within seventy-two hours after delivery, this amount is usually enough to protect the maternal circulation against the action of up to 30 cc of fetal blood entering the mother's bloodstream.

☐ *Can the Rh Disease Occur in a First Pregnancy?*   In a first pregnancy the risk of Rh disease is minimal because the baby is usually born before the mother's blood can produce enough Rh positive antibodies to harm the pregnancy. However, in some cases a phenomenon called *spontaneous immunization* occurs early enough in a first pregnancy to injure the baby. Spontaneous immunization, caused by fetal Rh positive blood leaking into the mother during the pregnancy, results in the production of Rh positive antibodies in the mother's blood, which in turn attack the fetus. This is why it is important for a woman with Rh negative blood to have repeated blood tests at certain intervals to screen her progress during each pregnancy.

☐ *Can Immunization Occur Only During a Delivery?*   The answer is no. An Rh negative woman can also develop antibodies to Rh positive blood if she receives a mismatched blood transfusion of Rh positive blood or if she experiences an abortion, miscarriage, ectopic pregnancy, or amniocentesis test during which enough Rh positive blood is allowed to enter into the bloodstream and begin the formation of antibodies. Because it is so important to safeguard the fetuses of later pregnancies, any woman with Rh negative blood should be given an injection of Rhogam within seventy-two hours after delivery or after an abortion, miscarriage, ectopic pregnancy, or amniocentesis test, even if the fetal blood type is unknown.

If the condition is detected, the fetus can be safeguarded before birth by early delivery or intrauterine transfusions, or a neonatal blood-exchange transfusion can be ordered immediately following delivery.

☐ *Why Are There Still Cases of Rh Disease?*   Unfortunately the widespread use of the vaccine has still failed to eradicate Rh disease. One out of every five American women who need the vaccine still do not receive it, either because a woman is not aware of her Rh negative status or because hospitals and other medical facilities have an insufficient understanding of the disease or neglect to protect women at risk. Often it is simply the result of carelessness. If you are being treated in a medical facility in which the caseload is unusually heavy and the doctor has prescribed the Rhogam vaccine but the nurse forgets to give you an injection, insist on proper treatment: go up to the nursing station to demand the Rhogam vaccine if you can't get one of the staff to come to you. Remember, you need a Rhogam injection only if you are Rh negative and not immunized (have not developed Rh positive antibodies) and the baby is Rh positive. As an additional precaution, make sure to mark down your blood type after a routine blood test and commit it to memory. An accurate knowledge of your blood type will enable you to correct any discrepancy in the hospital records.

Nonetheless, the immunization of all vulnerable women would still fail to eliminate Rh disease entirely. There is a small but persistent failure rate of approximately 1–2 percent with the Rhogam vaccine; in other words, a few women still develop Rh disease in a subsequent pregnancy despite immunization. Two main reasons have been suggested for this small group of cases: first, the injection of Rhogam is not always strong enough to bind all the Rh positive blood cells entering the bloodstream; and second, a few women seem to possess some unusual immunity to the injection.

☐ *If Every Woman Received the Vaccine, Could We Eliminate the Disease?*   Careful screening of all pregnant women and the scrupulous use of the injection would eliminate most of the remaining cases of Rh disease. The number of spontaneous immunizations would also be reduced by the routine use of Rhogam early in every Rh negative pregnancy, but this would be an expensive undertaking. The majority of American doctors feel that Rhogam should be given only after a blood test in the twenty-eighth week of gestation.

☐ *Is There Any Way to Get Rid of Rhesus Antibodies Once You Have Them?*   No. Although you don't feel any different and your body functions normally after Rh immunization, the antibodies become a permanent part of your immune system. Nevertheless there are ways to protect your child if you have been Rh-sensitized, and it is still possible to carry a child to viability. In a case of prior sensitization, the doctor monitors the pregnancy with amniocentesis and other procedures, and the baby may require blood-exchange transfusions at birth.

☐ *What Happens if You Are Carrying a Rhesus Negative Baby?*   There is no danger if you are carrying a Rhesus negative baby. Since it is impossible for positive Rhesus antibodies to develop in your immune system from the blood of a Rhesus negative child, you can carry the pregnancy all the way to term and experience a normal delivery without the need for a Rhogam injection or any other special treatment.

☐ *If You Are Rh Positive and the Father Is Rh Negative, Is That Dangerous?*   No. If you are Rh positive, you already possess the Rhesus factor and it is immaterial whether the father or the baby has Rh negative blood. Rh negative blood from the fetal circulation will not result in immunization if it enters your own bloodstream. You can get Rhesus disease only if you are Rh negative and the baby is Rh positive.

☐ *If the Man and the Woman Are Both Rh Negative, Can Anything Go Wrong?*   No. If both partners are Rh negative, the baby will also be Rh negative, and there is no chance that Rh antibodies will be produced.

☐ *How Can You Find Out What Blood Type You Have?*   You can have your blood type analyzed by sending a blood sample to a laboratory or a blood bank. This should be done routinely at the first visit to the obstetrician or during testing at a clinic or women's health center. Make sure to ask your doctor or the clinic personnel what type of blood you have and note it down in your own records; hospitals have been known to make mistakes.

☐ *How Often Does Rhesus Immunization Occur?*   About 10–15 percent of all Rhesus negative women become immunized by the delivery of the first Rh positive child, and women who escape immunization in the first pregnancy have a failure rate of 3 percent in the second pregnancy and in each subsequent pregnancy. In other words, the more times an Rh negative woman becomes pregnant, the greater is the chance of her becoming immunized and developing Rh antibodies, unless she received a Rhogam injection during an unaffected pregnancy.

☐ *How Are Rh Antibodies Produced After an Abortion or Miscarriage?*
When the placenta separates from the wall of the uterus, a small number of Rh positive blood cells may enter the woman's bloodstream. The Rh negative woman then responds to the foreign blood cells by producing antibodies.

☐ *Should an Injection Be Given After Amniocentesis?* There is a slight chance of bleeding if the needle comes in contact with the placenta. Given this small risk, any woman who is Rh negative should receive an injection of Rh antibodies when she undergoes the test, because the fetal blood type might well be Rh positive.

☐ *What Is Micro Rhogam?* Micro Rhogam is the mini injection of Rhogam that is frequently used after a miscarriage, abortion, ectopic pregnancy, or amniocentesis instead of the full dose. Hospitals like to use Micro Rhogam if they can because it is considerably cheaper than the full vaccine and it protects a woman against as much as 2.5 ml of packed red blood cells, an amount that is rarely exceeded in a miscarriage or abortion. The full dose is still given after delivery because higher amounts of fetal blood can be expected to enter the mother's bloodstream.

Unusually heavy bleeding after a miscarriage or an abortion, however, poses a much higher risk of immunization. A traumatic abortion or miscarriage requires the full dose, or more than one dose in a few exceptional cases.

☐ *Are There Any Adverse Reactions to Rhogam?* A few women experience temporary soreness at the site of the injection or run a slight fever for a few hours. A very few women experience an allergic reaction, with a skin rash at the injection site. This is similar to the allergic reaction some people experience after a blood transfusion. In general, any side effects are so mild that no woman should be afraid of asking for the injection. It has saved literally thousands of children from death and brain damage.

☐ *How Often Should an Rh Negative Pregnant Patient Be Screened for Antibodies?* The first visit to the obstetrician should include a blood test to establish a woman's blood type and detect the presence of antibodies. If she is not immunized, the same test should be repeated at approximately the twenty-fourth, twenty-eighth, thirty-second, and thirty-sixth week of gestation in the first pregnancy and in each subsequent pregnancy. This schedule helps to rule out the occurrence of a spontaneous Rhesus immunization. If immunization does occur, a woman must be cared for and the pregnancy safeguarded in every way possible. (See the material on the treatment of Rh immunization below.)

☐ *What Happens if You Are Immunized During Your Pregnancy?* Suppose you are an Rh negative woman who is not immunized at the beginning of your pregnancy, and at some later point you are told you have developed Rh antibodies, what does this mean to your baby? The degree of immunization is important. Low levels of Rh antibodies are not usually considered dangerous to the fetus. A higher level of immunization, on the other hand, indicates the need for special care.

Degrees of immunization are described by measurements called *antibody titers*—an indication of the level of immunization. Your doctor will take a *Coombs titer*—a blood test—at the beginning of your pregnancy and then at regular intervals (see above). If antibodies do show up in the blood at one of these routine screenings, treatment depends on the level of the titer, the number of antibodies in the blood. When the level is less than 1:8 (positive is a 1:8 detection) your doctor will take your blood pressure every week to exclude the development of preeclampsia and arrange for regular ultrasound screenings to monitor fetal growth. Any sign of toxemia or the development of polyhydramnios (excessive amount of fluid around the baby) should be acted on immediately. I also like to monitor my patients with a weekly nonstress test in the office or on the labor floor (nonstress testing is a relatively new device for gauging the well-being of the baby). Most doctors like to induce delivery if there is a noticeable drop in fetal activity.

The risk increases as the titer measure is higher. A titer of 1:16 or more is always a danger signal, and the doctor will begin intensive treatment right away. A mature baby, over thirty-five or thirty-six weeks old, is often induced immediately. A younger fetus is sometimes left for a week or two to gain more maturity before the delivery. When the doctor decides to wait, he usually performs an amniocentesis test to evaluate the condition of the fluid around the baby. The amniotic fluid provides a useful clue to the baby's condition, because the excretion of bilirubin from the blood of an affected fetus darkens its normal color, and the degree to which the fluid is discolored can be evaluated under an optical instrument called a *spectrophotometer*. If a perinatologist is not handling the case already, he is usually called in at this point to help determine the best time for delivery; babies at risk are delivered as soon as they are reasonably mature and are given blood-exchange transfers immediately after birth.

If your titer stays below the 1.8 level, you can expect to go to term or very close to term, as long as your weekly tests remain satisfactory. It is still a good idea to keep a close watch on the baby for any postnatal signs of Rh disease, and consequently the best place to deliver is a large university center where the nurseries are equipped to monitor the baby and perform an exchange transfusion if necessary.

☐ *If You Already Have Rh Antibodies Can You Still Have a Child?*   Yes, this is still possible, although the situation is more complicated once you are immune. The first step is genetic counseling and testing before conception takes place, including a blood test for both partners. If the woman's initial blood test shows a titer higher than 1:8, her husband's blood type is crucial. An Rh positive father will, of course, mean the chances of an untroubled pregnancy are far fewer.

One possible solution is artificial insemination with the sperm of an Rh negative donor. When a couple decides to go ahead with a pregnancy without artificial insemination, the immunized woman is classified as high-risk and will be put in the care of a perinatologist. Sophisticated pre- and postnatal treatment can now save babies who not so long ago died or suffered permanent injury, but it would be unrealistic to suggest that Rhesus disease is not even now a difficult or potentially dangerous condition. Because of the risks, you can see how important it is for a woman to get the proper screening before she becomes pregnant and to insist on a vaccination when she needs it.

☐ *What Happens During the Pregnancy of an Rh-Sensitized Woman?* Beginning early in the pregnancy, the perinatologist or obstetrician takes serial blood tests and monitors the progress of the pregnancy by ultrasound. (Blood tests by themselves do not give a clear indication of the health of the fetus.) After initially relying on ultrasonography and fetal-movement charts, he then usually orders an amniocentesis test at around the twenty-fourth week if the mother's titer is higher than 1:8. Analysis of the amniotic fluid establishes the extent to which the fetal red blood cells are breaking down in what doctors call the hemolytic process. Once your doctor has monitored the baby's blood, he will establish the baby's lung maturity by further amniotic fluid tests. He may perhaps elect to perform an *intrauterine blood transfusion* of Rh negative blood if he feels the lungs are still too immature to allow for delivery. The transfusion is usually fairly simple, although it should be performed only by a skillful perinatal team. Fetal position is established with an X-ray or ultrasound test and the blood is injected into a needle guided into the mother's abdomen and into the baby's peritoneal cavity. The transfusion is then absorbed into the fetal bloodstream and reduces the baby's anemia by increasing the oxygen-carrying capacity of the baby's blood. In most cases of Rh disease, a number of intrauterine transfusions are performed two weeks apart until tests indicate that the baby is strong enough to survive outside the uterus. Delivery is then induced, and the baby is taken to a premature nursery, where blood-exchange transfusions can take place.

A pregnancy in which the mother is already immunized can be difficult. It is not always possible to carry a baby through to term without the baby dying in the interim or suffering serious brain damage. Studies of babies who were treated by prenatal transfusions in the past also suggest that the frequent X-rays then used to monitor the transfusions resulted in an increased incidence of childhood leukemia. Fortunately more modern centers now use ultrasound.

☐ *Future Management of Rh Disease* In the future there may be new hope for women who are severely immunized and have failed to carry a child to term. One American research group has treated immunized women with a weekly plasmapheresis, a procedure in which a pint of blood is removed from the mother's bloodstream, the plasma is extracted and discarded to get rid of the antibodies, and the plasma-free blood is then reinjected into the mother. This proved effective in some cases but not in others. A group of French scientists has been experimenting with an oral extraction of Rh antigens given on a daily basis to immunized women. The seven women in the initial experiment were tested throughout pregnancy, and their blood titer remained low up to delivery. All of these women, who had previously lost babies to Rhesus disease, were carried safely up to the time of elective delivery and had healthy babies. One of the women delivered a fine set of twins.

☐ *Can Immunization Occur in a Woman Who Is Not Rh Negative?* Very occasionally sensitization to Rh antigens takes place in a Rhesus *positive* woman, usually as the result of a mismatched blood transfusion. A doctor is often alerted to the presence of unusual antibodies because a woman has lost a baby inexplicably or given birth to a baby with jaundice. After taking a past history and carefully screening any atypical antibodies in the mother, the doctor usually evaluates the father's blood as well to determine the seriousness of the condition. Blood disease caused by antibodies to minor red blood-cell antigens such as the K factor, the M factor, the FY factor, and the U factor, produce fetal symptoms similar to those found in Rhesus disease and require the same careful evaluation and treatment. Any woman at risk should have an initial blood test and further tests and screening at the twenty-eighth and thirty-sixth weeks of gestation. Prenatal screening to detect any ABO blood-type incompatibility (any immunological abnormality between the baby's and the mother's blood type) is also advisable.

Although sensitization in an Rh positive woman is unusual, the fact that it can occur is another strong argument for early screening and identification of *any* abnormalities. This can be done only if you go to your doctor as soon as you even suspect you are pregnant and have the routine blood tests carried out on the first visit.

21

Bleeding During Pregnancy

☐ **Bleeding in Early Pregnancy, Miscarriage, And Other Problems**   Bleeding during pregnancy can be an extremely upsetting and traumatic event, since bleeding of any kind is usually associated with the threat of losing the baby. Fortunately, this is a misconception. Of course, any bleeding should be treated as a warning sign, but most people don't realize that occasional bleeding occurs in approximately 30 percent of all pregnancies, and most of these pregnancies continue without damage to the fetus and end in the delivery of a healthy child. Even so, bleeding can be dangerous under certain circumstances. You should educate yourself to recognize the signs of a normal pregnancy and to act quickly if you detect some abnormal event. Since bleeding is considered one of the warning signals of pregnancy, bleeding of any kind should be reported to your obstetrician immediately. He can then evaluate your condition for himself.

This chapter will explore some of the many reasons why bleeding occurs during pregnancy.

☐ **Bleeding During the First Trimester**   In most cases, bleeding is associated with the first trimester of pregnancy, the period from the baby's conception to the end of the twelfth week, calculated from the first day of the last menstrual period. Occasional bleeding during the first few weeks of pregnancy is a common phenomenon, so common that I have reviewed it in Chapter 5, "The First Signs of Pregnancy." A woman may experience slight bleeding in the first day or two after ovulation takes place; at the time of implantation, the attachment of the fertilized egg into the uterus; or around the time of the missed period. The latter is occasionally mistaken for menstruation.

In each case, the slight spotting or staining associated with these stages of the

270 / *Childbirth with Love*

pregnancy is in no way harmful to the continuation of pregnancy, nor does it indicate an abnormality in the fetus.

☐ *Is Bleeding a Danger Sign?*   Occasional bleeding at the beginning of pregnancy is, as a general rule, distinguishable from bleeding associated with miscarriage, or the bleeding you normally experience during your menstrual cycle, by its quantity and appearance, and the symptoms that accompany it.

If you occasionally experience slight bleeding during the first trimester, and the bleeding is without cramping or pain, it is usually *not* a sign of fetal abnormality. This is actually true for any form of painless bleeding during pregnancy. Bleeding should, however, not be dismissed but reported to your doctor and evaluated further. Even harmless bleeding is a warning sign, a signal to rest in bed, and slow down your activities, including abstinence from sexual relations, bathing, and exercise for a few days until the bleeding has stopped, and your doctor is confident about your progress.

If at any point spotting or bleeding is accompanied by severe cramps, it could be a danger sign. Severe cramping can restrict the oxygen supply to the developing fetus. In such a case your doctor should carefully evaluate the progress of your pregnancy. Staining and cramping may be the first symptoms of a threatened miscarriage.

☐ *Is There a Difference Between an Abnormal Menstruation and Miscarriage?*   Sometimes abnormal bleeding associated with menstruation is, in fact, an early miscarriage. This frequently occurs without a woman being aware of the inception of pregnancy. If a woman is not using a reliable form of contraception and experiences abnormal bleeding or pain during her period, especially if the period is a few days late, these may be signs of early miscarriage. Heavy bleeding during a delayed menstrual cycle of any kind is due to the fact that more tissue has a chance to build up inside the uterus. Naturally, if conception has begun, there will also be more tissue than usual. It is difficult to tell the difference between a delayed period and a very early miscarriage from the events of menstruation itself, but if you are trying to conceive, it is useful to take your basal body temperature every day as a means of diagnosis (see Chapter 1).

If it is not a good conception, in the sense that the egg or the sperm is defective, the pregnancy may be sustained for a few days beyond the normal onset of menstruation, but the natural defense mechanism of the body will then take over and abort the conception. As I will explain later, an early miscarriage is often nature's way for the body to rid itself of a defective embryo.

☐ *Cyclic Bleeding During the First Trimester*   Occasional bleeding is usually confined to the first month or two after conception, but women occasionally continue to experience intermittent bleeding for several months at around the time of an expected menstrual period. A typical pattern is some spotting approximately two to three weeks after the first missed period and then once a month for three to four months. Some of the pregnancy charts actually have a little red dot each month when bleeding can occur. These episodes are completely different from menstruation; bleeding of this kind is usually slight, and the color is quite different from that of normal menstrual blood: light pink instead of dark red.

Bleeding episodes during early pregnancy may well be caused by some bio-rhythm in the body which scientists still fail to understand fully. It is generally not dangerous, although any type of bleeding should be carefully evaluated by your doctor.

☐ *Bleeding Caused by Low Progesterone Levels*   Many women miscarry or do not conceive because their progesterone level is not sufficiently high to main-tain pregnancy (the function of progesterone in the ovulatory cycle is described in Chapter 1). At the beginning of pregnancy, progesterone relaxes the uterus and aids the egg in implanting itself in the uterus. If the progesterone level is too low or the corpus luteum produces insufficient estrogen and progesterone, the uterus might contract and expel the egg from the uterine lining, preventing preg-nancy from taking place. Sometimes implantation occurs, but because the pro-gesterone level is too low, uterine cramping develops, and bleeding and miscarriage can take place.

In either of these cases, the level of progesterone can partly be determined by reading the BBT, which should remain one degree higher than normal in the two weeks after ovulation and during a healthy pregnancy. If a reading of the BBT shows fluctuations in the temperature in the two weeks after ovulation, a woman may be failing to become pregnant through what is known as an inade-quate luteal phase. Also, if heavy bleeding occurs within a few days after a missed period, it could be an early miscarriage brought on by a lack of proges-terone, even though in the majority of cases miscarriages are caused by the pres-ence of a defective fetus. Again, fluctuations in the basal body temperature may furnish a clue to the nature of the miscarriage. In cases where a progesterone de-ficiency is suspected, your doctor might recommend natural progesterone injec-tions or suppositories.

In a normal pregnancy, the placenta takes over from the corpus luteum the task of manufacturing progesterone by the fourth or fifth week after conception. However, if the placenta is not healthy enough, insufficient progesterone is pro-duced, and a woman might experience slight bleeding approximately two to three weeks after her expected menstrual period. If this occurs, complete bed rest is usually recommended to increase the blood supply to the uterus which, in turn, may increase the progesterone level and prevent a miscarriage. In some women the corpus luteum disintegrates before enough progesterone is produced from the placenta. In such cases a patient may need natural progesterone injec-tions or suppositories to keep the pregnancy going and prevent miscarriage until progesterone is produced in sufficient amounts by the placenta. In my own practice, I have seen several women with a history of early miscarriages who were able to sustain a pregnancy only after treatment with natural progesterone.

☐ *Bleeding Caused by Fibroid Tumors*   If a woman has large fibroid tumors, a fairly common condition among women in their thirties, the uterine cavity is often disturbed. This may lead to a failure to conceive, since the fibroid might make the uterine cavity too large for conception or separate the wall of the uterus. Even if implantation does take place, these two conditions can still result in miscarriage. If implantation occurs in the area of the tumors, there may be an insufficient blood supply for fetal growth, or premature labor could result.

In certain cases, progesterone suppositories or injections can help relax the uterus sufficiently to allow the placenta to grow normally inside the uterus and permit continuation of the pregnancy. But if a woman experiences repeated miscarriages due to fibroid tumors, she may need a myomectomy, a major operative procedure in which the surgeon enters the abdominal cavity and removes the fibroid tumors without removing the uterus itself. In certain cases of infertility, women have been able to conceive successfully only after a myomectomy operation was performed.

☐ *Bleeding Caused by Cervical Polyps*   A cervical polyp is a small growth just inside the cervix. It is usually caused by irritation or by an inflammatory reaction in the cervix itself. A cervical polyp, because it contains a rich blood supply and because it is very fragile, can cause periodic bleeding, particularly after sexual intercourse or the insertion of a tampon.

If you experience spotting during pregnancy, it is important for your obstetrician to evaluate the source of the bleeding. If the bleeding is coming from the cervix rather than the uterus, your doctor will simply remove the cervical polyp, and the pregnancy can continue uneventfully.

☐ *Cervical Infections and Erosions*   The vaginal area is a perfect medium for infections. It possesses exactly the right temperature and moist environment that bacteria thrive on. At any time, whether you are pregnant or not, there can be an irritation or inflammatory reaction on the cervix, which usually results in some of the blood vessels breaking and forming a small sore on the cervical area. Sometimes the sore will result in staining or bleeding, especially during sexual intercourse. Naturally, during pregnancy this can be mistaken for the beginning of a miscarriage.

Usually a cervical erosion is left alone during pregnancy. The usual methods of treatment in a nonpregnant woman, cautery (burning) or cryosurgery (freezing), are inadvisable during pregnancy. If you have a cervical erosion and your doctor suggests any of these procedures, make sure that you are not pregnant first. Treatment by heating or freezing the cervix could damage the embryo. Since cervical erosion does not affect the course of pregnancy, you can delay surgical treatment until after delivery and soothe the affected area locally with a vaginal cream. Most vaginal creams are safe for use during pregnancy (see Chapter 18). A Pap smear must of course be performed to rule out cancer.

☐ *Cervical Cancer*   Any irregular bleeding at any time should be evaluated immediately by your doctor since it could be a sign of cervical cancer. Fortunately, the early stages of cervical cancer are detectable by the Pap smear. Cervical cancer is a disease that progresses slowly, and the first symptom will usually be picked up by the smear several years before the onset of the disease. Every sexually active woman should have such a test at least once a year. A routine Pap smear is part of the first prenatal examination.

The reason a cervical erosion or sore should be evaluated with a Pap smear is that it usually can't be differentiated from cancer by the naked eye. Any suspicious abnormalities can be checked out by a technique called colposcopy. This is a procedure in which the doctor looks at the cervix through a colposcope, a large microscope pointed into the vagina. Colposcopy enables him to see the blood vessels and the blood cells more clearly, and to take a biopsy of any area that looks suspicious. In the very rare case in which a pregnant woman has advanced cancer of the cervix, it would be up to an oncologist, a cancer specialist, to determine how it should be treated or if it is wise to let the pregnancy continue.

☐ ***The Intrauterine Device and Pregnancy***   Occasionally a woman becomes pregnant when her intrauterine device is still in place. In such a case the IUD sometimes interferes with the implantation of the fertilized egg into the uterine wall, and bleeding may result. If the woman wants to continue the pregnancy, she must see her doctor immediately and have the IUD removed. Otherwise the tail of the IUD could act as a means of absorbing bacteria into the uterus, and a violent infection could result, particularly if the waters break prematurely. A few years ago the risk of this happening was greater, possibly due to the Dalkon Shield, a device which is no longer in use. Sometimes a doctor has difficulty finding the tail of the IUD, because the uterus grows in size in the first weeks of pregnancy and the tail is pulled into the uterus. Special instruments or ultrasonography may then be needed to locate and remove the IUD. While removal of an IUD does increase the risk of miscarriage, a doctor is forced into using these measures because of the high risk of infection.

Once the IUD is removed, the pregnancy can usually continue normally because the placenta generally is implanted into in an area unaffected by the IUD. Since the chance of miscarriage is slightly higher in the first few days after removal of an IUD, a woman should abstain from sexual relations until her doctor is satisfied by her progress.

☐ ***Trauma and Pregnancy***   A pregnant woman may occasionally experience slight bleeding if she has a fall or vigorous sexual relations. Either of these so-called traumas can result in increased uterine cramping, which, in turn, results in shedding blood from the placenta.

In general, the uterus is well protected from any bumps or falls. Although we tend to think of the uterus as a static organ, sitting in a firm position (like the nose), it is actually attached to the abdominal cavity by ligaments and moves freely from side to side. Its special qualities allow it to enjoy a freedom of movement which acts as a buffer if a woman is knocked or bumped during pregnancy. A bump or fall is usually sustained without injury. But if you do fall and the fall results in slight staining, see your doctor immediately. He will usually perform an ultrasonography test to evaluate any possible damage to the fetus or the placenta. If no damage is detectable, he will ask you to stay in bed for a few days to give the uterus and placenta a chance to heal.

Trauma commonly occurs after sexual intercourse when the thrusting of the penis is vigorous enough to push up the uterus and produce some uterine cramping. This in turn reduces the blood supply to the placenta and results in staining or spotting. Report any bleeding of this kind to your doctor, even though sexual activities are unlikely to harm the baby. Sometimes the onset of staining under these circumstances will lead your doctor to forbid sexual relations for a few days or longer until he is sure the fetus and placenta are healthy. Sexual relations during pregnancy should always be gentle, even if a woman is perfectly healthy.

☐ **Bleeding Disorders**   A few women of childbearing age suffer from what the medical profession call bleeding disorders. These include diseases of the blood in which there is an abnormality of the clotting mechanism. A woman with any of these conditions is a high-risk patient, and the pregnancy is usually monitored carefully by a perinatologist and a hematologist, a specialist in blood disorders. In a pregnancy of this kind, there is a higher risk of abnormal bleeding. Patients are often asked not to have sexual relations and are warned against the dangers of falls or strenuous physical activities. Of course, these women are well aware of their condition and know how important it is to contact their physician at the first sign of any bleeding.

☐ **Bleeding After Strenuous Exercise and Jogging**   In the last few years we have entered on an era of increased physical awareness, and there has been an enormous interest in jogging, bicycling, exercise classes, and other structured physical activities during pregnancy. In fact, many pregnant women increase their physical activity, especially in the second trimester, because they have more energy than usual. They are delighted by the way they feel, and they want to keep their bodies in good condition in preparation for labor. This new emphasis on fitness has its good and bad aspects. Most women exercise within their capabilities, but when a woman prolongs a strenuous workout, this decreases the blood supply to the uterus, just as a bump or fall does, by diverting the available oxygen to the muscles. Consequently, less oxygen reaches the uterus and the placenta, and the deprivation of oxygen can result in a spasm reaction in which the blood vessels are broken and there is bleeding from the uterus.

Any bleeding after exercise is a warning sign, particularly for women who are older. If you begin to bleed, arrange to see your doctor immediately and have ultrasonography performed; a sonogram will assure you that the placenta is in the proper position in the uterus, and the fetus is still growing. If everything is going well, it is still a good idea to cut down or eliminate sports activities for a few weeks after the bleeding has stopped, and to slow down in general. I would personally recommend a pregnant woman to cut down her usual exercise program and make some reasonable compromises during pregnancy. It's much better to play a quieter game of tennis or take up doubles instead of singles, or try to find another pregnant woman to play with than to put excessive pressure on your body. This is equally true of other popular sports. Remember: never push your body beyond its limits.

☐ **Early Miscarriage**   The word "miscarriage" is generally used by lay people to describe the premature birth of a fetus before it is sufficiently developed to survive outside the mother's womb. The age of viability is considered to be the twenty-fourth week of fetal development. Doctors usually use the term "spontaneous abortion" rather than "miscarriage." A spontaneous abortion is the same thing.

Miscarriage is a very common event and not always a traumatic one. In many cases, women miscarry without even realizing what has happened; a period which is delayed by a week or two and causes unusually heavy bleeding is often a miscarriage in disguise. Miscarriages after a clear diagnosis of pregnancy has been made are also extremely common; 15 to 20 percent of all known pregnancies end in miscarriage. Initially, this figure may seem high, but the successful continuance of pregnancy depends on such delicate factors that a doctor is often amazed by the number of successful pregnancies that end, miraculously, in the birth of a baby.

☐ *The Psychological Aspects of Miscarriage* It is very important to realize that a miscarriage is a natural event. The overwhelming majority of miscarriages occur when the egg or the sperm are abnormal in some way, and such severe abnormalities ensue that the body responds by cleansing itself of the defective embryo or fetus. Unfortunately, when a woman realizes that she has miscarried, she and her partner often feel tremendously guilty and blame themselves for injuring the pregnancy, not knowing that it is almost impossible to completely dislodge the fetus through physical exertion or a blow to the uterus. Again, in the great majority of miscarriages, the embryo or fetus is simply unable to survive the normal progress of pregnancy because of congenital abnormalities incompatible with life.

☐ *Why Does a Miscarriage Occur?* Most miscarriages take place very early in pregnancy. In 50 percent of miscarriages, the embryo is too defective to mature beyond the earliest stage. This pathological condition is known as "the blighted ovum syndrome" (although a defective sperm is just as likely to cause the event as a defective ovum). Despite its frightening name, a blighted ovum simply means that the embryo was so abnormal that growth was not possible from the very beginning of the pregnancy and disintegration followed. When miscarriage occurs under these circumstances, a woman usually passes nothing more than a small sac filled with fluid because there is no fetus. The second most common cause of miscarriage is a chromosomal or structural abnormality in the fetus. Chromosomal abnormalities are usually more common than structural ones. In one study, researchers discovered chromosomal abnormalities in 60 to 70 percent of the tissues from spontaneous abortions. *In most cases, a blighted ovum or an aborted fetus is a random event.* A woman can experience one miscarriage, and the next pregnancy will be completely normal. A single miscarriage is upsetting, but it does not necessarily jeopardize your chances of a successful conception and pregnancy the next time.

☐ *Signs of Miscarriage* When a miscarriage is threatening, a woman usually observes some initial spotting or staining. Then the bleeding increases and is accompanied by a degree of pain which is caused by the stretching and opening of the cervix as the uterus contracts. When severe pain occurs, it is usually a sign that the blood supply to the placenta is insufficient, and the fetus has been damaged.

☐ *Treatment of Miscarriage* If you experience the early symptoms of a miscarriage, you should alert your doctor immediately. If you are only spotting and there is no cramping or pain, this is termed a "threatened abortion," and the uterus may simply heal up. In this case, your doctor may decide to follow your progress with ultrasonography. By using sonography, he should be able to see the embryonic sac and the embryo itself. If the test reveals an empty sac, this is proof that the embryo has disappeared, and a miscarriage is inevitable. Usually a woman is admitted to the hospital for a D&C.

In cases where there is bleeding but the doctor can still see the fetus on an ultrasound machine, he can continue to monitor the patient with ultrasound. If he then detects some abnormality and the amount of tissue in the uterus starts to decrease, he may feel it is better to have a D&C or a suction abortion to empty the uterus immediately and enable a woman to plan for a new pregnancy. A doctor who does not have ultrasound can perform an initial quantitative measurement of the beta subunit level of human chorionic gonadotropin (HCG), the hormone which is produced in large quantities in the beginning of pregnancy, and then ask the patient to return for another test in a week. If the amount of beta subunit HCG decreases, he will probably presume that the fetus is not developing normally.

If pain or cramping is severe, see your doctor immediately. At this point it may be impossible to stop the miscarriage, and you should be admitted to the hospital at the first opportunity, because miscarriage can cause tremendous bleeding as the uterus empties itself.

If you have already miscarried, it is very important to see your doctor and have the uterus examined, even if you feel quite sure that the tissues have been completely expelled. In early pregnancy there is rarely a clear separation between the uterus and placenta, and the placenta often fails to detach itself completely from the uterine wall. Even the smallest amount of tissue can keep the uterus open and as the uterus continues to contract, bacteria can be sucked in and cause a serious condition called septic abortion. The only way to treat septic abortion is by massive doses of antibiotics, and it could do permanent damage to the uterus and Fallopian tubes. Nowadays most doctors like to use the suction procedure to treat patients who have miscarried rather than the old-fashioned D&C, because it is possible to injure the lining of the uterus through an overvigorous scraping of the placenta. After a poorly done D&C, too much of the uterine lining may be removed, and this can result in *intrauterine adhesions,* which could make it difficult to conceive in the future. Suctioning is a far gentler way to remove the tissues from the uterus.

☐ *One Miscarriage Is Very Common*   Remember, a single miscarriage is a common experience. Don't let it destroy your emotional life. Go to the doctor promptly, get the proper treatment, and try to regard it as a random event, although I know the emotional adjustment after a miscarriage can be difficult.

Most women want to know whether they can or should conceive again after a miscarriage. There is no reason for you not to do so, and the chances are that the second pregnancy will be a successful one. However, you can take some practical steps before conceiving again. Give yourself a few months to allow the body to heal so the uterus will become strong and healthy. In the meantime, have your thyroid function tested (the thyroid gland can be checked by a blood test of the T_3 and T_4). If your thyroid function is slightly below normal, this could mean that it is insufficient to stimulate the brain hormones which, in their turn, normally trigger ovulation and aid in maintenance of the pregnancy. Second, use the time to get your mind and body in good physical condition, and take extra vitamins, particularly vitamin B_6. Ask your doctor to prescribe prenatal vitamins; they are more nearly complete than the commercial brands, and at least one new study has shown the value of prenatal vitamins before conception in preventing birth defects (see Chap. 2). When the body is in good physical shape, there are likely to be fewer fetal abnormalities. Finally, when you do conceive, take your basal body temperature every day to make sure that your temperature remains at a consistently high level. If your temperature drops, indicating an insufficient amount of progesterone in the blood, your doctor can treat you with natural progesterone injections or progesterone suppositories to help avoid a miscarriage.

☐ *Repeated Miscarriages—What Do They Mean?* If a woman has experienced more than three first-trimester miscarriages, the couple should probably go to a genetic specialist for counseling. At this point, a full medical work-up of *both* partners is needed to help establish the underlying cause, if any. (See Chap. 21.) Once genetic factors have been ruled out through chromosomal analysis of both the husband and wife, most infertility specialists will recommend a thyroid function test, a biopsy of the endometrium to check for hormone deficiencies, and an X-ray examination of the uterus.

☐ *Incompetent Cervix* A miscarriage in the second trimester is often caused by a condition doctors call "incompetent cervix." It is more common among women who have had repeated abortions or who have an inborn abnormality of the uterus. This condition was often seen in the past after the cervix was ripped apart during an illegal abortion. A miscarriage due to an incompetent cervix usually takes place when the cervical muscle suddenly weakens, and the cervix dilates prematurely and painlessly without noticeable contractions. A woman may experience a slight discharge or a feeling of wetness, and the fetus is then expelled rapidly.

Since there does seem to be a connection between incompetent cervix and the number of abortions a woman has had before the pregnancy, any woman who had more than one abortion in which the cervix was damaged should be particularly careful during pregnancy and try to rest as much as possible. Furthermore, a hysterosalpingogram, an X-ray of the uterus and tubes, can usually determine whether or not there is a shortening of the cervix or any other abnormality. If necessary, the cervix is stitched up by the procedure described on page 389.

A woman who has experienced three or more miscarriages in the second trimester is usually considered to have a condition called *habitual abortion*. Very often this condition can be taken care of by a simple procedure in which the cervix is stitched together to prevent it from opening prematurely. The woman's doctor will try to establish the cause of the miscarriages before the next pregnancy by taking an X-ray of the uterus. If the problem is attributable to an incompetent cervix, a suture or stitch is placed around the cervix and then tightened to make sure that the cervix stays intact (a *Shirodkar procedure*). This is usually done immediately after the twelfth week of pregnancy. Once the cervix is stitched, the obstetrician will recommend increased bed rest, avoidance of sexual relations, and extra care at work or around the house. Women in demanding physical jobs where there is lifting or bending are usually asked to take a leave of absence from work. This simple operation has helped many women who lost babies in the past to carry their pregnancies successfully to term. At term, the stitch can be removed to allow for spontaneous labor.

☐ *Hydatiform Mole*   A hydatiform mole is a developmental abnormality of the placenta which results in miscarriage. It is rare in the United States and Europe—approximately one out of every two thousand pregnancies are affected—but Oriental and South American women, including Orientals and South Americans living in the United States, experience it in far greater numbers. The chances of it occurring are higher as a woman grows older. While a hydatiform mole is usually the result of benign (noncancerous) cell growth in the uterus, it can, under special circumstances, develop into a form of cancer called *choriocarcinoma.* Fortunately, this can now often be prevented by proper treatment.

A molar pregnancy is one in which pregnancy begins normally but the placenta begins to change for unknown reasons and forms small cysts (moles) which subsequently begin to replace the placenta and kill the fetus. Usually the placenta is damaged, and a miscarriage takes place. The first symptom is generally an episode of painless bleeding. Once the molar pregnancy has been diagnosed by ultrasound or a blood-level test (the blood level of HCG is much higher than normal in a molar pregnancy), the doctor will admit a woman to the hospital for a D&C or suction abortion. The uterine wall should be scraped carefully, and all the blood vessels removed. The patient's blood level will then be monitored intensively for about one year to make sure that the HCG has completely disappeared from the body, since an incomplete miscarriage from a molar pregnancy can turn into cancer in the twelve-month period after the D&C. Modern chemotherapy is now used to treat this condition with a reasonable degree of success.

If you have experienced a molar pregnancy, the safest form of contraception is the birth control pill, which does not interfere with the HCG levels. You will usually be advised to wait for a year before becoming pregnant again. After that time, there is no reason not to try for a second pregnancy, and, since the recurrence of molar pregnancies is low and the success rate of subsequent deliveries is high, you have every chance of enjoying a successful pregnancy the next time.

☐ *Placenta Previa*   Placenta previa is a condition in which the placenta lodges itself abnormally low in the uterus, usually close to or around the cervix. This condition, which is rarely seen in a first pregnancy, may cause irregular bleeding soon after the implantation of the egg, an occurrence that is described more fully in Chapter 25, "Serious Complications During Pregnancy."

☐ *Bleeding as a Sign of Labor*   Any bleeding in the later part of pregnancy should be evaluated since it could be a sign of impending labor.

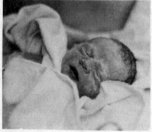

Figure 49: Sara Rachel a few minutes after birth, still covered with the greasy intrauterine vernix. A molar pregnancy is a frightening experience for any woman, but it can be successfully cured. Since the chance of recurrence is extremely slim, there is no reason why a woman should not try to conceive again, as soon as her doctor believes she can do so safely. Sara Rachel's mother had had a molar pregnancy just a year and a half before her birth.
Reproduced with permission from Sara's parents.

☐ *Ectopic Pregnancy*   An ectopic or extrauterine pregnancy is one that takes place outside the uterus. Instead of the egg's implanting itself in the lining of the uterus, it develops in one of the Fallopian tubes or one of the ovaries, or somewhere in the abdomen. This situation occurs only when a fertilized egg is unable to enter the uterus, and the environment elsewhere in the sexual organs is sufficiently favorable to allow implantation and development, at least for a short time. By far the most common location for an ectopic pregnancy is one or the other of the Fallopian tubes, which is why it is so often known as "tubal pregnancy."

Unfortunately, it is almost impossible to sustain a pregnancy outside the uterus (I have to say "almost impossible" because there have been instances of abdominal pregnancy that have come close to term). Within a few weeks of a tubal pregnancy, the embryo is pushed through the end of the tube or ruptures the tubal wall, causing a serious medical emergency and frequently loss of the tube itself. A woman can die if an ectopic pregnancy is misdiagnosed or treatment is delayed.

One in every hundred or so pregnancies is an ectopic pregnancy, and the incidence seems to be increasing. Because of the statistical possibility of such a pregnancy, all couples, whether they are planning a pregnancy or not, should be alerted to the characteristic symptoms of this very serious condition.

☐ *Symptoms of Ectopic Pregnancy*   If a pregnancy occurs outside the uterus, the symptoms will vary, depending on where the implantation takes place. If the embryo implants itself in the ovaries or the abdomen, there may be few symptoms. In the rare instance of an *abdominal pregnancy*, the pregnancy can come quite close to term. Then the only possible delivery method is by Cesarean section.

In the great majority of cases, the embryo implants itself in one of the Fallopian tubes. For the first few weeks of a tubal pregnancy, a woman usually experiences normal pregnancy signs: an absence of menstruation, increased hormonal levels, including the level of HCG, even morning sickness. Then, when the conception is about six weeks to two months old, it becomes large enough to strain the Fallopian tube, causing an increasing degree of pain which is often associated with vaginal bleeding (although this is not, by any means, experienced in every tubal pregnancy). The bleeding sometimes begins slowly during the night, and by the morning a woman may think she has had a miscarriage because of the clotting of the blood fractions in various layers; one of the layers will be white from the white blood cells and is easily mistaken for the fetus. If bleeding of this type occurs or you experience bleeding and pain in rhythmic contractions or a severe pain that is more acute on one side, *go to the doctor immediately.*

After a few days, the pain from an untreated ectopic pregnancy increases in strength to such a degree that a woman is almost incapacitated. At this point the Fallopian tube can burst and cause profuse internal bleeding. A woman often goes into shock if the tube ruptures, her pulse increases, and her blood pressure goes down. Since lack of emergency treatment can lead to death from internal bleeding, *go to the emergency room of the nearest hospital if you cannot locate your doctor immediately.*

☐ **What Is the Treatment for Ectopic Pregnancy?**   If a woman experiences bleeding and pain or pain alone, her doctor will first evaluate her condition with a pregnancy test. Sometimes a suspected ectopic pregnancy will turn out to be a ruptured ovarian cyst or internal bleeding during ovulation, and no surgery will be needed. If the pregnancy test is positive, he may decide to perform a laparoscopy, a procedure that will enable him to view the Fallopian tubes through a periscope; and at the same time, he may order a sonogram. By using ultrasonography, a physician can determine whether a pregnancy has occurred inside or outside the uterus. If the doctor judges that the tube is about to burst, he may perform a further test called a *culdecentesis,* a minor surgical procedure performed in the office. The woman's feet are placed in stirrups and a speculum is inserted into the vagina. A needle is then inserted through the vaginal wall into the abdominal cavity. If blood is aspirated through the needle, this indicates the presence of internal bleeding, and surgery must be performed immediately if the blood is ample in amount and does not show signs of clotting—another symptom of a ruptured ectopic pregnancy.

Once a tube has ruptured, exploratory laparotomy must be carried out under a general anesthetic so the surgeon can find the source of the bleeding and tie up the blood vessels. A blood transfusion is usually required to replace the lost blood. Unfortunately in an emergency procedure, the doctor may remove a large portion of the Fallopian tube, making it more difficult for the woman to conceive at a future time. This is one of the reasons for seeing a doctor at the onset of the initial symptoms of an ectopic pregnancy because, under certain conditions, a Fallopian tube can be saved if surgery is performed before the tube bursts.

☐ **Can the Tube Be Saved After an Ectopic Pregnancy?**   Yes, it can. Modern surgical techniques developed by a few specialists in the larger medical centers have pioneered the so-called conservative treatment of ectopic pregnancies. Conservative surgical treatment is a new procedure in which part of the tube is saved by the use of microsurgical techniques. Unfortunately, knowledge of these new techniques is still limited, and the majority of doctors are not specialists in this area. Ideally, you should always have a back-up doctor at one of the larger university hospitals whom you can use in an emergency. If an ectopic pregnancy is suspected and you are initially seen in a hospital that does not have modern facilities or doctors trained in the new techniques, you should, if possible, be referred to another hospital for surgery.

The new procedures are extremely delicate and require a high degree of skill. If the doctor can operate before the tube has burst, he can make a tiny incision in the tube, empty out the developing embryo, and sew the tube back together again, using a magnifying glass and special microsurgical techniques. This enhances a woman's future chance of conception, because the tube is still viable. In my own hospital, we have performed a number of these operations, and many of the women have subsequently given birth successfully. Even after the tube has ruptured, it is still possible for it to be saved if the doctor can salvage the unaffected portions of the tube instead of taking it out completely. This will enable an infertility specialist to evaluate the condition of the tube at a later date and perhaps repair it so that a pregnancy can occur more easily in the future.

It is not impossible for a woman to conceive even if she has lost one of her

Fallopian tubes. However, it does cut down the chances of a conception. We hope the new procedures will make it much easier for women to recover from the effects of a tubal pregnancy and raise the conception rate considerably in the future.

☐ *Why Ectopic Pregnancies Are Increasing* The number of ectopic pregnancies is rising, and in the United States the rate may now be as high as 1 out of every 130 pregnancies, or about 8 out of 1000 women who become pregnant. At the same time, the death rate for this condition is decreasing, thanks to better methods of treatment, although ectopic pregnancy remains a major health hazard.

There are probably good reasons for the recent increase. The risk of a tubal pregnancy is higher among women who have experienced an infection of the Fallopian tubes. Today, with increased sexual activity involving more than one partner, the infection rate is definitely higher than it used to be. Infections of the sperm or egg may possibly result in ectopic pregnancy as well. The introduction of the IUD in the last twenty years may also have had an effect; some researchers think the use of the IUD prior to pregnancy increases the risk of an ectopic pregnancy because it so often leads to infection or scarring of the tubes. Since an IUD can cause unsymptomatic infections or inflammatory reactions in the tubes and the *known* infection rate decidedly increases with IUD use, there may well be a connection between IUD use and the increase of tubal pregnancies in the last decade. If you have had an IUD, you ought to be even more alert to the signs of ectopic pregnancy.

☐ *How to Protect Yourself Against an Ectopic Pregnancy* First, the best way to prevent an ectopic pregnancy is to avoid a pelvic infection or treat it promptly. Most ectopic pregnancies occur in women who have had acute tubal infections. If you have lower abdominal pain, however slight, or you suspect you may have contracted gonorrhea or some other infection, go to your doctor immediately for treatment. Particularly in a case of gonorrhea, the sensitive time is the period during and after menstruation, when the bacteria can move into the Fallopian tubes and cause permanent damage. Any woman who is using an IUD should know that she is more sensitive to pelvic infections.

Second, if you plan to conceive and you know you had a serious infection in the past, it might be wise to schedule a hysterosalpingogram, an X-ray of the uterus and tubes, before conception to rule out any abnormalities (see Chap. 3). If there is significant scarring, it may be removable by microsurgical techniques. Once you conceive, inform your doctor of your past gynecological history and watch for any symptoms of an ectopic pregnancy. Even if you were never aware of a pelvic infection but you used an IUD in the past, be alert to the symptoms of an abnormal pregnancy. Finally, if you have had one tubal pregnancy and plan to become pregnant again, any symptoms, however slight, should be evaluated immediately. The likelihood of an ectopic pregnancy is higher among women who have already experienced one such pregnancy.

In any case of ectopic pregnancy, it is important to recognize the symptoms, to get medical help immediately, and, if possible, to have the pregnancy treated by conservative surgical techniques and thus protect your fertility for the future. As in every aspect of health care, an informed woman is her own best friend.

22

Genetic Counseling

When the knowledge of genetics was in its infancy, prospective parents with a family history of inherited disease were faced with a heartbreaking dilemma: should they try to have a child and run the risk of passing on the disease or should they avert a potential tragedy by avoiding childbearing altogether and thus deprive themselves of having a family? Because families and family doctors had little understanding of how genetic diseases were transmitted or how they affected the individual, the common fear of genetic disease deterred many people from marrying and having children, sometimes unnecessarily. Now that our knowledge of genetic disorders is increasing rapidly, parents and parents-to-be are still asking the same question, "Will my child have a genetic disorder?" but the difference is that some of the answers are being provided by a new medical specialty called genetic counseling.

Recent studies of genetics have revolutionized knowledge in this area: more than two thousand genetic and chromosomal disorders have already been identified and a number of them can now be detected prenatally through amniocentesis and other sophisticated tests. Couples who a few years ago would have refused to have a second child because their first child was born with a birth defect, or who would have hesitated to have a child at all because a relative had a crippling disorder or they felt they were too "old," are now being given counseling and testing that enable them to have healthy children or at least provide them with an informed option about childbearing. In the future, it may well be possible to treat successfully many affected children while they are still inside the womb.

☐ *What Is Genetic Counseling?* Genetic counseling is a service to families who are, or feel that they are, at risk for hereditary or genetic disorder. According to the American Society of Human Genetics, the aim of genetic counselors is to help the family or individual understand: (1) the medical background and the probable course of a particular disease; (2) the way heredity contributes to the disease and the risk of its recurrence within the family; (3) the alternatives for dealing with the recurrence of the disorder; (4) how to choose a course of action that best fits in with their personal circumstances and ethical and religious beliefs (i.e., when amniocentesis and other tests are called for and what they entail); and (5) how to make the best possible adjustment when a family member is already affected by a genetic disease.

□ *Who Needs Counseling?*

1. Anyone who is aware of a family history of inherited genetic disorders, or who has a genetic disorder or birth defect.
2. The parents of a child with a serious congenital abnormality or known genetic disorder.
3. A couple who have experienced more than three miscarriages, or a miscarriage in which the fetal tissue was analyzed and found to be chromosomally abnormal.
4. A pregnant woman over the age of thirty-five who, because of her age, has an increased risk of bearing a child with a chromosomal abnormality.
5. Prospective parents belonging to certain ethnic groups who are at high risk for particular genetic disorders: Tay-Sachs disease, thalassemia, and sickle-cell anemia.
6. A couple who is aware of prenatal exposure to an excessive dose of radiation, drugs, or other environmental agents that could result in congenital malformation.

□ *How Can I Find a Genetic Counselor?*   Genetic counselors usually work with physicians whose basic training is in internal medicine but who also have an advanced knowledge of obstetrics, pediatrics, and the study of chromosomal and genetic disorders. Most of the large medical centers now have genetic counseling and testing centers, and some more progressive states have also set up regional genetic consultation services to help people on a local basis. In addition, certain organizations, such as the National Tay Sachs and Allied Diseases Foundation, have developed screening programs to detect carriers of particular genetic diseases. Some states request premarital sickle-cell screening. If you, or another family member, would like to be screened for a particular genetic disorder or are aware of a family history of a particular genetic disease, you can ask your doctor to refer you to an appropriate center or organization, or you can write directly to the March of Dimes Birth Defects Foundation at 1275 Mamaroneck Avenue, White Plains, New York 10605 or the National Genetics Foundation at 555 West 57th Street, New York, New York 10019.

Both of these organizations help to fund clinical services to affected families and prospective parents and will supply you with a guide to services in your own area. If you are already pregnant, the first step is a consultation with your obstetrician *early in the pregnancy*. He can then refer you and your partner to a genetic counseling center where any prenatal tests can also be carried out. Be prepared to take the initiative. Many obstetricians unfortunately fail to give their patients information in appropriate cases, either because they don't like to add to a couple's anxieties, or because they feel that prenatal diagnosis encourages abortion.

☐ *The Stages of Genetic Counseling*   A genetic counseling session or sessions involves a number of stages. The first step entails assembling a complete family history, which can provide information about the genetic basis of any disorder which might be present. Even if you are considering prenatal diagnosis because of advanced maternal age alone, the family history is still important.

It is sometimes difficult to obtain an exact family history, but anything that might indicate a congenital problem should be written down. (It is also important to be aware of any negative information—an *absence* of a particular symptom or symptoms.) Go to your counseling session prepared to give dates of birth and death for your parents, aunts, uncles, and siblings, and a detailed medical history of each individual if possible. Any miscarriage or stillbirth within the immediate family should be listed as well; either event is sometimes an indication of genetic disease. Once the counselor has assembled the family history, she/he may recommend special blood tests or a complete chromosome count for you and/or your partner.

The second stage is the counselor's interpretation of the evidence. Each case is individual and any number of conclusions are possible. Establishing or excluding a genetic or chromosomal condition is often a complex undertaking, since birth defects are not always the result of genetic factors. A birth defect can be caused by a random or inherited chromosomal abnormality; it can be transmitted by a single gene from one parent or a matching gene from both parents; it may be caused by environmental factors; or it can result from what is called multifactorial inheritance—a combination of environmental and/or several genetic causes. Once the counselor has assembled the available evidence, she or he will try to arrive at a diagnosis of the disease and then attempt to calculate the chances of an occurrence or recurrence within a couple's immediate family by consulting statistics from other, similar cases. Many parents are relieved to find that the risk of bearing a severely defective baby is not nearly as great as they had anticipated, and the vast majority of patients who are referred for advanced maternal age can be comforted by the finding that they are carrying a chromosomally normal child.

Once the counselor has outlined the probable or possible risks and presented the available options to the parents, a couple is left to make their own decision. Some prospective parents with a heritable genetic disorder choose artificial insemination or try to adopt a child rather than chance an affected pregnancy; others take a calculated risk and the woman becomes pregnant, or they choose to continue an existing pregnancy, hoping that the child will not be seriously handicapped. Fortunately for many parents, the risk of bearing a child with a disease incompatible with normal life has been considerably reduced by new prenatal testing methods. Amniocentesis (the insertion of a needle into the amniotic fluid to withdraw a sample for analysis), ultrasonography (a scanning device that projects an image of the fetus), and a recent technique called fetoscopy (which enables the perinatologist to obtain a blood sample from the fetus) have now been used in thousands of pregnancies to establish the absence or presence of a genetic disorder or serious birth defect.

☐ *Types of Genetic Disorders*   Classically, genetic disorders are divided into three main groups: (1) single-gene disorders, in which there is a genetic error that is passed on to the next generation; (2) chromosomal disorders, in which the usual orderly chromosomal pattern is disturbed by the presence of an extra chromosome or chromosome fragment, the absence of a chromosome, the translocation, or rearrangement, of the genetic material within or between the chromosomes, or the presence of more than one cell line, each containing a different number of chromosomes; (3) multifactorial disorders, in which a number of small mistakes in the genetic information combine to produce the defect; or the defect has an environmental as well as a genetic origin.

These categories do not include the large number of birth defects that appear to have a purely environmental cause—those caused by rubella, for instance.

☐ *How Chromosomal Abnormalities Occur*   Chromosomes, the tiny chemical structures that are central to every cell in the human body, are the critical factors in determining heredity traits. In the normal human being the chromosomal structure is rather precise. Every human cell, with the exception of the cells found in the maternal egg and the paternal sperm, contain twenty-two matching pairs of autosomal chromosomes, each one of which is distinctly different in appearance from any other pair. The full human complement of forty-six chromosomes is rounded out by the two sex chromosomes: two X chromosomes for the normal female, and an X and a Y for the normal male—one inherited from the egg and one from the sperm.

Since each chromosome is made up of thousands of microscopic genes arranged in a precise order, it is not surprising that the ribbon of genes is sometimes broken or that whole chromosomes are occasionally missing or are accidentally doubled in number, or completely out of sequence. A significant break, or an extra or missing chromosome, changes the way in which the cells function, and the cells either fail to develop beyond an early stage, or the child is born with an obvious birth defect. Chromosomal abnormalities are usually random occurrences. A few otherwise normal parents possess an unusual chromosome pattern that produces a visible defect in their children, but by far the largest number of chromosomal abnormalities happen spontaneously when the egg or the sperm is damaged in some way before or during conception.

In the last few years it has become possible to detect chromosomal abnormalities prenatally through a special process known as karyotyping. Karyotyping, a relatively new technique perfected in the 1960s, enables the geneticist to analyze the chromosomes by arranging photographs of them in pairs and examining them for abnormalities. The use of a technique called banding has greatly improved the accuracy of the procedure. In banding the chromosomes, an enzyme is used to stripe the chromosomes in a characteristic way, so that smaller changes within them can be identified.

The first step in the chromosomal analysis of a fetus is amniocentesis, de-

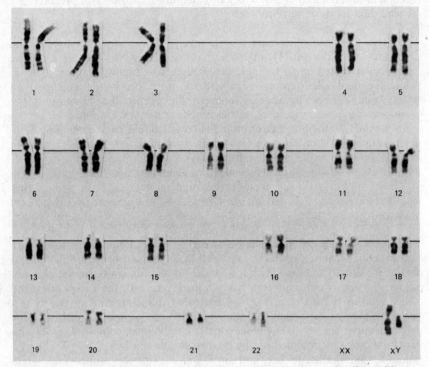

Figure 50: Normal Karyotype: This picture shows the twenty-two pairs of matching autosomal chromosomes belonging to a normal infant. Each one is distinctly different in appearance from any other pair. The child's sex (male) is indicated by one X chromosome and one Y chromosome.

Picture from Dr. Rina Schmidt, Director of Cytogenetics, Metpath, Teterboro, New Jersey.

scribed in detail beginning on page 299. The fetal cells obtained in the test are placed in an incubator. Here they are mixed with special agents that speed up their division and growth, and are left undisturbed for about two weeks until cell division has progressed far enough to allow for analysis. The resulting clusters of chromosomes are put under a microscope and photographed. The chromosomes from each of three or more cells are then painstakingly identified, cut out from the photograph, and placed with their appropriate partners (see Fig. 50). Any peculiarly shaped, missing, or extra chromosomes may be signs of abnormality, and the geneticist can usually identify the syndrome affecting the fetus by examining the pattern of the karyotype. Down's syndrome, for instance, is characterized by the presence of three instead of the normal two chromosomes, in the twenty-first position (see figure). The karyotype also establishes fetal sex—a piece of information that is important when a family has a history of sex-linked diseases. A family with a history of hemophilia, for instance, might choose to abort all male fetuses and have only daughters, since only males are affected by this disease.

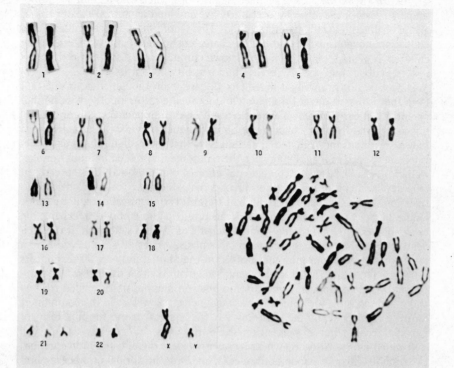

Figure 51: Karyotype Showing Down's Syndrome: As in Figure 50, photographs of the chromosomes, which are initially located in clumps, have been cut out and carefully matched, pair by pair. This karyotype shows three chromosomes instead of the normal two chromosomes in the twenty-first position, an indication of Down's syndrome (formerly called mongolism). There is one X and one Y chromosome, indicating a male infant. After this kind of careful analysis, a geneticist can inform the parents that a woman is carrying a child affected by Down's syndrome.

Here are the most common reasons for performing a chromosomal analysis on the fetus:

1. Advanced maternal age—the mother is already thirty-five or over, or expects the child at age thirty-five (in some centers thirty-seven is considered a more appropriate age to initiate analysis).
2. When the family already has a child with a chromosomal abnormality, such as Down's syndrome.
3. When either parent is known to be the carrier of a chromosomal problem.
4. If the mother is known to be the carrier of a sex-linked disease such as hemophilia or certain types of muscular dystrophy, in which only male offspring are at risk for the disease. Fetal blood sampling (see page 304) is another more sophisticated test that may be used to detect the actual presence of certain X-linked diseases.

☐   **Down's Syndrome**   The great majority of women who request a chromosomal analysis of the fetus are over thirty-five and are therefore at greater risk of giving birth to a Down's syndrome child. This syndrome, a defect that was once known as mongolism because of the characteristic facial appearance of these children, is by far the most common known chromosomal disorder, occurring as it does in about one out of every six hundred fifty live births.

Down's is not primarily a hereditary disease, even though there is one rare form that is passed down through a chromosomal error in an otherwise normal parent. Most cases of Down's are the result of an improper division of the fertilized egg shortly after conception. Some geneticists think the association of Down's with advanced maternal age suggests that some slight abnormality develops in the egg as it ages, but since the syndrome is also seen in much younger women, it could be just a coincidental error in chromosomal division early in fetal development, or the result of direct damage to the egg or sperm before fertilization. Normally, cells divide in half to form two identical daughter cells. A failure in the process of cell division can result in the embryo's receiving the extra number 21 chromosome so characteristic of Down's syndrome. If the accident has occurred before fertilization takes place, the resulting fetus will have a total of forty-seven chromosomes instead of the normal forty-six throughout its cells—an aberration that leads to mental retardation and a distinct physical appearance. This pattern of three chromosomes in one position is called *trisomy* and it is responsible for other chromosomal defects as well as in the commonest form of Down's syndrome. Trisomy 21, the medical name for this form of Down's, accounts for 95 percent of all Down's cases.

A much rarer form is known as mosaicism. Here the affected individual has two or more different populations of cells, one with the normal number of chromosomes, and one with forty-seven chromosomes. This unusual situation arises when there is an accident in the cell division shortly after fertilization.

The third and rarest form of Down's is an inherited defect; the result of a familial condition known to geneticists as translocation.

An individual becomes a Down's carrier when one of the two number 21 chromosomes is accidentally patched onto another chromosome. This apparently normal individual lacks the symptoms of the syndrome because he or she has the normal amount of chromosomal material present in each cell. However, during reproduction, there is a risk that an egg or sperm cell will receive the "free" number 21 chromosome *and* the chromosome that has another chromosome attached to it. Successful fertilization will then produce a child with three chromosomes, two of them free and one attached to some other chromosome—in other words, the child, unlike the parent, will receive an extra number 21 chromosome and will have Down's syndrome. Unfortunately Down's carriers are usually recognized only after the birth of a child with the disease, though their condition could have been detected through a simple blood test for chromosomal analysis.

☐   **Down's Syndrome and the Older Mother**   A number of common chromosomal defects are trisomy disorders, in which three chromosomes instead of the normal two are present in the cells. A trisomy disorder can be caused by a defect in either the sperm or the egg, but most accidents of cell division appear to originate in the egg rather than the sperm, probably because the eggs are present in the ovaries at birth and deteriorate over the years. Another theory suggests a relationship between the trisomy disorders and the onset of menopause: one possible explanation for the sudden rise in Down's children born to women over forty.

The risk of having a child with Down's syndrome increases slowly after thirty-five and quite dramatically after forty:

MOTHER'S AGE	INCIDENCE OF DOWN'S SYNDROME
UNDER 30	LESS THAN 1 IN 1000
30	1 in 900
35	1 in 400
36	1 in 300
37	1 in 230
38	1 in 180
39	1 in 135
40	1 in 105
42	1 in 60
44	1 in 35
46	1 in 20
48	1 in 12

The chances of a woman under thirty having a child with a trisomy disorder is so low that the slight risk of miscarriage associated with amniocentesis, as well as the time and expense, would make it impractical for every pregnant woman to have the test. So many more babies are born to women in the younger age groups, however, that younger women actually have more Down's babies than older women, a fact that conflicts with common belief. This means we will have to wait until there is a simpler prenatal screening test, similar perhaps to a Pap smear, before all pregnancies can be screened and the majority of chromosomal disorders are detected prenatally. One group of researchers are already experimenting with a vaginal smear test designed to detect abnormalities from the leakage of amniotic fluid into the vagina, and another group is working on the first stages of a simple blood test. Until such techniques become available, we can at least make amniocentesis available to more women in the high-risk group through education, counseling, and increased facilities for testing.

☐ **Genetic Disease in the Children of Older Fathers**   The average age of fathers whose children have chromosomal or genetic abnormalities is younger than one might expect, at least as far as certain abnormalities are concerned. Apparently this is due to alterations in the genes as a man gets older. Geneticists now believe that the number of new *autosomal dominant diseases* in children increases by about 1 percent once the father is forty years of age or older (see below). Since these are spontaneous mutations, few of these disorders can be diagnosed by amniocentesis. There is a greater risk of a *chromosomal* disorder if the father is fifty-five or older.

☐ *A New Prenatal Test to Curb Mental Retardation* (**The Fragile X Syndrome**)   A mental disorder that affects males is linked to a defective X chromosome passed down from mother to son. This is known as the *"fragile X syndrome"* because the long arms of the affected chromosome apparently have a tendency to break easily. This abnormality, the second largest cause of mental retardation after Down's syndrome, was not detectable through karyotyping until recently, when a test was developed accidentally in an Australian laboratory, where a researcher found a new way to culture the cells. Women with a family history of the disorder can now have their pregnancies screened prenatally through amniocentesis, while another, simple test will determine whether or not a woman is a carrier of the defective chromosome.

☐ *Miscarriage and Chromosomal Abnormalities*   Chromosomal abnormalities are a common cause of early miscarriage. About 15 percent of all recognized pregnancies end in miscarriage, 80 percent of them in the first trimester. The proportion of all early miscarriages that can be attributed to chromosomal defects is over 60 percent. A serious chromosomal defect is incompatible with life, and the embryo fails to develop beyond the earliest stages. Many parents blame themselves quite unnecessarily for a misfortune they can neither prevent nor are responsible for in any way.

Many of these early miscarriages are the result of autosomal trisomy disorders. This is why fetuses affected by Down's syndrome sometimes die spontaneously at a very early stage of development. Other trisomies commonly seen in miscarriages are Trisomy 13, 16, and 22. Trisomy 16 is so disruptive of normal development that the fetus is always aborted at an early stage. Trisomy 21 and 22 are equally common in miscarriage, but Trisomy 21 is more common among live births. The single most common chromosomal abnormality associated with miscarriage is a sex chromosome defect: Turner's syndrome (45, XO) which is compatible with life in only one out of every ten thousand affected pregnancies. Another sex chromosome defect is Klinefelter's syndrome, characterized by two X's and one Y chromosome. This syndrome, again, often results in miscarriage, but some individuals are born with the defect. It usually goes unrecognized before puberty, when the testes and the secondary sex characteristics are poorly developed. A person with Klinefelter's syndrome is considered a male.

One miscarriage is generally a random event. There is only a slight chance that a specific chromosomal abnormality will repeat itself in the next pregnancy; the great majority of chromosomal abnormalities are not hereditary but appear spontaneously. Most geneticists don't feel there is a need for counseling unless a couple has a history of three or more miscarriages in their present marriage, or in the previous marriage of either partner. At this point, blood karyotype studies of either partner can be valuable in establishing or ruling out carrier status, or in distinguishing a genetic disorder that has gone unsuspected since childhood.

☐ *Should I Have Amniocentesis?*   Testing is *always* an individual matter, and a decision should be made only after a consultation with a doctor or genetic counselor and a discussion between the couple. Many doctors do not recommend amniocentesis unless a couple is considering terminating an affected pregnancy, because of the risks associated with the test, even though a favorable result is a great relief to a couple concerned about the health of their offspring.

The risk versus the benefits is something you will have to take into consideration. Some couples decide against amniocentesis because of ethical, religious, or personal considerations.

Only a very few tests—about 3 percent—reveal a significantly abnormal karyotype. But if a serious abnormality is discovered, it is still the couple's right to sit down with their doctor or counselor and receive a careful evaluation before deciding on termination of the pregnancy. Certain chromosomal disorders affect the fetus far more severely than others, and even with Down's syndrome, the amount of physical and mental handicap can vary quite considerably from child to child. The couple's personal circumstances are obviously another important consideration; a couple with one handicapped child, for instance, is often unable to give much support to another.

After careful and supportive counseling, a decision regarding termination of pregnancy is the prerogative of the parents alone. Test results are usually returned within three weeks of the amniocentesis, allowing enough time to arrange for a legal and safe termination, if so desired.

☐ *How Genetic Diseases Occur*   The course of a genetic disease, as opposed to a chromosomal disorder, is decided by a defect in the genes rather than a disruption in the chromosomal pattern. Hundreds of thousands of genes make up a typical cell in the human body and store the genetic information that each human being passes down to his or her offspring. Most of these genetic characteristics are innocuous or even beneficent, but every human being possesses a few "faulty" genes that could theoretically result in a genetic disorder. The likelihood of this occurring in most families is remote because the majority of genetic disorders do not arise unless one defective gene from one parent is matched by a similar gene from the other parent—a statistically improbable happening—but the few faulty genes still carry a certain potential for damage. Then there are families in which there is a history of inherited defects or one child is already affected by a genetic disorder. Here the geneticist investigating the disease is dealing with a disorder that is already visible and in which the chances of another child inheriting the disease can often be calculated.

Genetic disorders are divided into three categories: dominant, recessive, and sex-linked disorders. If the gene in question is dominant, it does not require a matching gene from the other parent to pass on the trait or the disease to the next generation. Familiar examples of dominantly inherited disorders are Huntington's disease and certain forms of dwarfism. If the gene is recessive, it must be matched by a similar gene for a child to inherit the disease, although the child can become a heterozygote, or carrier, by inheriting the trait from one of the parents. The recessive-gene disorders, including cystic fibrosis, hypercholesterolemia, muscular dystrophy, sickle-cell anemia, and Tay-Sachs disease, are among the most common of the gene disorders. Finally, in the case of a sex-linked disease, the defective gene is carried on the X chromosome and passed down from mother to son, with a daughter acting as a potential carrier. Two well known X-linked genetic disorders are hemophilia and Duchenne's muscular dystrophy. In all there are about two thousand known genetic diseases.

Dominantly inherited disorders usually exhibit obvious and very characteristic patterns that can be traced through the family history. In a family in which one parent is affected by a dominantly inherited disease, there is a 50 percent chance that a child will inherit the disease and an equal chance that he or she will not. In a recessive disorder in which both parents are heterozygotes, there is a 25 percent chance of a child's inheriting the diseased genes from both the mother and the father and therefore the disease itself, a 50 percent chance of inheriting one defective gene and one normal gene and becoming a carrier like the parents, and a one in four chance of inheriting two normal genes and escaping the disorder completely. Heterozygotes may be completely asymptomatic, but in certain genetic disorders they may exhibit mild symptoms of the disorder.

The problem with genetic disease is that parents are usually unaware of their carrier status. Dominant diseases can sometimes be traced through the family history, but recessive disorders often appear without any prior warning. Most parents carry recessive genes without even considering their potential for harm, unless there is already one child in the family with a recessive disorder, or they have been tested because they belong to an ethnic group which is at higher risk for a particular disease.

☐ ***Biochemical Inherited Congenital Malformations***   One large group of inherited diseases are the result of changes within the structure of the cells. A number of different proteins are synthesized in the cells of the human body. These proteins, which can be either enzymes or what are known as structural components, are responsible for the proper development and the metabolic processes of all the organs and systems in our bodies.

The fundamental relationship between genes and proteins is their specific sequence in the DNA structure. Any alteration in the sequence of the genes results in alterations in the way the proteins are formed, and this change in the structure may, in turn, alter the way the protein functions before and after birth. This is the reason why a gene mutation can lead to a genetic disorder, although genetic changes do not always result in a detectable abnormality. Sometimes a mutation alters the amino acid sequence of an enzyme, resulting in what is known as a biochemical disorder, such as Tay-Sachs disease, or it may change the amino acid sequence within a structural protein such as hemoglobin. Inherited hemoglobin disorders include sickle-cell anemia and thalassemia minor and major.

A number of these defects can be detected prenatally, although little in the way of effective treatment is available for many of them. In most instances they are autosomal recessive defects, so the parents of one affected child face a one-in-four risk of having another child with the disorder. A few are dominant inherited disorders; in one or two rare cases, the disorders are sex-linked.

☐ ***Biochemical Disorders***   In an inherited biochemical disorder, the child inherits a malfunction in the amino acid sequence of the enzymes. This takes place in a number of different ways, according to whether the stability of the enzyme is disturbed or some other function is affected. Some of the deficiencies are correctable or relatively harmless, and allow the individual to live a normal or almost normal life; others are serious enough to cause death at an early age.

Inherited biochemical disorders include disorders of the lipid metabolism, of which familial hypercholesterolemia is the best known (this condition is a disorder in which the mechanism that normally regulates cholesterol production results in a build-up of cholesterol); disorders of the carbohydrate metabolism, including galactosemia, a hereditary condition that results in enlargement of the spleen, cataracts, and mental retardation if the affected child is not put on a milk-free diet; and disorders of the amino acid metabolism, including a rare condition called phenylketonuria (PKU), which results in profound mental retardation. With PKU, a disorder of the amino acid phenylalanine, a simple blood test after birth will detect the abnormality, although known carriers for the disease can have their children screened prenatally. Most hospitals do this test routinely. An affected child can be put on a special phenylalanine-free diet and will usually do well. Altogether, there are sixty biochemical disorders that can be detected through prenatal amniotic fluid testing, but most of them are so rare that amniocentesis is recommended only among families with a previous affected pregnancy or a family history of a particular disorder. The exception is Tay-Sachs disease, in which the disease is generally confined to a recognizable ethnic group and couples can be screened routinely to detect heterozygotes. A couple who are both found to be carriers can choose to have a pregnancy screened prenatally through amniocentesis.

☐ **Tay-Sachs Disease**   Tay-Sachs, a rare but inevitably fatal biochemical condition, is one disease that has already been brought under control through effective prenatal screening. A child with Tay-Sachs is deficient in a vital enzyme called hexosminidase, a substance that normally appears in a variety of tissue structures, and whose absence interrupts the normal metabolic function of the entire central nervous system. A baby with Tay-Sachs appears normal at birth, but at six months or a year the first signs of degeneration appear, to be followed by a rapid and progressive decline in the functions of the brain and the nervous system. Death usually occurs before the fourth birthday.

Tay-Sachs disease is generally confined to a relatively small ethnic group: Jewish couples of Ashkenazi, or eastern European descent. While Tay-Sachs occurs in approximately one out of every 360,000 births in the general population, its frequency among Ashkenazi Jews is about one in 2500, and the gene for the disorder is carried by one person in twenty-five among the American Jewish population. Both parents must be carriers for a child to inherit the disease, and the incidence within a particular family in which both parents are carriers follows the inheritance pattern for other autosomal recessive disorders: a one-in-four chance that the child will inherit the disease.

The relatively confined nature of the disorder, and the fact that there is now a simple blood test available to screen carriers, has made it possible to detect most couples at risk. Screening programs are available all over the United States and your doctor can probably take the blood for the test and send it to a laboratory.

Once you are pregnant the test will not be accurate. Your husband should have the blood test taken instead. If the test is negative, it does not matter if you are a carrier, since your baby will at most be a carrier himself. If the test is positive, you will need to be evaluated further to rule out your carrier status.

If you want more information about Tay-Sachs disease, you can write to The National Tay-Sachs and Allied Diseases Association at 922 Washington Avenue, Cedarhurst, New York 11516 (516-569-4300).

☐ **Cystic Fibrosis**   This is the most common inherited fatal disease among white Americans, affecting about one out of every two thousand Caucasian live births. It often makes an initial appearance at birth when the child is born with an obstruction of the small intestine and is generally small for its gestational age. The first signs of lung damage follow early in childhood—usually within its first year. The child suffers from coughing episodes and frequent lung infections, and in general fails to thrive. With modern treatment, children have grown up to become adults, but most victims of the disease die before they are twenty.

The defect appears to result from a disorder of the exocrine glands, the glands that secrete to the surface of the body. This defect produces the characteristic episodes of sweating that characterize the disease, which may end in shock from sodium depletion. A skin test can be used to detect carriers among affected families. The test is too complicated to be used for mass screening, but is invaluable in detecting carriers among families already at risk for cystic fibrosis. Prospective parents can be accurately informed of their chances of producing a cystic fibrosis child and saved the anguish of seeing that child die painfully over a period of years.

☐ *Hemoglobin Disorders*   Hemoglobin is an essential component in human blood because it contains the oxygen-carrying capacity of the red blood cells. The hemoglobin molecule is composed of a number of units, including two different types of amino acid chains known as the alpha and beta chains. These chains are coded by different genes, so a mutation may affect one but not the other. A change in the amino acid sequence in either chain could lead to an abnormality, but one which is not necessarily severe. However, sickle-cell disease and thalassemia major (Cooley's anemia) are both life-threatening disorders.

Sickle-cell disease is a hemoglobin disorder characterized by anemia, jaundice, and episodes of what is known as "sickle-cell crisis" (see Chap. 24). Life expectancy is usually short, less than forty years. In the United States the disease is generally confined to blacks and Hispanics; about 9 percent of the black American population are carriers, although only .25 percent of black American births are affected by the disease. (Among equatorial people the sickle-cell trait seems to offer protection against malaria, an advantage that becomes a disadvantage in a malaria-free environment.) Individuals with sickle-cell traits are usually asymptomatic and have a normal life expectancy, although the trait may encourage a tendency toward anemia and frequent urinary-tract infections.

☐ *Sickle-Cell Screening Test*   When the red blood cells of individuals with sickle-cell anemia are placed in an atmosphere of very low oxygen pressure, the cells will "sickle," or become distorted into sicklelike shapes. Sickling can be observed by placing a drop of blood on a glass slide and sealing it off from the air for as long as twenty-four hours. Sickling occurs more rapidly in affected individuals, but heterozygotes can be detected by a mixture of normal and sickle-cell hemoglobin. A faster, more accurate test is the hemoglobin electrophoresis test, in which the hemoglobin is split up into various bands and the bands can be read out to confirm the trait or the disease. A couple who are both carriers have a one-in-four chance of giving birth to an affected child.

☐ *Can Sickle-Cell Disease Be Detected Prenatally?*   Sickle-cell disease cannot be detected prenatally except by fetoscopy and fetal blood sampling, a new, selective technique that is available to only a very few couples at the present time. (Fetoscopy is described in detail later in this chapter.) A couple who know they are both carriers for sickle-cell anemia should consult a genetic counselor when the woman is pregnant. (It should be mentioned that routine screening of couples has been seriously questioned because carrier identification has, until recently, caused great anxiety without much benefit to the parents. This may change as fetoscopy becomes more generally available.) It is a serious disease that can be ameliorated only to a certain extent by modern forms of treatment, and counseling should be obtained.

☐ *Cooley's Anemia or Thalassemia Major* Cooley's anemia, or thalassemia major, is a hereditary blood disease that affects people of Mediterranean descent. The victim is seriously anemic, growth and other functions are affected, and death usually takes place in the early teens. This very serious blood disease occurs as a result of a reduced rate of synthesis in the beta plus amino acid chain. A related disease in which the beta chain is impaired, thalassemia minor, induces a mild form of anemia (see Chap. 24) and is not dangerous, although two parents with thalassemia minor do have a one-in-four chance of producing a child with thalassemia major. This hemoglobin disorder can be detected prenatally through fetal blood sampling, although as I have already said, the technique is available to only a few couples. Carriers can be detected through a simple blood test, but again, this may not be useful to you unless prenatal detection is available.

☐ *Sex-Linked Diseases* A number of genetic diseases are linked to a defective gene located on the X chromosome and passed down from mother to son. Typically, a female child born to a woman with an X-linked disorder has a 50 percent chance of becoming a carrier, while each of her brothers has a 50 percent chance of inheriting the defective X chromosome and the disease itself. By far the most common X-linked disorder is color blindness, a condition that affects about 8 percent of American men. Many of the other 170 known X-linked disorders are equally minor, but certain rare X-linked disorders are so crippling that affected families are having the sex of their children screened prenatally through amniocentesis. One of the most famous is hemophilia, the bleeding disease inherited by the son of the last czar of Russia through his mother, a granddaughter of Queen Victoria; another is Duchenne's muscular dystrophy, a fatal muscular disease in which life expectancy is less than fifteen years.

One of the most promising aspects of the new fetal blood sampling technique is its ability to distinguish male fetuses affected by hemophilia from healthy male fetuses. In the future, fetoscopy and fetal blood sampling will undoubtedly be used far more in the detection of biochemical X-linked diseases.

☐ *Multifactorial Defects* There is a large group of birth defects that can be attributed to a combination of genetic and environmental causes. (There are also a number of normal characteristics that appear in humans through the same combination of causes: height, for example, is usually the result of genetic and environmental factors mixed; so, often, is intelligence.) Most multifactorial defects are caused by a failure in development early in pregnancy. They are difficult for the genetic counselor to predict, since a number of complicating factors are involved, but information is continually being collected on the frequency of defects in the general population and among specific families, and this may be helpful if you have had a previous affected pregnancy. Neural-tube defects are one group of multifactorial defects that can be detected prenatally through ultrasonography, amniocentesis, or a special blood test.

☐ *Neural-Tube Defects*   Neural-tube defects are among the most common of all birth defects, second in the United States only to cerebral palsy. The two most common forms of the defect are anencephaly, in which a part of the brain is missing, and spina bifida, in which a section of the spine is absent or improperly closed. Anencephaly is inevitably fatal, before or immediately after birth, but spina bifida is compatible with life, although life expectancy is often short. The defect causes a protrusion of nerves through an area of the spinal cord; in some cases this is not associated with much difficulty, but sometimes the nerves are damaged and the child never develops the use of its lower limbs. In certain instances the child is also born with the complicating factor of hydrocephalus.

The cause of neural-tube defects is not exactly known. Genetic factors are assumed to exist because a family with one affected pregnancy has a 5 percent chance of the defect's recurring, but this does not mean that the defect does not occur spontaneously. Certain ethnic groups are affected more than others; neural-tube defects are less common among black and Oriental populations than among whites, and the British and Irish have a far higher incidence than Americans. They are so prevalent in Ireland that one widely held but not very convincing theory links neural-tube defects to the consumption of potatoes. Dr. Renwich proposed in 1972 that neural-tube defects were caused by factors present in potato tubers, possibly a teratogenic antibiotic induced by the potato-blight fungus *Phytophthora infestans*. Other studies confirmed this theory, but recent research has not been able to verify the correlation between blighted potatoes and neural-tube defects. Among the white American population, parents of Irish and Welsh descent, young parents (under twenty-one), and middle-aged parents are statistically more likely to have a neural-tube-affected pregnancy. Neural-tube defects are also more common on the east than the west coast, perhaps because pollution levels are higher in the East. Although the cause is unknown, researchers feel it could well be an abnormality of the sperm or the egg, caused, perhaps, by some genetic factor or by a substance such as LSD or caffeine that has the power to alter the genetic makeup of the cells.

☐ *Cleft Lip, Cleft Palate, and Other Common Birth Defects*   Cleft lip with or without cleft palate is perhaps the most common of all the multifactorial defects. Cleft lip and cleft palate result from a failure of development in the seventh week after conception when the upper portions of the fetal jaw fail to fuse correctly. It is often difficult to isolate the factor involved since the defect sometimes occurs as part of a larger group of chromosomal abnormalities. In other cleft-lip cases, evidence points to some teratogenic agent, possibly a drug such as Dilantin or Valium, or a viral exposure occurring at the crucial point of development.

Cleft lip occurs in one out of every thousand white babies, and is found in slightly higher numbers among black and Japanese Americans. There is a familial factor, although the chances of either cleft lip or cleft palate reappearing in the same family is low: about 2 percent. Fortunately these are both defects that can now be treated successfully through surgery and special therapy.

A number of other common multifactorial birth defects caused by drugs or environmental factors, including *heart defects, clubfoot, congenital dislocation of the hip,* and *pyloric stenosis* (a congenital blockage of the stomach, which is five times more common in boys than in girls) can also be corrected by postnatal surgery. The success rate is high. Seventy-five percent of children with major defects of the heart or gastrointestinal tract are now being saved by surgery in comparison with less than half that number only twenty years ago, and the outlook for these children in later life is usually untroubled.

☐ *Environmental Defects and Genetic Counseling*   If you have knowingly been exposed to a serious viral condition, abdominal X-rays, or a teratogenic drug during early pregnancy, a genetic counselor can help you by carefully evaluating the amount of exposure and calculating the effects on the fetus. An infection or an exposure to a teratogen is most serious in the first four weeks after conception, when there is a 50 percent chance of a major malformation. After the first trimester the chance is close to zero.

A genetic counselor might also determine that no judgment can be made from the available information. It would then be up to the parents to make the decision themselves. Amniocentesis is rarely helpful, but sonography could be useful in detecting a major structural abnormality.

The effects of exposure to drugs or radiation at work or in the environment is often difficult to estimate since it depends on the amount of the exposure and its coincidence with gestation. If a couple is concerned, genetic counseling is again advocated as a way of eliminating unnecessary fears. It is important to remember that serious abnormalities are relatively rare and that 95 percent of births result in normal, healthy babies.

☐ *Antenatal Detection of Hereditary Disorders or Congenital Defects*
After the genetic counselor has collected a complete family and personal history and determined whether or not your unborn child runs a substantial risk of an inherited disease or a congenital defect, the counselor and your physician will, with your consent, arrange for appropriate prenatal evaluation and testing. The major tests and technologies used to detect a fetal abnormality or the presence of a hereditary disease are:

1. The use of amniocentesis to obtain and analyze the amniotic fluid.
2. The use of ultrasonography and real-time ultrasound scanning.
3. Fetoscopy with direct vision of the fetus, and fetal blood sampling, for use in genetic evaluation.
4. Serum and blood analysis of alpha fetoprotein and/or the measurement of alpha fetoprotein in the amniotic fluid to detect the presence of neural, nerve, or brain abnormalities (neural-tube defects).

It is important to recognize that these methods of detecting fetal abnormalities or inherited diseases are not required in a normal pregnancy in women under age thirty-five. *Only* those pregnancies in which the fetus is considered at high risk for a chromosomal abnormality or some other congenital malformation should be considered for these antenatal testing procedures, with two possible exceptions. The first is ultrasonography, a scanning device capable of a rough evaluation of fetal development that is now used routinely by many private doctors. The second is the alpha fetoprotein blood test, which is presently available on a limited basis and could, in the future, be used to monitor all pregnancies. The other procedures are unlikely to be recommended except in certain controlled situations.

Your doctor or counselor should point out and discuss the pros and cons of each test with you and ask you to sign appropriate consent forms. A typical amniocentesis consent form describes the reason for the test in plain language and briefly explains the risks associated with the procedure.

☐ *Genetic Testing Does Not Mean Abortion*   It is also important for parents thinking about prenatal testing to understand that consenting to the use of a screening technique does not mean they must automatically consent to the elective abortion of a handicapped fetus. Elective termination of pregnancy is a private decision made by the couple in consultation with their doctor and is not the immediate concern of the hospital or clinic where the prenatal test takes place. Although many parents do choose elective termination in these circumstances, a prenatal test can just as well be used to help the family understand the nature of a defect and prepare to meet the specific needs of an affected newborn.

We hope that one day our technology will be so advanced in this area that many of the abnormalities that now cripple children physically or mentally will be correctable *in utero*. A few successful attempts have already been made to treat fetuses with serious birth defects, including the work of a team of surgeons at Harvard University who have saved several fetuses with hydrocephalus by installing drainage shunts to divert fluid from the brain. These are exciting developments, although intrauterine surgery is limited at present to a few very skilled groups of doctors and won't be generally available for many years.

☐ *What Is the Function of Amniocentesis?*   Amniocentesis, an important tool in prenatal genetic diagnosis, involves the sampling and analysis of the amniotic fluid. A typical amniotic sample can be used for a number of different analyses that contribute vital information about the health of the fetus, including the presence or absence of a hereditary disease. If a serious inherited condition or a birth defect is discovered, parents can, if they wish, arrange to have the pregnancy terminated. In the great majority of cases the results are favorable and the parents can be assured of the baby's health, at least as far as the disorder under investigation is concerned.

At the present time, amniocentesis can detect three hundred chromosomal conditions, and about sixty hereditary defects of biochemical origin. Many of these conditions are extremely rare, though a few, like Down's syndrome, are to be found among a fairly large group of the population. A large number of inherited diseases, including cystic fibrosis and muscular dystrophy, are not yet detectable prenatally through amniocentesis. We may have to wait for many years before the majority of hereditary diseases or structural birth defects can be determined *in utero*. Nor is the test infallible; a favorable result does not guarantee that the fetus is free from all defects, it simply means that the baby will not suffer from a particular crippling or life-threatening disorder. A test guaranteeing a "perfect" baby is an unlikely development, even in the future.

A number of questions have been raised about the accuracy and safety of amniocentesis, but the most recent studies confirm a low rate of serious complications for both the mother and the baby. There have been very few mistaken diagnoses. As laboratory facilities and diagnostic testing continue to improve, there is the possibility of almost 100 percent accuracy in the future. At the same time, it is very unlikely that amniocentesis will be used to monitor *every* pregnancy, as some people have suggested. Besides the risk factors involved, the facilities to run millions of tests and analyze the results are simply not available at the present time. Amniocentesis remains, and probably will remain, a test for families who have some good reason to be anxious about their age or family history.

☐ *How the Test Is Performed*   Amniocentesis is usually performed between the sixteenth and eighteenth week of gestation, calculated from the first day of the last menstrual period. Doctors wait until this point in pregnancy before attempting the test because the amniotic fluid volume is generally sufficient to allow for the removal of a small sample without damaging the baby, and the placenta no longer obstructs access to the amniotic sac.

In the more advanced medical centers, the first stage is preliminary ultrasound diagnosis to delineate the outline of the fetus and placenta and identify an area of the sac where there is plenty of fluid for the needle to enter without damaging the fetus or the placenta. Some amniocentesis tests are performed with a special device under the direct beam of the ultrasonogram; in other hospitals, the ultrasonographer marks a place of entry on the woman's abdomen, and notes the depth to which the needle should go to avoid any contact with the fetus or the placenta. The abdomen is then carefully washed with an iodine solution in preparation for the test. Some hospitals administer a small shot of novocaine to numb the skin tissue, but testing centers are increasingly omitting the use of local anesthetics because the anesthetic is about as painful as the procedure itself. The prick of the amniocentesis needle is no worse than that of the average blood test.

The small, slender, hollow needle is inserted through the skin of the uterine wall and into the amniotic sac (See Fig. 54). The amniotic fluid usually flows directly into the needle. Then a syringe is attached and the fluid is carefully aspirated and withdrawn. The syringe is then removed from the needle and the needle in turn is drawn from the woman's abdomen. This is not painful, but it is sometimes associated with a slight cramping.

The amount of fluid in a typical amniotic fluid sample is small, about twenty to thirty milliliters. Approximately 250 milliliters of fluid are present in the fetal sac in the fifteenth to eighteenth week of pregnancy, so the remaining fluid is ample to protect the fetus, and in any case the lost fluid is replaced within a matter of hours. The doctor will run another ultrasound test after he completes the tap to make sure that the fetus is unharmed and the fetal movements and heart rate are normal. After the second ultrasound test, the patient is asked to sit in the laboratory for half an hour to an hour to rest, and is then allowed to go

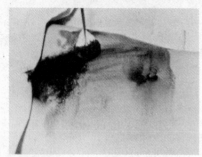
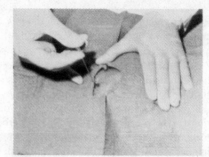

Figure 52

Figure 54

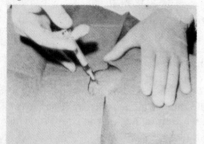
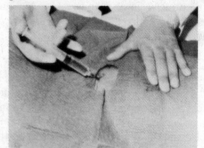

Figure 53

Figure 55

Figure 52: Preparation for Amniocentesis: The abdomen is carefully washed with an iodine solution as the first step.　　*Figure 53: Local Anesthetic:* Some physicians prefer to administer a small amount of novocaine to numb the skin tissue before the amniocentesis.　　*Figure 54: Amniocentesis:* A thin "spinal" needle is inserted through the numbed skin into the pocket of amniotic fluid. The depth to which the amniocentesis needle is inserted depends on the results of the preceding ultrasound examination.　　*Figure 55: Aspiration of Amniotic Fluid:* Clear amniotic fluid is seen in the syringe held in the doctor's right hand. The physician often gives gentle pressure with the other hand as the amniotic fluid is aspirated. Amniotic fluid is mostly comprised of fetal urine, but it also contains cells from the fetal tissue which can be cultured and used for chromosomal analysis. (See Figures 50, 51.)

home. Since there is a slight risk of miscarriage associated with the test, her doctor will suggest that she take it easy for a few days to allow the uterus time to heal completely.

The most serious complication associated with amniocentesis is rupture of the fetal membranes and miscarriage. The risk can be minimized by using ultrasonography and taking certain precautions during the tap itself. An experienced doctor usually takes the sample from an area in the upper part of the uterus (with a test performed in the lower section there is more likelihood of the amniotic fluid's leaking out from the cervix), and is careful to hold the needle steady throughout the tap; a needle twisted from side to side sometimes results in bleeding and a weakening of the membranes. Occasionally the needle does come into contact with the fetus, but fetal injuries are rarely more serious than a scar or slight puncture visible at birth. In general, the risk of hitting the fetus or placenta or weakening the membranes is considerably lessened by the routine use of ultrasound, since fetal position can be accurately established before a tap is attempted. Under ideal conditions, a test would be done only in combination with ultrasound and by a doctor who performs a number of tests regularly. In the hands of a skillful doctor, the risk of a serious complication is small.

The initial ultrasound test has a number of other diagnostic functions besides establishing the best location for amniocentesis. It establishes fetal gestation by the measurement of the fetus' head; it indicates the presence or absence of multiple births; and it locates the position of the placenta within the uterine cavity, a piece of information that is important in ruling out placental abnormalities such as placenta previa (see Chap. 25). In addition, ultrasonography can often distinguish a serious structural or internal abnormality of the fetus, or detect uterine abnormalities such as large fibroid tumors that might require special care.

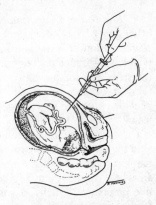

Figure 56: Amniocentesis: Approximately 250 milliliters of fluid are present in the amniotic sac in the fifteenth to eighteenth week of pregnancy. Thus there should be sufficient fluid to protect the baby even after the physician removes 20–30 milliliters for analysis. Furthermore, the amniotic fluid quickly regenerates itself.

If you have Rh-negative blood there is a possibility that the fetus will develop Rh blood disease (see Chapter 20) after an amniocentesis test. A special injection of Rh-positive antibodies (a Rhogam vaccination) within seventy-two hours after the amniocentesis is performed will protect both the fetus and you. Otherwise you might develop antibodies and endanger your present or future pregnancies.

☐ *What Is Done with the Amniotic Fluid?* The fluid is sent to a laboratory that specializes in genetic evaluation. When it reaches the laboratory it is placed in a centrifugal unit to separate the fetal cells from the fluid itself. The fluid is used to study alphafeto protein, enzymes, and other metabolic functions that indicate a genetic disease or a neural-tube defect in the fetus, while the cells go through the karyotyping process to prepare them for an evaluation of the fetus' chromosomal structure.

☐ *How Long Before the Results of the Test Are Known?* The alphafeto protein analysis takes only a few days. A biochemical analysis or a karyotyping take much longer, sometimes as long as three or four weeks. Your doctor will call you as soon as he gets the results from the laboratory and arrange for a consultation.

Many women say that the time spent waiting for the test results is by far the hardest period of the pregnancy. Some women even refrain from purchasing maternity clothes until the test results are in. Fortunately, in more than 95 percent of all cases, the results are completely reassuring.

☐ *Fetal Sex* If you have a karyotype performed, the test will establish the fetal sex. Fetal sex is incidental unless you have a history of sex-linked diseases in your family, and your doctor will either tell you the sex of your child or withhold this information, depending on your preference.

☐ **How Much Does Amniocentesis Cost?**   The cost of amniocentesis and other genetic services varies from hospital to hospital. The initial genetic-counseling session or sessions usually cost between $200 and $300. Although some people's insurance policies pick up some of the cost, insurance companies often refuse to pay for preventive medicine, so it is important to discuss the counselor's fee before becoming involved in enormous expenses. Even so, if you suspect the presence of a congenital malformation in your family, the expense is usually well worth while.

An ultrasonogram generally costs about $50 to $70. This is usually reimbursable by your insurance carrier, because ultrasonography is considered an essential procedure in determining fetal condition. Amniocentesis itself costs anywhere from $100 to $200, and again this is usually reimbursable as an operative procedure. Finally, a complete chromosomal analysis is another $100 to $200. So as you can see, counseling and tests are rather expensive, and might cost from a few hundred up to a thousand dollars or more. The best way to deal with these expenses is to inquire in advance, find out specifically what each form of genetic counseling will cost before any procedures are performed, and be sure to check with your insurance company about their reimbursement policies.

☐ **Can Amniocentesis Be Performed on Twins?**   The answer is yes. Among fraternal twins, it is possible for one twin to have a chromosomal abnormality or a genetic disease while the other twin is completely normal. Amniocentesis can be performed successfully on both twins by locating the twin fetal sacs with ultrasound and performing the test on the first fetus. Then, once the amniotic fluid has been withdrawn, red or blue dye is injected into the sac to use as a marker. If the doctor inadvertently enters the first sac when he is attempting to test the second twin, the needle will pick up the dye. Otherwise, if the fluid is clear, he will know he is tapping the second sac. This simple device means that each child can be evaluated separately.

In a case in New York City that attracted a great deal of attention from the press, a set of twins was screened by amniocentesis, and one of them was found to have Down's syndrome. Rather than abort both twins, the woman's doctor used ultrasound to locate the affected twin's heart and punctured it with a needle. The affected twin succumbed, but the other normal twin lived.

☐ **What Is the Risk of Amniocentesis?**   Potential risks include bleeding and infection for the mother, and a number of hazards for the fetus. The superficial skin wound heals quickly and it is usually impossible to distinguish the needle mark after a week or so, but the risk of internal bleeding is altogether more serious. Although bleeding from the uterine wall seems to occur only when there are a large number of varicose veins in the wall of the uterus, the needle can accidentally stab an artery in the uterus, or puncture a vein or artery in the bladder, bowel, or abdominal wall. Nonetheless, these potential hazards can usually be avoided if the doctor performs a careful evaluation and internal examination before proceeding with the test, and serious problems are normally encountered only in women who have had extensive pelvic surgery or an acute abdominal infection.

Risks to the fetus include trauma, bleeding, and infection, but these can be minimized by careful timing of the test. By the fifteenth week, the placenta should cover about 50 percent of the surface area of the uterus, allowing enough room for the needle to be inserted safely without puncturing the placenta or the fetus. If the initial ultrasound examination shows a large placenta still covering the front portion of the uterus, the test should be postponed and the patient asked to return in a week or two to allow time for the uterus to expand and diminish the area covered by the placenta. By the fifteenth week, the volume of amniotic fluid is also sufficient to protect the fetus during the test. In the early days of amniocentesis, tests were performed earlier in the pregnancy, and the amniotic fluid loss led to a much higher rate of miscarriage, and increased chance of hitting the unprotected fetus and causing bleeding or scarring.

☐ *How Safe Is Amniocentesis?*   When a government-funded study looked at the safety of the test in 1976, it found no significant difference between a group of one thousand women who had undergone the test and a matching control group whose pregnancies were in other ways similar but who had not been offered the test. The two groups had almost identical rates of miscarriage and other serious complications, and the physical examination of the babies immediately after birth revealed no important differences in birth weight or in rates of congenital abnormalities. When the same groups of children were tested at one year of age, their growth, development, and intelligence levels were essentially similar. After looking at the results of this study and a similar one in Canada, a special task force appointed by the United States government concluded that the risk of a serious complication after an amniocentesis test in an experienced center is less than .5 percent.

☐ *Your Doctor's Responsibility for Amniocentesis*   Many doctors still fail to advise their patients of the availability of the test even in instances in which a woman's age or family history would make the test advisable. In the future, though, doctors may be more careful about warning women at risk because of a number of law cases, including a ruling handed down by the New York State Court of Appeals, which seems to support families against negligent doctors. In the case heard in New York State, the court reviewed the complaint of two couples whose obstetricians failed to advise them of their risk of bearing a defective baby, and ruled that any doctor who neglects to inform a patient at clear risk can be required to pay the lifetime costs of caring for the affected child. Meanwhile in California, a woman has successfully sued her hospital for neglecting to offer her amniocentesis. She was thirty-six years old when she gave birth to a son with Down's syndrome.

☐ *How Ultrasound Detects Genetic Abnormalities*   Ultrasonography is being used with increasing frequency in the detection of genetic and other fetal abnormalities. The form of ultrasound you are most likely to encounter as a patient is real-time ultrasound, a unit with a hand-held scanner and a small screen resembling the screen of a television set. Real-time ultrasound is capable of picking up an image of the fetus in motion and can be used to visualize the pregnancy at several critical stages of development.

The outlines of the embryo and placenta first show up clearly on the screen at the eighth or ninth week of gestation. Visible fetal development at this point is the sign of a normal pregnancy. Absence of a visible fetus—the so-called empty sac—means there is some kind of serious genetic abnormality, and a miscarriage is imminent. Four weeks later, at the end of the first trimester, a normal pregnancy has usually progressed sufficiently for the obstetrician to see fetal movement, and detect a multiple birth or a large structural abnormality of the placenta or the fetal organs. Then as the pregnancy moves into the second and third trimester, ultrasound can be used to measure the fetal head and the size of the placenta to get some idea of whether or not the baby is growing in the normal range. A fetus that is undersized for its gestational age may be suffering from malnourishment or may have some unsuspected chromosomal abnormality; Trisomy 21 (Down's) and other chromosomal disorders often affect fetal growth as well as its intelligence and general health. Thus, if a normal growth curve can be traced with ultrasound, this is another assurance of normalcy. As the fetus develops further, ultrasound can also be used to monitor the fetal heartbeat and respiration rate, other signs that help tell whether the fetus is growing and developing well.

Now that ultrasound is generally available in the office or medical center, it can be used to detect the presence of a number of serious structural defects of the limbs, internal organs, and central nervous system, including gross malformations of the heart, brain, lungs, kidneys, and bladder. One of the disorders that can now be successfully diagnosed prenatally through this technique is a fatal hereditary condition called polycystic kidney disease. Others are anencephaly and certain cases of spina bifida (both described on page 296), although smaller spinal defects are too tiny to show up well on the screen, and hydrocephaly, a serious birth defect in which fluid collects in the fetal brain and causes severe mental retardation. Few of these evaluations can be made by X-rays, the only other available technology. Ultrasound is not only more sensitive than X-rays but preliminary studies on ultrasound have failed to connect its use with any visible malformation, chromosomal disorder, or childhood illness, including leukemia. The present data suggest there is no reason to be apprehensive about the effect of ultrasound on your health or that of the fetus.

☐ *Fetoscopy and Fetal Blood Sampling*   Fetoscopy, the most recent and by far the most delicate of the current prenatal screening techniques, enables the physician to view the fetus directly and take blood and skin samples that can be used for further analysis. The technique has made it possible to perform a number of essential tests that cannot be carried out through any other prenatal screening technique. Amniotic-fluid tests detect many biochemical disorders, but they are not capable of giving information on the fetal blood or body cell type, information that is needed to detect certain genetic diseases prenatally. This is a function that fetoscopy can perform through fetal blood sampling and fetal skin biopsies. The geneticist who has a blood sample can use it to diagnose certain hemoglobin disorders, including sickle-cell anemia, beta thalassemia, hemophilia, and disorders of the white blood cells and the serum proteins. Skin sampling can be used in tissue culture for karyotyping, or to measure the level of drugs and other teratogens in the immediate fetal environment.

The procedure requires great skill and precision. Once the targeted area has been established by ultrasound, the specialist makes a tiny skin incision in the patient's abdomen and inserts the fetoscope, a slender periscope-like instrument, through the abdominal wall and into the amniotic cavity. The patient is given

Demerol or another mild tranquilizer, but the procedure is relatively painless and does not require a general anesthetic. The fetoscope has a light source and visual optics that allow a limited but direct view of a two- to four-centimeter-square area of the fetus, and with patience a doctor can gather information about small areas that do not show up clearly on the ultrasound screen—the eyes, ears, mouth, fingers and toes, the major joints, and different areas of the spine.

Visualization of the fetus, however, is secondary in importance to fetal blood sampling. Once the fetoscope is in place, the doctor inserts a small blood-sampling needle through the fetoscope and directly into the placental blood vessels, aspirating a tiny amount of placental blood for further testing. The placenta is the preferred area because a placental blood sample is equivalent to a sample taken directly from the fetus, and it avoids disturbing the fetus itself. When a skin biopsy is required, a small fragment of skin is taken from the fetal scalp or trunk. Both samples are sent to the laboratory for further testing.

Fetoscopy is a specialized technique, and only two centers in the United States are presently working in this new area: the University of California at San Francisco, and Yale University. Two centers in Canada and several others in Europe have also developed fetal blood sampling capabilities. Once more medical centers offer fetoscopy, many families at risk for hemophilia, sickle-cell anemia, beta thalassemia, and other serious blood disorders will be able to have their pregnancies screened prenatally instead of gambling with a pregnancy or choosing to abort all male fetuses, as they do now.

☐ *How Safe Is Fetoscopy?* Because fetoscopy requires great skill and precision, it is associated with a much higher rate of serious complications than amniocentesis, including an increased risk of bleeding, ruptured membranes, and miscarriage. When doctors began using fetoscopy a few years ago, centers experimenting with the technique reported an increased miscarriage rate of 5 to 10 percent, a substantial proportion of cases. Now, with further experience, the rate has fallen to under 5 percent, and will probably be reduced in the future as doctors gain more knowledge of the technique.

Even with the present risk of miscarriage, fetoscopy has incredible potential. The widespread use of fetoscopy would help reassure many couples that now face the possibility of bearing a child with a crippling blood disease or a serious birth defect, and one can look forward to a future in which fetoscopy is used with other techniques to treat the fetus prenatally—an area of genetics that is now barely in its infancy.

☐ *The Alpha Fetoprotein Test* The presence of high levels of alpha fetoprotein in the amniotic fluid or in the mother's bloodstream can be used to detect a common group of birth defects—the neural-tube defects.

Alpha fetoprotein is a substance normally found in fetal blood. In the first month after conception it is manufactured in the embryonic yolk sac, but as the fetus develops it is increasingly produced by the fetal liver. After birth it disappears rapidly from the newborn's bloodstream and its place is taken by a substance called albumin, the most important protein found in human blood. Because alpha fetoprotein is secreted only by the fetus, its presence in the maternal blood always indicates pregnancy.

A certain level of alpha fetoprotein is a sign of normal development. A higher than normal level suggests a number of possibilities, including a multiple birth, a threatened miscarriage, or a neural-tube defect. The alpha fetoprotein level is abnormally high in the latter case because fluid containing alpha fetoprotein leaks from the brain or the open spine and enters the amniotic fluid, where it can be detected through amniocentesis. A woman with a family history of neural-tube defects or a previous affected pregnancy can arrange for an amniocentesis test after the fifteenth week of the pregnancy, or a woman who is having the test for another purpose can arrange to have the alpha fetoprotein analysis performed for a modest extra fee, just in case.

Amniocentesis, however, is an expensive and selective way to screen a common birth defect, and in certain other countries, including Great Britain, where the incidence of neural-tube defects is four times higher than in the United States, a simple, inexpensive blood test is used as a first stage in alpha fetoprotein analysis. All pregnancies in Great Britain are routinely monitored by the test, which is now becoming available on a limited basis in certain areas of the United States. Testing begins with an initial blood sample taken early in the second trimester of pregnancy. A woman who is found to have a high level of AFP in her blood is then asked to take a second test. If the level is still high, she can arrange to have an ultrasound examination to rule out a multiple pregnancy or a visible neural-tube defect such as anencephaly. A negative result leads to the next stage: amniocentesis. If a very high level of AFP is found in the amniotic fluid, this is invariably caused by an open lesion in the fetal spine, and at this point it is necessary for the parents and their doctor to discuss the prospects for the fetus and make the decision regarding termination of pregnancy or special care after birth.

The use of the alpha fetoprotein blood test has just been approved in the United States, after years of public debate and over the strong opposition of right-to-life groups and certain members of the medical profession. There has been a mixed reaction to the test among American doctors. Some have welcomed it as a simple, safe method of screening large numbers of women who might otherwise never suspect that they were carrying a child with a neural-tube defect; others think there are potential hazards because the sophisticated procedures that should accompany the test—amniocentesis, ultrasound, and proper counseling—are available to relatively few American women. If you have a family history of neural-tube defects or you are aware of a higher incidence of tube defects in the area in which you live, you can ask your physician to obtain the test for you or to direct you to a medical center where the test is already in use. In the future, the test will undoubtedly be available to all women as testing facilities are developed commercially.

☐   *Genetic Engineering—Is This the Future's Answer to Genetic Disorders?*
Some scientists have claimed that genetic research will one day be so advanced that the individual's genetic makeup will be irrelevant. This is perhaps a possibility, although it is many years away. Most genetic diseases are caused by a single abnormality and it should be theoretically possible to regulate genetic deficiencies by transplantation or some other method. Scientists can already transplant fragments of DNA into bacterial cells, using an incredibly skillful splicing technique, the so-called "chemical knives," known by scientists as restriction en-

zymes. This has enabled them to produce experimental substances in the laboratory that are normally produced only in the body. Human insulin for the relief of diabetes is one of them. Other experiments have successfully introduced foreign genes into mouse embryos and seen the mice pass down the gene successfully to the next generation.

A few attempts have already been made to introduce compensatory genes into humans whose genes have failed to carry out their normal functions. If a technique like this is successful at some point in the future, it should be possible to cure a disease such as thalassemia major, which is now fatal at a tragically early age. One day genetic engineering might well become so advanced that a great number of diseases that today are incompatible with life will disappear.

23

Monitoring the High-Risk Mother and Baby: Modern Testing Techniques

One of the reasons for the increasing number of successful high-risk pregnancies in the last few years is the recent development of a series of testing procedures that can be used to evaluate, and protect, the development of a healthy child. These sophisticated biophysical and biomedical tests—which include ultrasonography, amniocentesis, fetal monitoring, and a group of blood and urine tests—have enabled obstetricians and perinatologists to identify normal prenatal patterns, and use this information to detect fetuses at high risk before irreparable damage has occurred. Since you might well be exposed to any one of these tests if your pregnancy has a complicating factor, the most common procedures will be described separately in this chapter, together with information on the safety and accuracy of each test. I must emphasize that none of these tests should be carried out by a physician who is not a well trained obstetrician familiar with the care of high-risk patients. The aim of all of these new procedures is to make an accurate determination of which babies and mothers are at risk and to deliver as healthy a child as possible with as little harm as possible to the mother.

☐ **Ultrasonography During Pregnancy**   Ultrasound waves are sound waves that vibrate at an extremely high frequency, about thirty thousand cycles a second. These sound waves are far too high-pitched to be heard by the human ear but can be reflected on a televisionlike screen when they bounce off the surface of a nonmoving object. By using a technological analysis of the frequency of these sonographic waves, one can measure the distance between two objects as the waves reflect off them.

Ultrasound technology was invented by a Scottish researcher in the 1960s and first developed commercially in the early 1970s. One of the industries that initially exploited ultrasound most successfully was commercial fishing, in which ultrasound was used to measure the depth of the ocean bed and locate schools of fish. Then medical researchers, interested in the similarities between the fetus, floating in its fluid-filled sac, and a fish in water, began experimenting with the same technology to determine the size of the baby. Out of this research, a form of ultrasound that uses low-intensity ultrasonic waves was developed for use in obstetrics and other fields of medicine, and diagnostic ultrasound has now become one of the most valuable devices available to the obstetrician.

☐ *How an Ultrasound Unit Works*   Ultrasound waves are transmitted to and from the mother's abdomen through a cluster of quartz crystals placed inside a small hand-held transducer. When this transducer is moved over the surface of the skin, the ultrasound waves are directed against the placenta and the amniotic sac containing the baby. Once the waves hit a permanent organ they will be deflected outward and can be picked up through a special receptor, which, in turn, feeds the transmitted impulses of sound into a scanning machine that prints them out onto the ultrasound screen. A clear picture of the various fetal organs can be put together by moving the transducer over different areas of the abdomen. The size, location and contour of various organs can then be measured and analyzed.

ULTRASOUND EXAMINATION

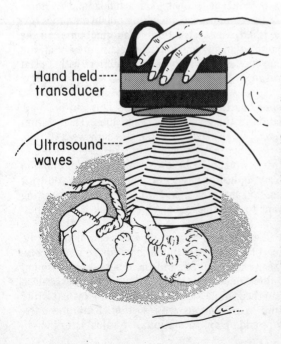

Hand held transducer

Ultrasound waves

Figure 57: Ultrasound Examination: The ultrasound waves are transmitted to and from the mother's abdomen through a cluster of quartz crystals placed inside a small hand-held transducer. In this instance the ultrasound waves are directed against the baby's head, which will appear on the ultrasound screen (not shown). Ultrasound therefore can be used to determine fetal head measurements, but the sound waves can also be directed against the placenta to determine its location and configuration. The amount of amniotic fluid can also be determined by ultrasonic examination.

☐ **Ultrasound for Determination of Fetal Age**   If a woman is unsure of her due date because she has an irregular ovulation pattern or a poor record of her first missed period, her obstetrician can use ultrasound to measure the diameter of the gestational sac or the fetal skull, or the length of the fetus, and arrive at an estimated date of delivery. Ultrasound is capable of delineating the fetus at a very early stage. At six to eight weeks the fetal sac is already visible, and a complete fetal outline and fetal movement can be detected on the screen by the tenth to twelfth week. Later on in gestation, the fetal head is large enough for the doctor to estimate fetal maturity by measuring the size of the fetal skull, just above the ear (the biparietal diameter, or BIP) and plotting it against a growth curve (see Chapter 8). Two measurements derived on two successive visits will usually give an accurate enough reading to confirm a woman's due date or set a new due date. Fetal measurements can also be plotted against the curve to make sure that a fetus is growing at the normal speed and to identify a fetus suffering intrauterine growth retardation.

☐ **Location of the Placenta**   The outline of the placenta will show up quite clearly on the ultrasound screen, enabling the obstetrician to locate the exact position of the placenta during an amniocentesis test or a fetoscopy test (see pages 298–305). A placental complication such as placenta previa, in which the placenta obstructs the cervix, can also be determined by the use of ultrasound.

☐ **Can Ultrasound Determine Congenital Malformations of the Fetus?**   Modern ultrasound techniques have reached such a high degree of sophistication in the last few years that a number of serious abnormalities now can be determined *in utero* by doctors who specialize in this technology. Abnormalities of the heart and central nervous system (anencephaly, spina bifida, and hydrocephaly), certain abnormalities of the amniotic sac, including polyhydramnios (excessive amounts of amniotic fluid), and structural malformations can be detected at a relatively early point in pregnancy. Ultrasonograms are not always 100 percent conclusive, because the fetus' position might interfere with a clear picture of the different fetal organs.

☐ **Can Fetal Sex Be Determined by Ultrasonography?**   This can be done, but it requires direct visualization of the genital area—and luck. The scrotum and penis are visible on the screen by the sixteenth to eighteenth week of fetal development, but sometimes the labia on a female fetus will be enlarged and look enough like a scrotum for a woman to be given the wrong information about her baby's sex. Only if very sophisticated technology is used can you trust a sonogram for sexual determination and even then I would recommend waiting until after the birth if you want to buy traditional blue or pink baby clothes.

☐ **Real-Time Ultrasound**   Two types of ultrasound are in common use: the B-mode scanning device, which provides a two-dimensional image in cross section and is used when static scans are required, and the diagnostic ultrasound technique known as real-time ultrasound. Real-time ultrasound uses gray scale, a narrower image of the fetus than the B-mode device, to capture a moving picture of the uterus' internal structure in continuous cross section. Real-time ultrasound's ability to pinpoint limbs and organs in motion is so valuable to the ob-

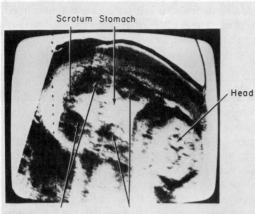

Scrotum Stomach

Head

Legs bent   Arms flexed

Figure 58: Fetal Sex Determination Through Ultrasonography: Parents are often anxious to know the sex of their baby. Frequently they will ask the doctor doing an ultrasound examination to determine the fetal sex. This, however, is extremely difficult. This ultrasound picture shows a baby lying on its back. The baby's legs are spread apart and a genital enlargement simulating male organs is visible. The parents were told that this baby was a male. Much to the surprise of the doctor, what was thought to be the scrotum was an enlarged labium, and a baby girl was delivered.

stetrician that this is the type of ultrasound you will usually find in the high-risk specialist's office, even though the picture itself is somewhat poorer in quality than the one produced by the static B-mode scanning device. If you have a real-time ultrasound scan taken, you will be able to see the fetus's image move on the screen as your doctor passes the transducer over your abdomen.

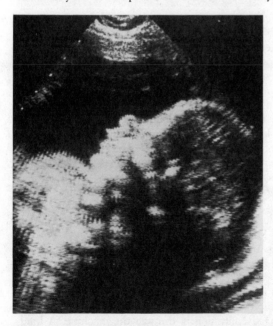

Figure 59: Ultrasound of a Five-Month-Old Fetus: Ultrasound can pinpoint limbs and other organs. Occasionally it will outline the baby's profile. A nose, mouth, and chin are seen here in the middle of the picture. Ultrasound is an important tool in evaluating the fetus and in excluding fetal abnormalities.

☐ *How Safe Is Ultrasound?* Very high levels of diagnostic ultrasound, levels far more intense than those used in clinical practice, are capable of producing tissue or cellular damage in laboratory animals. It is difficult to predict how brief exposures, at much lower levels, affect the fetus, but preliminary studies of children exposed to diagnostic ultrasound prenatally do not suggest that there are any permanent effects from its use. An intensive government-funded study is now following the progress of a group of children over a five-year period. However, according to our present knowledge, ultrasound appears safe and effective.

☐   *Nonstress Testing and Stress Testing of Fetal Well-Being*   The fetal heart rate is a valuable clue to fetal well-being. Ultrasound techniques have enabled doctors and the hospital staff to monitor the fetal heart rate during labor or before labor begins with two types of fetal monitors: an external monitoring unit using what is known as a Doppler technique, and an internal type of monitor that attaches an electrode directly to the baby's scalp. The latter can be done only if the membranes have ruptured.

External forms of fetal monitoring are now frequently used in stress testing and nonstress testing. Stress testing is the type of fetal monitoring that is probably most familiar to you because so many contemporary hospitals use fetal monitors in their labor and delivery suites to obtain a continuous record of the fetal heart rate under the stress of labor. Nonstress testing is a newer technique that high-risk specialists use to monitor the fetal heart rate in the final weeks of pregnancy. Both nonstress and stress testing devices differ from real-time ultrasound units because they do not visualize the fetus but instead use a phenomenon known as Doppler ultrasound to gain a record of the fetal heart rate during fetal movement or during labor.

☐   *The Doppler Technique*   When ultrasonography is used to obtain a picture of the placenta or of the fetal skull, the beams are aimed toward a static object and the reflected sound waves can be picked up on a special electronic receptor, the ultrasound screen. Nonstress and stress testing, however, are designed to monitor a moving object—the fetal heart. An ultrasound wave that bounces off a moving instead of a static object is likewise reflected back but at a different ultrasound frequency from the one in which it was originally transmitted. This is the phenomenon known as the *Doppler* ultrasound principle, after the famous Austrian mathematician Christian Doppler, who first described the way sound is reflected and changed in pitch as a moving object comes toward the listener and then moves away (a natural occurrence he observed when trains passed him on a railway station in Vienna). Because these differences in frequency can be detected audibly or recorded graphically, a monitoring unit using Doppler ultrasound is capable of picking up and constructing a continuous record of the fetal heart rate. This information is so valuable during labor and delivery that fetal monitoring units have become standard equipment in the more advanced medical centers, even for women whose pregnancies are not considered high-risk.

Once the ultrasound signal has been sent out and returned to the unit, it is transmitted through a highly sophisticated apparatus that records the fetal heart rate on a long strip of paper fed continuously through the machine. A loudspeaker in the monitoring unit simultaneously provides the patient and the obstetrician or hospital staff with a steady, continuous sound reflection of the heartbeat. Some of the new and/or more sophisticated fetal monitors are so finely tuned that each single beat is audible, giving a very clear idea of the way the fetal heart is behaving.

☐ *Analysis of the Fetal Heart Rate*   By watching the fetal heart rate, it is possible to determine the well-being of the fetus. A normal fetal heart rate is like that of healthy adults—it exhibits a slight but noticeable alteration between each beat, a pattern that is known as variability. Variability indicates that the body is functioning normally. Exactly the opposite phenomenon occurs if the heart is put under tremendous stress; the natural variability is lost, and one beat follows the next at exactly the same interval, in the classic flat pattern seen during a heart attack or in adults with severe heart disease. The same pattern is observed in the fetus *in utero*. Some variability between each heartbeat indicates that the baby's environment is healthy, whereas a lack of variability might mean that the baby is not receiving enough oxygen. In this instance plans for delivery should be initiated immediately to prevent fetal brain damage or fetal death.

Fetal heart rate monitoring can also determine whether the fetal heart is behaving normally. Usually a baby's heart rate is twice that of its mother, normally around one hundred forty beats per minute at rest. As the physician watches the baby's heart rate on the fetal monitoring paper he will notice the heart rate responding to the baby's movements—another sign of a healthy cardiovascular response. If the heart rate does not increase by about fifteen beats and remain elevated for fifty seconds when the baby moves, it could indicate that the regulatory mechanism of the heart is not functioning correctly.

Another phenomenon he will look for is an occasional drop in the heartbeat that is not related to an external cause. If what is known as a spontaneous deceleration does occur, this is also a disturbing symptom which must be evaluated further.

☐ *Nonstress Testing*   Nonstress testing is a newer external fetal monitoring technique that has been found to be extremely useful in high-risk cases. Women with diabetes or hypertension or a number of other high-risk disorders are often asked to take a nonstress test or series of nonstress tests beginning at the thirty-fourth week of gestation, when the baby is close enough to term to survive delivery successfully. A nonstress testing device monitors the heart rate by using an external Doppler technique. In the first part of the test, the obstetrician places a transducer over the skin of the abdomen and reads off the heart rate from the strip of fetal monitoring paper. Then the woman is given a signal indicator and asked to press it every time she feels the baby move. The signal in turn is marked directly on the fetal monitoring paper to identify periods of movement. During the next twenty to thirty minutes, the normal duration of the test, a healthy fetus can be expected to move at least two or three times, and, as it moves, the heart rate should increase by at least fifteen beats a minute and remain elevated for about fifty seconds before it goes down again (see figure 60). This acceleration pattern is a normal, healthy response to movement; children or adults show a similar heart-rate increase when they walk briskly or break into a run.

A so-called "positive" nonstress test, one in which the fetal heart rate behaves normally, is usually followed by another test no more than a week later to keep a

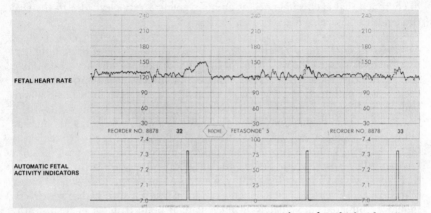

Figure 60: Nonstress Testing: A nonstress test is a test performed on high-risk patients before their due date or on patients who have passed their due date. A Doppler ultrasound unit, which traces the fetal heart rate, is placed on the mother's abdomen. A pressure transducer will also be placed on the mother's abdomen to indicate each time the baby moves. This can be done automatically, or the patient can be asked to press a button each time she feels fetal movement. With a healthy infant, the baby's heart rate should increase in response to fetal movement (as the tracing indicates in the picture). More than three fetal movements within a twenty-minute period with a satisfactory increase in fetal heart rate during each fetal movement indicates a "positive" response. If the baby's heart rate does not increase in response to movement, it could be a sign that the baby is not receiving enough oxygen or the nervous system is not functioning well. The patient might then have to be admitted to the hospital for additional testing or labor induction.

continuing check on the fetus' progress. A so-called "negative" test is cause for concern since it could indicate that the fetus is in jeopardy. A woman whose first test is found to be negative should be asked to take a further test, *the oxytocin challenge test*, described below.

☐ *Oxytocin Challenge Test*   This is a slightly more complicated fetal monitoring technique that is usually employed after a nonstress test is judged to be "nonreactive"—in other words, there is no heart-rate increase in response to fetal movement. The patient is placed in her hospital's labor unit, where she is given an intravenous infusion of Pitocin (a synthetic form of oxytocin, the labor-inducing hormone) and the baby's heart rate is simultaneously recorded on a fetal monitoring unit. Enough oxytocin is used to induce three fairly strong labor contractions within a ten-minute period; this provides a reasonable simulation of the stress placed on a baby in normal labor. If the heart rate remains stable during this time (that is, there is no sudden deceleration—decrease or a persistent pattern of depression—under stress; see Chapter 28), the obstetrician can be sure that the placenta is strong enough to supply the baby with a continual supply of oxygen during labor, and the patient will usually be sent home to wait for labor to begin spontaneously or asked in for another test within twenty-four to forty-eight hours. A decrease in the heart rate, on the other hand, is a danger sign, because it indicates a serious insufficiency in the placenta. After a so-called "positive" oxytocin challenge test, a doctor who decides that a fetus is in jeopardy will arrange for an immediate delivery either by labor induction or by cesarean section. Because of the nonstress test and oxytocin challenge test, we can now recognize fetuses at risk and save many babies who would otherwise have been brain-damaged at birth or stillborn.

☐ *What Does Fetal Movement Mean?*   When the fetus moves, it is sending out signals to the outside world that can be intercepted and interpreted by the pregnant woman or her doctor. You can usually feel movement from the fourth or fifth month of your first pregnancy, although the early movements are faint and infrequent and grow strong enough to be distinguished clearly only as pregnancy progresses.

Daily movements increase considerably as the baby becomes more mature. When the fetus is about 20 weeks along in gestation there are about 200 movements daily, although you will not be able to sense anything like that many yourself. By 32 weeks of gestation there might be as many as 500 separate incidents of movement in a 24-hour period. After the 32nd week, movements seem to decrease gradually until they reach an average of 280 to 300 movements daily at the time of delivery. These are only average daily totals, of course, and each pregnancy can be expected to have its own rhythm. Movements might well fluctuate from around 200 one day to 700 or so the next, although a woman can often sense a characteristic pattern. Movements are dependent on the woman's eating habits. Women who prefer to eat their main meal in the evening usually sense more movement at night, when the blood sugar reaches a peak.

☐ *Does the Fetus Ever Sleep?*   Yes, it does. The fetus usually moves in a rhythm between sleep and wakefulness, and a long period of sleep is usually followed by a quick flurry of fetal movement. Fetuses, like newborn babies, tend to experience longer periods of sleep than they do of wakefulness. These periods of deep sleep are often picked up by monitoring equipment, so you should not be frightened if the baby shows no signs of movement during a test as long as the heart rate is steady.

☐ *Fetal-Movement Alarm Signal*   A woman who is high-risk, or a woman who has passed her due date, may be asked to keep a continuous record of her baby's movements by noting each period of activity on a fetal-movement chart. A useful record can be invaluable in the last critical weeks of a diabetic pregnancy or a pregnancy complicated by toxemia. For example, if the baby *slows down or stops moving* altogether, this is often a sign that labor is about to begin—or a danger signal. If you have some reason to be concerned about the baby's well-being because your pregnancy has been difficult, act immediately if you experience either a pronounced decrease in movement or a complete cessation of movement. Test the baby's responsiveness by drinking a beverage containing sugar, such as orange juice, or tea with sugar added, sit down quietly for a few minutes to allow the blood sugar to reach the baby, and then call the doctor or the medical center once the baby fails to respond. You will need further evaluation and testing if the baby is judged to be in danger.

Women with high-risk pregnancies are already using fetal-movement charts in a number of medical centers in the United States as well as abroad. One hospital where doctors rely highly on monitoring fetal movements is Haddassah Hospital in Jerusalem, where a noted researcher, Professor Eliahu Sadovsky, has made a number of in-depth studies of fetal movement and concluded that a significant decrease in movement often precedes fetal death in high-risk cases, particularly toxemia and diabetes. After he and his colleagues began educating women to the meaning of fetal movement, an increasing number of babies in their hospital survived birth.

A sudden cessation of movement is not the only sign of distress. If you sense a violent increase in fetal movement that is not related to any external factor, particularly a series of convulsive movements, as if the baby were struggling inside you, report this to your doctor immediately. The baby could be suffering from oxygen deprivation and will need help. Any dramatic change in movement should, in fact, be reported to your doctor; a sudden or violent variation in movement patterns might indicate a critical need for delivery.

☐ *Amniocentesis*   Amniocentesis, a procedure in which a fluid sample is taken from the amniotic fluid around the fetus and used for analysis, has already been described in the chapter on genetic counseling. The amniotic-fluid sample can be subjected to a number of different tests, including the chromosomal and biochemical analyses described in the same chapter. It is also used to evaluate the fetus in cases of Rhesus disease (see Chapter 20) where analysis of the fluid will determine whether or not the baby is sick enough to need an intrauterine transfusion of Rh-negative blood. Finally, amniocentesis can be performed just before an elective delivery to determine whether or not a baby's lungs are mature enough to allow it to survive the birth. This step is taken in a high-risk case in which the baby has shown distress during a nonstress test or an oxytocin challenge test, or where fetal movements have decreased so disturbingly that an early delivery seems desirable. The test is also used before an elective repeat Cesarean section. (This test, the L/S ratio, is described later in the chapter.) Amniocentesis, in fact, has become one of the most valuable tools that a perinatologist or obstetrician has at his command, and in the future it will undoubtedly be used to detect, and treat, other serious conditions.

☐ *What Are Estriols?*   Estriol is a special pregnancy hormone whose precursor is produced in the baby's brain, or more precisely, in the fetal pituitary, which stimulates the fetal adrenal glands to produce a hormone called dehydroepiandrosterone (DHEA). This estriol precursor is then metabolized in the fetal liver, is passed through the placenta, and enters the mother's circulatory system via the umbilical cord. Finally the estriol is excreted through the mother's urine.

☐ *Estriol Testing*   The high-risk patient, particularly the diabetic patient, is often at special risk in the final weeks of the pregnancy, when many babies die unexpectedly. This critical time can be monitored by tests on the mother's urine and blood that determine the amount of estriol being excreted from the fetus.

The level of estriols increases as the size of the fetus increases. When a blood or urine estriol analysis is performed, the level of estriols is determined and then plugged into a normal growth curve similar to the one used to measure fetal growth with ultrasound. If the estriols in a particular pregnancy follow the curve, this is a reassuring sign. An unusually high level of estriols means the mother is carrying twins or the baby is abnormally large for its gestational age. A lower than average level, on the other hand, could mean that the fetus is not receiving enough nutrition or has some congenital abnormality.

A doctor who suspects that a fetus is in danger can take an estriol test every few days to detect any sudden drop in the estriol level—a sign that the fetus has ceased to grow or the blood supply to the brain is insufficient to trigger proper brain function. If the level drops, the patient will be sent to the hospital immediately for further analysis, usually with a nonstress and a stress test.

Estriol analysis is a test that high-risk centers frequently used in the past, and many centers continue to regard it as one of the best methods available to determine fetal well-being. The problem is that the accuracy of estriol analysis cannot always be relied on unless the hospital has a good laboratory and an experienced staff, because it is easier to derive a false negative test result with estriols than with some of the other, more precise tests. For this reason, some centers use fewer estriol tests and are now relying more on fetal heart rate monitoring tests. Nonetheless, you might be referred to a center where the testing standards are high and the laboratory is sophisticated enough to analyze the estriol level correctly. Remember: if your estriol level falls, your obstetrician should order further testing immediately.

☐ *Human Placenta Lactogen Analysis*   Human placenta lactogen (HPL), also known as human chorionic somatomammotropin, is an important pregnancy hormone that is produced by certain cells in the placenta. In a normal, healthy pregnancy, the placenta secretes more HPL as the fetus continues to grow and develop. If, however, placental growth is retarded, as it often is in a pregnancy in which the woman has chronic hypertension or develops toxemia, the detectable level of HPL in the woman's blood will be unusually low.

Detectable levels of HPL can be picked up by a human placenta lactogen analysis carried out on a woman's blood serum, usually in conjunction with an estriol analysis. This is a relatively new test, devised in the 1960s after research teams first isolated human placenta lactogen and began to study its special role in pregnancy. Not all high-risk centers use it, even though some obstetricians feel the test adds important information on the well-being of the baby, especially in the case of a woman with hypertension and intrauterine growth retardation.

☐ *The L/S Ratio: Evaluation of Fetal Lung Maturity*   Tests that doctors rely on in high-risk cases, such as estriols, nonstress, and stress tests, can indicate the need to start labor artificially because the fetus is beginning to suffer or is struggling inside the uterus. The problem that any obstetrician then faces is the question of the baby's maturity: is the baby ready to be born, or is the baby at least mature enough to avoid a severe case of hyaline-membrane disease—a disorder of newborns in which the baby's immature lungs fill up with fluid and the baby dies a few days after birth in the premature nursery? Hyaline-membrane disease is less of a threat now than it was in the 1960s, but a great number of premature babies still suffer from the disease, and some of them still die despite the new oxygen therapy now used in premature intensive-care units. Thus, when researchers came up with a test which they thought could be used to predict the maturity of the fetal lungs, it was a major breakthrough in high-risk obstetrics.

This test is the so-called lecithin-sphingomyelin ratio (known generally as the L/S ratio), a method pioneered by Dr. Louis Gluck of the University of California, San Diego. The test, as its name suggests, measures the ratio of two lipids, lecithin and sphingomyelin, which are present in the normal fetal lungs. The ratio of these important lipids changes as pregnancy progresses; sphingomyelin is the lipid that is found in the highest quantities early in fetal life, but around the thirty-fourth week of gestation the sphingomyelin begins to decrease as lecithin, the component that prevents the newborn's lungs from collapsing outside the uterus, increases in readiness for delivery. Both of these lipids drift out of the fetal lungs during fetal respiration and circulate in the amniotic fluid. By using amniotic-fluid samples derived at different stages of the pregnancy, Dr. Gluck developed a ratio of the amount of lecithin over sphingomyelin in the mature fetal lungs. This is the ratio now used when a doctor aspirates amniotic fluid during an amniocentesis test and sends it for an L/S ratio and other laboratory tests before deciding to induce labor by oxytocin or perform a Cesarean section. The test which is now also routinely used before a repeat Cesarean section can analyze a variety of phospho lipids in the amniotic fluid.

☐ ***Does a Mature L/S Ratio Always Mean a Safe Delivery?***   Although the L/S ratio may indicate that the baby's lungs are mature enough to support it outside the uterus, this does not always mean that the other organs, including the liver and the brain, are fully developed. A satisfactory L/S ratio only guarantees that the baby will be free of hyaline-membrane disease, and the full maturity of all the organs is so important to the newborn that a good obstetrician will try to keep the baby in the uterus for as long as possible. That is why we try to do everything we can to avoid premature labor by increasing bed rest and using new medications like ritodrine and other drugs to arrest premature labor. The lungs, the brain, and the other human organs are really mature only when nature intends them to be, at term.

☐ ***Steroid Therapy for Lung Maturation***   Certain doctors are currently giving a potent steroid preparation to hasten the maturation of the fetal lungs. The mother of a baby at risk is given the steroid betamethasone, which enters the baby's bloodstream. The exact mechanism is not understood fully, but it seems to work via a stress factor in the fetus which results in a maturation of the lung tissue with a change in the L/S ratio, and increases the baby's pulmonary function so it can survive more successfully after birth.

☐ ***Is Steroid Therapy Harmful?***   Steroids have been proven efficacious in a number of tests. No one is completely sure, however, about their safety. Steroids are extremely potent hormones that have produced decreased brain and body growth and problems of carbohydrate metabolism in laboratory animals, and appear to inhibit nerve development in fetal animals. Groups of children treated with steroids *in utero* have been tested and pronounced healthy, but there is still a possibility that dyslexia and other communication disorders might become obvious once these children enter school. The fact that steroids hasten lung maturity does not give any obstetrician the right to deliver a baby prematurely without taking all the other factors into account. Certainly, if a premature delivery is imminent and the only way the baby can possibly survive is by its being given dexamethasone or betamethasone, then steroids should be used. But if they are being given indiscriminately, just because there is nothing else that can be done, or are being used to allow the doctor to deliver a premature baby who could survive for a longer period without delivery, then either is an improper and unethical use of the obstetrician's power. Your doctor should always explain the risks as well as the benefits of any drug or procedure before he goes ahead with any treatment. Every drug you are given can have both positive and negative results, and there is a certain element of risk in almost any procedure or test.

□ *No More Guessing Games*   A few years ago all a doctor could do in a high-risk pregnancy was to examine the mother at close intervals and monitor the fetal heart rate by a fetoscope (a special stethoscope). An experienced doctor might then be able to make an educated guess as to the fetus' health, but it was often little more than that. With the introduction of specific tests, much of this guesswork has been eliminated in high-risk cases because we now have relatively simple and reasonably safe methods of estimating the fetal health and maturity. While one test alone may not offer a conclusive diagnosis, these new tests can be used in sequence to help determine the precise nature of the difficulty, and enable the obstetrician to make informed judgments that were simply not possible twenty years ago. In another ten years, there will probably be other, even more sophisticated tests that will make our present advanced monitoring methods look old-fashioned, and will help to deliver healthier babies with fewer problems.

24

High-Risk Pregnancy

"High-risk pregnancy," a term that has become familiar in the last few years, describes a pregnancy that poses an increased risk to the mother or the fetus because it is associated with a complication or possible complication; in other words, a pregnancy that is more difficult than usual because of some complicating factor not found in the normal pregnancy. "High-risk" is often contrasted with "low-risk," a pregnancy in which there are no problems with conception and no difficulties or complications during pregnancy itself. However, this distinction is somewhat misleading since doctors do encounter apparently low-risk pregnancies that, due to unforeseen circumstances, end up in the high-risk category. Some medical specialists say that *every* pregnancy is high-risk at the moment the woman goes into labor because unforeseen problems are always possible. Even a healthy woman can experience heavy bleeding, or strong uterine contractions that cut down the blood supply to the baby, or a sudden rise or fall in blood pressure during labor. Serious complications like these usually occur quite unexpectedly, making a hitherto low-risk pregnancy suddenly high-risk.

Pregnancies that start off in the high-risk category have a clear element of difficulty. These include pregnancies in which the woman has some past or present medical or obstetrical complication or is having a first baby at a very young or a relatively advanced age. Any woman who is diabetic, has high blood pressure, has a history of infertility due to pelvic abnormalities, or endometriosis, has fibroid tumors, is asthmatic or has a history of tuberculosis, heart problems, thyroid disorders or severe allergies, or is simply having a first baby at 35 or older, should be considered high-risk and receive additional care. This group also includes women with problematical obstetrical histories, including a previous Cesarean section or a miscarriage or stillbirth. Women who are very high-risk should be seen by a perinatologist rather than an ordinary obstetrician; he not only has the special training to handle high-risk cases but he usually has better backup facilities to take care of specialized tests and laboratory analysis. In addition, certain women have a family history of genetic disorders or are inadvertently exposed to drugs, radiation, or infections at the beginning of the pregnancy and are, therefore, classified as high-risk, even though they are otherwise in good health.

Certain other high-risk factors become apparent during the pregnancy itself. If a woman develops high blood pressure, the first sign of toxemia of pregnancy, or her monthly urine sample contains traces of sugar, or she comes down with a severe viral infection or an attack of herpes, any one of these would immediately place her in the high-risk category. Another group of hazards that arises during the pregnancy is obstetrical rather than medical. A woman who is found to be pregnant with twins or triplets is considered high-risk, and so is a woman with an incompetent cervix or a placental complication. The next chapter, Serious Complications During Pregnancy, deals with some common pregnancy-related complications, including toxemia and premature labor.

As you can see from this rather formidable list, a large number of pregnant women each year are likely to find themselves in the high-risk group, and with better medical care we can expect their number to grow rather than diminish. At the same time modern technology has allowed obstetricians and perinatologists to follow and care for high-risk women far more successfully than was possible even a few years ago. Any woman in the high-risk category should be fully informed about her progress and have a special understanding of the physiology of pregnancy, and any unusual problems that could arise in her own case, since she needs extra care from her doctor and may not be free to enjoy the same activities as a woman in a low-risk pregnancy. You might well be expected to stay in bed for long periods of time, or you might require tests or early hospitalization if the complication is a more serious one. In any high-risk pregnancy the best way to achieve a successful outcome is through education, understanding, and the guidance of a physician who specializes in difficult pregnancies and is affiliated with a good, well equipped hospital; and this is certainly the way to have healthier babies, and mothers, in the future.

☐ *Age and Pregnancy*   Regardless of the many traditional beliefs about the timing of parenthood, the best time might well be when it is right for you. The two fundamental considerations are: How possible is it to have a baby later in life, and does pregnancy later in life pose unacceptable hazards to the mother or the baby?

☐ *Later Childbearing*   Many doctors were trained to think and still believe that childbearing should be completed before a woman is thirty, because it is dangerous or somehow "wrong" to have a child at a later age. Some of the medical textbooks still refer to a woman having a first child at thirty as an elderly primigravida, and presume that obstetrical complications begin immediately as a woman enters her third decade. This attitude is gradually changing, as increased understanding, better women's health care, and more advanced monitoring systems, including genetic counseling and amniocentesis, are making it easier and easier for women to have babies at a later age. Sophisticated doctors, who are used to caring for primigravidas of thirty-five or forty, are helping to create a more hospitable and flexible environment for the so-called "older mother." Hospitals are seeing an increasing number of women over thirty-five in their maternity units; recent birth statistics reveal that women aged thirty-five or older produce about 7 percent of the newborn babies in the United States, or about 250,000 babies a year, and many of these births go well. But, at the same time, it would only be fair to say that a gynecologist or obstetrician does have some right to caution a couple delaying childbirth because unexpected complications can develop as a woman gets older.

By thirty-five or forty a woman is usually less fertile than she was in her late twenties. Fertility in women drops slowly between thirty and thirty-five, and then declines precipitately: by forty many once-fertile women are infertile. The same is true of the woman's partner: male fertility drops quite rapidly after forty, and if the man is in a high-pressure or stressful job, this can also have an adverse effect on his fertility.

If a woman can become pregnant successfully, there is *no time* when she is *too old* to have a child, unless she suffers from some serious medical complication which would make it difficult for her to go through with the pregnancy. Age itself does not contraindicate pregnancy, and if you find yourself pregnant in your late thirties or even your early forties, don't let anyone tell you that you shouldn't have a child because it is dangerous, or suggest you have an abortion just because you are older.

Look for a doctor who seems open enough to treat you as he would any woman having a baby—and if he is insensitive or technically unable to care for your pregnancy, go to a second doctor, preferably a younger perinatologist who is used to seeing women who are having a first baby at an older age. You should have no problems going through pregnancy if you are willing to follow the doctor's advice.

There are a few caveats, however. Older women have a higher rate of hypertension and toxemia than younger women, and a higher number of growth-retarded infants. Because the body tissues become stiffer as you grow older, you will probably need more bed rest before and after birth, and the lack of elasticity in the uterine and vaginal tissues results in a higher Cesarean rate among women over thirty-five. But even a Cesarean section is much easier today than it used to be, and, under the care of a competent physician, the chance of a serious complication is small.

As to a second or third child, there is really no age limit once you have conceived, because the uterus is already enlarged and the body has made other subtle adjustments to pregnancy and labor. Women who are multipara (women who have given birth to at least one child) can have a child successfully at an even later age—in their mid- or late forties—than a primipara (women who have never given birth) as long as they get plenty of rest, eat properly, and take proper care of themselves. Doctors often presume that a woman who already has one or two children won't continue with a pregnancy if she conceives in her forties, but on medical grounds at least, there is no need to rush into an abortion because of age.

☐ *Pregnancy After Thirty-Five*   Once a woman over thirty-five has become pregnant, she may well face an uncomplicated pregnancy. A woman in good health who is having a first child at a later age, and who has no complicating factor with her pregnancy, is not going to find the nine months too difficult despite her high-risk status. A first pregnancy at this age is automatically put in the high-risk category because this is good preventive medicine—not because every woman will necessarily meet with a serious complication. "High-risk" here simply alerts the obstetrician to difficulties that occur more frequently in this age group so that he will keep a particularly careful watch over the pregnancy.

Statistically, there is a higher chance of certain pregnancy-related complications with increasing age, including toxemia, placenta previa, gestational diabetes, hypertension, and premature labor. A woman pregnant with her first child in her late thirties is twice as likely to develop toxemia as a woman in her early twenties. Cases of placenta previa are also much higher in this group, occurring in about seven out of every hundred births among older first-time mothers. A sonogram in the second trimester will detect a placenta which has attached itself in an abnormally low position in the uterus. Other complications, including gestational diabetes and hypertension, are more likely to be found in high-parity women who are overweight or already have a history of high blood pressure or some other medical complication. Any woman with an existing medical problem such as diabetes or a cardiovascular disorder is going to find pregnancy at a later age that much more difficult, and should to go a perinatologist early in the pregnancy to ensure skilled high-risk care.

A first pregnancy at thirty-five or older is, medically speaking, perfectly feasible as long as a woman is healthy. The contemporary American woman is still healthy, active, and energetic well into her forties, and many of these women feel they are in better shape physically and emotionally, as well as better prepared for childbearing and child-rearing, than they were in their twenties; I have found, too, that their attitude toward the pregnancy is often more realistic. An older woman who has waited so long to become pregnant and is aware of her declining fertility has far more invested in her pregnancy than a woman half her age, and is not going to jeopardize her chances of having a child.

☐ *Monitoring the Pregnancy*   Most mature women know their menstruation patterns better than younger women and are less likely to need ultrasonography to estimate the probable date of delivery, because they probably have kept records of the time of conception. Women over thirty-five, however, have a higher proportion of babies with intrauterine growth retardation, and may require a few serial ultrasonograms to check the healthy growth of the fetus. Furthermore, because there is an increased rate of complications, particularly a higher risk of stillborn babies in this age group, women over the age of thirty-five should have a nonstress test twice a week from the fortieth until the forty-second to forty-third week of pregnancy or up to the time the baby is born. Postmaturity (a pregnancy that has passed the due date and shows signs of disintegration of the placenta) seems to be associated with a higher rate of fetal death among older women. A disaster such as this late in pregnancy can often be prevented by inducing labor. In general, there is an increased need for monitoring the pregnancy of an older woman, not because something will necessarily go wrong, but to prevent any mishaps from occurring.

□ *Is Labor More Difficult for the Older Mother?*   There is a higher incidence of abnormal or dysfunctional labor later in life, although many women in
their thirties and forties deliver early and spontaneously. Often women who are
older do not seem to have good labor patterns, and labor either has to be induced or encouraged by labor-stimulating hormones, or ends in a Cesarean section. It is almost as if the uterus does not respond quite as well as it does in a
younger woman. A recent study from Harvard Medical School, where a large
group of first-time older mothers were compared with a matching group of
women in their twenties, indicated an increased frequency of prolonged labor
and labor that stopped after the initial contractions in older women having their
first pregnancies. It was felt that the uterine muscles might not be as sensitive or
effective in a woman in her late thirties or early forties. However, this slight labor
dysfunction can often be overcome by the careful use of a small amount of oxytocin under the continuous surveillance of a fetal monitor. If this Harvard study
is a fair survey of older mothers in general, the likelihood of prolonged labor, and
therefore an increased chance of Cesarean section, is something that an older
woman ought to consider when preparing for labor. It is also true that doctors
are quicker to resort to a Cesarean when the mother is older because they are
more nervous than usual about the patient. If you are having a first baby and you
are thirty-five or older, make sure that you find out, well in advance of labor, how
often your doctor initiates Cesarean sections in his patients and for what reasons. No doctor should rush into an elective Cesarean without making sure that
a woman is close to her due date, or perform an emergency Cesarean when a
woman is capable of laboring on her own.

Labor problems are experienced primarily by first-time mothers. Older
women who have had a child within the previous five years tend to have shorter,
easier labor, and a much lower Cesarean rate. A second or third birth preceded
by a longer interval is not always so comfortable, because the muscles have stif-
fened since the previous labor, although problems are always fewer after one natural delivery. This is true of a woman at any age.

While recent studies do seem to confirm that labor is more difficult among
older women, many women having their first baby at thirty-five or even forty still
experience uncomplicated and enjoyable deliveries. Today, with fetal heart rate
monitors and more understanding of labor and delivery, it is more than possible
for an older woman to deliver comfortably, and she often has an advantage over
a much younger woman because her emotional maturity and greater understanding decrease fear and anxiety in the labor room. I have personally delivered
a number of babies to women in their mid-forties and usually without any difficulties. Epidural anesthesia is generally a good form of analgesia at that time,
and if the obstetrician is not rushed, a spontaneous delivery can easily be performed if fetal heart rate monitoring indicates that the baby is doing well. Thus,
birth after forty does *not* mean that a Cesarean section is a must.

□ *Is There an Increased Chance of Twins When I Am Older?*   There is a
slightly increased risk of twin gestation when you are older, but if this is your
first pregnancy, the chance is only a little higher than in any other first-time
mother. As a rule, multiple births increase with age and the number of previous
pregnancies. The only group of older first-time mothers with a much higher likelihood of giving birth to two or more babies are women with infertility problems

who have ovulation induced by Pergonal, a potent fertility drug. The use of Pergonal increases the possibility of a multiple birth by 20 percent or more.

☐ **Genetic Counseling After Thirty-Five**   Genetic counseling and amniocentesis are now recommended for any woman who will be thirty-five or older at the time her child is delivered. After thirty-five, the statistical probability of Down's syndrome and other chromosomal abnormalities in the fetus increases by several percentage points (see Chap. 22) and rises sharply once a woman reaches forty or more. With its increased safety record, amniocentesis is rapidly becoming a routine part of pregnancy care for women over thirty-five, and the test is now available at many medical centers.

Another group of common defects that occur more frequently among older couples are the neural-tube defects. A woman having amniocentesis can arrange for an alpha fetoprotein test to be run coincidentally with the fetal karyotype to detect spina bifida or anencephaly prenatally. The incidence of certain other birth defects, particularly cleft lip and cleft palate, and congenital heart defects, are also higher in this age group. Unfortunately, these are not detectable prenatally with our present methods of screening, although many children can be operated on successfully after birth. In general, the risk of giving birth to a congenitally malformed child is greater as the parents grow older, but the numbers are not large enough to deter couples from later childbearing.

☐ **Babies After Forty**   Just a few years ago, women knew that having a child after forty would be risky and difficult. After all, in the past there was an old belief that a child born after forty was either extremely bright or mentally retarded, and this reflected a certain reality. People observed more medical complications as women grew older, and more chromosomally abnormal babies among children of older mothers. Both are still true, but the risks of childbearing after forty have been mitigated now that women of forty are in much better general health than they used to be and prenatal chromosomal analysis is available to detect Down's syndrome and other chromosomal disorders in the fetus.

Studies of the older mother are inconclusive, but a group of studies published a few years ago concluded that the chance of a low-birth-weight or abnormally high-birth-weight infant was greater among women giving birth after forty. Certainly, the general stiffness of the tissues and the prevalence of toxemia among older mothers would contribute to the number of growth-retarded babies born to this group. A woman of forty should rest more, so that more oxygen and nutrition reach the baby. Since toxemia occurs in as many as a quarter or a third of these pregnancies, perhaps because the stress to the body is more severe, bed rest is important to the older mother, and she may have to stop working earlier than she had intended. One also needs to be seen frequently by the obstetrician, or preferably the high-risk specialist.

The number of abnormally large babies found among women in this age group is related to the higher incidence of pregnancy-related diabetes after a woman reaches forty, although this is more likely to occur in a second or third pregnancy in which a woman has retained much of the weight from the previous pregnancy. (Gestational diabetes is one of the high-risk situations discussed later in the chapter.) Women in their first pregnancy whose weight is within normal limits are not at any particular risk. But for any woman in this age group who is overweight, it is important to decrease her weight and get herself into the best possible physical condition before she conceives, and to rest and eat well throughout the pregnancy. The threat of premature labor—more common among all groups of older women—can be eliminated by resting, avoiding physical strain, and restricting sexual intercourse in the last trimester.

☐ *Teenage Pregnancies: What Happens to the Very Young Mother?* The huge number of postwar baby-boom children reaching adolescence in the 1970s and the increase in sexual activity among adolescent women has resulted in a marked increase in teenage pregnancies and births. One in every ten teenage women becomes pregnant each year, and six in every ten teenage pregnancies end in a live birth. The number of teenage pregnancies has increased to such an extent that teenagers now give birth to almost one-fifth of all births in the United States, and according to the latest figures, three-quarters of these births are out of wedlock.

It is not difficult to see why. A study conducted in 1976 showed that 40 percent of all seventeen-year-old teenagers (male and female) were sexually active and so were 18 percent of all fifteen-year-olds. At the same time, only about half of the teenage women aged fifteen to nineteen received any kind of contraceptive services, and perhaps only 7 percent of sexually active girls under fifteen used birth control. In 1976, 83 percent of unintended first pregnancies among teens occurred in the absence of contraception.

Unfortunately there seem to be more risks associated with teenage pregnancies than there are with a pregnancy at any other age, except those after the age of forty-five. Girls younger than fifteen have particularly troubled pregnancies. The death rate from complications of pregnancy and childbirth is small among all groups in the United States, but a girl of fourteen is still 60 percent more likely to die from pregnancy-related complications than a woman in her twenties. And the babies born to teenagers are vulnerable also—these babies are two to three times more likely to die in their first year than a baby born to a more mature woman. Often the higher risk to the baby is the result of insufficient care and nutrition during pregnancy—a teenager may not realize or may refuse to admit that she is pregnant and will eat poorly or continue smoking through most of the pregnancy, and the resulting prematurity or a low birth weight (also high in teenagers) increases the risk of cerebral palsy and mental retardation. After birth, the baby of a very young mother is at special risk because often she is too much of a child herself to become an adequate mother.

The great increase in problems seems to be related to the physical and mental immaturity of the mother. A girl of fifteen is not fully grown. She doesn't always know how to take sufficient care of herself, and fails to get enough vitamins and iron to support the pregnancy. If she is seriously anemic, the baby will have intrauterine growth retardation. Her body might be stressed so that the kidneys fail to function properly, and toxemia (blood poisoning) occurs. Young girls under age fifteen are a special risk for toxemia; they are over three times more likely to die from this serious complication than women in their twenties. Toxemia increases the blood pressure, and the baby, deprived of oxygen and nutrition, grows at a slower rate. The extra stress of the uterine environment may lead to premature labor. In other words, we are talking about a major problem—a dramatic one for the teenage mother herself, and also for her family and for the child she is bringing into the world.

One hopeful study has recently come out of Denmark, where young mothers given proper prenatal care in a Copenhagen hospital did so well in childbirth that their rate of complications was even lower than that of women in their twenties. Although this finding has been disputed, the American researcher Dr. Brian Sutton-Smith of the University of Pennsylvania has stood by his research and has concluded that society, not biology, has made it difficult for younger mothers to give birth successfully. This study also found that while the young mothers had an easy time during pregnancy and delivery, they were not better at mothering. At one year of age, their babies were beginning to show signs of stress, while the babies of older mothers who did not have such a good start had improved considerably. Perhaps in the future, if we can help teenagers better, their children will have, at least biologically, a better start in life, although we are not going to overcome the social problems associated with teenage pregnancies easily.

☐ *Anemia in Pregnancy*   Anemia is one of the most pervasive of all pregnancy-related complications, because women of childbearing age are particularly prone to anemia at all times, and partly because pregnancy itself imposes an increased need for iron on the body. Anemia, in fact, is such a persistent problem that as much as 75 percent of all pregnant women (according to one medical authority) may be affected to some extent by a lack of iron.

A woman becomes anemic when the number of her red blood cells or the level of hemoglobin in the blood is reduced sufficiently to hinder the normal transportation of oxygen throughout the body. A low hemoglobin level (hemoglobin is the substance that colors the red blood cells and enables them to transport oxygen) leads to an insufficient level of oxygen in the body and brain cells and a reduction in the amount of oxygen reaching the fetus. A woman with anemia is often tired, dizzy, and experiences frequent loss of appetite and abdominal pain.

Pregnancy increases the production of the red blood cells because the body is circulating an increased amount of blood, but at the same time the total hemoglobin level usually decreases together with the expansion of the fluid volume. This means a pregnant woman needs to increase her iron intake quite considerably, especially during the second half of pregnancy, to avoid becoming seriously anemic. A low oxygen-carrying capacity in the blood reduces the amount of oxygen in the fetal circulation, causing intrauterine growth retardation and increasing the possibility of toxemia.

☐ *Iron-Deficiency Anemia*   This is by far the most common type of pregnancy-related anemia; but it is the easiest to treat. Perhaps as many as 95 percent of women who have anemia in pregnancy have it because of iron-deficient diets, or because they have exhausted their iron reserves through the increased requirements of pregnancy. If you suffer from iron-deficiency anemia, you might well have begun your pregnancy with a depleted store of iron and experienced a continuing loss of iron as pregnancy progressed. The body absorbs iron more efficiently during pregnancy, but this is not usually sufficient to meet the fetus' needs. Again, as I mentioned earlier in this book, one of the best ways to prepare for pregnancy is to increase your iron stores before pregnancy begins; this will not only make you feel better, it will make pregnancy much less exhausting and do much to promote the baby's good health.

The initial prenatal visit should include a simple blood test to determine your hemoglobin level and the ratio of the red blood cells to the total volume of blood (hematocrit level in the blood). A woman with anemia has a hemoglobin level of ten milligrams or less and a hematocrit level of 30 percent or below.

☐ *Iron Requirements During Pregnancy*   A woman's iron stores normally range from 200 to 400 milligrams. (During pregnancy close to 1000 mg. of iron are required—400 to 500 mg. for the fetus. An infant at birth contains a total body iron content approximately equal to that of a grown woman.) The recommended daily intake of iron during pregnancy increases to 60 mg., which is about four times the amount needed by a nonpregnant woman.

The capacity to absorb and store iron is increased during pregnancy, and a pregnant woman usually absorbs about 1.5 mg. of iron daily over the nonpregnant woman. However, this is not sufficient to offset the loss of iron to the fetus without a change in diet or special iron supplementation.

☐ *Treatment of Iron-Deficiency Anemia*   Iron-deficiency anemia can normally be prevented or corrected by supplemental iron tablets. Most doctors give their patients ferrous sulphate or ferrous gluconate tablets in doses of 300 mg. three times daily. The response to iron supplementation in a woman with iron-deficiency anemia can be constantly checked by a series of blood counts.

In addition, you can increase your absorption of iron by increasing the number of iron-rich foods in your diet, including organ meats and green leafy vegetables. (Chapter 16, "The Pregnancy Diet," contains a comprehensive list of iron-rich foods and more information on iron supplementation.) It is important to remember that the body is incapable of absorbing more than 40 percent of the iron in your diet, even during pregnancy. You can help ensure a sufficient level of iron by avoiding certain compounds that interfere with the body's capacity to absorb iron, and increasing others that retain iron for the body's use during pregnancy. Phosphates and oxalates, for instance, bind with iron and thus cause the iron to become insoluble. (Soft drinks are a common source of phosphates in the modern diet, another good reason to avoid them during pregnancy.) You can counteract this potential iron loss by increasing the amount of calcium and vitamin C in your normal diet, since foods that are high in calcium and vitamin C tend to counteract the binding effect of phosphates and oxalates and free iron for the body's use. Spinach, for instance, which contains both iron and oxalates, could be cooked with milk instead of water to preserve its high iron content.

If you have never used an iron supplement before becoming pregnant you may be alarmed by a sudden bout of constipation or the unexpected color of the stool. Don't worry if the stool looks much darker than usual; the stomach problems that many women experience with iron supplementation can be partially counteracted by drinking extra milk or fruit juice with the iron supplement to hasten its absorption. Your doctor may suggest switching to another brand of supplement if you become very uncomfortable with the first compound, since tolerances vary from brand to brand. If you have a malabsorption for iron you might need iron injections.

☐ *Folic-Acid Anemia*   This is a much rarer form of anemia that is caused by a folic-acid rather than an iron deficiency. Folic-acid anemia accounts for about 2 to 4 percent of the women suffering from anemia in pregnancy, although a woman with iron-deficiency anemia can have folic-acid anemia in addition, further reducing her already low hematocrit level. This form of anemia is sometimes the result of a natural inability to absorb folic acid properly, but it is more often caused by the increased demand for the vitamin during pregnancy itself.

Foods that are a good source of folic acid are listed in Chapter 16. Folic acid is naturally stored in the liver, but the reserve is sufficient for only one month at a time and will be rapidly depleted by the fetus' increased need. Most brands of prenatal vitamins include folic acid, or a special folic-acid supplement can be added to the diet.

☐ *Vitamin-B_{12} Anemia*   Deficiencies of Vitamin B_{12} cause the type of anemia commonly known as *pernicious anemia*. A woman who suffers from pernicious anemia usually experiences tingling and numbness of the hands and feet in addition to the other classic symptoms of anemia. This is a rare complaint in pregnancy and can be treated effectively by B_{12} supplementation. Prenatal vitamins usually contain enough B_{12} to counteract the deficiency.

☐ *Inherited Forms of Anemia*   Although iron-deficiency anemia is responsible for the great majority of anemia cases in pregnancy, inherited forms of anemia do exist and affect a certain number of pregnant women every year. The two most prevalent forms of inherited anemia in the United States are *sickle-cell anemia* and *thalassemia,* both serious hereditary blood diseases.

☐ *Sickle-Cell Anemia*   Sickle-cell anemia is a chronic form of hemolytic anemia frequently seen in the United States among certain black and Hispanic families. This inherited blood disease causes a number of painful and often crippling symptoms, including joint pain and swelling, an enlarged liver and heart, and recurrent crises requiring repeated blood-exchange transfusions. The onset of the disease begins in early childhood and many of its victims have a short life expectancy: few survive up to or beyond the age of forty.

A very small number—about .25 percent of black and Hispanic Americans—are born with the disease but 8 percent of the black population carry the sickle-cell trait. These individuals are usually asymptomatic and have a normal life expectancy, although the presence of the trait may affect a woman's pregnancy in certain subtle ways.

Pregnancy is rare among sickle-cell victims because so many of them do not reach childbearing age. For many years doctors thought that the sickle-cell disease itself decreased fertility in women, but with better medical care, more women with sickle-cell anemia are now becoming pregnant and carrying their pregnancies to term. The disease certainly has a grave effect on the mother. Women with sickle-cell anemia suffer tremendous bone and joint pain during pregnancy, and the only way to curb it is by heavy doses of pain-killers and repeated blood transfusions. Even if the condition is well controlled, there can still be a sickle-cell crisis that requires exchange transfusions and other emergency treatment. Hospitalization, frequent blood checks, and folic-acid supplementation to counteract the rapid breakdown of the red blood cells remain the best ways at present to bring a woman with sickle-cell anemia through a pregnancy, but the miscarriage rate is high, and the perinatal mortality among the babies of these women is between 25 and 50 percent.

☐ **Sickle-Cell Traits**   A woman who has inherited the sickle-cell trait but not the disease has normal fertility and will usually have very few problems during pregnancy. Nonetheless, two potential complications are common to these pregnancies: one is an increased susceptibility to urinary-tract infections and the other is a greater chance than usual of persistent anemia. If you have inherited the trait, your blood count should be checked frequently to detect any serious iron deficiency before it begins to affect the pregnancy.

Take extra folic acid and extra iron, and try to eat as nutritiously as possible. Some women with the sickle-cell trait are anemic, although others are not. Also, there is a higher likelihood of morning sickness and other related complaints during pregnancy, partly due to an improper absorption of food.

The major problem is the recurrent urinary-tract infections experienced by women with the trait—for reasons that are, at present, unknown. If you feel any pain on urination, see your doctor immediately and have a urine culture made, because if you do develop a serious urinary-tract infection, the high temperature that often accompanies these infections could trigger premature labor. Drink plenty of fluids, especially cranberry juice, which helps to keep the urine more acid, and have routine urine cultures run several times during the pregnancy.

If both you and your husband possess the sickle-cell trait, you would be well advised to have genetic counseling to find what can be done, since there is a 25 percent chance that your child will be born with sickle-cell anemia.

☐ **Thalassemia Major and Minor**   The thalassemias are a group of hereditary disorders of hemoglobin synthesis in which the basic defect results in a reduced rate of synthesis in either the alpha or the beta chains. Thalassemia major, or Cooley's anemia, the most severe form of the disease, usually manifests itself in early childhood when the affected child becomes seriously anemic and fails to grow. Symptoms in the older child include weakness, fatigue, growth retardation, and an enlarged spleen and liver. Most of the victims die early in life, between the ages of six and twenty. A pregnancy is almost unknown among women with thalassemia major because their life expectancy is so short.

The related disease, thalassemia minor, which is found among a much larger group of people, also of southern Mediterranean background, is a milder form of iron-deficiency anemia. It is not incompatible with a normal life span. Women with this disease need to be on a specific diet rich in folic acid, but can otherwise carry a pregnancy with very few problems. If you know you have this inherited form of anemia, you will probably need no more extra attention than good nutrition, extra folic acid, and a normal iron intake. You should not anticipate any unusual problems during pregnancy, but your obstetrician will follow you carefully and possibly run an ultrasound test a couple of times to assure the good healthy growth of the baby.

If you are pregnant, or hoping to become pregnant, and you and your husband are both of southern Mediterranean descent, you might want to contact the Cooley's Anemia Foundation, or have your doctor check you for thalassemia traits. It is easy for an individual to carry the trait without being aware of it, and unless you have been tested there would normally be no reason for you to know your carrier status. An occasional mild degree of anemia is usually not enough of a clue. Any child born of parents who both carry the trait for thalassemia major has a 25 percent chance of inheriting the disease.

☐ *Asthma in Pregnancy* Women with severe asthma tend to become worse during pregnancy, particularly in the second half of the pregnancy, while mild asthmatics usually improve or remain at the same level. Certain women do experience very severe complications, and need emergency-room treatment during an asthma attack to stabilize their oxygen level. Occasionally a fetus dies during a crisis of this kind. The possibility of a severe attack makes it important for any woman with chronic asthma to go to a specialist before she becomes pregnant and review her general health and current medication (see Chap. 19).

Asthma attacks are usually triggered by an allergen or an allergic reaction associated with an infection. A severe attack is characterized by wheezing, coughing, and laborious breathing, as the asthma victim tries to clear away the bronchial spasm blocking the airway passages, and deflate the lungs. Eventually the airways may become permanently blocked. Most people with severe asthma develop the first symptoms before the age of ten, but a substantial number of asthmatics, 30 percent or more, have no sign of the disease until their thirties, so it is possible for a woman to develop asthma quite unexpectedly while she is pregnant.

Why some women with the disease experience acute attacks in pregnancy and some do not is unknown; but we do know that progesterone, one of the hormones naturally produced by the body during pregnancy, stimulates the respiration rate, probably by increasing sensitivity to carbon dioxide. Since progesterone levels vary greatly from woman to woman, this might influence the individual's susceptibility to asthma during pregnancy. A certain number of women with asthma have such difficult pregnancies that they need hospitalization and intensive care. Other women have uneventful pregnancies and then develop a sudden, severe attack only during labor and delivery. In addition, asthma probably increases a woman's chances of experiencing certain pregnancy-related complications; there is, apparently, more morning sickness, toxemia, and irregular bleeding among asthmatics than among nonasthmatics, and women who suffer from a severe form of the disease have an increased chance of premature delivery and miscarriage. Babies of asthmatic mothers also seem to have a somewhat greater than usual risk of dying just before or just after birth.

☐ *Treatment of Asthma* Asthma requires the care of an obstetrician and a specialist in pulmonary diseases. A severe asthmatic needs particularly careful watching in the last weeks of pregnancy and during and after delivery, when asthma attacks often become more virulent. Any pregnant woman with a bronchial condition or asthma must try to avoid viral infections or exposure to environmental agents that could worsen her condition, and any respiratory-tract infection should be immediately treated with antibiotics. If you have a tendency to asthma and you experience difficulty in breathing or fever symptoms, call your internist or obstetrician immediately.

Although women who need anti-asthma drugs must exercise caution because of the possible effects on the fetus, certain forms of asthma relief are effective and reasonably safe. A mild asthma attack can usually be controlled by a bronchial dilator such as epinephrine. Your obstetrician may also recommend ampicillin if there are signs of pulmonary infection. A very severe attack, or one that is not brought under control quickly, is best dealt with in the hospital where intravenous injections of corticosteroids are often favored. Corticosteroids are highly effective in the treatment of asthma, but they should be used only in an emergency situation, because the fetus may be affected. But if your physician feels that the only possible treatment is a daily dose of steroids, then you would be well advised to take the medication, under your doctor's supervision.

☐ *Bleeding Disorders During Pregnancy*   Certain bleeding disorders are hereditary conditions. While women are only the carriers for hemophilia, they can inherit other coagulation and platelet disorders, including Von Willebrand's disease, a blood disorder that is seen as frequently as classic hemophilia. During pregnancy and delivery, these bleeding disorders can pose a great risk to the mother, especially if the disease is unrecognized or only poorly understood.

Bleeding disorders do not always follow a clear course. A woman may suddenly experience abnormal bleeding after many years that are free of symptoms. The coagulation factor increases in pregnancy, so a woman might even deliver a child without any problem and then begin to bleed in later life. A known bleeding disorder would, however, put a pregnancy in the high-risk category. A woman's medical history should be carefully evaluated before pregnancy begins and the pregnancy followed by a hematologist in association with a high-risk perinatologist.

☐ *Hemophilia Carriers and Pregnancy*   Carriers for both types of hemophilia (hemophilia A—classic hemophilia—and the Christmas disease) have certain blood-clotting abnormalities associated with their carrier status. While these are generally not serious enough to interfere with a normal life, approximately 25 percent of these women can be expected to have some bleeding symptoms with the majority of these bleeding incidents associated with trauma, surgery, or dental work. This means that a spontaneous or induced abortion, particularly one followed by a D&C, might be dangerous. Amniocentesis can also be a problem, since several known carriers have experienced severe bleeding after the amniocentesis tap.

The risks to the hemophilic fetus are generally low, although severely hemophilic children occasionally develop intracranial bleeding—bleeding underneath the scalp—during delivery. Up to a half of hemophilic infants show the first signs of bleeding problems in the first week of life.

☐ *Von Willebrand's Disease*   Von Willebrand's disease is a hereditary blood-clotting disorder affecting both men and women. The disorder can be distinguished from classic hemophilia by its inheritance pattern and its clinical course. The disorder was named after a Finnish physician, Dr. Eric von Willebrand, who first described it in 1926 after a family within his practice had lost five out of seven of its young daughters to an unknown bleeding disorder.

The disease is characterized by a prolonged bleeding time. The severity of the disease varies greatly from individual to individual. Before medical treatment was available, a family with Von Willebrand's disease might well include a young woman who bled to death when she began her first menstruation or after childbirth. On the other hand, some women are unaware of their blood-clotting deficiency because they have accepted nosebleeds and heavy menstrual bleeding as normal. Some affected individuals experience nothing abnormal until they undergo surgery or a D&C.

During pregnancy, the critical time is after labor and delivery. A pregnant woman with a coagulation disorder should be tested before surgery or delivery to determine what bleeding factors are missing. If adequate laboratory facilities are available, factor 8 or platelets can be administered before delivery to enhance the coagulation as long as the delivery is carried out carefully and the uterus massaged to diminish postpartum bleeding. Nonetheless, an unexpected emergency can be dangerous; a case of placenta previa, for example, might cause heavy bleeding requiring blood transfusions to save the mother's life.

There is still no information on the effect of Von Willebrand's disease on the fetus. The risk of intracranial bleeding is no greater than among mildly hemophiliac infants. In both cases, the bleeding disorder might first show up in a routine circumcision a few days after birth.

☐ **Blood-Clotting Disorders** A woman with a past history of *thrombophlebitis, pulmonary embolism*, or some other blood-clotting disorder is at increased risk during pregnancy. Other women develop blood clots unexpectedly during the pregnancy or in the postpartum period.

The most serious vascular complication that might occur in pregnancy is a thrombophlebitis with a pulmonary embolism. This complication is potentially fatal.

The pregnant woman is at increased risk for vascular complications because the blood-coagulation system undergoes some dramatic physiological changes in pregnancy. This is why blood-clotting diseases, primarily thrombophlebitis, increase five to six times over in the pregnant woman. Not only does the clotting mechanism change, leading to formation of more blood clots, but the blood itself tends to become thicker. Finally, the blood flow alters temporarily, restricting the circulation of the blood returning to the heart from the legs and the pelvic area. Even women with normal pregnancies develop varicose veins and hemorrhoids because their circulation becomes so sluggish in the last trimester.

☐ **How to Prevent Pulmonary Embolism** One of the best ways to prevent a vascular disorder is by knowing the warning signs of thromboembolism: pain, especially pain behind the calf of the leg, and swelling (typically, one leg is more swollen than the other). Swelling occurs because a blood clot forming in the deep veins of the leg prevents a free flow of blood back to the heart. If a woman neglects the warning signs, a small blood clot could break loose and travel back to the heart; or it could move from the heart and into the lungs, causing a pulmonary embolism. The other vulnerable area is the brain; a blood clot traveling to the brain can result in death or brain tissue injury.

Certain women are at particular risk. Thromboembolism is found more frequently in pregnant women with cardiovascular abnormalities, a heart prosthesis, or some other abnormality in which there is known to be a higher risk of blood clotting. There is also a higher risk of thrombophlebitis and embolism after surgery, and particularly after Cesarean birth. If a woman gets out of bed and moves around as soon as possible after delivery, this will help eliminate the formation of blood clots in the legs and may prevent a serious problem from pulmonary embolism. But every pregnant woman should take certain precautions whether she is a high-risk patient or not. First of all, drink plenty of fluids to counteract the natural rise in temperature and the consequent loss of fluids from the body. Second, do not stand still in one place for long periods—keep walking, or at least move your feet around if you do have to stand—and when you sit down, elevate your legs to allow the blood to flow to the heart. If you habitually sit with crossed legs, the venous blood could form small circulatory movements, eventually forming a localized blood clot.

Note: Do not sit with crossed legs for more than a short time during pregnancy or the postpartum period.

At the first sign of swelling or discomfort, consult your obstetrician immediately. Anticoagulation treatment will usually relieve the blood flow and prevent a clot from forming.

☐ *Anticoagulation Therapy*   Anticoagulation therapy is carried out by oral medication (warfarin/Coumadin) or with intravenous injections of heparin. Most nonpregnant women who need steady anticoagulant therapy for a heart or vascular condition will be on Coumadin, because oral forms of anticoagulation medication are much easier to administer than injectable forms. This presents a dilemma during pregnancy. An anticoagulation therapy such as warfarin (Coumadin) that works as an antagonist to vitamin K is a substantial hazard to the unborn child, particularly if it is given in the first trimester and just before delivery. A decreased level of vitamin K in the fetus has been associated with a characteristic pattern of abnormal fetal development, which includes changes in the appearance of the nose and eyes, undersized fingers and toes, and mental retardation. Warfarin (Coumadin) given late in the third trimester will also cause anticoagulation in the baby, with the danger of intracranial hemorrhage or other bleeding, particularly during birth. A woman who is on anticoagulation medication because she has a heart or blood-clotting disorder should always seek skilled genetic counseling before she begins a pregnancy, and have her medication and general health evaluated.

Heparin, the injectable anticoagulant, is not associated with fetal anticoagulation because the heparin molecule is too large to pass through the placenta easily. Like any other potent drug, it cannot be considered completely safe for use during pregnancy, but most perinatologists prefer to place a woman with a history of vascular disease or a woman who develops thromboembolism in pregnancy on heparin solution for the duration of the pregnancy. Of course, injections are inconvenient, but some women on anticoagulation can give themselves low-dose heparin injections at home.

☐ **The Diabetic Pregnancy**   Before the discovery of insulin in 1921, the onset of juvenile diabetes usually resulted in death within three to four years. Pregnancy among diabetic women was virtually unheard of and was certainly not encouraged, because most pregnant diabetics died before they could be delivered. But the introduction of insulin injections, which enabled many juvenile diabetics to survive into their childbearing years, still did not solve all the problems of the diabetic pregnancy. Fetal and maternal mortality remained high— only twenty years ago 50 percent of the babies of diabetic mothers died just before or just after birth—and it was only recently that newer technologies and more advanced medical care increased the survival rate to over 90 percent. Still, a diabetic pregnancy remains a problem, and it needs to be understood and carefully supervised.

Diabetes is one of the areas of pregnancy in which high-risk specialists throughout the country are beginning to do some innovative work. If you are diabetic, this means a local obstetrician might not be the best doctor to care for you, and you should look for a high-risk center that has advanced facilities to monitor your progress. Although pregnancy among diabetic women is often no more hazardous than among nondiabetics, all diabetic women need careful surveillance, and a few diabetic women are too ill to attempt pregnancy at all.

☐ **Does the Type of Diabetes Matter?**   The severity of diabetes usually depends on when it begins. This also affects the method of treatment: juvenile diabetes is normally controlled by insulin, while other forms of diabetes can be effectively treated by diet therapy rather than drugs. It helps to clarify the different forms of diabetes because they do vary so much in severity and in methods of treatment. The following classification system was developed by Dr. Priscilla White of Boston, who has spent her entire professional life caring for diabetics, and in particular, diabetic women.

Class A: Class A diabetes is also called gestational diabetes, the form that some women develop during the later months of pregnancy. This can often be controlled by diet alone, although careful supervision and, in many cases, elective induction of labor, are called for. However, there are some women with a more severe form of gestational diabetes who require insulin as well as diet therapy.

Class B: A Class B diabetic is a woman whose diabetes began after she was twenty years of age and has had diabetes for less than ten years. Because there are no signs of vascular disease, a safe and healthy pregnancy and delivery are possible if she is carefully followed by her doctor and the diabetes is controlled by insulin.

Class C: A Class C patient develops the disease between the ages of ten and nineteen, and the duration of the disease is anywhere from ten to twenty years. In these diabetic patients no overt abnormalities of the vascular system or the eyes have yet developed, and a carefully supervised pregnancy can take place without too much of a problem.

Class D: Class D patients have had diabetes for the same length of time as Class C patients, but have begun to experience deteriorating eyesight. A woman who is a Class D diabetic has a considerably greater risk of developing complications such as retinal detachment. She also needs more intense genetic counseling and special consultations with a diabetologist and a perinatologist before beginning a pregnancy, since there is a much greater chance of serious complications for her and the baby.

Class F: Women with Class F diabetes have developed early kidney damage plus other damage to the organs. These women have had diabetes for so many years that the body has begun to change, and this makes pregnancy all the more difficult because the kidneys and other organs no longer function efficiently. The extra load on the heart alone makes pregnancy questionable. Any woman with Class F diabetes needs expert genetic counseling before going ahead with a pregnancy.

Class R: A woman with Class R diabetes has developed retinal damage and damage to the heart and other organs. Women in this diabetic group are usually so ill that pregnancy is considered inadvisable.

It is important to be realistic about diabetes, despite the advances of the last few years. With all the promising new research, the outcome is not always satisfactory in every pregnancy. Miscarriage rates are higher for diabetics than nondiabetics, there are problems during labor and delivery and a greater chance that the baby will be stillborn or born with a congenital abnormality. If you are a diabetic, particularly a juvenile diabetic, seek skilled genetic counseling before going ahead with a pregnancy. You need to know how dangerous pregnancy would be in your case.

☐ *Congenital Fetal Malformations Caused by Diabetes*   Diabetic women have a higher incidence of birth defects in their children than women who are not diabetic. A principal reason for this higher rate of congenital malformations is the unusually high blood sugar level in diabetic mothers. Recent studies have directly linked the blood sugar level in the first three months of pregnancy to the appearance of specific birth defects in the baby.

The congenital malformations that are known to appear in a diabetic pregnancy, heart malformations, cleft lip and palate, missing kidneys and lungs, are all linked to problems with erratic blood-sugar levels in the first trimester. When a nondiabetic pregnant woman takes in sugar with her diet, her pancreas responds by pumping a sufficient amount of insulin into the bloodstream to bring the blood sugar down to a proper level, the level that is healthiest for fetal development. This natural control mechanism is missing in the diabetic woman, whose pancreas fails to stimulate the production of insulin quite as easily as the normal individual's. Insulin injections are designed to increase the insulin blood concentration to a steady level which, in turn, enables the body to use the energy from the fatty tissues more effectively.

The demands of early pregnancy, however, place an additional strain on the diabetic woman's pancreas. Low blood-sugar reactions are common in the first trimester since the diabetic woman is experiencing morning sickness, or eating less than usual, and losing glucose to the developing fetus and placenta. Frequent attacks of hypoglycemia affect the formation of the organs and central nervous system of the fetus and endanger the mother herself. Thus it is very important for a diabetic woman to plan ahead and have her blood sugar under complete control in the first three months, through insulin, and a good diet.

Frequent small meals will help avoid hypoglycemia and the development of ketones in the urine (acute hypoglycemia eventually results in the mother's burning up her fatty acid reserves, and producing a state of acidity that could endanger the fetus).

Recently some innovative work in diabetic pregnancies has come out of large medical centers. There are new monitors that a patient can even use at home that check the blood-sugar concentration in one drop of blood, helping her to keep a much more normal blood-sugar level.

At the universities of Washington (Seattle), Cornell, Pittsburgh, Harvard, and Northwestern, groups of diabetic patients are taught to recognize the time of conception by constant monitoring of their own basal body temperatures. Once pregnancy is confirmed, they are hospitalized for a few weeks to bring their blood-sugar level completely under control, and taught how to monitor their blood sugar on a day-to-day basis. After a woman has been released from the hospital, she makes a weekly visit to her obstetrician and is monitored by ultrasound and other tests to assure the normal, healthy development of the fetus. Another group of hospitals in Boston, the Boston Hospital for Women and the New England Deaconess Hospital, are fitting pregnant women with a battery-operated insulin pump that can be worn on a belt. The pump injects a carefully controlled supply of insulin through a needle implanted under the skin of the abdomen, providing the patient with additional insulin at mealtimes when a healthy pancreas would normally perform this function. A woman wears the device constantly through the first critical months of fetal development.

☐ **Diabetes in the Middle Months**   In the second or third trimester, insulin requirements rise sharply, and most diabetic women require double or triple their normal dose to avoid becoming hypoglycemic or developing ketones in the urine. Uncontrolled blood-sugar levels and ketoacidosis are serious conditions; in the past they often resulted in diabetic coma and fetal death, tragedies that are, fortunately, far less common today. Your doctor will monitor your urine frequently for signs of ketoacidosis. Any symptoms of a urinary-tract infection should be reported to him immediately.

The growing fetus is at risk as pregnancy progresses. Elevated fetal blood-sugar levels derived from the mother's hypoglycemia lead to stimulation of the fetal pancreas, whose cells produce a huge amount of a growth hormone called chorionic somatomammatropin, and the fetus becomes abnormally large for its gestational age. Overgrowth, known by doctors as macrosomia, is probably responsible for the difficulties these babies often have after birth and the risk of sudden fetal death just before birth. Many diabetic pregnancies used to end abruptly in the final weeks when the baby suddenly stopped moving. Once again, with better care before delivery, the survival rate of these babies has increased tremendously.

☐ **Timing of Delivery**   A woman with diabetes should be followed throughout her pregnancy by a high-risk specialist and a diabetologist. A high-risk specialist is capable of monitoring the critical first and third trimesters with modern techniques and deciding the optimum time of delivery.

Why or how labor is triggered is still a mystery, but it appears to have something to do with the natural deterioration of the fetal environment at the end of pregnancy. However, in a diabetic pregnancy there is more amniotic fluid and an increased blood supply that continues to reach the fetus beyond the point normal in most full-term pregnancies. This lack of stress in the fetal environment results in delayed labor, and the macrosomatic baby continues to grow inside the uterus. The timing of delivery then becomes critical, since the baby cannot be allowed to remain in the womb too long. The diabetic patient is followed closely in the final weeks with nonstress fetal monitoring tests and estriol levels to detect the amount of fetal growth (see Chap. 23). If either of the tests shows serious abnormalities, labor will be induced immediately. Otherwise the obstetrician might wait until the patient is one or two weeks overdue and then begin labor artificially.

In a case in which the diabetes is under control and the baby seems healthy, it is advisable to induce labor only if the doctor is certain of the due date and the baby's maturity. One of the problems in the past was that doctors, deceived by the baby's size, induced labor prematurely, and a number of these premature babies died soon after birth. Here again, a perinatologist who uses the L/S ratio test and monitoring equipment (see Chap. 23), can estimate the baby's maturity with far more accuracy than an obstetrician who is relying on estimates and physical examination alone. Don't allow a doctor to induce labor without adequate testing. You are perfectly within your rights as a patient to ask for a second opinion before undergoing elective induction or any other major procedure. Unfortunately, too many babies die after premature inductions, due to a miscalculation of their real gestational age.

☐ *Gestational Diabetes* Gestational diabetes is the pregnancy-related form of the disease that usually shows itself in the second half of the affected pregnancy. Its onset is often unpredictable, since a number of women with incipient gestational diabetes have a history of uneventful pregnancies and then develop diabetes with a third or fourth child. One clue is the increasing size of the baby in each successive pregnancy. Women who are more likely to develop gestational diabetes are over twenty-five, have delivered a large baby (over nine pounds) in a previous pregnancy, have suffered an unexplained stillbirth or miscarriage, are overweight, hypertensive, or have experienced recurrent bouts of moniliasis, a common yeast infection that thrives in an environment with increased blood-sugar levels. Gestational diabetes is usually detected by an abnormal-urine test. When sugar turns up in the urine at a routine monthly examination, the obstetrician will order a glucose-tolerance test—a test in which the woman is given a glass of sugar water and the blood-sugar levels are then checked hourly for three to five hours. If the blood-sugar level is abnormally high, this confirms the suspicion of gestational diabetes and immediately places a woman in the high-risk category.

If you develop gestational diabetes, you will be placed on a special diabetic diet for the duration of the pregnancy and given frequent urine and blood tests to monitor your blood-sugar levels. Also, you should be seen more often by your doctor at the medical center because sugar in the urine is a sign of excessive sugar in your diet. Some women with gestational diabetes are now being taught how to monitor their urine with litmus paper and modify their diet accordingly.

What you eat is important; you need extra protein, vitamins, and iron just like any other pregnant woman, and you need to eat regularly, because otherwise the fetal environment might become acidotic. The diet suggested by the American Diabetes Association has a careful balance of 45 percent carbohydrates, 25 percent protein, and 30 percent fat. A steady intake of the right combinations of food would result in a weight gain of about twenty-five pounds during pregnancy—a sufficient gain to safeguard fetal growth.

☐ *Is Insulin Needed to Control Gestational Diabetes?* Gestational diabetes can usually be controlled by diet alone. But there are women with the condition whose blood-sugar levels are so elevated that the baby's growth is overstimulated, leading to complications just before or just after birth. These women are frequently placed on insulin injections for the duration of the pregnancy. More insulin in the body will result in lower blood-sugar concentrations and smaller and healthier babies with a much more normal birth weight. If you are being followed in a high-risk diabetic center, or by a perinatologist, they will usually have developed their own system, and if they believe that insulin is the best therapy for some of their patients, I recommend you follow their advice. In my hospital, we have seen many women who have lost a previous baby and are carried to term successfully in the next pregnancy with insulin. A normal-sized baby is rarely stillborn.

☐ *What Happens to the Gestational Diabetic After Pregnancy Is Over?* A gestational diabetic's labor and delivery is usually managed by the methods I have already described earlier in the section. Women with gestational diabetes also need tests to determine the baby's health and maturity in the weeks before delivery. Today, when we try to control diabetic patients with insulin and special diets, the babies seem to be somewhat smaller than they used to be and a woman might be able to go into labor on her own. If you are more than two weeks overdue and the baby is still growing, your doctor may decide to induce labor, which is probably a good idea.

After delivery, the blood sugar usually drops to a normal level. There is, however, the likelihood of the condition's returning with a subsequent pregnancy, and gestational diabetics also run a greater risk than the general population of developing adult diabetes later in life.

☐ *Heart Disease and Pregnancy* There is a definite change in heart functions during a normal pregnancy, labor, and delivery, and a woman with heart disease must be aware of the extra work load if she wants to become pregnant. In women with very severe heart conditions, the strain is such that pregnancy is usually considered inadvisable. In milder cases, the extra burden is only temporary and there is no evidence that pregnancy has any long-term effect on the course of the disease. If you have heart disease, your cardiologist will usually be able to estimate your chances of a successful pregnancy.

A woman with any form of heart disease should be followed throughout her pregnancy by a cardiologist and an obstetrician associated with a large medical center. She will need more visits, more tests, and more patience than most pregnant women—increased bed rest is one palliative that all doctors recommend—so she must be prepared to invest heavily in her pregnancy. Genetic counseling may also be recommended in difficult cases.

☐ *Heart Changes During Pregnancy*   The fetal heart rate increases early in pregnancy and continues to rise until the seventh month; it then remains at a relatively steady level until labor and delivery. The maternal heart rate itself increases by ten to fifteen beats a minute, reaching its highest point close to term. Blood pressure changes too in a normal pregnancy; it is higher at the beginning of the first trimester, drops in the second trimester, and increases again in the third, contributing to the load on the heart at the end of pregnancy. The most critical stage for a woman with heart disease is labor and delivery, which can impose such a burden on a woman with a serious heart disease that there is a risk of dying from pulmonary congestion or heart failure during, or just after, delivery.

☐ *Pregnancy and the Cardiac Patient*   Today when we have more knowledge about heart conditions and corrective surgery is frequently successful, many women are able to become pregnant and deliver healthy children even if they have a heart defect or a surgically corrected heart condition. Generally, the outcome of pregnancy in a woman with a history of heart disease depends on her ability to function in the nonpregnant state.

Heart disease patients have been classified by the New York Heart Association into four distinct classes. In Class I, the disease is asymptomatic; in Class II, the patient experiences fatigue, palpitations, or anginal pain with ordinary physical activity; Class III patients have palpitations or pain from less than normal physical activity; and Class IV patients are unable to carry out any physical activity without pain, and have symptoms of the disease even at rest. The babies of women who have nonexistent or only mild symptoms of heart disease have about the same chance of doing well as other newborns; but the mortality rate rises to about 30 percent among the babies of Class IV patients. A woman in Class III or IV is often advised against pregnancy altogether, and will need prolonged hospitalization and very careful supervision if she does become pregnant. Heart disease is still one of the leading causes of maternal death in the United States.

A woman who has no problem with her heart condition and has no physical limitations with it will probably have a normal or almost normal pregnancy and delivery, although there is a higher chance of growth retardation and prematurity among the children of asymptomatic or mildly symptomatic patients. These women have a lower cardiac output than the normal pregnant woman, which seems to affect fetal growth. Nor does open-heart surgery necessarily make pregnancy inadvisable; a number of women with mitral-valve replacements now enjoy successful pregnancies. The most common and most serious complication is the onset of congestive heart failure between the twenty-fourth and thirty-second week, when the volume of the blood is circulating at peak levels. Any signs of stress will mean immediate hospitalization and complete bed rest.

☐ *The Stress of Labor*   Labor and delivery are critical times for women with chronic heart conditions. Because the changes in cardiac output and heart rate are greater during labor than during pregnancy, the patient labors lying on her side to take the pressure off the uterus and is carefully monitored with frequent blood-pressure checks and a heart monitor. In the second stage of labor the patient is given an epidural anesthetic to stop her bearing down with each labor contraction, and the baby is usually delivered by forceps as soon as it is safe to do so. Cesarean section increases the risk to some cardiac patients and is not favored except in special circumstances. During and after delivery, women on regular antibiotic therapy require extra antibiotic coverage for at least three or four days to avoid any spread of infection to defective heart valves. Antibiotic therapy with broad-spectrum antibiotics is recommended for all patients with cardiovascular disease.

☐ *Cardiac Drugs in Pregnancy*

Anticoagulant Drugs: Many women with artificial heart valves are on regular anticoagulant therapy. The safety of different anticoagulant drugs is discussed in the special chapter on drugs in pregnancy and earlier in this chapter.

Antiarrhythmic Drugs: Women with severe rhythmic abnormalities are either on a well known group of drugs, the digitalis drugs, or a lesser-known drug, called quinidine. Digitalis is considered a safe drug for use during pregnancy and is often prescribed for normal women who have suddenly developed tachycardia (rapid heart beat) or other heart problems during labor. Quinidine also appears safe for use during pregnancy under carefully controlled conditions. Propranolol (Inderal) is a drug that is extensively used among cardiac patients. Propranolol is a beta-blocking agent that works directly on the heart through its beta receptors (cell membranes in the cardiovascular system which when stimulated will speed the heart rate, and when blocked will lower the heart rate and blood pressure). So it is effective in treating hypertension and certain arrhythmia disorders, since it decreases the heart function and lowers the blood pressure. The drug must be used with caution during pregnancy because it has the potential of initiating premature labor through its beta-blocking action on the uterus. It also has a depressant effect on the baby's respiration and lowers the fetal heart rate. Because of its potential ill effects, it must be prescribed only after a careful evaluation and, if possible, digitalis or quinidine should be used instead for the duration of the pregnancy.

☐ *Hypertension*   Hypertension is one of the more serious complications of pregnancy. Unchecked or uncontrolled, it can result in fetal damage or fetal death, so it is important for chronic or pregnancy-related high blood pressure to be followed carefully.

A number of women who become pregnant already have chronic hypertension, particularly if they are black or overweight. Blacks in America in general have a far higher rate of hypertension than whites, for reasons that are not fully understood, but that seem to be familial. A woman is found to be hypertensive when her diastolic pressure is higher than ninety to one hundred mm of mercury at two or three different weekly examinations at close intervals. Severity and treatment varies from individual to individual; women with mild hypertension are placed on a diet and asked to watch their salt intake or are given blood-pressure medication (the type of treatment depends on whether the doctor feels that the blood pressure can be controlled by diet and exercise, or is unlikely to come down to an acceptable level without medication as well). With hypertension, like any other medical complication, it is important for a woman to see the doctor before becoming pregnant and have a complete physical examination with a blood-pressure check and a full set of tests to establish the underlying cause of the hypertension. (High blood pressure has several possible origins, from overweight to kidney damage to cardiovascular disease.) If a woman has been carefully evaluated and placed on proper medication and diet, if her blood pressure is under control and her weight is down to a level at which she feels comfortable, then she is ready for pregnancy.

☐ *The Risks of Pregnancy in a Hypertensive Woman*   An obstetrician treating a hypertensive patient will become concerned when the diastolic (lower) pressure exceeds ninety mm because that means the resting blood pressure is not high enough to allow a sufficient blood supply to reach the fetus. The fetuses of mothers with chronic hypertension face the greatest risk during the third trimester, when the baby's rapid growth demands a steady supply of nutrition from the mother. Intrauterine growth retardation not only results in a smaller baby who is at more risk because of its low birth weight, but it may also mean that the fetal brain is incompletely developed because it has been deprived of oxygen and other forms of nutrition during the critical period. Furthermore, there is a higher incidence of premature labor among these babies, possibly because the baby is so deprived of oxygen that its extreme discomfort triggers birth several weeks prematurely. This adds another risk—that of brain damage. The third and most serious complication is the premature separation of the placenta, a condition called placenta abruptio, in which the fetal membranes separate from the placenta and cause fetal death or brain damage, besides the threat of severe hemorrhage in the mother.

A woman with unchecked chronic hypertension during pregnancy is also placing herself at risk. High blood pressure has led to strokes, seizures, and death: hypertension and a pregnancy-related complication, toxemia, is one of the leading causes of maternal death in the United States at the present time.

☐ *How Blood Pressure Changes During Pregnancy*   A rise in the diastolic pressure greater than twenty mm of mercury and in the systolic (upper) blood pressure of fifteen mm of mercury is significant, and should immediately alert your doctor to begin further treatment. If a woman with hypertension then develops toxemia, she needs immediate bed rest, possibly a sedative, and careful evaluation with monitoring techniques. Toxemia is a somewhat mysterious but extremely serious pregnancy-related condition in which the kidneys and other organs retain excessive amounts of fluids and the blood pressure becomes so elevated that shock and seizure can result. The reason why toxemia occurs is unknown, but among women who have chronic high blood pressure it may be that the kidney is already working poorly and the extra blood supply required during pregnancy causes it to malfunction. Not all hypertensive women develop toxemia, but it is prevalent among patients with uncontrolled chronic hypertension, as well as older women and overweight women.

☐ *Gestational Hypertension*   Certain women whose blood pressure is within normal limits at the beginning of pregnancy develop a form of hypertension known as gestational hypertension in the second half of pregnancy. This may or may not be accompanied by other symptoms of toxemia.

☐ **Treatment of Hypertension During Pregnancy**   Because most of the fetal problems result from a reduced blood supply to the placenta, the main aim is to restore or increase the uterine blood flow to the baby, and at the same time prevent the mother's high blood pressure from going completely out of control and causing a stroke or convulsive seizure. Unfortunately there is no known medication that can improve the blood supply to the uterus, and the classic treatment for high blood pressure is, therefore, complete bed rest. Once a woman is in bed, less blood goes to the muscles in the legs and more flows directly to the uterus. If the patient is also given a sedative like phenobarbital, a medication that has been used for years without discernable ill effect to the fetus, she will probably rest better and enhance the blood supply to the placenta. The care of hypertension requires frequent blood pressure and weight checks and periodic evaluations of the electrolyte balance in the liver and kidneys. A low-salt diet is recommended to keep the weight down and reduce the amount of fluid in the tissues. A patient with high blood pressure is usually given a more intensive evaluation of the fetus, so serial ultrasonography is a must to determine intrauterine growth retardation at an early stage and to allow the obstetrician to begin treatment with increased bed rest and perhaps antihypertensive blood medication if the patient needs it. From the thirty-second week on, when the baby is considered mature enough to permit delivery if necessary, doctors with nonstress testing equipment are now choosing to monitor the baby's movements and the heart rate variability on a week-to-week basis to estimate its growth and general health. If testing indicates a serious abnormality at this point of the pregnancy—a significant drop in the fetal heart rate, for instance, or the development of an uncontrollable bout of toxemia—the obstetrician may decide to deliver the baby before irreparable damage occurs. Usually one has time to do an amniocentesis test first to obtain a sample of the amniotic fluid and subject it to the L/S ratio test (see Chap. 23). A relatively mature baby can be delivered safely before the placenta breaks away from the uterus or some other catastrophe endangers the baby or the mother.

With modern techniques and careful surveillance, it is possible to carry a woman with high blood pressure to term and deliver a healthy baby. However, a woman who has high blood pressure and does nothing about it may well end up with a stroke or permanent damage to the kidneys, and possibly a dead fetus. It is important in any high-risk pregnancy to take advantage of preventive medicine, and take care of yourself if you do become sick.

☐ **Multiple Births**   A multiple birth was once a rare event. A twin birth in the ancient world was so unusual that it was considered either ill-omened or a favorable sign from heaven. In certain cultures the event was regarded as unnatural, and only one twin was allowed to survive.

Before the 1960s, multiple births in the U.S. held at a steady rate for over half a century. Birth statistics from the end of the nineteenth century and information on births collected between 1928 and 1955 showed that quadruplets occurred once in every 490,000 births; triplets once in every 9,300 births; and twins once in every 90 births. The introduction of fertility drugs in the early 1960s led to a sudden upswing, and quadruplets, quintuplets, and even one set of sextuplets were born and survived. In recent years, multiple births generally have begun to decline as the number of fraternal twins has dropped markedly. In

Figure 61: Quadruplets: Linda Schreiber, an incredible woman and the author of *Marathon Mom* (Houghton Mifflin, 1980), is seen with her three daughters and one son only a few weeks after she gave birth to the quadruplets in a natural delivery. She is surrounded by the proud nurses and doctors who cared for her and her babies. Mrs. Schreiber spent several weeks in the hospital before the babies were born, but recuperated extremely rapidly. With early diagnosis and proper treatment and bed rest, multiple births can be managed successfully in a hospital with high-risk facilities.

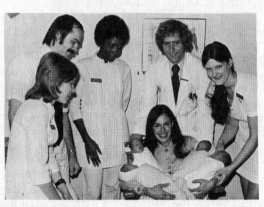

part this is because women over thirty are having fewer babies and women in general are having fewer births (the likelihood of fraternal twins tends to increase with age and parity). One other possible factor is the widespread use of oral contraceptives, since contraceptive steroids depress the pituitary activity of the brain directly, with a prolonged suppression of multiple ovulation. Interestingly, the rate of identical-twin births has remained steady.

☐   *Who Is Likely to Have Twins?*   Twin pregnancies that occur in the absence of fertility drugs often follow a family pattern. If your or your husband's family has in it one or more sets of twins, this doesn't mean that you will necessarily have twins yourself—it often skips a generation or two—but the tendency is inherited.

Black women have a higher number of twin pregnancies than whites and white women have almost twice the number of twin pregnancies that are found in Oriental populations. The incidence of twins in Japan is one in every 156 births, and triplets are so rare that they occur only once in every 17,200 births. Age is one other important factor. Teenage girls have few multiple births. After the age of twenty the incidence rises steadily and peaks between the ages of thirty-five and forty, when twins are born to one out of every sixty women. Frequency declines sharply after the early forties, and women who give birth when they are forty-five or older have a likelihood of a multiple birth equivalent to that of a teenage girl.

Hormones may influence a predisposition to twinning among certain women. Mothers of twins in western Nigeria, where the twinning rate is almost 60/1000 live births, have been found to have an unusually high level of the FSH hormone during their normal ovulatory cycle, perhaps as a result of some traditional foodstuff. This would be consistent with the artificial administration of FSH in fertility drugs. Mothers of twins in America have been found to have shorter menstrual cycles and an earlier menarche, also suggesting some hormonal influence in multiple pregnancies.

☐ *Twins: Identical or Fraternal?*　　Identical or monozygotic twins originate from a single egg fertilized by one sperm and then divided into two at some very early stage of its development. The two offspring of the resulting pregnancy are identical in sex, facial features, coloring, height, build, blood type, and often in personality as well. Psychiatrists who have made a special study of identical twins have noticed striking similarities in speech patterns, mannerisms, tastes, and posture among identical twins, and have traced a remarkable pattern of similarities among identical twins separated by adoption at an early age. One such pair of brothers, who were adopted by two different families at the age of one week and first met thirty-nine years later, were both named James, had married and divorced women named Linda, and had called their firstborn sons James Alan and James Allan.

Twins that result from the fertilization of two different eggs by two different sperm are known as *dizygotic* or fraternal twins. Fraternal twins are either of different sexes or the same sex, depending on the chromosomes carried by the two different sperm, and have as much similarity or as little similarity as any other sibling pair.

The frequency of identical and fraternal twins is interesting because it varies among ethnic groups. In the United States only 34 percent of all white twins and 29 percent of all black twins are identical—in other words, two-thirds of American twins are fraternal. Among Orientals, the opposite tendency prevails: two-thirds of all twins born are identical, and only one-third are fraternal. The reason for this notable variation is unknown, but it must have some genetic origin.

☐ *How Can Identical Twins Be Distinguished from Fraternal Twins?*
Twins of different sexes are always fraternal. If they are of the same sex, the placenta can be examined immediately after birth to distinguish fraternal from identical twins. When the two children are born with a single placenta, and the two sacs around the fetuses are separated by only two layers of membranes, the twins have developed from one egg. On the other hand, if each twin has a separate placenta, or the partition wall in the single placenta has four membranes instead of two separating the babies, the twins are fraternal. Further testing and genetic analysis can be carried out if there is any doubt. A simple blood test will show whether or not the two blood samples are alike in all respects, including the Rhesus and blood groups as well as the subgroups, as they must be if the twins are identical. Genetic analysis can also be performed to compare the twins' karyotypes. A final, definite test is performed through skin grafting. A small piece of skin grafted from one identical twin to another will not be rejected—a sign that the immune systems are the same. This extraordinary phenomenon has made it possible for one identical twin to donate a kidney to the other twin without the kidney's being rejected after surgery.

☐ *Why Do Twin Gestations Occur?*　　The origin of identical, or one-egg twins, is not understood, but it is felt to be genetic in origin. One theory suggests

346 /   *Childbirth with Love*

that some specific influence on the ovum immediately after fertilization, perhaps decreased oxygenation, causes the fertilized ovum to divide in two and create two identical human beings. There are no studies to back this up, so the exact mechanism remains a mystery. A simple explanation exists for fraternal twins; the two eggs are released from both ovaries or from the same ovary at the same time and are fertilized simultaneously. The release of two eggs is, theoretically, so possible that it is amazing it does not happen more frequently in nature, although one egg that begins to mature usually inhibits the growth of any other egg. If two or more eggs, however, have matured to the same extent, one might not be able to suppress the other, and double ovulation occurs. This is more common when fertility drugs are used, leading to the simultaneous release and fertilization of two or more eggs at the same time.

☐ *Superfecundation*   Superfecundation is a rare but not unheard-of phenomenon that occurs when two eggs are fertilized within a short period of time by two different ejaculations of sperm from the same father or from two different fathers. In other words, superfecundation refers to a conception that takes place after a woman has already conceived, an event that is statistically improbable but biologically possible.

One authenticated case of superfecundation occurred in Germany, when a woman delivered a black and a white child simultaneously. She later told her doctor she had had intercourse with her husband and another man on the same night. Other women have delivered babies weeks or even months apart who appeared to be the children of two separate pregnancies. A woman in Australia is said to have given birth to one twin weighing four pounds and delivered the second twin, weighing six pounds, two months later. Both twins survived, the first weighing six pounds when the second was born. This was later attributed to the *twin transfusion syndrome*, in which one twin receives most of the blood supply from the placenta and grows much faster than its twin. Naturally, it could look as though one twin were older than the other, although they were conceived at the same time.

☐ *Diagnosis of Twin Pregnancy*   A recent study from the Twin Care Study Center in Oakland, California, has suggested that mothers are considerably better at diagnosing their own twin pregnancies than their obstetricians. Fifty-three women, over half the group interviewed, reported predicting their twin pregnancy three months before their doctors did. Not only were they larger and heavier than they had expected by the end of the first trimester, but many of them noticed two distinct patterns of fetal movement as early as the fifth month. Several of the women experienced premonitory dreams around the midpoint of pregnancy.

In fact, this guessing game is no longer needed since a conclusive diagnosis can be made as early as the third month by using ultrasonography. At that point of development the fetus, or pair of fetuses, are already capable of movement, and the head, arms, and legs, together with the fetal sac or sacs, are clearly outlined on the screen. Multiple gestations are even easier to identify once pregnancy has progressed beyond the third month. Since ultrasonography is so readily available, there is no longer any reason for a woman to walk around for months uncertain of whether she is carrying twins or not. If you feel bigger in your second pregnancy than you were in your first, if you have a familial history of twins, or you have any other reason to suspect you are carrying two babies rather than one, ask your doctor to run a sonogram in his office or refer you to the hospital sonography unit. The test is reimbursable by your insurance company. Early diagnosis is valuable: it helps reduce the risk of premature birth and enables you to plan your nutrition better. And your family will be given time to find extra help if a multiple pregnancy is diagnosed in advance.

☐ *The Twin Pregnancy*   If you find out you are carrying twins, you need to take better care of yourself than if you were carrying one child. First of all, you will be bigger and your nutritional needs greater because you have to feed two babies. You will probably have to double up on your prenatal vitamins and iron, and you may need folic-acid supplements. You must watch your calcium intake carefully, and in general eat more. Sometimes it is better to eat six small meals in the last trimester rather than the usual three because the stomach is often constricted by the extra bulk of the uterus.

Rest is very important. One of the problems with multiple births is prematurity. If you are expecting twins, you might not be able to work quite as late in the pregnancy as a woman who is carrying a singleton. You should try to get at least an hour's rest in the middle of the day, lying on your side to increase the blood flow to the uterus, and plan for as much rest as possible in the evening. Try to have someone help you with the chores at home. As soon as you get home from work, lie down for at least one hour before carrying on with your normal activities. Some women with a multiple gestation enter the hospital early and are put on complete bed rest for a few weeks before birth, or you may be asked to rest at home. It is well worth taking the time to stay in bed and rest because weeks gained in a twin pregnancy may make a lifelong difference in the health of your children. Children born at term, or almost at term, have a far higher survival rate and less serious problems than children born before thirty-six weeks.

This increased risk of prematurity is the reason why you may be asked to abstain from sexual intercourse in the final trimester when you are expecting twins. The cervix often begins to efface (thin out) prematurely in a multiple gestation, and intercourse could cause the uterus to contract, increasing the dilatation of the cervix and causing premature labor. In the last trimester, your doctor will watch the cervical activity carefully, and increase your bed rest if effacement occurs.

Any woman with a twin pregnancy can expect more discomfort and minor problems than other pregnant women, if only because of the extra weight. You are more likely to experience varicosities, excessive fluid retention, breathlessness, and insomnia, as well as difficulty in moving around in the final weeks. A more serious problem is the increased likelihood of developing toxemia in the final trimester. The abnormal size of the uterus seems to contribute to the prevalence of toxemia in multiple births, and this can be serious for both the mother and the babies (see Chapter 25 on toxemia of pregnancy). A woman with toxemia may need hospitalization, but it can often be controlled at home with increased bed rest. Because the first stage of toxemia, preeclampsia, sometimes worsens rapidly you need to be especially alert to symptoms of toxemia in a multiple pregnancy. Consult your doctor immediately if you experience any noticeable swelling of the hands or face. Urinary infections are also more likely if you are carrying twins. In general, the number of prenatal visits is increased in a multiple pregnancy, and your obstetrician will probably ask that you refrain from being away for extended periods of time during the pregnancy because of complications that may develop while you are away. Twin pregnancies require careful attention in order to detect possible problems early; they are not always easy and you need to take extra good care of yourself.

☐ *Twin Deliveries*   Delivery of twins is usually more complicated than the delivery of a singleton. When it comes to a twin gestation it is important for you to see a doctor who is familiar with twin deliveries, although most twins can be delivered by a natural, vaginal delivery, as long as they are delivered close to the due date. In the weeks before delivery, you need to be followed by ultrasonography to assure you and your doctor that the babies are in the right position for an easy delivery. Twin presentations vary from birth to birth. In almost 50 percent of twin deliveries, both babies are in the vertex position, which makes delivery relatively simple, but about 40 percent of second twins are breech, and in 10 percent of twin births, both babies are in the breech position. If the first baby is a vertex, the doctor can simply await spontaneous labor and deliver the first twin as a normal head-first delivery. He should then monitor the second twin carefully before its birth. (There might be an interval of several minutes between the two births, since the uterus needs time to contract and readjust itself before it begins to contract for the second birth.)

When the second baby is ready to be born, the obstetrician will rupture the amniotic sac of the second twin and insert his hand inside the uterus to guide the second baby down into the birth canal. If the second baby is in the vertex position, delivery should be easy and natural. If the second baby is a breech, the presenting part can be guided down with one hand while pressure downward is put on the uterus from the other, or the doctor can find the legs and deliver the baby by a vaginal breech delivery. Sometimes this is impossible, due to the baby's position, and the second twin is delivered by Cesarean section. There are other times when the uterus contracts severely or the placenta separates itself suddenly, between the two births, and again, delivery of the second twin requires a Cesarean. When both babies are in the breech position, it is often safer not to try to deliver the babies vaginally.

After the delivery of twins, the uterus sometimes relaxes instead of contracting, causing hemorrhaging and other difficulties, so your doctor and the nursing staff need to observe you carefully in the first twenty-four hours to make sure that your uterus is firm and well contracted and no unusual bleeding is occuring. But as long as the delivery takes place close to the due date and you have taken good care of yourself during the pregnancy, there is no reason for the birth not to go well. An experienced doctor can usually take care of any complication that might arise.

A high proportion of twin pregnancies terminate naturally before the thirty-eighth week, and a number of them before the thirty-sixth week. The average twin pregnancy is twenty-two days shorter than the average singleton. Sometimes this is the result of a premature rupture of the membranes, a complication that is more frequent in multiple pregnancies than single pregnancies. By the eighth month there is a good chance of the babies' being in a healthy condition, although both twins are relatively disadvantaged nutritionally and usually weigh less than the average singleton at any stage of prenatal development. With a very premature birth there is naturally the risk of a serious problem because the babies are often so tiny, and a doctor will usually try to halt the onset of labor by uterine relaxant drugs (pages 370–372) or complete bed rest.

Male twins usually weigh more than female twins, and fraternal twins weigh more than identical twins. The second fraternal twin is often smaller than the firstborn and may have more difficulties in the first year because of this difference in size and relative maturity.

☐ *Neurological Disorders in Pregnancy*   A surprisingly large number of neurological diseases affect women of every age, including women who are pregnant or hope to become pregnant. Epilepsy and other seizure disorders, severe migraine headaches, and neurological conditions that affect the voluntary muscles are all to be found among women of childbearing age. Neurological disorders not only complicate what might otherwise have been an uncomplicated pregnancy, but pregnancy itself can influence the course of a neurological disease, and certain disorders are particularly likely to make a first appearance during a pregnancy. This makes it important for any pregnant woman to understand more about neurological disorders and their effect on pregnancy.

☐ *Epilepsy and Seizure Disorders*   Pregnancy tends to alter the normal course of the disorder, at least temporarily. An epileptic woman who usually experiences more than one seizure a month often finds that her condition grows worse during pregnancy, especially during the first trimester, and then reverts to the prepregnant pattern once pregnancy is over. A woman who has a mild case of epilepsy (less than one seizure every nine months) is much less likely to experience an increase in the disorder. However, there are women who have not had a seizure for years and then suddenly suffer an attack once they are pregnant. This is why any woman who has had a seizure disorder in the past must give her obstetrician a full medical history at the first visit. If she is not being currently followed by a neurologist he can then send her to a specialist for an evaluation and an electroencephalogram to detect any abnormalities in the brain pattern.

Increased susceptibility to seizures during pregnancy is probably caused by the metabolic and hormonal changes of pregnancy itself, including the marked change in fluid retention that all pregnant women experience. Pregnant women whose epilepsy is serious enough to require medication may find it more difficult than usual to control their seizures with the normal drug prescription, increasing their chances of experiencing more frequent attacks. The main concern is that loss of oxygen during a seizure can have a dangerously adverse effect on the baby, and with a very severe seizure, there is the risk of fetal death, or placental separation followed by fetal death.

☐ *Treatment of Seizure Disorders During Pregnancy*   Women who need seizure-disorder medication run a much higher risk of congenital malformation of the fetus than occasional epileptics who do not require medication. The reported number of live births affected by congenital malformations is eighteen out of every thousand births to epileptic women who are medication-free. This is somewhat higher than among the general population, perhaps because the seizures tend to cause hypoxia (low blood-oxygen concentration) in the fetus.

Among women under treatment, this figure rises to sixty or seventy per thousand. Many of these births are affected by congenital heart disease or cleft lip and cleft palate. It is not known exactly why some antiseizure drugs have teratogenic effects, but it may be that they lower the mother's folic-acid level, a deficiency that can be remedied to some degree by folic-acid supplementation throughout pregnancy. Another possible explanation is the development of chromosomal abnormalities in the ova after prolonged exposure to antiseizure medication.

☐ *What Is the Safest Drug to Control Seizure Disorders During Pregnancy?*
The two drugs most commonly prescribed for epilepsy and other seizure disorders are phenytoin (Dilantin) and phenobarbital, singly or in combination form. Dilantin, a widely favored antiseizure medication, has been directly associated with the typical congenital malformations I have just mentioned, and is not recommended for use during pregnancy for that reason. Combinations of phenytoin and phenobarbital are equally suspect. Phenobarbital itself, however, is an old medication that is not 100 percent safe but has, at least, been around for many years, and hundreds of thousands of women have used it in early pregnancy without apparent harm to the fetus. If you do suffer from seizure disorders and are on medication, it is important to plan ahead and review your drug use with your doctor before you become pregnant.

Since phenobarbital has fewer side effects, it should be the drug of choice during a pregnancy. There is, however, one problem with it when given in high amounts just before delivery: the baby might be somewhat depressed and harder to take care of the first few hours of life, although this is rarely seen on the normal therapeutic doses. Phenobarbital is not excreted from the bloodstream until a few days after delivery, so it is likely to pass into the baby's bloodstream and depress its neuromuscular system.

☐ *Migraines During Pregnancy*   Chronic migraine headaches often lessen in intensity and frequency once the first trimester of pregnancy is over, but a few women experience more migraines than usual during the second and third trimester or suddenly develop a severe attack quite unexpectedly. One patient of mine was seven months pregnant when she had a migraine attack in a department store. The attack was so intense that her whole body was affected. She told me later she had numbness in her hands and her right side, the room began moving around her, and for a few moments she was unable to see the woman standing beside her at the counter. After that she had no clear idea of what happened, although, fortunately, she remained conscious. I felt she might have had an intracranial hemorrhage or a blood clot in the brain and immediately rushed her into the hospital, but after extensive testing we managed to exclude any brain damage, and the electroencephalogram revealed the most likely cause, an attack of migraine. She was of course followed in the hospital in the next few weeks but went into labor naturally and delivered a healthy child. As you can see from this story, the symptoms of migraine can be very strange at times; so if you are susceptible to migraines and experience a similarly unusual or disturbing incident during pregnancy, always have it evaluated by your obstetrician or a neurologist. When it comes to neurological diseases, it can be very difficult to make an accurate diagnosis.

Migraine in pregnancy is not a dangerous disease, but it may be serious enough to require attention. An occasional aspirin or Tylenol is reasonably safe, but the best treatment is to learn to relax; or try to avoid the episode altogether by eliminating tension. Lying in a darkened room is helpful during an attack. Do not, under any circumstances, taken antimigraine medications containing ergotamine while you are pregnant, because ergotamine has uterine contracting effects, and may precipitate a miscarriage. Once again, whenever you feel you need medication, check with your obstetrician before refilling a prescription written for you before you became pregnant.

☐ ***Myasthenia Gravis in Pregnancy***   Myasthenia gravis, a neurological disease of voluntary muscles, might well present itself for the first time during pregnancy or immediately after delivery. Among women who already have symptoms of the disease, a relapse is not uncommon in the first trimester, followed by a remission in the later stages of gestation, but other variations have also been seen in pregnant women.

Muscle weakness is the first symptom. This can be so severe that it restricts movement, and women with myasthenia gravis sometimes find it difficult to walk more than a few minutes at a time. However, the disease does not interfere with the involuntary, as opposed to the voluntary muscles, and labor and delivery usually proceed spontaneously. During pregnancy, women with myasthenia gravis are usually given Prostigmin to increase the secretion of an enzyme that helps the voluntary muscles recover from fatigue.

Labor and delivery in a patient with myasthenia gravis are usually not a problem, but the weakness of the voluntary muscles contributes considerably to a woman's sense of fatigue during labor, hindering the second stage and making forceps delivery likely. After delivery the uterus contracts normally, and prolonged bleeding is unusual. Since the baby of a mother with myasthenia gravis has a 25 percent chance of inheriting the disease, a neurologist will examine the infant for signs of muscle weakness and general feebleness. The disease can be treated with anticholinesterase drugs.

☐ ***Polio and Pregnancy***   Women who were polio victims in childhood or adolescence have no special problems with conception and if the polio has caused only a minimal degree of impairment, there should be no difference between these pregnancies and any other pregnancy. A woman left with more severe paralysis has, of course, more of a problem, including the difficulties she may already experience taking care of herself. During labor, however, the uterus usually contracts by itself even in women who are paralyzed, and if a woman does not have enough force to push, her obstetrician can help deliver the baby with forceps. A polio victim has a good possibility of having a healthy pregnancy and a healthy child, but the situation should be evaluated carefully so that everyone in the family as well as the doctor is aware of the pros and cons before conception takes place.

☐ ***Multiple Sclerosis in Pregnancy***   There is conflicting information about the effect of pregnancy on a woman with multiple sclerosis. Cases in which the condition worsened during the pregnancy or after delivery are on record, but the risk of a serious aggravation of the disease appears to be small. A woman with multiple sclerosis who is otherwise healthy enough to carry a child can generally expect a successful pregnancy as long as she is followed by an obstetrician experienced in high-risk cases and a neurologist. There should be no contraindication to a normal labor and delivery, or even natural childbirth, in women with multiple sclerosis. The treatment, if any, is usually steroid drugs.

☐ ***Thyroid Disease During Pregnancy***   In a case of thyroid disease the thyroid gland is either overactive or underactive. A woman with acute hyperthyroidism or hypothyroidism may well fail to conceive, since the thyroid gland has a close interaction with the hormones in the brain that release the FSH and LH hormones, which trigger ovulation. Pregnant women occasionally develop hyperthyroidism or hypothyroidism during the pregnancy, or begin pregnancy with a milder form of either thyroid abnormality. Thyroid disease can be dangerous during pregnancy, and it is important to treat any symptoms before the condition runs wild and injures either the mother or the baby.

☐ ***Hyperthyroidism: Overactive Thyroid Gland***   The incidence of severe hyperthyroidism in pregnancy is rare, less than .5 percent, but a pregnant woman can have a milder case of hyperthyroidism that goes undetected until she becomes pregnant. Women with severe uncontrolled hyperthyroidism who manage to become pregnant have a very high rate of miscarriage, stillbirth, and neonatal death. The babies that survive are often growth-retarded, since the placenta fails to develop properly during the pregnancy.

In general, a woman with an overactive thyroid gland has a few minor symptoms, which are often masked by pregnancy itself. The symptoms of hyperthyroidism are often similar to those of early pregnancy: fatigue, heat intolerance, nervousness, palpitations, increased appetite combined with unexpected weight loss, and diarrhea. A physical examination may reveal an enlargement of the thyroid gland, but this is not always conclusive; the gland is often larger during pregnancy because it supplies the fetus with some essential hormones.

The similarities between a normal pregnancy and hyperthyroidism have led doctors to rely on laboratory analysis; specifically a blood test to evaluate the level of T4 (serum thyroxine) and the T3 uptake (the resin triodothyronine uptake) in the blood. Patients with a common form of thyroid disease known as Graves' disease usually have a triad of symptoms: hyperthyroidism, exophthalmos (protrusion of the eyes alone) and an enlarged goiter. A hyperthyroid woman can be treated by medication or by surgery followed by medication. Most doctors would prefer to use medication during pregnancy rather than risk surgery, although the final decision depends on each physician's experience and the patient's condition. The most widely used antithyroid medications are propylthiouracil (100 mg) or methimazole (Tapazole; 10 mg three times a day, decreasing to a lower dose if the disease appears to be under control). The problem with either of these drugs is their tendency to block fetal production of thyroid hormones and cause thyroid goiters in the fetus or the newborn. This is why some doctors give a thyroid medication such as Cytomel (25 mcg daily) together with the antithyroid drug. A third form of treatment—the use of radioactive iodine—is contraindicated during pregnancy because of the serious risk to the fetus, and you should not allow your doctor to take any radioactive tests if you are pregnant or think you might be pregnant.

In many cases of hyperthyroidism, treatment can be successfully discontinued in the last two or three months of pregnancy to reduce the risks to the fetus, or the patient can be maintained on a very low dose of medication. Symptoms of hyperthyroidism usually improve after only two or three weeks of therapy.

☐ *Hypothyroidism: Low Thyroid Function in Pregnancy*   Acute hypothyroidism in early pregnancy can interfere with fetal development by preventing a normal rise in the levels of other important hormones, including progesterone and HCG. This deficiency leads to a high rate of miscarriage among hypothyroid women. Consequently, any woman who has had a history of repeated miscarriage should have her thyroid function checked during an infertility work-up.

There are certain signs that a physician can look for if he suspects hypothyroidism. Women with acute hypothyroidism usually have a marked intolerance to cold, move slowly, and have coarse hair and puffiness around the eyes. They are often somewhat overweight. But many women show only minimal external symptoms of the disease, and a conclusive diagnosis can be made only by a T4 and T3 thyroid test. A low amount of T3 indicates a case of hypothyroidism.

The preferred method of treatment is desiccated thyroid medication or Cytomel or Synthroid, with the dose monitored by the T4 level. If hypothyroidism is left untreated, there is a strong possibility of early miscarriage, since the fetus relies on the mother's thyroid function in the early weeks of pregnancy before the fetal thyroid begins producing its own hormones. Thyroid medication crosses into the fetal circulation, but does not block thyroid production or produce abnormalities in the newborn.

☐ *Toxoplasmosis*   Toxoplasmosis is one of the viruses that causes subclinical or very mild symptoms in children and adults but affects the unborn child in a far more dramatic fashion. An adult who contracts toxoplasmosis might have a fever, or a slight rash, or general cold symptoms. An affected fetus, on the other hand, might suffer from an enlarged spleen, infection, and damage to the eyes, and possibly, microcephaly. The virus can also result in premature birth, with all its associated problems.

The most common sources of the virus are *cat feces and undercooked or raw meat.* As I have already mentioned in Chapter 2, a true house cat is unlikely to harbor the virus because it does not usually eat live prey, but precautions should still be taken during pregnancy to avoid contamination. Any meat, including beef, should be thoroughly cooked. Practical suggestions for avoiding toxoplasmosis infection can be found in Chapter 2.

Fortunately congenital toxoplasmosis, the form that affects the fetus, is rarer than you may have been led to believe; according to some authorities, it occurs in only one out of every eight thousand live births, although other researchers put it as high as one out of every eight hundred. The presence of antibodies correlates with increasing age—40 percent of the adult women in the United States whose antibody titer is on record possess them, and a positive titer is twice as frequent among black women as it is among whites. The fact that few women can recall any specific group of symptoms would suggest that the disease is so mild, or so easily mistaken for another viral infection, that any woman planning a pregnancy should have a titer done before conception or early in the first trimester to establish her susceptibility to the disease. Take the proper precautions if you are found not to possess antibodies. Then if you develop a sudden fever or virallike disease, ask your doctor to take another blood titer. A higher titer confirms the active phase of the disease, with the possibility of teratogenic effects on the fetus.

A number of researchers have tried to develop therapies for toxoplasmosis, but as yet no treatment is available for women who are pregnant. If the virus is detected early enough in the pregnancy, the parents should be given the option of interrupting the pregnancy. When the disease is diagnosed at a later stage, the infected infant should be treated as soon as possible after birth because the virus will continue to damage the brain and eyes in the postnatal period. A high-risk center with an experienced pediatric staff is the best place to deliver. Usually the baby will be treated with a combination of folic acid and sulphur, but some hospitals like to try corticosteroids instead.

☐ *Urinary-Tract Infections* Urinary-tract infections, particularly cystitis, are very common in pregnancy. Persistent infections can be caused by bacteria entering the bladder or by some kind of kidney abnormality. A number of abnormalities of the kidney are also associated with abnormalities of the uterus, so if you have ever had problems with kidney or urinary-tract infections in the past, you are more likely to develop a similar infection during pregnancy.

☐ *Cystitis During Pregnancy* Cystitis has several quite unmistakable symptoms: a frequent need to urinate, pain over the bladder area, pain during urination, and often blood in the urine. In a serious case of cystitis, the patient runs a high fever and the upper urinary tract becomes tender and painful. About 2 percent of all pregnant women develop a urinary-tract infection during pregnancy, but perhaps as many as 10 percent of all pregnant women have bacterial growths in their urine without, however, developing overt symptoms of the disease. You are more likely to come down with cystitis if you are anemic or the balance of the body is upset under the stress of pregnancy.

If you have any of these symptoms of cystitis, see your obstetrician immediately. A urinary culture will establish the presence of infection in the urinary tract. Simple cases of cystitis can be treated effectively with antibiotics, particularly ampicillin, Negram and Macrodantin (the sulphur antibiotics which are often favored in urinary-tract infections are contraindicated in pregnancy).

Large amounts of fluids, especially extra cranberry juice, which helps to make the urine more acidic, will clean out the system and create a hostile environment for the bacteria.

Women with sickle-cell traits or any other type of anemia in pregnancy have a much higher incidence of cystitis and other urinary-tract infections, and would be well advised to have a series of bacteria cultures run at monthly intervals during the pregnancy to detect any infection as soon as it occurs. If treatment is not begun in time, the bacteria might travel up through the bladder to the kidney and cause a kidney infection or a severe urinary-tract infection that would be much more difficult to treat than simple cystitis. Urinary-tract infection during pregnancy can, furthermore, trigger premature birth.

☐ *Upper-Urinary-Tract Infections*   When the bacteria spread to the upper urinary tract, there is a chance that the infection will attack the kidneys. This is a potentially serious situation, since an infection in the kidneys usually causes fever. A classic pattern in upper-urinary-tract infections is high fever at night and a lower degree of fever in the morning. In an acute case, the woman will run such a high fever that there is danger of seizures or of premature labor. The patient should in this case be hospitalized immediately and given intensive antibiotic therapy. If you experience fever and pain in the urinary tract, *call your doctor immediately.*

☐ *Recurrent Urinary-Tract Infections*   With prompt treatment, cystitis rarely occurs more than once in a pregnancy. If a woman experiences a recurrence, it is important to find out why she is unusually susceptible. She may, for instance, have anemia, or the sickle-cell anemia trait, which might contribute to the reinfection. If other causes can be excluded, her doctor may suspect that a congenital urinary-tract malformation is involved. A malformation of this kind is best detected by an IVP, a form of X-ray known as an intravenous pyelogram. However, a responsible doctor does not like to use X-rays during pregnancy, and he is more likely to keep a woman on antibiotics throughout the pregnancy to prevent a recurrence and wait until after the delivery of the baby to arrange for an IVP. Certain effective medications are felt to be safe for use during pregnancy, including Macrodantin, Negram, and all types of penicillin.

☐ *Venereal Disease and Pregnancy*   Apart from the common cold and the flu, venereal disease is the most common infectious disease in the United States. Indeed, it is so common that someone contracts a venereal disease every fifteen seconds. The two most infamous sexually transmitted diseases are gonorrhea and syphilis, with herpes now a close third, but a surprisingly large number of other infections are also considered to be venereal diseases, including fungal infections, trichomonas, hepatitis B, cytomegalovirus, and salmonellosis. Some of these common viral infections have little or no effect on pregnancy, and with some of them the effects on the fetus are devastating.

☐ *Gonorrhea and Pregnancy*   One of the difficulties with gonorrhea, in women at least, is that it is virtually symptomless in the early stages. There might be a discharge from the vagina, or possibly a minor irritation that comes and goes, but this can easily be mistaken for some other problem. Once the *Neisseria gonorrheae* organism has taken hold, however, it can spread quickly up into the uterus and Fallopian tubes, causing abdominal pain, fever, pain on urination, and tenderness in the pelvic area—a group of symptoms that usually appear just after a menstrual period. A serious pelvic infection often leads to sterility. Untreated gonorrhea will eventually result in crippling arthritis and even death.

Gonorrhea of the mouth and throat can be acquired through oral/genital sex. There are people who have gonorrhea of the mouth or throat or lungs but not of the sexual organs. A culture of the throat should be taken in suspected cases. Both types of gonorrhea can be treated successfully with heavy doses of antibiotics, but there are some bacteria that prove resistant to penicillin. Gonorrhea of the mouth could, theoretically, be passed on to the infant after birth.

☐ *What Happens in Pregnancy*   In pregnancy, the unruptured fetal membranes and the mucous plug blocking entry to the cervix form an effective barrier against a gonococcus infection up until the time of delivery. But once the membranes have ruptured, the bacteria can spread up into the sexual organs and infect the mother or the child, with the consequent risk of a gonorrhea-induced pelvic infection in the postpartum period, or a case of septicemia in the newborn. Gonorrhea in the postpartum period must be treated immediately with antibiotics to prevent a crippling infection.

The other risk is an eye infection in the newborn when the soft tissues in the baby's eyes come into contact with the gonorrhea virus in the birth canal. Infection in this sensitive site often results in complete or partial blindness. As a preventive measure, all state authorities in the United States require the application of silver nitrate drops to both eyes after the birth, a simple routine precaution that has virtually eliminated gonorrhea as a source of congenital blindness in the United States. A few hospitals prefer instead to give the baby an injection of penicillin or use antibiotic creams rather than the silver nitrate. (See Chap. 27)

Gonorrhea can be treated safely during pregnancy with an intramuscular injection of 4.8 million units of procaine penicillin, plus oral pobenicid tablets (1 gram). A total of 3.5 grams of oral ampicillin are also useful. If the bacteria prove resistant to certain penicillins, as they sometimes do, a further culture must be obtained and the disease treated with the most sensitive antibiotics available.

☐ *Monilia Vaginitis*   Pregnant women are particularly likely to experience yeast infections because the increased estrogen levels stimulate glycogen production in the vagina. For the same reason it is harder to control during pregnancy, and treatment with vaginal antiyeast medications (see Chap. 19) should be continued for at least double the usual time, ten to fourteen days instead of five to seven. The only effect that monilia has on the baby is a chance that thrush, a skin irritation, will develop in the first days after birth. Antiyeast creams and jellies can be used to soothe the skin.

☐ *Syphilis and Pregnancy*   Syphilis, the most dreaded of all the venereal diseases, is passed from the infected woman's bloodstream into the circulation of the unborn child. Children with congenital syphilis are seriously affected with skin, bone, liver, and spleen abnormalities, and normal growth is often stunted. As the disease progresses in the adult years it leads to blindness, brain damage, heart disease, and death. Many babies infected with syphilis do not show any symptoms for the first two years or more, but develop overt symptoms in childhood or in puberty.

☐ *How the Disease Is Detected and Treated*   Syphilis is caused by a microorganism called treponema pallidum. The disease is particularly difficult to identify in a woman since the initial symptoms are often invisible. The first sign is a hard, painless sore called a chancre that usually appears at the site of the original infection. A woman who contracts syphilis vaginally can easily have a chancre hidden in her vagina and not notice it because she experiences no discomfort. Three or four weeks after its first appearance, the sore often disappears by itself; then, several weeks later, a rash will appear on the body and the victim might experience a mild fever. After the rash, too, disappears, the disease goes into a long latent phase when there are no overt symptoms, only to return again years later. In the last, active stage of the disease, it damages the eyes, the brain, and the cardiovascular system, and finally leads to death.

In the earliest stages when the chancre sore is present, syphilis can be diagnosed through physical examination and microscopic evaluation.

After the chancre disappears, the only sure method of diagnosis is a blood test. This can be carried out either with a VDRL (venereal disease research laboratory) test or an STS (serological test for syphilis). Treatment with penicillin injections at an early stage of the disease is extremely easy. A diagnosis at a later stage is also followed with penicillin, but in much higher doses. The treatment should be given only by a specialist in venereal diseases.

☐ **Congenital Syphilis**   Syphilis can cross the placenta as early as the sixth week of gestation but recognizable symptoms in the fetus do not usually show up unless infection occurs after the sixteenth week. The outcome of the infection depends to a large extent on the stage the disease has reached in the mother. Syphilis in its active primary or secondary stages results in a late miscarriage, a stillbirth, or a premature or full-term baby affected with the disease, but a child conceived and born during a latent period may have no congenital abnormality of any recognizable kind. Affected babies are often born with a distinctive "saddle nose." The child with congenital syphilis is usually in poor health, does not gain weight well, is jaundiced, and suffers from enlargement of the liver and spleen. The skin has a raised brown coloration, and small lesions may appear on the hands and feet, or around the mouth. Untreated congenital syphilis ends in irreparable damage to the eyes and brain.

Because congenital syphilis is usually contracted in the last five months of the pregnancy, it is important to recognize the disease with a VDRL or an STS blood test at the first prenatal visit and begin prompt treatment with antibiotics. If a woman then has sexual relations late in the pregnancy with a man she suspects may have syphilis, she must ask her doctor to run another test to exclude any chance of the disease developing and harming her and the fetus. Penicillin, which is generally safe for use during pregnancy, remains the preferred method of combating syphilis in all its stages.

☐ **Virus Infections and Pregnancy**   The danger of viral infections during pregnancy has recently gained far more attention because the congenital malformations and other problems caused by viruses can be even more devastating than those caused by genetic disorders. Anyone who intends to become pregnant should take certain important precautions against viral disease in the pre-pregnancy period, including a blood test to establish rubella and toxoplasmosis antibodies (see Chap. 2) and should try to avoid unnecessary exposure throughout pregnancy. Particularly in the first three months, a viral disease such as rubella can have a terribly damaging effect by attacking the fetal nervous system and the vital organs.

In addition to the breakthroughs such as a recent rubella vaccine, we have learned more about the effects of such persistent viruses as herpes and cyto-megalovirus in the fetus and newborn, although we are still a very long way from preventing the recent dramatic rise in genital herpes virus infections or the con-genital defects associated with cytomegalovirus. More is also being discovered about the effects of influenza and other common viral infections on the fetus and newborn.

☐   *Cytomegalovirus and Pregnancy*   Cytomegalovirus, a virus whose name is derived from its gargantuan effect on the body cells, is harbored as a parasite within the body and triggered into activity by stress or some other unknown fac-tor. It usually fails to cause an identifiable disease in adults or children, although 80 percent of the adult population of the United States are believed to possess the virus or its antibodies. (One-third to two-thirds of adult women have anti-bodies, confirming widespread exposure to cytomegalovirus.) Although the symptoms, if any, are mild among adults, fetuses and newborns are uniquely sensitive to the effects of this virus because they are too young to have developed the full human immune system, which matures only a few months after birth.

The virus crosses the placenta and attacks the fetus, or the newborn baby ac-quires the virus as it passes through an infected birth canal or in its mother's breast milk. Intrauterine infections usually involve the firstborn of an infected mother, although there are documented cases in which a second pregnancy was affected. Every year, about one out of every one hundred newborns is affected with the disease and close to four thousand of these children are born with mi-crocephaly (an unusually small brain) or other severe forms of brain damage. Many others show a more limited degree of brain impairment or develop hear-ing problems later on in life. Other babies are stillborn. The degree of damage depends on the time in pregnancy in which the infection occurred. Cytomega-lovirus in the first trimester might result in damage to the central nervous system or miscarriage; in the second trimester, central nervous system damage is likely; while infection in the third trimester may produce no clinical signs of the dis-ease. Consequently, damage from this virus is not inevitable; about 50 percent of children born to women infected during pregnancy show some cytomegalo-virus symptoms, but only 10 percent of these affected children suffer mental re-tardation, blindness, deafness, or other severe abnormalities.

☐   *Detection of Cytomegalovirus*   Cytomegalovirus has been isolated from the vagina and the cervix in 5 percent of pregnant women. Women who are in poor health or live under stressful conditions are primary targets. Since a cyto-megalovirus infection is often asymptomatic, except in women who have never been previously contaminated, or in newborns, a pregnant woman may well not realize that she has the infection and neither may her doctor. Some doctors do suggest a therapeutic abortion if a known infection occurs in the early months, but a cytomegalovirus infection is most likely to occur in the last trimester of pregnancy rather than the first. There is no documented effective treatment. After birth, certain advanced hospitals, including Grady Memorial Hospital in Atlanta, are now routinely screening the urine of newborns to detect cases of cy-tomegalovirus in the postnatal period. Any serious brain damage is irreversible, but an early detection of the disease could help the parents and pediatrician to begin early treatment of hearing and learning disorders. This virus has become a major problem in obstetrics, one that is greater in effect and certainly in frequency than many genetic disorders. Since there is no vaccine available, the best way to prevent an attack of cytomegalovirus is to eat well and take extra rest—a healthy woman has a stronger immune system and therefore greater resistance to this dangerous disease. Other than taking preventive measures, there is little, unfortunately, that a pregnant woman can do to protect herself at the present time.

☐ *Hepatitis During Pregnancy*   Hepatitis in general is on the increase among the American population. While the number of pregnant women with hepatitis is still very small—less perhaps than .5 percent of all pregnant women—150,000 hepatitis cases are seen each year in the United States, and their number is rising so fast that in the future the number of pregnant women affected can be expected to go up as well.

Traditionally, viral hepatitis, the B strain, and serum hepatitis, the A strain, were treated as if they were two separate forms of the disease. Type A, associated with drug addiction and contaminated needles, was believed to have an exclusively intravenous origin, while type B hepatitis was known as virus-infectious hepatitis because it was transmitted orally or sexually. This rigid distinction between infectious hepatitis and serum hepatitis went back to the early days of hepatitis research just after World War II, and is no longer tenable now that we know that hepatitis is basically the same disease, but is created by two different viruses, the so-called A and B viruses. Serum hepatitis can occasionally be transmitted orally, and infectious, or B, hepatitis via a needle.

Hepatitis symptoms usually show themselves within a month after exposure. The first symptoms are often mild fatigue and a general lack of energy. Then the initial feeling of lethargy develops slowly into a degree of jaundice, complicated by nausea and vomiting, followed by increasing fatigue and increasing jaundice. Often the initial symptoms go unrecognized, and the first time the hepatitis sufferer becomes alarmed is when nausea and vomiting begin. During pregnancy, of course, recognition of the disease may take even longer than usual because nausea and vomiting are so common in the early months. Another complicating factor is the confusion of hepatitis with the mild jaundice that affects certain women when the extra weight of the abdomen presses on the gall bladder, creating a pool of bile in the liver. This means that a pregnant woman who goes to her obstetrician with nausea or jaundice should always undergo a battery of tests before a specific diagnosis can be made. Liver disease, gall bladder and gallstone, a drug allergy or drug toxicity, and infectious mononucleosis have all been mistaken at different times for hepatitis. Today, the presence of the serum hepatitis antigen in the blood (the sign of the active disease) can be accurately established by a group of blood tests.

☐ *Will Hepatitis Affect a Pregnancy?*   Contrary to all past beliefs, the latest research has suggested that hepatitis in an otherwise healthy woman does not alter the course of the pregnancy, nor will she find it more difficult to recover from the disease than a woman who is not pregnant. Doctors who have observed pregnancies affected by hepatitis report no increase in stillbirth, congenital malformations, or growth retardation among infants born to women with hepatitis, and not even an increase in premature labor among women suffering from type

A or type B hepatitis. A pregnant woman with hepatitis will be put in the hospital immediately and placed in isolation, but there is no reason for the pregnancy not to continue to term. The hepatitis virus cannot be conquered by drugs, so complete bed rest remains the only way to treat the disease, with the body being allowed time to heal and build up immune antibodies to the hepatitis virus, as it would against any other virus. During the period of rest and isolation, the patient will be followed with repeated blood tests. Once they indicate that the liver function has begun to normalize, she will be allowed to go home and rest in quiet isolation for a few more weeks.

Labor and delivery are likely to progress normally. Hepatitis does not increase the need for a Cesarean section or a forceps delivery, and a woman with hepatitis can still have natural childbirth if she wishes. The main concern is the health of the baby, since neonatal hepatitis infection is a grave disease. Experiments with antihepatitis B globulin vaccinations have proved unsuccessful with newborns, and so have vaccines prepared with the plasma of hepatitis B carriers. All that the modern hospital can do is simply to place the baby immediately in an isolation unit until the mother is declared free of the disease. One day, perhaps, efforts to achieve a live virus vaccine for all hepatitis sufferers will be met with success, but until then understanding and prevention are our most useful tools against this unpleasant and damaging viral disease.

☐ **Herpes Infection in Pregnancy**   Herpes simplex, or herpes type I, is an infectious viral ailment that usually shows up on the lips in the form of a cold sore. Herpes type II is commonly known as venereally transmitted herpes, and occurs more frequently in the vagina, penis, and lower body. The two strains are slightly different in the way they produce antibodies and develop, but there can be a cross reaction of the two, and they are not always confined to one specific area or areas.

Herpes type I is annoying but harmless. Herpes type II often produces a fairly serious disorder and is highly contagious. The sores are persistent; they cause fever and pain; and they heal slowly. Furthermore, there is no known treatment, and recurrence is common. The parasitic virus is located inside the cell tissue, where it begins to multiply under certain conditions—particularly during stress situations—and as it spreads it forms small fluid-filled vessels that eventually break a group of the host cells. This causes an open sore that can spread to other areas.

☐ **Herpes Infection During Conception**   No harm should result to the fetus if the mother or father has an active herpes lesion at the time the woman conceives. A past history of herpes infection is not a factor either. There is no proof that active herpes before or at the time of conception affects fetal development or the baby's health before birth. Stories about herpes are mostly false, or at least greatly exaggerated. Any active herpes infection in the mother is usually confined within the genital area, and the intact fetal membranes and the mucous plug blocking the entry to the cervix act as an effective barrier against all types of vaginal infections. Delivery, not pregnancy, is the critical time with herpes, because these barriers to infection are removed, and the baby is passing through the birth canal.

☐ *Herpes During Pregnancy* An attack of genital herpes could be contracted during sexual intercourse with an infected partner, or might become active during a period of pregnancy when you are run down or your body is weakened by some other infection. An active herpes lesion produces a sore that heals so slowly that your doctor should be able to take a culture from it and identify its nature. Though the infection is prevented from traveling into the uterus by the fetal membranes, certain studies do suggest that pregnant women with active herpes have a slightly higher rate of miscarriage than other women. Once you go into regular or premature labor with an active virus present in the vagina, the risk to a baby born vaginally is very high. A neonatal virus infection contracted from the open blisters in the vagina can be so severe that it results in death within a few days. A fatality is all the more likely because there is no treatment available, and a young baby has no immune system to fight off the virus.

If any sores resembling the herpes lesions appear in the vaginal area during the last days or weeks of your pregnancy, see your doctor immediately and get him to take a herpes culture. If the lesion is positive for herpes, a Cesarean section should be performed. There are even some hospitals that perform routine cultures on all pregnant women in the final weeks to screen out herpes cases that might have gone undetected by the mother or her doctor, or that might be dormant inside the vagina. However, other medical authorities feel that screening is necessary only if there are open sores or blisters present. If a woman has had herpes in the past and the blisters have already healed, there is no reason why she cannot have a vaginal delivery.

☐ *Rubella* Congenital rubella is a cause of miscarriage, infant death, blindness, deafness, heart damage, and mental retardation. Many of its victims suffer from multiple defects. During the last great rubella epidemic, in 1964–65, about 30,000 infants died before birth, and another 20,000 American babies were born with congenital defects.

If a woman is exposed to rubella and becomes infected, she may or may not develop the typical skin rash (30 percent of rubella cases have no recognizable symptoms of the disease). In either case, the initial phase of the disease develops into a viral infection of the blood, which lasts anywhere from a few days to four weeks. Toward the end of the incubation period and during the acute stage, the virus is shed from the throat. This period of acute infection is the time when the fetus is affected as the virus passes through the placenta. Since the fetal tissue has no immunity to the effects of the rubella virus, the virus either interferes directly with the normal patterns of development or produces a chronic infection; either mechanism results in a pattern of severe birth defects. Once a case of rubella has been diagnosed in the first four months of pregnancy (see Chapter 2 for an explanation of the rubella titer), a pregnant woman and her partner should seek genetic counseling and either have the pregnancy interrupted or at least be given that option, since the chance of the fetus' contracting congenital rubella syndrome at this point of the pregnancy is high.

☐ *Varicella Infections in Pregnancy* In 1947 an infant whose mother had developed chicken pox in early pregnancy was born with growth- and motor-retardation problems, atrophic limbs, and eye damage. This was the first recognized case of congenital varicella syndrome; it can occur with herpes zoster (shingles) as well as chicken pox contracted before the sixteenth week of pregnancy.

Tests will reveal varicella or herpes zoster antibodies by the second or third week of the rash. These antibodies persist for a long time. Research figures indicate that about 50 percent of women of childbearing age in the United States are susceptible to varicella infection, although perhaps only 5 percent of the women who become infected before the sixteenth week of gestation in fact bear a child with congenital defects. A varicella infection that occurs later in pregnancy might produce characteristic skin lesions, or a case of pneumonia in the postnatal period. No reliable vaccine exists at the present time, so the best prophylaxis is prevention. If you are pregnant or are planning to become pregnant, try to be alert to your surroundings. If you know someone or someplace where there is chicken pox or shingles, stay away—there is always the risk of the virus damaging the baby.

☐ *Venereal Warts*   Venereal warts are caused by a virus and spread by sexual intercourse. They appear as small growths clustered on the penis or the vaginal area. During pregnancy the vaginal environment is particularly conducive to their growth, and a small group of such warts, or condylomas, can sometimes become so large that they obstruct the birth canal, necessitating a Cesarean section.

The best treatment is to leave them alone and hope they will disintegrate spontaneously after birth. Localized treatment with podophyllin resin can be dangerous because the medication is absorbed through the vaginal tissues and then circulated through the placenta. Electrocautery or cryosurgery, methods normally recommended to remove condylomas, are difficult, and dangerous during pregnancy with the increased vascularity of the vaginal area. There are even cases in which severe bleeding has resulted from such treatment. It is probably better to leave the condylomas alone and observe the patient carefully during labor and delivery. In the case of one patient of mine, the vagina was completely obstructed and the woman was so nervous that it was impossible to examine her, but before a decision as to the mode of delivery was made, the baby had made its way through the mass of warts and a Cesarean was avoided. In this instance, the condylomas disappeared spontaneously after the delivery.

☐ *Warts Can Spread to the Baby's Vocal Cords*   One undesirable side effect from a vaginal delivery in a woman with venereal warts is contamination of the baby. There have been times when the newborn has contracted venereal warts from its mother and they have spread into the baby's lungs. The resulting laryngeal condylomas (venereal warts of the vocal cords) are an extremely serious problem that is very difficult to treat. Babies often need microlaryngeal surgery to correct the problem, and even then the disease can reoccur.

☐ *Uterine Abnormalities and Pregnancy*   A few women have inborn uterine abnormalities—a double uterus and cervix (uterus didelphys) or two uteruses joined by one cervix (uterus bicornis) or a uterus with a large uterine septum, for instance. Other women develop uterine abnormalities such as fibroid tumors over the years that make pregnancy more complicated. Whatever the problem, it is important to be aware of it before conception because it may affect the woman's fertility or her pregnancy.

☐ *Congenital Uterine Abnormalities in Pregnancy* Some women with uterine abnormalities have difficulty in conceiving or maintaining the pregnancy. If a woman with a uterine abnormality has miscarried, she would be wise to arrange for a hysterosalpingogram, an X-ray of the uterus, to delineate the exact configuration of the abnormality. In certain cases, the abnormality can be corrected by surgery (see Chapter 3 for more information on surgical infertility techniques).

Many women, however, do get pregnant successfully even though they have a bicornuate uterus or other abnormalities. The main problem here again is miscarriage if implantation occurs in an area that does not have enough blood supply to support the pregnancy.

The other problem is that the uterus itself is smaller and stretches faster— leading, possibly, to premature birth. Here again, women are expected to cut back on their physical activities and rest in bed, especially in the last trimester. Yutopar (ritodrine) tablets are sometimes helpful in relaxing the uterus.

☐ *Fibroid Tumors* Fibroid tumors are benign growths on the uterus. They present little problem if they are located in the uterine wall or on the outside of the uterus, but a tumor or tumors growing inside the uterine cavity (submucosal myomas) might interfere with the placenta and cause a miscarriage. Another problem with fibroid tumors is premature birth, since the uterus is often more irritable and may contract more easily. In most cases they do not cause major problems, and are not contraindicative to pregnancy.

A diagnosis is best managed by ultrasonography. Serial ultrasonographies during pregnancy will locate the fibroids and measure their position in relation to the placenta and fetus. The chance of premature labor is higher when a pregnancy is complicated with fibroid tumors, and the patient will be expected to rest more, especially in the last two months, and avoid heavy physical work. Less sexual activity is particularly recommended in the last trimester because any stretching of the uterus can lead to premature labor. A new uterine relaxant medication, commercially called Yutopar (ritodrine) is often given to relax the uterus when a woman with fibroids experiences pain or uterine cramping during pregnancy (see Chapter 24 on premature labor and other pregnancy-related problems). But if you are careful, there is usually little difficulty in reaching term successfully.

Fibroid tumors are associated with more bleeding postpartum. Otherwise a major problem is likely to arise only if the tumors are exceptionally large—large enough to obstruct the birth canal. In this case a Cesarean birth must be performed to avoid injuring the baby.

☐ *How Healthy Will the Baby of a High-Risk Pregnancy Be?* Of course your pregnancy will require special care if you are high-risk, but there is no reason why you cannot have a normal, healthy baby. Often high-risk pregnancies result in the delivery of an unusually healthy child because the mother received extra care and rested and ate well before the birth.

In any case, a high-risk pregnancy need not be a frightening event. Doctors have more knowledge today than ever before and can monitor the high-risk pregnancy meticulously with special techniques. As far as the woman herself is concerned, she must inform herself as fully as possible and be willing to follow her obstetrician's directions carefully. She also needs complete support and understanding. Above all, she should be aware of the specialized treatment now available from high-risk specialists—perinatologists—whose practices are usually to be found in major medical centers. This might of course mean travel, but it is probably worth it.

The delivery of a child to a high-risk woman is one of the greatest moments in the life of the family and a happy event for the doctors and nurses caring for the mother and baby. In many ways I think these children do unusually well as they grow up because they are born into loving homes where they are really wanted and are therefore given a rare degree of care and affection.

25

Serious Complications During Pregnancy

Although most pregnancies proceed uneventfully, certain pregnancies do end up with a problem; a problem serious enough to pose a real threat to the mother or the infant. Sometimes difficulties can be anticipated because the pregnancy starts off in the high-risk category, but other pregnancies may well start out normally and then develop a pregnancy-related complication such as premature labor or toxemia, or a pregnant woman may require surgery or some other emergency procedure that puts a hitherto low-risk pregnancy into the high-risk group. Most low-risk pregnancies remain low-risk; but the possibility of a sudden complication does exist for many women.

An awareness of potential problems is invaluable in any pregnancy, even a low-risk pregnancy, since many of the problems that are encountered during a pregnancy could be avoided, or at least mitigated, if more women were familiar with the early signs of trouble. For instance, I think we would see a decline in the number of premature labors each year if women at higher risk of prematurity understood their bodies, avoided activities that could increase the chances of prematurity, and knew the early signs of labor well enough to seek treatment quickly.

If all pregnant women were familiar with the major complications that can blight a pregnancy, and were encouraged to take more responsibility for their own health care, we doctors would benefit considerably, because a pregnancy-related complication always is most serious when it is misdiagnosed or neglected, and treatment is delayed or comes too late.

☐ **What Is Premature Birth?**   Premature birth is defined as the delivery of an infant between the twentieth week of gestation and the thirty-sixth week of gestation, when the birth weight is likely to range between 500 grams (1⅛ pounds) to 2500 grams (5½ pounds). Before the twentieth week, premature labor is known as spontaneous abortion or, more familiarly, as a miscarriage. The great majority of spontaneous abortions take place in the first trimester and are the result of some serious defect in the embryo or fetus. After the thirteenth week of gestation, the aborted fetus is usually normal. There is almost no hope of survival before the twenty-fourth week of gestation, the point that is now considered the age of viability. The lungs and other vital organs are so profoundly immature that even the advanced respirators available in neonatal nurseries are incapable of keeping the fetus alive for more than a limited period.

Once the fetus passes the twenty-fourth week, survival becomes possible, although the chance of survival is only slim before the twenty-eighth week of pregnancy. One is also worried about the quality of life with such a tiny premature, given the risks of brain damage to the nervous system.

After the twenty-eighth week of gestation the lungs and other organs are still profoundly immature but the chance of survival is increased and continues to increase with each week until term. A baby born from the thirty-sixth week on is no longer considered premature, unless the birth weight is under 5½ pounds. At that time a baby is likely to do almost as well as a baby born at full term. Since there is often only a few weeks' difference between a seriously premature birth and one in which the baby's prospects are reasonably good, the aim of the obstetrician and neonatologist is to gain as much time as possible when premature labor threatens, in the hope of increasing the baby's maturity.

☐   *What Causes Premature Labor?*   The phenomenon that triggers premature labor is not presently understood, but some stimulation seems to occur within the uterine environment that puts the baby under stress. During this period of stress, the fetus appears to send certain hormonal signals via the placenta that stimulate the beginning of contractions in the uterus, as though nature were telling the baby it would be better off delivered. The same mechanism operates at term, when the uterine environment begins to deteriorate and prepare for the expulsion of the baby. If the stress could be removed and the uterus relaxed, it might be possible to reverse this mechanism and prolong the pregnancy to a point closer to term. The focus of the present efforts to halt premature births is, therefore, to educate women about the causes and signs of premature labor and to begin early treatment.

☐   *Risk Factors for Prematurity*   Although the exact mechanism that stimulates premature labor is not understood, certain factors are known to predispose women to prematurity. All pregnant women should be aware of these risk factors and be prepared to deal with a problem, should it arise. Many women feel so pressured by their jobs and household duties, or so determined not to let pregnancy disturb any of their normal activities, that they stubbornly ignore the first signs of trouble and refuse to slow down, even though their bodies may be telling them that something is wrong.

Risk factors for prematurity are: (1) multiple gestation; (2) a past history of premature labor; (3) incompetent cervix; (4) uterine abnormality; (5) fever or an elevated temperature; (6) urinary-tract infection; (7) cervical infections; (8) malnutrition; (9) severe stress; (10) hard physical labor; (11) more than one previous abortion; (12) a previous traumatic abortion; (13) previous uterine surgery; (14)

advanced maternal age; (15) hypertension or toxemia during pregnancy; (16) severe anemia during pregnancy; (17) severe heart disease during pregnancy.

A woman whose pregnancy is a high-risk for prematurity should try to be aware of the warning signs and be enough in tune with her body to know when to slow down and when to seek medical help.

☐ *Exploring the Risk Factors Further*   With a *multiple pregnancy*, the likelihood of prematurity is higher because the uterus is expanded more than usual. When the uterus is stretched unduly, there is an abnormal degree of friction that could release the prostaglandin hormones and trigger labor. A woman with a multiple pregnancy is expected to stop working earlier and rest in bed as much as possible, preferably lying on her left side to allow more blood to reach the uterus and nourish the fetuses.

With a previous history of *premature birth*, the chance of a premature labor recurring is rather high. Among certain women in this special group, the mechanism that normally allows for the expansion of the uterus seems to function inadequately; in other women, the problem may well have a genetic origin. A woman with a prior history of premature birth should be seen more frequently than usual by her doctor, and rest as much as possible during pregnancy. She might even be admitted to the hospital from the beginning of the last trimester until the baby is born. Some women in this high-risk group seem to benefit from the new uterine relaxant drug, ritodrine, which is now frequently prescribed from the fifth month of gestation on. A combination of ritodrine (Yutopar) therapy and complete bed rest often relaxes the uterus sufficiently to carry the pregnancy to term.

If the problem is an *incompetent cervix*, the damaged cervical muscle fibers are unable to bear the weight of the uterus, and the cervix begins to dilate in midtrimester, months before the baby is due. If a woman has a clear history of incompetent cervix, a cervical stitch or a Shirodkar suture (see page 389) can be placed around the cervix to hold the uterus firmly in place and prevent premature dilatation. Once the band is in place, the woman must rest more, give up work earlier, and avoid sex during the rest of the pregnancy, since there is always the risk of sexual intercourse's precipitating labor by hastening the contraction of the uterus.

Women with congenital *uterine abnormalities,* or fibroid tumors, have a higher risk of prematurity because the uterine cavity itself is not free to expand, or the fibroid tumors irritate the wall of the uterus and release the labor hormones, the prostaglandins or oxytocins. Again, the best prevention is bed rest, a general reduction in physical activities, and a longer period away from work.

A temperature *elevation* or *viral infection accompanied by a fever* have been known to trigger labor prematurely by releasing prostaglandins into the maternal bloodstream. If you run a high fever (over 101°) for a prolonged period, this release of labor-inducing hormones could begin a chain reaction that ends in full labor.

Common causes of fever during pregnancy are urinary-tract infections, upper respiratory infections, and pulmonary infections, including chronic bronchitis. These infections can be promptly and safely treated with antibiotics. Contact your doctor immediately if you have any symptoms of fever, and take antibiotics and possibly aspirin to bring your temperature back to normal. At the same time, you should be especially alert to the warning symptoms of premature labor. Some women with urinary or other infections are admitted to the hospital and put on complete bed rest and uterine relaxant medications to prevent the inception of premature labor contractions.

An *infection* of the *cervix* or *uterus* is sometimes enough of an irritant to cause a premature rupture of the fetal membranes and labor. Vaginal infections have been known to crawl into the cervix, irritate the membranes, and precipitate rupture. This usually leads to labor, although in some cases a woman can be monitored carefully in the hospital and brought closer to term despite the loss of the protective membranes. The risk of infection is real, and is especially prevalent in a high-risk patient, in whom rupture may result from an infection's being pushed up into the vagina during sexual intercourse. This is why sexual intercourse in the last trimester is now considered inadvisable for women at risk for premature labor.

Malnutrition during pregnancy and a low *prepregnancy weight* have a dramatic effect on birth weight. A prepregnancy weight of less than 112 pounds has been linked with a threefold increase in the prematurity rate compared to weights over 126 pounds. From the point of view of prematurity it is, in fact, better to begin pregnancy somewhat overweight than chronically underweight, since heavy women rarely have premature babies. A good weight gain during the pregnancy itself is another factor essential to proper fetal growth. Other social factors, including heavy smoking and drinking and drug use, contribute to prematurity by weakening the mother's resistance to infection and increasing the stress on the fetal environment. Worldwide, there would be far fewer premature or growth-retarded babies if women had proper nutrition throughout their lives and did not use substances harmful to their unborn children.

Physical stress cuts down the oxygen reaching the fetus and contributes to a premature degeneration of the fetal environment. Pregnant women should avoid heavy physical work, especially if they are older or have some chronic medical problem. In general, cut back on your activities in the last few months of pregnancy, try to take an early leave of absence if your job requires heavy lifting or is otherwise physically taxing, and don't allow yourself to become overtired. Regular resting periods throughout the day will help reduce fatigue and muscle strain.

Recent studies on *emotional stress* in pregnancy have confirmed suspicions that this is a causative factor in prematurity (see Chap. 14). In a pregnancy in which the baby is unwanted, or the woman is under constant emotional stress, the body tenses up and cuts down the free flow of blood to the uterus, stressing the fetus in turn. These babies are often growth-retarded, or delivered prematurely. On occasion, a severe emotional shock or extreme stress is enough to trigger labor quite abruptly, and over the years I have treated a number of patients whose labor began prematurely after a violent quarrel erupted at home.

More than *one previous elective abortion* or a *complicated abortion* in which the cervix is torn will all contribute to the weakening of the cervix and an increased risk of prematurity. Although a woman with one or two abortions performed without noticeable trauma might feel no subsequent ill effects, the chances of prematurity increase rapidly with the number of abortions she has undergone. This is the general conclusion of a number of studies from European countries where liberal abortion laws have existed for many years. A woman at risk would be well advised to cut down on her physical activities and rest more during the pregnancy.

Women at high risk, because of *advanced maternal age,* or the presence of some physical problem such as *heart disease, severe anemia,* or *hypertension* have a much higher likelihood of premature birth and must plan accordingly. More bed rest, extra care, more visits to the obstetrician and good nutrition are all required in any high-risk pregnancy, and so is extra alertness to the signs of premature labor.

☐ *Is Sexual Activity a Risk Factor in Prematurity?* Sex during pregnancy is an area in which there are a number of conflicting theories and recommendations, and this is consequently an area of great concern to the expectant couple (see Chapter 13 on sex and pregnancy). Although recent studies linking sexual intercourse with an increased incidence of premature labor and infection rate have been disputed by other researchers, there is no doubt that forceful intercourse could, in some instances, induce premature labor by stimulating the cervix to release prostaglandin. Since we cannot always predict who will go into premature labor, a woman whose pregnancy is in any way sensitive should be aware of the evidence and consider decreasing her sexual activity in the latter months of gestation. Women with infertility problems or women who show warning signs of prematurity, or are in a high-risk category for premature birth, probably should avoid intercourse during the pregnancy, or a part of the pregnancy. Avoidance of intercourse is particularly important in the last trimester when the cervix sometimes softens prematurely, increasing the risk of infection and ruptured membranes. Bacteria can be pushed up into the vagina and through the softened and dilated cervix, causing irritation and rupture of the membranes, and premature birth.

☐ *Does Orgasm Lead to Premature Birth?* One or two studies have attempted to link frequency of orgasm with a higher incidence of premature birth. This has not been verified by other investigations of the subject, although theoretically it would be possible for orgasm to lead to extrauterine contractions, or even to the secretion of prostaglandins. Both phenomena *could* result in increased uterine contractions, effacing the cervix (that is, thinning the normal shape of the cervix) and triggering premature labor. As an extra safety precaution, a woman in a high-risk group for prematurity probably should try to avoid orgasm after the twentieth week of gestation until the birth.

☐ *Recognition of Premature Labor* A woman who recognizes the warning signs of premature labor may help save her baby's life.

The first symptoms are often mild and can be mistaken for constipation or backache. However, a woman who feels regular uterine cramping with or without pain should suspect premature labor. The inception of premature labor contractions is not always painful, but it can be distinguished from other painless uterine movements by a simple test you can perform yourself. If you feel an apparent contraction of the uterus, place your hand on your abdomen and try to follow its movements. A uterus that rhythmically tightens and relaxes may be going into premature labor. On the other hand, if a woman has *irregular* labor contractions without cervical dilatation, she could be in *false labor* with what are known as Braxton Hicks contractions. Only a doctor can distinguish the two clearly.

A woman who thinks she is experiencing premature labor contractions should contact her doctor immediately without waiting for the symptoms to increase or decrease. If the doctor is unobtainable, go to the labor unit of your hospital (ask your doctor to give you this number, or a hotline number you can call in an emergency). Once you are in the labor unit you can be evaluated, because most hospitals with trained staffs have doctors on call around the clock when premature labor is suspected. Your obstetrician or the hospital staff will look for cervical changes indicating uterine activity and will begin an intravenous infusion of ethanol or a uterine relaxant such as ritodrine, to try to stop the labor from progressing further. A gain of even a few days is valuable if you are at a crucial point in the third trimester. If no significant cervical or uterine activity is detectable, you may be asked to stay in the hospital for observation and then sent home to rest.

With early recognition and early treatment, there is a good chance of stopping premature labor in time to save the pregnancy. Once labor has been allowed to progress beyond a certain point, it is irreversible.

☐ *Treating Premature Labor*   In certain situations, the obstetrician or hospital staff will not attempt to stop the full onset of labor. If the placenta has separated from the uterus, necessitating an immediate Cesarean, or the mother is seriously ill, or the fetus severely distressed, it is better to allow labor to continue rather than risk injury by trying to prolong the pregnancy. But if labor can be halted safely, several courses of action are open to the physician.

The traditional treatment is complete bed rest, at home or in the hospital, with or without sedatives or uterine relaxant drugs. Bed rest is effective because it reduces the pressure on the cervix by shifting the full weight of the baby away from this vulnerable area. At the same time, oxygen and blood are free to reach the uterus in larger quantities and increase fetal growth. A side lying position

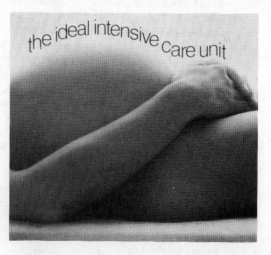

Figure 62: Treatment of Premature Labor: The ideal intensive-care unit is the uterus itself. A woman can learn to recognize symptoms of premature labor and contact her doctor immediately if she detects something untoward. Today there are drugs that successfully stop premature labor and often allow the patient to come successfully to term.
Reproduced with permission of Duphar Laboratories, Southampton, England.

will help reduce the uterine pressure on the vena cava, the large vein in the back of the abdomen, and assure a better return of blood to the heart.

If signs of premature labor are evident to the physician, powerful drugs are now available to halt preterm labor. These are the beta-mimetics, a group of relatively new drugs that act by stimulating the beta cells in the uterus, the cells that naturally relax the myometrium muscles in the uterus and slow down the labor contractions. Several types of beta-mimetic drugs have been used in Europe and in other countries around the world for a number of years, and one, ritodrine, has recently been approved for general use in the United States. This drug is available in intravenous and oral forms under the trade name Yutopar.

☐ *Ritodrine Treatment for Premature Labor*   If you enter the hospital with a suspected case of premature labor and are treated with ritodrine, the first stage is a period of observation designed to establish the amount of uterine activity. If labor is ongoing, but the fetal membranes are still intact and the cervix is less than four centimeters dilated, the chance of stopping labor is high—greater than 80 percent—and with less dilation the prognosis is even more favorable. When the cervix is more than four cm dilated, your doctor might still try to stop labor, although his chances of success are less. Once the decision has been made to use the drug, ritodrine is then given intravenously to relax the uterus and halt the contractions.

Stabilization is often achieved within ten to twenty minutes. After the cramps have stopped, your doctor will most likely continue with an intravenous infusion for the next twelve hours to make sure that the uterus remains relaxed and to give the body time to metabolize and excrete the hormones responsible for the premature contractions. Then, once the initial period of treatment is over, you will be kept in the hospital for another day or two for observation and started on a regimen of oral ritodrine, a 10-mg dose every four hours, until the staff is certain that labor has been halted and the cervix is no farther dilated. A reasonably normal schedule is possible for the rest of the pregnancy, but you will certainly be advised to rest more, and refrain from sexual intercourse. Ritodrine therapy should continue, with a 10-mg ritodrine tablet every four to six hours around the clock, until you reach the thirty-sixth or thirty-eighth week of gestation and the baby's chance of survival has increased greatly. In a group of studies conducted by our own research group at New York Hospital and Mount Sinai Hospital in New York, we found that women could successfully postpone labor for at least six weeks by resting and taking a uterine relaxant—sufficient time for the fetus to grow and mature into a baby capable of an independent existence.

☐ *Is Ritodrine Safe?*   The beta-mimetic drugs stimulate the heart and pulse rate at the same time that they slow down the uterine contractions. Your pulse and heart rates should, therefore, be followed carefully throughout the period of the intravenous infusion. At the same time, the systolic blood pressure tends to increase slightly, while the diastolic pressure decreases, causing palpitation, headaches, or occasional nausea. Side effects with oral doses of ritodrine are the same as during the intravenous infusion but much less severe—most women tolerate oral ritodrine administration well. Intravenous ritodrine can lower the potassium levels, which should be checked and regulated if necessary.

☐   *The Effects on the Fetus*   Ritodrine is generally considered a safe drug for the fetus. It does increase the baby's heart rate, and also its blood sugar, which are relatively minor side effects.

☐   *Alcohol Treatment for Premature Labor*   In the past, we treated premature labor with alcohol given in intravenous form. Alcohol (ethanol) has the ability to block the oxytocin released from the pituitary gland in the brain as well as directly relaxing the uterus itself. Before the FDA released ritodrine for general use in the United States, thousands of women were given intravenous alcohol and had their labors successfully postponed through the use of this drug. Today, fewer hospitals are using ethanol for the majority of their patients, although women with heart disease and other contraindications to ritodrine are still given an alcohol drip because it is less hard on the cardiovascular system. The one unpleasant side effect of intravenous alcohol is the state of complete inebriation it induces in the patient, who often becomes irrational under its influence. Effects on the fetus or newborn seem to be temporary and apparently do not contribute to fetal alcohol syndrome.

☐   *Prostaglandin Inhibitor in the Treatment of Premature Labor*   Another group of drugs used experimentally in the treatment of premature labor are the prostaglandin-inhibiting agents: aspirin, indomethacin, and mefenamic acid. Since the prostaglandin hormones are known to initiate labor, experimental studies in the United States, Israel, and Sweden have used these prostaglandin blockers to prevent the prostaglandin level from rising. However, there is one serious problem: the ductus arteriosus, the artery that shunts blood away from the fetal lungs, is very sensitive to prostaglandin-blocking agents, and fetuses have died when this vital artery has been closed by indomethacin or some other inhibitor. For this very good reason, the prostaglandin-inhibiting agents are not considered safe for use during pregnancy.

☐   *Even if Ritodrine Fails, the Baby May Have Been Helped*   Even if ritodrine treatment fails to prevent premature labor, as it does in some cases, studies would indicate that it has some positive effect by hastening lung maturity in the fetus. When women have been on ritodrine for one or two days and subsequently deliver, the premature infant often has less respiratory distress than might have been expected, because ritodrine appears to cause a maturation of the surfactant, the substance responsible for initiating lung maturity before birth. This is a phenomenon I have seen myself in many premature births. Given the positive effect of ritodrine on the newborn child, one should always attempt to stop labor with ritodrine when possible.

☐   *Premature Rupture of the Membranes*   A premature rupture of the membranes is a serious complication since no artificial means are available to close up the sac, and the chance of imminent delivery is therefore rather high. A woman who suspects that her membranes have ruptured should call her doctor or go to her hospital's labor unit, where a physician will examine her under sterile conditions. Although a conventional internal examination is avoided with a suspected rupture because of the risk of infection, a test can be performed using a pH-sensitive litmus paper, and a sample of fluid from the vagina. Amniotic fluid is highly alkaline and a drop placed on litmus paper will turn it blue immediately.

The patient with ruptured membranes is placed in the hospital on complete bed rest. Her temperature is checked several times a day; the fetal heart rate is monitored carefully, and blood samples are taken daily to assure a low white-cell blood count. This type of intensive treatment often makes it possible to gain a few more weeks before the delivery. Here once again, it is important to know what to do in a case of emergency. As soon as the membranes rupture, go to the hospital as quickly as possible; walking around with ruptured membranes will cause the baby to rest against the cervix, resulting in stretching of the cervix and a greater risk of premature labor, infection, and possible brain damage.

Unfortunately, some women with prematurely ruptured membranes do develop fever, despite precautionary measures. If fever and infection occur, the doctor might have to induce labor to prevent the baby from becoming infected *in utero*. At least with a rupture of more than twenty-four hours, the chance that the baby's lungs have matured somewhat under the stress of the rupture increases its potential for survival.

If the membranes rupture closer to term, the possibility of spontaneous labor occurring within twenty-four hours is greater than 80 percent. This is beneficial, since the rapid onset of labor is associated with less infection and other problems. Otherwise, a woman whose rupture is several weeks premature is best cared for in the hospital where sterile surroundings will help protect her against infection, and labor can be induced immediately if the fetus becomes endangered. If your local hospital is too small to manage a premature birth sucessfully, the hospital might elect to transport you by ambulance or helicopter to a larger hospital with more specialized facilities.

☐ *Delivering the Premature Infant* The gentlest form of delivery is the best, since the skull of a very premature infant is fragile and susceptible to intracranial hemorrhage and bleeding. A baby who shows signs of distress is often delivered by Cesarean section; otherwise the hospital might favor a vaginal delivery. Labor with these tiny prematures often proceeds easily and rapidly, although the mother will probably be asked not to push quite as hard as she would at term. If a woman is admitted with a premature baby in the breech position, then most hospitals would prefer to initiate a Cesarean section because the unripe cervix in a vaginal birth often closes around the head, causing trauma and intracranial hemorrhage.

☐ *Toxemia in Pregnancy* The term "toxemia" is derived from two Greek words, *toxikon*, poison, and *haima*, blood. Toxemia was, therefore, historically regarded as the condition of having a toxic substance in the blood, which suggests that doctors had no clear idea of how the disease developed. Toxemia takes two distinct forms, known as preeclampsia and eclampsia. Preeclampsia is the milder form of the condition, in which no eclamptic activity (seizures) has yet occurred. Since most cases of toxemia do not progress beyond the preeclamptic stage, the terms "toxemia" and "preeclampsia" are often used synonymously.

Symptoms of preeclampsia are edema or weight gain, hypertension, and proteinuria (protein in the urine, a sign of kidney damage). A case of preeclampsia is often well established before the patient notices any symptoms, although she may be aware of some puffiness of the fingers and face, the first signs of an unusual amount of fluid retention in the tissues. But if the other symptoms of preeclampsia appear, and the condition is not treated promptly, preeclampsia can develop into a classic case of advanced preeclampsia, with severe kidney damage, unremitting headaches, nausea and vomiting, elevated blood pressure, and seizures. The full eclampsia syndrome could be deadly to the fetus and severely damaging to the mother.

Preeclampsia affects many pregnant women, especially women in their first pregnancies, so it is important for a woman to become familiar with the disease and learn to detect the early warning signs before the problem becomes serious. With early treatment and a good understanding of the disease, preeclampsia can usually be brought under control in time.

☐ *What Are the Causes of Toxemia?*   Toxemia is still a mysterious condition, although several recognizable mechanisms have been identified that apparently contribute to its onset. It is most often seen in a first pregnancy, particularly toward the end of the third trimester when the uterus is at its full height, or in a pregnancy in which the uterus is extended prematurely by a multiple gestation. Social factors are often suspected of playing a part, since poor women whose diets are inadequate are far more likely to develop toxemia than well nourished women. Women with chronic hypertension or diabetes are also more likely to become preeclamptic as pregnancy advances.

One favored theory suggests that uterine ischemia (a decrease in the blood supply to the uterus) is the underlying cause. The theory postulates that this decrease is due to a mechanical insufficiency because the uterus is overextended and the blood flow is unable to compensate for the deficiency. This less than sufficient amount of blood then triggers the production of what are known as pressure polypeptides—thromboplastins or thromboplastin-like substances. These polypeptides in turn cause the kidneys to secrete the enzyme renin, which will increase the blood pressure and encourage more blood to reach the uterus. In other words, the increase in blood pressure is a compensatory mechanism in the body functioning to overcome the insufficient supply of blood to the overextended uterus. At the same time, the increase in blood pressure leads to a general increase in the blood flow, which in turn leads to edema, kidney damage, and subsequently to the appearance of protein in the urine (proteinuria). Hence, the first toxemia symptom is usually edema, followed by elevated blood pressure, and finally proteinuria. When that occurs it is usually a sign of serious damage, so extensive that it might be difficult to reverse.

☐ *Convulsions and Coma*   With a neglected case of preeclampsia, the sequence of events could well continue and become aggravated into the full eclampsia syndrome: increased stimulation of the central nervous system, muscle spasms, extreme irritability, rapid reflex movements, and finally, seizures.

Eclamptic seizures are intense muscle contractions that resemble the *grand mal* seizures seen in epileptic patients. When the body goes into an eclamptic seizure, the limbs go rigid, the respiration ceases to function, and there are violent intermittent contractions of the muscles of the head, the limbs, and the tongue. A severe incident is often followed by coma in the postseizure period. Unremitting seizures can result in kidney injury severe enough to require dialysis; or they have been known to end in brain damage, prolonged coma, or maternal and fetal death.

Eclampsia is preceded by several characteristic symptoms—severe headache, disorientation, somnambulation, visual disturbances, and epigastric pain. These are symptoms that should always be heeded, whether your doctor has diagnosed preeclampsia or not. A number of women who go into seizures do so unexpectedly, and by the time they reach the hospital the damage is often irreversible.

☐ **When Does Toxemia Occur?**   Toxemia can occur at any time after the twenty-fourth week of pregnancy, but it is more likely to develop close to term, after the thirty-seventh week of gestation. At this point it is usually possible to bring it under control quickly, or to protect the baby by hastening the delivery. The biological changes characteristic of toxemia regress after delivery, and there is no equivalent condition in the nonpregnant woman, although if the condition is not caught and treated early, it could lead to chronic hypertension later in life.

If toxemia develops early in pregnancy—at the end of the second trimester, for instance—it is associated with a significantly higher incidence of fetal growth retardation and death of the baby, either before or just after delivery. In one study of 2500 preeclamptic women in Australia, fetal growth retardation occurred in 18 percent of the pregnancies, and there was a high level of perinatal mortality, higher than 10 percent.

☐ **Edema: A Normal Part of Pregnancy**   Despite its association with toxemia, fluid retention *is* normal in pregnancy. The amount of fluid circulating in the mother's bloodstream increases by up to 45 percent during pregnancy, helping to meet the extra demands placed on the body by the growing fetus. The greater volume of circulating liquids and the extra pressure on the uterus lead to a number of circulatory problems familiar to pregnant women, including varicose veins and hemorrhoids. Some of this excess fluid tends to move from the intravascular space into the extravascular space (the space outside the blood vessels), creating another characteristic sign of pregnancy: *pregnancy-related edema.* As the pregnancy progresses and the fetus grows larger, many women experience swelling in the feet and ankles, especially if they have been sitting still for long periods, or notice stiffness and swelling in their fingers. Sometimes the entire hand is numb, a complaint known as carpal tunnel syndrome. You may find that the swollen tissues make it difficult to remove your rings, particularly in the morning when the hands have retained extra fluid overnight.

Up to 40 percent of all pregnant women experience some form of edema and all pregnant women can expect to gain as much as ten to fifteen pounds through fluid retention in the tissues, whether they show overt signs of edema or not. According to a British study, many of the women who experience edema have unusually healthy pregnancies, with larger babies and a lower rate of premature labor than other women, which would suggest that a certain amount of edema is a favorable sign. At the same time, this does not mean that *excessive* water retention is desirable or healthy. A woman with severe edema is in danger of developing the full triad of toxemia symptoms and should seek medical help as quickly as possible.

Do not allow your doctor to treat a case of edema with diuretics and a salt-free diet, a form of treatment that was popular years ago. A reasonable amount of salt is an essential element in a healthy pregnancy, a subject that is discussed fully in Chapter 16, "The Pregnancy Diet."

☐ **Prevention of Toxemia** A woman in her first pregnancy can help prevent toxemia by planning ahead, eating well, taking vitamins, and getting her body into good, healthy condition before she conceives. Chronic kidney disease or hypertension increases the risk of developing preeclampsia in pregnancy, so a woman in these high-risk groups should be evaluated carefully before she becomes pregnant to eliminate serious problems during gestation.

Once you are pregnant, see your doctor as early in the pregnancy as possible and arrange a schedule of follow-up visits at frequent intervals (most obstetricians like to see new patients every three to four weeks at the beginning of pregnancy, and every two to three weeks as pregnancy progresses.) The routine work-up at each prenatal visit is designed to detect preeclampsia at an early stage. The doctor will look for an excessive weight gain between two visits, a sign that edema or water retention has begun; a significant rise in blood pressure; and finally, traces of protein in the monthly urine sample. Protein in the urine usually indicates that the kidneys are already damaged and that toxemia has set in.

In general, a woman is less susceptible to toxemia if she is careful about her diet. Proper nutrition means sufficient proteins and vitamins, and a reasonable amount of sodium without excessive intake of salty foods. According to some new evidence, women who have a plentiful supply of calcium during pregnancy have a lower rate of toxemia than women who are calcium-deficient, even if both groups eat about the same amount of protein, so an increase of calcium is essential. Finally, make sure to drink plenty of liquids; they are valuable in reducing edema and improving the efficiency of the kidney functions. In this way the body will achieve a balance and problems will be lessened.

A good understanding of the nature of toxemia is the second line of defense against its worst effects. If you begin to experience an unusual amount of puffiness especially in the face, around the eyes, or at the joints of the fingers, make a special appointment with your obstetrician rather than wait for the next scheduled visit. The early symptoms of toxemia can usually be controlled effectively by generally cutting back on your normal activities and resting in bed, preferably in a side-lying position. Bed rest is effective because less blood is used by the voluntary muscles, and more reaches the involuntary muscles in the uterus. A free flow of blood often washes away the toxins in the kidneys and urine, preventing the onset of kidney damage and the possibility of hypertension. A number of normally healthy women develop mild symptoms of toxemia in a first pregnancy, particularly when the baby is fairly large, but you are unlikely to experience a severe form of the disorder if you rest and take care of yourself.

☐ **Treatment of Preeclampsia and Eclampsia** If toxemia sets in, or the patient begins to complain of headaches or epigastric pain, or becomes unusually irritated, the doctor should check her reflexes for hyperreflexia (brisk tendon reflexes), the precursor of a full eclamptic episode, and hospitalize her to prevent the condition from becoming worse and leading to a dangerous seizure. A hospital patient with toxemia is kept in a quiet environment under the careful supervision of the nursing staff and monitored by frequent blood pressure evaluations and weight checks. A mild sedative, such as phenobarbital, helps relax the body and also decreases the chances of seizure activity. A period of rest in the hospital is often enough to reverse a case of milder preeclampsia without further treatment. If, however, toxemia symptoms continue to increase, with visual disturbances, rapidly rising blood pressure, and brisker reflex activity, the doctor will evaluate fetal maturity, and then deliver the baby if the pregnancy has reached a point close to term. As soon as the baby and placenta are removed, the toxins that have been allowed to build up in the body will disappear, and the condition will reverse itself naturally.

When the baby is still too young to be delivered safely, a woman with severe toxemia will be kept in the hospital, given a mild sedative, and placed under careful supervision for a few weeks with frequent nonstress testings. Amniocentesis can then be performed to see whether or not the L/H ratio (see Chap. 22) has matured sufficiently; if it has, the physician might elect to induce labor or perform a Cesarean section.

A patient admitted close to term whose reflex activity is pronounced is usually treated with an intravenous infusion of magnesium sulfate. This powerful anticonvulsant drug controls the symptoms of eclampsia by decreasing the tremors in the muscle fibers and depressing the central nervous system. A patient can be kept on magnesium sulfate and delivered when her condition has stabilized. If the blood pressure continues to rise, even with the intravenous infusion, the hospital staff will initiate labor immediately, since the mother and the baby are in danger. Women with toxemia respond well to induction of labor and usually encounter less stress with a vaginal delivery. However, if toxemia has occurred early in the pregnancy and the baby is premature, blood pressure medication should be used to gain time until the baby has reached maturity. If the combination of rest, antiseizure and antihypertensive medications all fail and it is judged that the baby, although premature, should be delivered, a Cesarean birth might be preferred. Normal labor is sometimes too hard on a tiny baby. Even after the baby is born, the risk of seizure activity continues for at least twenty-four hours postpartum, and intravenous infusion of magnesium sulfate should be continued until the eclamptic condition is reversed. The baby too will need careful watching, because there is the possibility of magnesium intoxication, characterized by a weak or absent cry and respiratory distress. But this is only a minor possibility; in most cases the magnesium sulfate is excreted rapidly by the mother before magnesium levels have had time to build up in the infant.

☐ *Will Toxemia Occur in the Next Pregnancy?* A first pregnancy complicated by toxemia is not necessarily followed by a second pregnancy with toxemia. Once again, it would depend on the circumstances of the individual pregnancy. If a woman still has high blood pressure after the birth, it could imply some underlying hypertensive condition that should be corrected before the woman becomes pregnant again. If the problem is underlying kidney damage, signs of toxemia might develop in a second pregnancy, but more often than not it is the form of hypertension known as pregnancy-related hypertension, a condition less severe than toxemia because it is not associated with seizure activity. It is, however, likely to result in a growth-retarded fetus. Any woman who has had toxemia in her first pregnancy should make sure to consult with her regular doctor after delivery and have her general health evaluated carefully in the postpartum period to safeguard herself for the future.

☐ *Placenta Previa*   Placenta previa is a condition in which the placenta or a part of it covers the internal cervical os, the opening of the vagina to the uterus. There are various types of placenta previa; one is a *complete placenta previa*, in which the placenta completely covers the cervical canal and a vaginal delivery is impossible because the cervix cannot open. Then there is a *partial placenta previa*, a condition in which a portion of the placenta partially covers the internal opening of the cervix—the so-called internal os. Finally, there is a *low-lying placenta previa*, in which the placenta's edge reaches down into the lower portion of the uterus, but does not completely cover the internal os itself. A complete placenta previa is a reasonably rare complication, occurring as it does in approximately six out of every thousand pregnancies. The incidence of partial placenta previa is more difficult to estimate.

As pregnancy progresses, the degree of placenta previa often changes. A placenta previa diagnosed early in pregnancy, may change as the uterus enlarges and the placenta moves upward and out of the way of the cervical os. Doctors describe this phenomenon as "placental migration." Some women initially diagnosed as placenta previa patients might have no problem at all later on in pregnancy.

Modern ultrasound techniques have made it possible to locate the placenta much more accurately than in the past and follow its movement throughout the pregnancy. This has helped decrease the high fetal and maternal mortality rates that used to be associated with placenta previa when the woman either hemorrhaged in labor or the membranes ruptured early in the pregnancy.

☐ *The Causes of Placenta Previa*   A placenta previa occurs when the fertilized egg enters the uterus and fails to attach itself immediately to the upper portion of the uterus. This phenomenon is not completely understood, but it seems to occur when the uterine cavity is larger and the egg drops down in the uterus, implanting itself in the lower uterine section where the growing placenta eventually partially or completely covers the internal opening of the cervix. Therefore, the chance of experiencing a placenta previa increases with the natural expansion of the uterus after each pregnancy, and is rarely seen in a first pregnancy, unless the woman has had a number of abortions. Uterine scars from a previous Cesarean section or uterine surgery also increase the risk of placental abnormalities.

Recent studies have also shown that the incidence of placenta previa is increased by 25 percent in moderate smokers and 92 percent in heavy smokers; another problem associated with smoking and pregnancy.

☐ *Diagnosis of Placenta Previa*   If you develop painless vaginal bleeding at any time during your pregnancy, contact your doctor immediately, even if the bleeding stops by itself. A thorough evaluation is necessary. If a woman continues to bleed, or bleeds very heavily, she will be admitted to the hospital, where blood transfusions are made available and careful observation and diagnosis are required.

The best way to determine placenta previa is with the aid of ultrasonography rather than conventional vaginal techniques. A gentle vaginal examination can sometimes be performed with a speculum, but a finger caught in the placenta has been known to precipitate a bout of near-fatal hemorrhaging. The initial ultrasound examination will determine where the placenta is located and check the amount of amniotic fluid protecting the fetus. The natural migration of the placenta can then be watched closely by sonograms performed at weekly intervals.

Typically, a placenta previa produces what is known as the "three bleeds." The first bleeding symptoms are usually the least severe and often stop spontaneously. A period of heavier bleeding may then follow at an interval of a few weeks or even a few months. This "second bleed" is usually more prolonged than the first, although, once again, it often regresses without the need for a blood transfusion or other emergency treatment. Nonetheless, once a woman has experienced the "second bleed" a third bleeding episode is bound to follow within days or weeks, and at this point the patient is usually put in the hospital and followed by careful observation and ultrasound up until the time of delivery. The choice of a vaginal or abdominal delivery depends on whether the placenta is partially or completely covering the cervical os. If the placenta covers the cervix, a Cesarean birth is the only choice; however, if the placenta migrates away from the cervix, a vaginal delivery should be possible.

☐ *Caring for Placenta Previa Episodes*   Bleeding in early pregnancy can usually be cared for at home, as long as the patient rests, avoids sexual intercourse, and is followed carefully by ultrasound. Many of these early bleeding incidents need no further treatment except patient information and a decrease in physical activity.

Bleeding later in pregnancy or in the second trimester is often more severe, and the patient will need hospital treatment, with blood transfusions and intravenous infusion on hand. If the bleeding stops, the patient might be sent home to rest, with the understanding that she contact the hospital at the first sign of a third bleed. Once a third bleed does occur, similar emergency procedures are instituted to prevent serious hemorrhaging or the loss of the fetus. Sometimes this third bleed is so severe that the doctor is forced to perform an immediate Cesarean, but, once again, it may well regress spontaneously, and with careful monitoring a doctor might be able to watch the patient in the hospital for a few more weeks or until the pregnancy comes to term. When the placenta previa is known to be complete, a Cesarean section will be performed once the baby's maturity has been established by amniocentesis and L/H ratio. If the doctor is still unsure of the placenta's position, he might choose to perform what is known as a "double set-up," in which he makes his examination in the delivery room with an anesthesiologist and surgical nurses standing by for an immediate Cesarean should it prove necessary. In other words, with modern monitoring methods it is possible to treat each case of placenta previa individually, and wait for many of these babies to mature rather than doing emergency surgery at a relatively early stage of the pregnancy.

Once again, this is an area in which an informed woman can do much to help herself and her baby. The worst aspects of placenta previa can often be mitigated by intelligent medical care and information given the patient.

☐   *Abruptio Placentae, or Premature Separation of the Placenta*   The term "abruptio placentae" was coined by a distinguished Chicago doctor, Dr. Joseph De Lee, and is now used worldwide. This is a type of placental complication in which the placenta separates itself from the uterine wall at any point during pregnancy. The condition is different from placenta previa, where the placenta remains attached to the uterus despite the bleeding episodes.

Milder cases of abruptio placentae occur more often than is generally believed, but complete separation of the placenta is rare—occurring in fewer than one out of every five hundred pregnancies.

☐   *What Causes Abruptio Placentae?*   The causes are largely unknown, although some recent evidence points to folic-acid deficiency playing some part in this condition. (However, since the problem is one of malabsorption, folic-acid supplementation might not prevent the occurrence of the problem.) Abruptio is quite often associated with chronic hypertension, and other high-risk pregnancies in which the placenta is unusually small or the mother poorly nourished. It can happen accidentally; trauma, automobile accidents, and falls have been known to separate the placenta partially or completely from the uterine wall. Furthermore, smoking increases the risk of abruptio placentae to a significant degree. The chance of abruptio increases by 24 percent in moderate smokers and 68 percent in heavy smokers.

The time when the abruptio occurs differs in single and multiple pregnancies. *In single pregnancies*, about two-thirds of all abruptios occur just before the onset of labor. *In multiple births*, the onset is normally in the second stage, between the delivery of the two babies. Uterine abnormalities that seem to predispose a woman to this condition include a larger than normal amount of amniotic fluid and elevated venous blood pressure in the uterus.

☐   *Signs of Abruptio Placentae*   Slight, repeated attacks of bleeding and a painful, tender uterus are signs of some disturbance in the placenta. The uterus is tender because bleeding takes place behind the placenta and irritates the uterus itself, which then goes into hard, painful spasms. This in turn leads to increased shedding of the uterine lining, which eventually causes a partial or complete placental separation. A complete abruptio cuts off the blood supply to the fetus and the baby will die if immediate delivery is not carried out. There are milder cases in which the fetus shows no evidence of distress as long as the mother's cardiovascular state is good.

Since this complication can be fatal, a case of bleeding associated with a strong, painful, unyielding contraction should be dealt with only in the hospital. I remember the experience of one patient of mine who thought she was simply in early labor, and the bleeding was the "show." I asked her to come into the hospital immediately. Fortunately I was there when she arrived, because she was screaming with pain as she walked in, doubled over by the persistent uterine contraction caused by the placental separation. We performed an immediate

Cesarean—minutes ahead of the death of the fetus, who fortunately was delivered in good condition—but if this woman had not been alert enough to call me directly she experienced some unusual symptoms, her baby would probably have died.

☐ *Treatment of Abruptio Placentae*   The condition can be diagnosed by the clinical symptoms of bleeding and a rigid uterus, sometimes accompanied by a barely perceptible fetal heartbeat. With a complete abruptio, the doctor has no choice but to initiate an immediate Cesarean section to save the baby's life, and remove the placenta to stop the bleeding. If the fetal heart rate is stable when the woman enters the hospital, most doctors would prefer to wait and use ultrasonography to distinguish any bleeding behind the placenta. A vaginal delivery may be possible if vaginal bleeding is not too serious and the fetus' condition remains stable. There are even cases in which the separation is marginal enough to allow the physician to prevent premature labor by the use of an alcohol drip or a beta-mimetic such as ritodrine. The woman can then be watched in the hospital until the baby is mature enough for delivery.

Placental separation is seen frequently enough, especially among high-risk patients, to make it important for any pregnant woman to recognize the symptoms and contact her doctor as soon as she detects some abnormal sign. This is particularly true of women with high blood pressure and women who are heavy smokers.

☐ *Postterm Pregnancy*   A postterm pregnancy is defined as a pregnancy lasting for more than forty-two weeks from the onset of the last menstrual period—two weeks beyond the normal forty-week gestational span. About 5 percent of all deliveries are postterm, a lower proportion than one might expect, given that some women do not know exactly when they conceived or have a menstrual history of long, irregular cycles. While postmaturity is not in itself a dangerous situation, a postterm pregnancy in which the fetal environment has begun to degenerate and endanger the fetus is hazardous and must not be treated lightly. In this lies the difference between a *postterm* and a *postmature* pregnancy.

☐ *Differences Between a Postterm Pregnancy and Postmaturity*   A postdate or postterm pregnancy is one that has passed the forty-second week of gestation, calculated from the first day of the last menstrual period. Postmaturity refers to a much more serious condition in which the pregnancy is not only postterm but the abnormal length of gestation has led to the degeneration and shrinkage of the placenta and a decreased production of amniotic fluid. As the placenta grows old, it fails to provide sufficient oxygen and nutrition to the baby, who is left behind in the uterus without the proper nourishment. One is reminded of the apple that remains on the tree in late fall, wrinkled and rotten because the tree is no longer providing it with sustenance. In those cases in which the trigger mechanism that normally starts labor is missing, the baby might well die or be severely damaged if no attention is paid to the situation, or is not paid in time. Also, once the placenta ages, it shrinks, reducing the production of amniotic fluid and exposing the umbilical cord to harm. This places additional stress on

382 /   Childbirth with Love

the baby. Overall, postterm pregnancies are associated with double the perinatal mortality rate of term pregnancies: 15 percent of newborns that die just before or after birth are postmature.

☐   *The Postmature Baby*   If the oxygen supply from the placenta decreases, the first sign of mild distress in the fetus is a relaxation of the sphincter muscle in the anus. This causes portions of the stool to enter the amniotic fluid (meconium staining of the amniotic fluid), a condition that can be dangerous because the aspiration of meconium-stained fluid into the fetus' lungs might result in the collapse of the lung. Amniocentesis will determine whether or not meconium staining has occurred. A baby whose lungs contain significant amounts of meconium will need resuscitation at birth. Another sign of chronic placental insufficiency is an unusual form of fetal growth retardation in which the baby is large but has a somewhat malnourished appearance.

When a postmature baby is born, the skin is pale and parchmentlike, the fingernails and toenails are unusually long, and the scalp is covered with hair. The scanty supply of amniotic fluid will be meconium-stained. Some postmature babies are dehydrated and show signs of hypoglycemia. While only a small number of the babies born after the forty-second week display acute symptoms of a postmature syndrome, the problem is serious enough to make the postdate pregnancy a difficult one for the obstetrician, who must decide whether to leave the pregnancy alone or induce the birth.

☐   *Who Is Likely to Have Problems from a Postmature Baby?*   Most postterm pregnancies end with a normal delivery and a normal newborn. This fact, and the trend away from beginning labor artificially wherever possible, are among the reasons why most American hospitals have stopped doing routine inductions after the forty-second week and prefer to wait for labor to begin spontaneously in the postterm pregnancy. Certain women, however, have been identified as being at special risk. A woman having her *first baby at a relatively advanced age, 35 or older,* is more likely to lose a baby who is postterm than a younger woman, and so is a woman with toxemia or diabetes whose pregnancy goes beyond the forty-second week. Certain women must then be very alert to signs that the baby needs to be delivered. Once the forty-second week of pregnancy is passed, a woman in the high-risk group should be followed by serial nonstress tests and other fetal monitoring tests (see Chap. 23). Any changes in fetal movements should be observed carefully. If the baby's movements slow down, a postterm woman must immediately contact her doctor and be seen in the hospital for observation and fetal monitoring. Please understand the seriousness of passing your due date and make sure that you are checked with a nonstress test at least twice a week.

☐   *The Psychological Impact of Postterm Pregnancy*   A pregnancy that goes well past the estimated due date, for whatever reason, can be a very difficult time for a woman and her family. Mixed feelings of fatigue, frustration, nervous anticipation and even anger at the baby are not uncommon once the pregnancy has exceeded its expected limits. Some women become so worried and depressed that they find it difficult to get out of bed; others put on so much extra weight that normal movement is all but impossible. The feeling of frustration only increases once a woman and her partner realize there is nothing they can do to change their situation or force an end to the pregnancy. Unfortunately, the obstetrician often shows little understanding of the parents' emotions, and only adds to their frustrations by his apparent lack of sympathy.

☐ *Why Do Postterm Pregnancies Occur?*   Why certain women go into labor later than other women is unknown, in part because the exact mechanism of labor itself remains a mystery. We do, however, know that labor is more likely to be delayed in pregnancies where the baby is larger and does not push against the cervix as it would in the normal full-term pregnancy, thus failing to release the hormones that trigger labor. The uterine environment also remains favorable for a longer time in a pregnancy in which the infant is unusually large. Hereditary factors, too, may be involved; the mother who goes late often has a daughter who goes late, and a woman overdue in her first pregnancy might go late with the second.

☐ *Medical Management of Postmaturity*   If the patient has passed her due date by two weeks or more, the first step is a careful review of the medical records to resolve any discrepancies in her menstrual and gestational history. Manual examination and a sonogram will help establish the baby's size and confirm or disprove the original estimated due date. A number of tests, including estriol analysis, can then be performed to make sure that the postterm baby is doing well. Estriols, the estrogen precursors secreted by the baby into the maternal blood or urine, usually give a good idea of the baby's maturity and health (see Chap. 23). Once the estriol level begins to drop, this is often a sign that the baby is under stress and needs further evaluation, or induction of labor.

☐ *Nonstress Testing*   Nonstress testing (see Chap. 23) is now used routinely in high-risk cases after the forty-second week, when the test can be repeated every forty-eight hours to keep a constant check on the baby's well-being. If the fetal heart rate fails to increase with fetal movement, or the amount of fetal movement decreases suddenly, a further test, the oxytocin-challenge test, is usually given in the labor unit to check the heart rate under the stress of artificially induced labor. A detectable abnormality usually results in a decision to continue the oxytocin drip and induce the onset of full labor.

Another valuable test is one you can perform yourself. If you are well past your due date and you feel the baby's movements decrease, try the simple glucose test described on page 315 and contact your doctor immediately if the baby fails to respond. A sudden lack of movement in the postmature baby is often a sign of serious trouble.

Note: Some doctors will order nonstress tests only once a week. This is not sufficient. According to most studies, the test is capable of determining fetal well-being for only forty-eight hours and should, therefore, in this very high-risk situation, be repeated at least every two days.

☐ *Postmaturity After Thirty-five*   A postmature pregnancy appears to pose a high risk to the baby if the mother is thirty-five or older. If you are in this high-risk category, you should be aware of the extra risk to your baby and insist on careful monitoring in the postterm period, preferably with nonstress testing, fetal monitoring, and the other sophisticated modern tests designed to follow your progress. Your obstetrician might even elect to induce labor once you pass the forty-second week rather than wait for it to begin spontaneously. (In some countries, labor is always induced if it does not occur at forty-two weeks.) Women who are older need to be especially alert during a first pregnancy.

☐ *When Should Labor Be Induced in the Postterm Pregnancy?*   Labor must be induced when the patient goes beyond the forty-second week and a nonstress test or oxytocin-challenge test reveals an abnormal reading or a lack of fetal movement. Any other abnormal fetal sign or a worsening of the mother's condition would also call for elective induction. Some doctors like to induce women routinely once they have passed their due date by two or three weeks, regardless of the baby's condition. This is probably justified if the cervix is ready and ripe, the patient's history is known, and she lives at a distance from the hospital, because there is a risk of delivering before she reaches the hospital, particularly if she has already had one baby before.

☐ *Fetal Death* **in Utero**   Unfortunately, this is a tragedy that still strikes a number of pregnancies each year. Fetal death often occurs for no discernable reason, although a number of fatalities can sometimes be attributed to an accident or some factor associated with the pregnancy. Occasionally there is an accident in which the fetus strangles on the umbilical cord, or the uterus is penetrated or jolted severely enough to cause a complete displacement of the placenta. Certain babies seem to die *in utero* because the environment is so hostile that they fail to thrive; a severely growth-retarded fetus is sometimes seen in a pregnancy in which the mother has serious hypertension or toxemia. Diabetic pregnancies are another high-risk group. A greater tragedy is a death close to term or in the postterm period because the obstetrician failed to perform the necessary tests and the baby died just before delivery.

Fetal death is usually detected at a routine office visit, although a woman often experiences a prolonged pattern of diminishing or absent fetal movements before she visits her obstetrician. When the manual examination reveals no audible fetal heart rate, the obstetrician can schedule a sonogram to examine the fetal condition more accurately. (With modern real-time scanning, the doctor can obtain an instantaneous, clear picture of the fetus and the fetal heartbeat.) One can assume the baby is dead if the sonogram shows no sign of fetal movement or fetal heart rate, but further confirmation can be obtained from an X-ray of the uterus to determine the Spalding's sign, a characteristic overlapping of the fetal skull bones associated with fetal demise.

Once a couple has fully accepted the obstetrician's diagnosis, plans should be made for immediate induction of labor, if possible. There are physical as well as psychological problems involved in waiting for labor to begin spontaneously. Although most women go into labor within two to three weeks, in 25 percent of cases labor fails to take place and the patient is exposed to a significant risk of coagulopathy, a bout of abnormal blood-clotting behind the placenta that could endanger the woman's life through uncontrollable bleeding. The threat of physical harm, and the desire to spare the family as much grief as possible, has recently changed the way hospitals manage fetal demise.

☐ *Prostaglandins for Labor Induction*   The more advanced hospitals are now using a new method—prostaglandin E2 suppositories—to induce labor in a case of fetal demise, rather than waiting for the woman to go into labor naturally or inducing labor with pitocin. As soon as a diagnosis has been made, the patient is admitted to the hospital and the uterus emptied with the aid of these labor-inducing prostaglandins. Suppositories inserted in the vagina every two or three hours will initiate uterine contractions, open up the uterus, and result in the delivery of the fetus in less than ten hours. Once the uterus is empty, it will heal faster.

Prostaglandin suppositories are a relatively new method of induction that some obstetricians might not be familiar with, even though most major university hospitals throughout the world are now using them to initiate labor. Consequently, an obstetrician who is less familiar with modern methods might advise a patient to wait rather than giving her the option of inducing labor immediately. In this case, I think a woman would be fully justified in seeking a second opinion in a large institution. I have personally conducted a number of studies on fetal demise and have helped many couples through the emotional trauma and grief associated with this experience. In my opinion, the best cure is immediate termination of the unsuccessful pregnancy, followed by conception within a few months. Many of these women have beautiful healthy children in their subsequent pregnancies.

☐ *Changes in the Amniotic Fluid Volume*   The supply of amniotic fluid is not, as was once thought, an inert, stagnant pool of liquid but a continually changing stream of fluid carried by ongoing interchanges between the amniotic sac and the maternal and fetal circulation. The fluid is thought to be partly produced by the fetal urine and partly secreted by the maternal circulation across the placenta and the fetal membranes, although the umbilical cord and the fetal lungs do produce a small amount of it. It is present very early in pregnancy, even in pregnancies in which the ovum fails to develop into a fetus, which would suggest that it is first secreted from the fetal membranes.

The fluid circulates and is replenished constantly; most of it is swallowed by the fetus and subsequently excreted as urine; some is reabsorbed through the fetal membranes and the umbilical cord. A total turnover of amniotic fluid is believed to occur once every few hours.

☐ *How Much Amniotic Fluid Is There Normally?*   The amount of amniotic fluid varies greatly from one pregnancy to another. In very early pregnancy, the amount of liquid exceeds the size of the embryo, but by the twelfth week the fetus is slightly bigger than the total amount of fluid present in the sac. There are approximately 30 cc of fluid at ten weeks' gestation; this increases by about 25 cc per week to reach 800 at term, although there are considerable differences among term pregnancies. It is this change in the amniotic-fluid volume that the physician must observe carefully, since it could alter the outcome of the pregnancy.

☐ *Oligohydramnios—Too Little Amniotic Fluid*   Too little amniotic fluid could present a dangerous situation, since the amniotic fluid is there to help buffer the baby and protect the umbilical cord. With an insufficient amount of fluid, there is a chance of the cord being strangulated and cutting off the oxygen supply to the fetus. More attention has recently been paid to this problem, and ultrasonography is now frequently used to monitor the supply of amniotic fluid.

In certain cases of fetal abnormality, particularly with kidney or urinary-tract malformations, oligohydramnios can occur. A physician who observes a decrease in the amniotic-fluid volume by manual examination should perform a sonogram to determine whether a kidney is missing or there is some other kidney or urinary-tract abnormality. This can be done with sophisticated ultrasound machines designed to focus on specific organs. At least one baby with a urinary tract obstruction has been saved by fetal surgery performed *in utero*, and other successful attempts will surely follow.

Oligohydramnios is also found in women with chronic hypertension whose pregnancies are often complicated by intrauterine growth retardation and unusually small placentas. A smaller placenta produces less amniotic fluid, causing another problem, since the fetus is not that well protected. Once again, a woman should be followed by ultrasound and fetal monitoring to determine the best time for delivery, before the baby is damaged or succumbs *in utero*. The same problem has been detected in the pregnancies of heavy smokers in which the blood supply to the placenta is considerably less than normal. Women at risk need extra bed rest to assure a freer flow of blood to the placenta and a greater production of amniotic fluid to protect the baby.

☐ *Polyhydramnios—Too Much Amniotic Fluid*   Polyhydramnios is associated with several abnormalities. Too much amniotic fluid detected early in pregnancy could be a sign of fetal congenital malformation, since obstructions of the esophagus, trachea, or fetal digestive channels would prevent the fetus from swallowing the usual amount of fluid. Polyhydramnios detected early in pregnancy should be followed carefully with ultrasound examinations. There are, however, other conditions aside from congenital malformations in which excessive amniotic fluid is produced. It is particularly common in diabetic pregnancies, because a larger baby produces more urine and the larger placenta and umbilical cord secrete a greater amount of fluid. On the other hand, the baby may simply be a large baby in an otherwise normal pregnancy. Polyhydramnios is also found in multiple births, which, once again, is understandable because each fetus is surrounded by fluid.

An excess of fluid within a certain level is generally not as dangerous as too little fluid, since the umbilical cord is properly protected. The extra fluid does, however, add a considerable amount of weight, which makes it much harder for the woman to walk around. Where there is more amniotic fluid there is also more pressure on the uterine walls, so the chance of stimulating the uterus into premature labor is much higher.

A physician who detects polyhydramnios must send the patient for immediate evaluation with ultrasound and other special tests, and try to reach some conclusions on the origin of the condition. Sometimes no abnormality is found, or only a mild one, and in certain cases a child has subsequently been delivered with a slight malformation of the cardiovascular or fetal digestive system that was believed to be the cause of the polyhydramnios. In other words, the condition could mean a congenital malformation, but very often it simply indicates a large baby or a prediabetic state. Occasionally the reason for the excess fluid is never discovered, and a normal baby is born in good health. This does not, however, mean that your doctor can safely ignore the condition if you are much larger or heavier than you should be. When your regular obstetrician fails to do the necessary tests, you should get a second opinion. It might require making a special appointment at a university medical center where there is sophisticated testing equipment, but it is well worth the extra travel and expense.

☐ *Amniotic-Fluid Infections*   The amniotic fluid rarely gets infected before the fetal membranes rupture. Even then infection might not occur, since the fluid has bacteria-destroying properties, which vary in effectiveness from person to person. A woman in good health, particularly a woman with sufficient zinc intake, is usually better able to fight infection than a poorly nourished woman.

Infections of the amniotic fluid are usually introduced by sexual intercourse or by the physician's finger during an internal examination. The latter makes it advisable to have as few internal examinations as possible once the membranes have ruptured. Fortunately, the time between rupture at term and the onset of labor is short in most cases—80 percent of women go into full labor within twenty-four hours. If labor does not occur spontaneously, most physicians will elect to induce labor rather than risk infection attacking the uterus or the baby itself.

When the membranes rupture prematurely (what is known as PROM—premature rupture of the membranes), a doctor might either decide to induce labor or, if possible, await further fetal maturation. An infection that sets in at this point can be very dangerous, and will require aggressive antibiotic treatment. (See discussion earlier in this chapter.)

☐ *Trauma in Pregnancy*   In early pregnancy, the uterus is small enough to be sheltered by the pelvic bones and is rarely penetrated when injury occurs. But as the uterus increases in size, it becomes much more susceptible to damage. An automobile accident or fall in which the uterus forcibly comes into contact with a hard object can result in the placenta's separating from the uterus and causing fetal demise. You can reduce the risk of injury in the car by wearing a shoulder harness or lap belt at all times.

Another type of accident in which the fetus is vulnerable is a direct assault on the uterus with a penetrating object. An accident involving the penetration of the uterus by a bullet or sharp instrument often results in fetal death in the latter months of pregnancy when the uterus takes up the greater part of the abdominal cavity and protects the mother's vital organs from the full force of the blow. In these circumstances the fetus is likely to die and the mother to survive.

☐ *Management of Trauma in Pregnancy*   When a pregnant woman has suffered a serious accident and arrives in the emergency room with abdominal trauma, the emergency room physician must immediately evaluate her general condition and then call in an obstetrician. If the fetus has sustained direct damage, an emergency Cesarean is usually performed, although a few cases are on record in which an injured baby was born alive at term. In a case of placental separation due to an accident, however, the baby's heart rate may be so severely depressed that the physician cannot await delivery and a quick Cesarean section is called for. Each trauma case is special and different and should be treated individually.

An Important Note: The obstetrician's office is not equipped to deal with severe trauma. A woman who sustains injury during pregnancy should go to the emergency room of the nearest hospital if she cannot get in touch with her doctor right away. Immediate care can be given in the hospital, and the obstetrical unit is always at hand if obstetrical care or delivery is indicated.

☐ *Ovarian Cyst and Pregnancy*   Ovarian tumors are rare during pregnancy, although pregnant women have no specific mechanism to prevent their development. Nevertheless, the occasional cyst is found during a pregnancy, and the woman could experience problems. A cyst sometimes causes internal bleeding, or turns malignant, requiring specialized treatment. Furthermore, it could twist, causing tremendous pain and the formation of blood clots.

A modern diagnosis is usually obtained by ultrasonographic techniques, although it often is impossible to determine whether the cyst is benign or malignant. This is, naturally, a difficult situation since one is always afraid of malignancy. A suspicious cyst found early in pregnancy is usually removed surgically and biopsied. If the cyst is found later in pregnancy, the uterus is so large that it might be better to wait until fetal maturation and then deliver by Cesarean section and at the same time biopsy the cyst. If vaginal delivery is possible, it may be advisable to wait until after the delivery to evaluate the cyst. In the end, each case must be treated individually. However, an occasional cyst is so large that it obstructs the birth canal, and a Cesarean section is the only mode of delivery.

☐ *Cryosurgery During Pregnancy*   Noncancerous cervical abnormalities are often treated by cryosurgery, a freezing technique by which the cervical cells are destroyed. This is a common procedure, but it is not one that should be encouraged during pregnancy. The freezing could reach into the uterus and could directly harm the developing fetus or interfere with the blood supply to it. Although there are physicians who have performed cryosurgery on pregnant women whose babies have survived, a woman whose doctor suggests cryosurgery during pregnancy (as many do) should refrain and seek a second opinion at a university hospital from a perinatologist. A specialist is highly unlikely to recommend cryosurgery during pregnancy because there is a marked increase in cervical bleeding after the operation and a likelihood of continued bleeding, infection, and other serious complications in the period following the procedure.

☐ *Surgery During Pregnancy*   On occasions surgery becomes necessary during a pregnancy. The safest time for a surgical procedure is in the first half of pregnancy, when there is less risk of premature labor and the uterus is small enough to allow for an abdominal procedure, should that be necessary. If a woman does need an emergency surgical procedure in the last half of pregnancy, the higher risk of premature labor can be counteracted by a uterine relaxant medication such as ritodrine. Even an abdominal procedure such as *appendectomy* during pregnancy can be performed with very little problem if proper anesthesia is available, although the patient must be watched very carefully in the postsurgical period to prevent the onset of premature labor.

Penicillin can be used routinely after various forms of surgery or to combat certain infections during pregnancy, as it would in the nonpregnant state. If you are allergic to penicillin, keflex can be used instead, with no adverse effect on the baby.

☐ *Shirodkar Suture*   A Shirodkar suture, or drawstring of the cervix, is a surgical procedure that is often performed in pregnancy to secure the cervix and prevent its dilating prematurely. The suture is usually inserted at the thirteenth or fourteenth week of gestation. The patient is first anesthetized and then placed in the stirrups. The cervix is visualized and grasped with an instrument while a small incision is made in the front and back of it. The suture, or drawstring, which is made of nonabsorbable suture material, is then placed under the cervical mucosa, the outer layer of the cervix, and tied down firmly to keep the cervix closed. Once the drawstring is in place, the cervical mucosa is closed with catgut so that no part of the suture is exposed. A modification of this technique, the *McDonald suture*, is a simpler procedure in which the suture is placed around the cervix on the outside of the cervical mucosa and then tied down. In both procedures, the suture is removed at term to allow labor to proceed normally.

Either technique effectively prevents the onset of premature labor in up to 80 percent of cases in which the initial procedure is performed successfully. One potential problem during placement of the suture is the risk of triggering labor. The patient should, therefore, be observed for some time after the procedure and even given Yutopar (ritodrine) or some other uterine relaxing medication if the uterus does begin to contract. A woman with an incompetent cervix who has had a Shirodkar suture placed has a much higher chance of carrying to term, but she still needs to take it easy—get extra bed rest and she might even have to be placed on Yutopar for several months. But a careful evaluation of the initial problem should always be made before a doctor goes ahead with the procedure; when the procedure is performed too late in pregnancy or is done inappropriately, premature labor can result.

☐ *It Need Not Be That Serious!*   Many potentially serious problems can come up in pregnancy, but if a woman is alert and knows her body, she might well be able to prevent a disaster by avoiding situations known to trigger complications. Taking extra good care of yourself, with proper nutrition, prenatal vitamins, and plenty of rest, is certainly one of the most important steps toward a good pregnancy.

If a serious problem does occur, seek help immediately. Sometimes you will appreciate the seriousness of your problem more quickly than your doctor. Your knowledge of the problem might then help your doctor identify and treat a complication before it threatens you or the baby, in time to make the rest of the pregnancy a healthy one.

26

Preparation for Childbirth

Appreciating the pleasures of pregnancy and childbirth is a new phenomenon. We have only to look back to childbirth practices a few years ago when the woman was routinely separated from her family in the hospital, and routinely separated from her child after birth, to realize how much and how quickly childbirth practices have changed. It is only in the last few years that childbirth has even been considered the sphere of both parents. Births at home had always been the business of the midwife and the woman's female relatives, while the husband waited outside. This tradition persisted into modern life when deliveries were moved from the home and into the hospital, where women were left alone with the hospital staff and their doctors. Only in the last decade have both parents been allowed in the delivery room. The change has been so successful that new parents are no longer willing to put up with hospital rules or cultural taboos that separate them during the birth of their child.

A new, revolutionary view of childbirth has emerged. Rather than a traumatic, painful necessity, childbirth is now seen as a normal, joyful event in a couple's life. No one knows how the majority of women in the past felt about childbirth, because their experiences are not recorded, but culturally, childbirth has been considered a fearful event. In Western countries at least, this fear was handed down from generation to generation and was reinforced by myths, history, and religion. According to the English translation of the Old Testament, God himself ordained the pain and hazards of childbirth, as a punishment for Eve's original sin in the Garden of Eden. "Unto the woman he said, I will greatly multiply thy sorrow, and thy conception: in sorrow thou shalt bring forth children"; Genesis 3:16. (There is controversy among biblical scholars as to whether or not the original Hebrew referred to "hard work" rather than "sorrow.") Throughout the Middle Ages and beyond, the churches taught that childbirth was painful and dangerous, and there is no doubt that the fear of childbirth was shared by many people, since birth was indeed one of the most dangerous times in a woman's life. Pain in childbirth was, therefore, invested with great significance, and even in the nineteenth century, pious women were known to don shrouds at the first sign of labor. It is only in the last half century that modern obstetrics has diminished this fear to the point that, though a woman may be apprehensive about labor, it is no longer considered fearful. That has made it possible for us to consider childbirth in a very different light from that of a hundred years ago. Part of this change is our approach to what has been traditionally known as the "pain of childbirth."

☐ *History of Pain Relief in Childbirth*   History deals with the extraordinary rather than the ordinary. The standard histories of almost any Western country inevitably include horrifying stories of women who suffered agony during labor or died in childbirth but little information about the thousands of women who had easy, safe, natural deliveries and suffered little or no discomfort in the process. Our perception of childbirth has naturally been affected by these cultural associations of pain and suffering with birth, associations which do not exist as powerfully in other cultures.

In the past, women were generally looked after by older women who had themselves borne children and who therefore understood the emotions of the laboring mother and provided her with a degree of sympathy and understanding. This in itself probably acted as an effective method of pain relief. (The tradition is continued in the granny midwives of Africa, Asia, and South America, who still attend most of the births taking place today.) Many of these births were, and are, unmedicated. But there must always have been a minority of births in which labor was not easy, and the birth attendants sought to alleviate the mother's pain by more potent substances.

Various civilizations have used their own means to control the pain of labor; with the majority calling on supernatural forces to aid them in their efforts. Hence we find the use of charms, witchcraft, and the creation of special gods whose function it was to take care of pregnant women or women in labor. Among certain North American Indian tribes, this took the form of ritual chanting as the midwife and the woman's family attempted to lure the recalcitrant baby out of the womb. Other cultures favored herbs and salves as forms of pain relief.

Then in 1847, after thousands of years in which no effective pain relief was available, the Scottish physician Dr. James Young Simpson administered ether to a woman in labor in Edinburgh. Although different anesthetics, including opium in the form of laudanum, had been used by European physicians, Dr. Simpson must be credited with the first effective obstetrical anesthesia. Later in the same year he used chloroform, also for the first time, and began a fashion for "painless" birth among those women, like Queen Victoria, who were able to afford a private physician. Chloroform was followed by a number of other forms of relief: scopolamine, "twilight sleep," and the general anesthetics routinely administered to women in labor only twenty-five years ago when women were told the birth of a child was so painful it was better to be unconscious during the delivery rather than suffer the agonies of the birth. These forms of pain relief persisted despite the obvious disorientation suffered by mothers who were removed from any active participation in their children's delivery.

In the last two decades, greater interest has been shown in various methods of relieving or controlling pain during labor and delivery, while restoring the mother's active role. Different forms of pain relief fall broadly into four categories: (1) psychoprophylaxis and hypnosis; (2) drugs to alleviate either anxiety or pain; (3) regional and local anesthesia; (4) general anesthesia. The first category is the subject of this chapter.

☐ *Understanding Pain*   Pain is difficult to understand, in part because it varies so greatly from one person to another. There is no way to measure pain; one cannot think of pain in ounces or pounds, since pain is merely the way our cerebral cortex, the nerve center located in the brain, interprets certain stimuli in various parts of the body. However, there is no doubt that we do perceive pain, and it can vary greatly in intensity.

As human beings, we fear pain, but pain is a real and vital part of our body's protective mechanism. The ability to feel pain is important because pain sends out signals to the brain that prompt us to evaluate what the pain means. Unfortunately, if there is too much pain, it can be impossible to cope with it.

Recent studies have shown that *beta-endorphin,* a hormone released naturally by the body, is a self-made natural pain-killer. Since beta-endorphin is produced in larger quantities by some people as they anticipate a higher degree of pain, you might well encourage your body to release more beta-endorphins as you go into stronger labor. If you are generally frightened and confused, but are not prepared specifically for pain, beta-endorphins will not be released in such large quantities and the pain will be unalleviated. By anticipation and preparation, a relaxed person in control of her own body might produce her own anesthetic during labor and delivery.

No one knows how he or she will react to pain before the pain occurs. Often fear of pain makes it worse, since the person becomes disoriented. Then as the pain gets worse, a vicious circle often begins: the pain is followed by fear, and fear by pain, with each stage growing more intense and more intractable. If, in such a circle, the subject could stop, reevaluate the pain and start self-hypnosis, psychoprophylaxis, or some other relaxation technique, one could possibly begin to decrease the amount of pain by mind control alone.

☐ *Childbirth Pain—Is it Real?*   There are certain forms of pain we have been taught to fear more than others. One is the pain experienced in the dentist's office and another is pain in childbirth. Anticipation and fear are associated with both of these procedures, although both of them are much easier now than in the past.

Most women approach childbirth as they would a visit to the dentist. They have been told that childbirth will hurt, and they expect it to hurt. There is more than a chance that it will hurt when fear and tension are present, as this increases a woman's discomfort and retards her labor. As Dr. Grantly Dick-Read said in his book *Childbirth Without Fear**: "Tense woman, tense cervix." By a

* *Childbirth Without Fear,* by Dr. Grantly Dick-Read (Harper & Row, 1978).

realistic anticipation of pain and proper preparation it might be possible to control it better.

No one can describe exactly how painful labor is, since the experience varies from one person to another. Most childbirth educators feel there is some degree of discomfort during labor that cannot be taken away simply by understanding the process. Even Dr. Dick-Read, who believed firmly in a natural labor and delivery, never spoke of "childbirth without pain" but only "childbirth without fear." Pain, however, increases with anxiety and fear. A woman who understands the process of labor and delivery is well prepared to demystify and consequently diminish labor pain. There are relaxation exercises as well that will help the body cope more easily with the discomforts of labor. Still, there is some pain in normal labor, and abnormal labor can result in considerable pain.

☐ *Do the Contractions Cause Pain?*   Labor contractions are simply constrictions and relaxations of the uterine muscles, similar to the movements you make when you contract and relax your biceps muscles. They change in intensity in the different stages of labor. Uterine contractions in early labor are meant to prepare the uterus and cervix for childbirth and are not usually painful unless a woman is tense. They can last for a few hours to a few days. During this early stage, the contractions will release hormones that change the nature of the cervical tissue. First it becomes softer and then it begins to efface itself in preparation for the active stage of labor. This initial stage is generally not painful. Pain is usually associated with progressive dilation of the cervix (see Chapt. 27). A few women in early labor do complain of pain when they experience a prolonged uterine contraction, causing a decrease in oxygenation in the uterine muscle. This is felt as a constrictive pain, rather like a charley horse. Though rare in the first stages of labor, if it does occur, it causes real pain. Generally a woman who experiences pain at this point of labor has an unusually low pain threshold, or she is so fearful of labor that she tenses up all the pelvic muscles, working against the natural contractions of the uterus and the softening of the cervix. This will cause longer labor as well as emotional and physical pain.

As labor progresses and the contractions become harder, some pain is likely; how much depends again on a woman's pain threshold or on her attitude to labor. As the cervix dilates from five to ten centimeters, the most intense period of labor, most women will experience some pain, although it can be diminished by a confident attitude and relaxation and breathing techniques. If labor has been induced with oxytocin (Pitocin), the labor is artificial and is much harder and therefore more painful. One woman whose second baby I recently delivered, and whose previous labor had been induced, could not believe the difference between the two experiences. She used no medication at all in her second labor, relaxed completely through breathing techniques, and had almost no pain. A second labor is almost always easier, but a second induced labor or the second labor of a frightened mother is likely to be as painful as the first.

☐ *Suggestion for the Control of Pain*   Alleviating pain during labor without drugs depends first of all on removing psychological worries about the unknown through education and understanding. What is known as suggestion is a very powerful factor in controlling discomfort and pain in labor, but suggestion can also do harm by perpetuating myths about the agony of labor. Think of the disastrous psychological damage that might be inflicted on a small girl who listens to her mother's account of the agonies of labor and who is unlikely ever to think of labor except with fear. When a woman has grown up with the fear and anxiety of her mother's experiences, it will naturally be difficult to eliminate all her fears and tensions later on as she goes into labor herself. Horror stories about labor and delivery heard in early childhood are often difficult to eradicate in later life.

Methods of suggestion introduced during a childbirth preparation course are based on a positive attitude to labor and delivery. The complete elimination of apprehension and fear is the first step toward understanding pain and the control of pain. Otherwise fear will produce tension, and tension inevitably will produce pain. This is the triad known as *the fear-tension-pain syndrome*. A woman who is fearful in labor naturally tenses her muscles and, whether she is aware of it or not, fights every contraction instead of allowing the cervix and uterus to perform their natural function. Labor then becomes painful. The vicious circle continues and only becomes more acute as labor progresses and the contractions become longer and harder. Once labor is accepted as a natural function, one that should be desired, not feared, a powerful suggestive force in the labor experience has been established. An educated woman whose fears of exaggerated suffering during birth have been allayed is free to concentrate on other facts of the labor experience besides physical discomfort. She need no longer anticipate unbearable pain.

Conditioning is derived from other sources besides the woman's preconceived ideas of childbirth. The woman's family, her obstetrician, and the place in which she gives birth are all powerful influences. This is one of the reasons why fathers are encouraged to join their partners at the labor and delivery times and why enlightened hospitals are trying to make the hospital environment more homelike. A woman in labor is more likely to do well if she is given support. Even if the woman herself is initially relaxed, insensitive handling of the birth can produce such tension that cervical dilation is affected—a phenomenon also seen in animals, whose labors often stop completely if they are disturbed.

Certain childbirth methods, notably the *psychoprophylactic (Lamaze) method,* go beyond understanding and realization and introduce various exercises designed to create a new area of concentration during labor. These consist of breathing techniques, which change according to each stage of labor, accompanied by a fingertip massage known as *effleurage.* A certain amount of distraction is thus built into the pattern of labor to remove the laboring woman's attention from the pain of the uterine contractions and thereby reduce their intensity. This is an acknowledgment that labor is not and cannot be truly painless even though certain women testify to nothing more than mild discomfort during their own deliveries. It would be foolish to promise any woman a painless labor and delivery. But even though there is some residual pain in labor and delivery, modern techniques should help make pregnancy, labor, and delivery unforgettable and beautiful events rather than the fearful occasions of the past. It is important for us to have a complete understanding of what happens through the phases of childbirth. I hope to give you and your partner a good preparation for childbirth in the following pages.

☐ *The Use of Pain Relief* There is still said to be some antagonism between people who believe in a completely unmedicated childbirth and those who feel that pain-killers during labor and delivery are necessary. Both approaches are too dogmatic. Any responsible childbirth education class talks about abnormal labor, which no woman can be expected to go through without assistance, and about the different perceptions of pain among different women. However much a woman wants to be in control, she should never be ashamed to accept analgesics or anesthesia at some stage of labor and delivery if she experiences pain. This does not mean she is a failure; it simply means that her perception of pain makes it too difficult to cope with. Excessive anxiety in labor and delivery could be worse than asking for some kind of medication.

☐ *Hypnosis* Hypnosis or hypnotic aids for the relief of pain during childbirth have been used for centuries by many cultures and are simple enough to be practiced by the modern laboring woman. They do have disadvantages as well as advantages. Since the pregnant woman is particularly susceptible to hypnotic influences, she might be very receptive to hypnosis. But the use of hypnosis does alter the labor experience in ways that might not be beneficial.

Despite the mystique of hypnosis, there is nothing mysterious about the techniques that are used, even though the exact mechanism that produces it is unknown. Any interested person can easily learn it. First of all, the subject lies down and makes herself comfortable. (The room should be quiet and the subject mentally as well as physically relaxed.) The hypnotist will then suggest a state of deeper relaxation, leading to a trancelike condition in which the subject experiences amnesia and drifts into what is known as a fugistic stage. The subject is now highly susceptible to commands from the hypnotist. A pregnant woman is told that labor will be relatively pain-free or much less painful than she previously believed. In this respect there is a close comparison between the principles of hypnosis and the underlying principles of most childbirth relaxation techniques. Research with willing subjects has shown that about 50 percent of them can be trained in hypnotic techniques and hypnotized to a level at which they no longer experience pain during labor.

There are three major problems associated with hypnosis during labor. First of all, it is a time-consuming discipline because the hypnotist can work successfully with only a comparatively small number of patients. The second disadvantage is the occasional state of deep self-hypnosis it induces, which can lead to a serious and prolonged emotional disturbance. Neither of these two, however, is as important as the third: the state of dissociation experienced during hypnosis. Psychologically as well as physically, it is important for a woman consciously to push her child out into the world and bond with the child after birth. Alleviating the pain with hypnosis effectively removes the woman from participating in one of the great events of life. Only a very few women would regard a complete loss of consciousness a reasonable compensation for the loss of pain.

☐ *Prepared Childbirth* Childbirth education has changed the way many women feel about labor and delivery, decreased their anxiety, and resulted in a much healthier birth for the baby. By now there are at least an estimated 7500 practicing childbirth educators in the United States. It should be possible for every couple to find an educator in prepared childbirth. A good class gives a basic knowledge of the physiological changes during pregnancy, preparation for labor, and includes open discussions on childbirth and hospital techniques. Organization of classes differs, but a course of six classes is most often given in the last trimester, frequently preceded by one or two classes in the early months of pregnancy to deal with physical changes, fetal development, and emotional adjustment.

The emphasis in most classes is on what is known as "prepared childbirth" rather than "natural childbirth," the phrase originally used by Dr. Grantly Dick-Read, the British doctor who pioneered the natural-childbirth approach to labor and delivery. Prepared childbirth tends to emphasize a thorough preparation for hospital birth, including information on Cesareans, anesthesia, and active methods of pain relief in labor (the psychoprophylactic method). Many classes in the United States follow the basic methods of Dr. Fernand Lamaze, an obstetrician who introduced the psychoprophylactic method in France. A more recent approach to childbirth education, the Bradley method, which combines elements of Dick-Read's with those of Lamaze, is gaining increasing popularity. Organizations to contact for information on childbirth education are:

1. *The American Society for Psychoprophylaxis in Obstetrics, Inc.* (ASPO), 1411 K Street N.W., Washington, D.C. 20005
2. *The International Childbirth Education Association*, Box 20048, Minneapolis, Minnesota 55420
3. *The American Academy of Husband-Coached Childbirth*, P.O. Box 5224, Sherman Oaks, California 91413.

The principles of both natural childbirth and psychoprophylaxis have been known and practiced for many centuries throughout different civilizations. It was not until the twentieth century, however, that either approach was taught to women through formal instruction.

☐ *Childbirth Without Fear* When the famous British physician Dr. Grantly Dick-Read wrote the first draft of his book *Childbirth Without Fear* in the 1920s, his revolutionary theory of natural childbirth was based on observations of hundreds of women in labor, some under extremely adverse conditions. Experiences with frightened women and women who remained unexpectedly calm and free from pain had convinced him that women who had not acquired a fear of labor did not experience the pain or apprehension that is normally associated with childbirth in a civilized society. Consequently, he believed that normal childbirth need not be a pathological event; instead he spoke of the naturalness of labor and the inherent joyfulness of birth. This was quite contrary to the medical teaching of the day, which regarded labor as painful and difficult, and led to considerable opposition to his book by contemporary doctors. His natural-childbirth methods were based on the principle that fear, tension and pain are inextricably linked. Fear, according to Dick-Read, produces mental and physical tension; and physical tension then causes muscular pain. He believed this affects the natural relaxation of the muscles in the uterus, particularly the cervix, prolonging labor and intensifying the pain. A vicious circle of fear, tension, and pain is then established that can be broken only by removing the fear of labor. This he accomplished by simple instruction during pregnancy and a

able aspects of psychoprophylaxis is its realistic approach to obstetrical difficulties such as abnormalities that are out of your control; labor can be painful and you should not feel guilty if you need some form of analgesia or anesthesia. Even then, trained mothers are less tense and usually need less medication than an unprepared woman. Since the mother and father are well educated in the physiology of the labor process as well as the effect of drugs in general on labor and delivery, a couple can become active partners even when medication is called for.

☐ *Does Lamaze Work?*   This is a question that doctors have asked ever since the Lamaze method of childbirth education became popular. Over the years a number of medical concerns have been voiced, from the potential dangers of minimum or nonexistent anesthesia to the tendency of Lamaze training to induce hyperventilation. Obstetricians have even questioned the safety of the father's presence in the delivery room. Of course, part of the problem is that the more conservative members of the profession have had to adapt their methods to accommodate their patients—a compromise many of them have resented. There are still no definitive answers, but a few studies have been done that generally show that Lamaze has scientifically measurable beneficial effects on maternal attitude, maternal anxiety, as well as the amount of anesthesia and analgesia used in delivery. Patients taking Lamaze courses have been compared with groups of unprepared women and have been found to have one-quarter the number of Cesarean sections and one-fifth the amount of fetal distress of the unprepared group. Similarly, a group of Lamaze-prepared women in Chicago had fewer perinatal lacerations, postpartum infections, and other serious postpartum problems than a matching control group. Inexplicably, the unprepared women also had three times the number of toxemia cases and twice as many cases of premature labor. Some members of the medical profession may still feel that childbirth education is unproven, but the studies conducted in Chicago and elsewhere have clearly shown its medical benefits. The emotional benefits are probably immeasurable, in part because they can be estimated only by the couple themselves.

☐ *The Bradley Technique: Husband-Coached Childbirth*   In the 1960s Dr. Robert Bradley's technique of childbirth began to gain popularity in the United States. Dr. Robert Bradley was one of the first American obstetricians to follow Dick-Read's pioneering work with his own method of giving birth without drugs. He attributed his firm belief in a natural approach to childbirth in part to his boyhood in Kansas, where he saw horses, cows, and other animals give birth easily and the newborn struggle to its feet immediately, alert and responsive, not drugged and depressed. As a medical student a few years later, he could only contrast birth in nature favorably with the way humans were born. When he started doing deliveries himself, he began teaching women to approach labor with the instinctive natural behavior of animals.

What was later to be known as the Bradley method was an unmedicated labor and delivery, using slow natural breathing (in contrast with the Lamaze method) and complete relaxation. At the same time Bradley adopted the Lamaze concept of the labor coach wholeheartedly, encouraging fathers to enter hospital delivery rooms and act as labor coaches for their wives. He encouraged other unconventional practices, including immediate breast-feeding of the newborn on the delivery table or in the recovery room. He was also one of the first obstetricians to insist that the baby remain with the mother at all times rather than be isolated from her in the hospital nursery. Dr. Bradley has, perhaps, had a greater influence on modern hospitals than many people who know his name are aware of, an influence which is still continuing among modern parents. He always believed in hospital deliveries, although he saw the need to create a homelike environment for parents.

The Bradley method places the husband in a central role rather than as a supporting figure in the birth experience, a concept suggested by "husband-coached childbirth," the other name for the Bradley method. Unlike the Lamaze classes, a Bradley class is taught by a husband-and-wife team who are trained childbirth educators and have been through a Bradley birth themselves. Bradley teachers, certified by The American Academy of Husband-Coached Childbirth, are more commonly found in the West rather than along the East Coast of the U.S. They differ from the Lamaze instructors in stressing the entire childbirth experience rather than labor and delivery, and in promoting somewhat different techniques during the delivery itself. Instead of intricate breathing patterns, Bradley classes emphasize complete relaxation and natural breathing without acceleration or effleurage. The idea is for the woman to become aware of her body and learn to work with it in labor rather than create distractions to deal with discomfort.

The use of medications is actively discouraged in a Bradley class, in comparison with the moderate approach of the Lamaze classes. The husband is trained to coach his wife through labor and delivery and to allow her to maintain her concentration by himself dealing with the distractions of the hospital routine. In this area the Bradley method has been criticized, because it takes away a part of the woman's responsibility and gives it to the husband and the obstetrician. Nonetheless, the Bradley courses do strongly emphasize effective communication between both parents and the doctor and hospital staff to achieve an individual birth experience. (This is certainly a part of the changes that have been going on in hospitals in the last few years, now that hospitals understand the greater demands of the public.) Finally, labor and delivery are viewed, not as an isolated experience, but as a part of the whole experience of bearing and raising children. This is also, in my opinion, a concept we should focus on more emphatically: the total childbirth experience, which begins even before the baby is conceived and includes proper care before birth, a safe, natural delivery, as well as plans for the child's future.

☐ *Preparation for Childbirth Techniques*   Any one of the modern childbirth techniques is effective, but since a majority of childbirth educators and the women in my own practice follow a modified form of Lamaze, a group of Lamaze relaxation exercises and breathing techniques are included here to act as a guide for Lamaze-trained women.

☐ *The Stages of Labor*   Labor is divided into three different stages. *The first stage* is timed from the onset of labor when the uterus begins to contract and continues until the time the cervix is fully dilated (see Chapters 27 and 29 on labor and delivery). *The second stage* begins when the cervix is fully dilated and ends with the actual delivery of the baby. This is the period of labor in which the laboring woman can actively expel the baby by pushing. *The third stage* is the period of up to twenty minutes after the delivery of the baby, which ends with the delivery of the placenta.

☐ **Relaxation Exercises**   The object of any relaxation exercise is to learn muscle control and the conscious relaxation of muscle groups. During labor a woman uses certain muscle groups actively, particularly those found in the uterus, while others must remain relaxed. Relaxation assists the work of the uterus by allowing it to expand and dilate in an unhindered way. Even the simple tension expressed in the woman's facial expressions, or the clenching or un-clenching of the fingers can contribute to tension within the uterus. The following *tension-relieving exercises* will help you become aware of the different muscle groups so you can bring them under voluntary control. This will conserve the energy you need during labor and delivery and prevent unnecessary tension, which might otherwise lead to pain.

FIRST: Relax completely; your coach should check your relaxation before and during the following exercises to help you relax more effectively.

EXERCISE 1: Contract right arm, release it. Contract left arm, release it.

EXERCISE 2: Contract right arm, release it. Contract left arm, release it.

EXERCISE 3: Contract right arm and right leg and release them. Contract left arm and left leg and release them.

EXERCISE 4: Contract right arm and left leg and release them. Contract left arm and right leg and release them.

Your daily practice session should include various commands to contract and release combinations of muscle groups, including the abdomen, neck, shoulders, buttocks, and vaginal-floor muscles as well as the arms and legs. While you are practicing, make sure that the other muscles are completely relaxed. Daily practice is important. Your partner can assist you by giving commands and by checking your relaxation, making sure that you remain perfectly relaxed between contractions, and during contractions. These are not easy exercises; they demand practice and absolute concentration before you can learn to isolate muscle groups and relax on command.

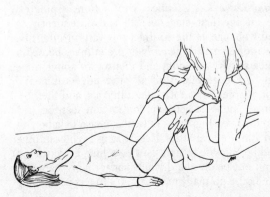

Figure 63: The Coach's Role: As your pregnancy draws closer to term, you can begin a close collaboration with your labor coach. The work of the coach is important in building strength and suppleness as well as in developing the breathing and relaxing exercises used during labor. In this illustration the woman is strengthening her leg muscles by applying pressure against her coach's hands—a good way to learn to control the voluntary muscles in collaboration with your coach.

☐ *Muscle-Building Exercises*   This group of exercises is used to improve the general well-being of muscle tone and circulation. The lying-down exercises should be performed on a flat surface (a carpeted floor or a mat is recommended). The legs should be bent at the knees, with the feet flat on the floor. Begin each exercise after a cleansing breath.

EXERCISE 1: Inhale slowly through the nose while raising the right leg slowly, with the toes pointed (do not point the toes if you have a tendency to leg or foot cramps). Then exhale slowly through the mouth as you lower the right leg slowly, foot flexed, until the leg is flat on the floor. Inhale slowly as you slide the leg back to the starting position with the knee bent. Then exhale. Repeat the exercise with the other leg.

EXERCISE 2: While still in the knee-bent position, do the pelvic rock. Begin with a deep inhalation and then slowly exhale as you pull the abdominal muscles in tight and allow the small of the back to press against the floor. Then slowly inhale as you relax the abdominal muscles and see the abdominal muscles rise while your back moves away from the floor. This should be repeated at least ten times.

EXERCISE 3: Pelvic floor concentration and relaxation. Contract the vaginal floor muscles (sphincter, vagina, and urethra) slowly to the count of six; then release slowly to the count of six. Repeat ten times.

EXERCISE 4: Slowly contract the abdominal muscles to the count of six. Relax slowly to the count of six. Repeat ten times.

EXERCISE 5: Sit on the floor in a cross-legged position (tailor or Indian fashion) for the pelvic stretch or the stretching of the thigh muscles. Next place the soles of your feet together, pull the feet as close to the body as is comfortable, using your thigh muscles, and press the knees gently toward the floor while adding opposite pressure under the knee with the palms of your hands.

EXERCISE 6: To rise from the lying position you should bend the knees, turn from your back to your side, and push up with both arms until you are on your knees. Then rise slowly.

☐ *Breathing Techniques During Labor*   Uterine contractions progress through three distinct phases in the first stage of labor. Consequently, a woman's approach to labor must change as the contractions vary in intensity. The beginning of the first stage is often called the *early* or *preliminary phase,* in which the cervix begins to efface slowly, softening and dilating to about three centimeters, or what is known by the hospital staff as "1½ fingers dilated." During this phase the contractions come first at irregular intervals, and then become regular enough to be timed. Intervals between contractions can be anywhere from five to twenty minutes (see Fig. 64). This first phase of labor, in which the contractions are mild and irregular, often lasts as long as eight or nine hours in a first labor, and it would be unwise to start your breathing exercises too early because they could tire you out before the difficult part of labor has even begun. Instead, walk around the house normally or, better, try to rest in the long

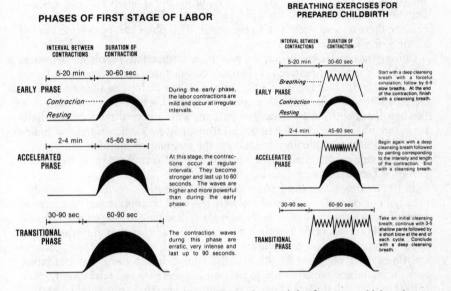

PHASES OF FIRST STAGE OF LABOR

BREATHING EXERCISES FOR PREPARED CHILDBIRTH

INTERVAL BETWEEN CONTRACTIONS / DURATION OF CONTRACTION

5-20 min / 30-60 sec

EARLY PHASE

Contraction

Resting

During the early phase, the labor contractions are mild and occur at irregular intervals.

INTERVAL BETWEEN CONTRACTIONS / DURATION OF CONTRACTION

5-20 min / 30-60 sec

Breathing

EARLY PHASE

Contraction

Resting

Start with a deep cleansing breath with a forceful exhalation; follow by 6-9 slow breaths. At the end of the contraction, finish with a cleansing breath.

2-4 min / 45-60 sec

ACCELERATED PHASE

At this stage, the contractions occur at regular intervals. They become stronger and last up to 60 seconds. The waves are higher and more powerful than during the early phase.

2-4 min / 45-60 sec

ACCELERATED PHASE

Begin again with a deep cleansing breath followed by panting corresponding to the intensity and length of the contraction. End with a cleansing breath.

30-90 sec / 60-90 sec

TRANSITIONAL PHASE

The contraction waves durng this phase are erratic, very intense and last up to 90 seconds.

30-90 sec / 60-90 sec

TRANSITIONAL PHASE

Take an initial cleansing breath; continue with 3-5 shallow pants followed by a short blow at the end of each cycle. Conclude with a deep cleansing breath.

Figure 64: A diagrammatic illustration of three phases of the first stage of labor, from the early phase with its irregular, mild contractions, through the transitional phase, the most intense period of labor. As you can see from the illustration, contractions become longer and closer together as labor progresses.   *Figure 65: A diagrammatic interpretation of the Lamaze exercises for prepared childbirth.* The specific breathing patterns for each phase of labor are shown above the darker areas illustrating the strength of the contractions. Techniques for dealing with the contractions change with each phase of labor, as you can see from the text accompanying the diagrams. These prepared-childbirth breathing patterns should be practiced over and over again with your coach so that the techniques will be totally routine the moment you enter into labor.

intervals between contractions and save your energy for later. When the contractions are strong and regular enough to need assistance, Lamaze instructions recommend beginning your breathing techniques.

The first phase of labor requires a pattern of chest breathing, which should be used only when it is impossible to move or speak during a contraction. When you feel a contraction beginning, focus on some inanimate object, then take a deep cleansing breath and blow the tension away as you exhale. Use slow, rhythmic chest breathing, inhaling through the nose and exhaling through the mouth *very slowly.* Six to nine breaths a minute would be considered ideal. At the same time, massage the abdomen gently with your fingertips as you breathe. These circular movements act as a distraction during labor and thereby help alleviate pain. When you feel the contraction is over, take another deep cleansing breath to blow away any residual tension. This emotionally and physically marks the end of the contraction.

The second part of the first stage is called the *accelerated phase.* The contractions are longer and stronger now, lasting for 45 to 60 seconds and occurring every 2 to 4 minutes. This is a more active phase of labor, when the cervix dilates from 3 centimeters to 7 or 8 centimeters and a woman needs to be actively involved in her breathing exercises and other forms of psychoprophylaxis. Particularly once the cervix is dilated 5 centimeters, discomfort usually increases because there is more stretching to the cervix. This phase can be expected to last about 3 or 4 hours in a first labor.

During the accelerated phase, the pattern of contractions makes steeper waves with shorter intervals between. When the contraction begins, focus and take a cleansing breath, blowing the tension away. Make sure to relax the various muscle groups to allow the uterus to work unhindered. Then pant quietly and slowly through the mouth, in a steady 4/4 pattern, with an equal number of exhalations and inhalations. Accelerate the breathing pattern as the contraction builds to a peak and then gradually decelerate as the contraction subsides, while all the time continuing a slow abdominal massage. When the contraction is over, take a cleansing breath and relax (see Fig. 65).

In the *transitional* or *third phase* of labor, contractions occur at erratic intervals, but one contraction is usually closely followed by another, and the interval between may be as short as 30 to 90 seconds. These long, strong contractions no longer build up smoothly and then diminish; instead they may surprise you because each contraction may build up to full strength quickly and then peak several times over. They last 60–90 seconds. Transition is a tiring phase of labor, and a woman needs to concentrate fully on her exercises and relaxation to cope with this, the hardest part of labor and delivery. Once the cervix has dilated from 7 to 10 centimeters (full dilation) the transitional phase is over, no more stretching is needed, and a woman can begin to push. After this there is usually less pain.

During the transition, the strength and frequency of the contractions must be borne in mind. A woman in the transitional phase needs to focus carefully on one point, concentrating on her breathing and relaxation, to keep abreast of the contractions and eliminate pain. When each contraction begins, immediately focus and release all tension in the other muscles. Then begin a pattern of 3 to 5 panting breaths followed by a forceful exhalation through pursed lips; continuing this pattern until the contraction is over, and slowing down only as the contraction diminishes. The labor coach can help you by looking at the monitoring strip on the fetal monitor or by feeling the contractions with his hand on your abdomen. When the contraction reaches a peak, he can signal this information and encourage you to continue breathing through the rest of the contraction by breathing along with you until you reach the point where the contraction is over.

Then take a deep breath and exhale the tension. Do not use the abdominal massage during this period of labor but use your hands to support your abdomen or keep them in place beneath the pubic bone.

At a certain point during this transition period, a woman often feels the first impulse to push. This is prompted by the increasing pressure of the baby's head against the vaginal walls and the pelvic floor. However, the impulse is premature before full dilation of the cervix is reached, and should be resisted. Otherwise you will experience unnecessary pain as the baby's head pushes up against the resisting cervix. Instead, at each urge to push, blow out forcefully through the lips several times, and then continue the pant-blow pattern when the urge to push is over. In the short intervals between each contraction, release all muscle tension and conserve your strength for the next one. This is an arduous stage that may be accompanied by other difficult symptoms, including backache between contractions, nausea, irritability, trembling, or chills, but it is by far the shortest of the three stages, lasting as it does an average of 30 to 60 minutes for a primipara and 15 to 30 minutes for a multipara.

☐ *Hyperventilation* A woman may experience hyperventilation either during a practice session or during labor itself. Hyperventilation sometimes occurs with improperly performed Lamaze breathing techniques, for the simple reason that the rapid breathing washes out carbon dioxide in large quantities from the body and takes in excessive amounts of oxygen. This imbalance causes dizziness, lightheadedness, and a tingling sensation in the extremities or around the lips, and the fingers often become rigid and inflexible for a few minutes during labor. The sensation is unpleasant. It is also potentially harmful, since prolonged hyperventilation could upset the baby's acid balance. Cup your hands over your mouth and breathe into them for a few moments, so you do not lose excessive CO_2 to the air, or ask your labor coach to bring a brown paper bag into the labor room and breathe into the bag.

☐ *Back Labor* A substantial number of women experience the pressure of the contractions in the back rather than in the area of the lower abdomen. Severe back pain can be associated with any fetal position but is frequently experienced with a particular type called the posterior position, in which the baby's head faces the abdomen and the back of the head puts pressure against the spine. Back labor can be difficult and painful. One way to eliminate the worst of the discomfort is for a woman to lie on her side while her husband massages or puts pressure on the lower portion of her back. Pressing the fists firmly into the small of the back will not damage the uterus and will give instantaneous relief. Back labor is discussed in more detail in Chapter 27, "Labor."

☐ *The Second Stage of Labor* As soon as the difficult period of transition is over, the bearing-down impulse can be used to help deliver the baby. At this point, a woman having her second baby is usually moved into the delivery room, unless she is laboring in a birthing room where the labor bed can be simply converted to a delivery table.

The initial stage of the expulsion period pushes the baby down inside the birth canal to the point where a small portion of the head will show during a contraction. A woman having her first baby is now moved into the delivery room. The rest of the second stage allows the cervix and vagina to stretch sufficiently under the pressure of the head and to release the head gradually, followed by the baby's shoulders and the rest of the body. In a sense the uterine contractions accomplish this without assistance, but the second stage of labor is shortened, as well as made more rewarding, if the woman helps to bear down with each contraction. Preferably you will be placed in a semisquatting position for this stage of labor, with the back propped up on a backrest and the knees wide apart. This gives you freedom to lean forward during a contraction, gripping the knees with your hands and pulling them outward and upward—a position that enables you to use the force of gravity in pushing the baby out. The conventional delivery table position—flat on the back with knees wide apart—

*Figure 66: The pushing exercise for
the second stage of labor:* The aim
in the second or expulsion stage of
labor is to help push the baby out
with the most economical and effective effort on your part. The woman
is lying with her upper back and
head supported by pillows and her
legs drawn up toward her chest and
knees wide apart. Her partner has
placed a relaxed opened hand just
above the pubic bone. During this
exercise you must learn to bear
down slowly without exerting all
your energy, then take a short breath
and again hold your breath and push
downward in the same direction and
with the same pressure as you would
during a bowel movement. Your
partner should be able with his hand
to feel if you are pushing correctly.
Important note: Don't push too hard
during the preparation exercises.
Overvigorous pushing can result in
damage to the fetal membrane or in
some other fetal damage.

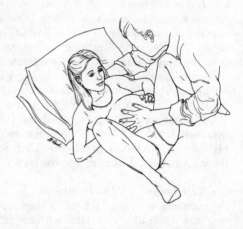

has advantages for the hospital staff but it works against the woman, who must
push harder to get the baby out. If you must use a conventional delivery table,
put pillows behind you to support the head and lower back. The hospital may
have one of the newer delivery tables with a back rest. Birthing beds also have
adjustable backs. Ask your labor coach to bring pillows in with him from the
labor room and help support your back and legs during delivery.

   The exercise for use during the second stage of labor is designed to exert force
on the uterus from the lungs and the diaphragm. (One of the advantages of the
semisquatting position is that it reduces the intraabdominal space and increases
the pressure you can bring to bear on the uterus.) This is the point at which
labor does indeed become work since it requires real physical exertion. Practice
the exercise by lying on the floor with your head supported by pillows and your
knees bent upward and outward. Hold your legs beneath the knees and pull
them toward your abdomen, keeping the knees bent away from the body. Then
take a deep breath and hold it for as long as possible, keeping the mouth closed.
The pressure on the diaphragm and hence the uterus will be increased if you
raise the head and the upper part of the body slightly with each breath. Use the
contracted muscles to push down on the diaphragm, but allow the pelvic muscles to remain relaxed. Finally, direct the force of the pushing toward the vagina.
Do this *gently* during the practice session.

   During an actual second-stage contraction, it is important not to hurry but to
let each contraction reach its most effective point before you begin to push.
When you feel a contraction begin, focus, and take a deep cleansing breath, followed by a second deep breath. Then, on the third breath, hold the breath and

bear down with a strong steady push, assisting the force of the contraction with your upper body, but keeping the pelvic muscles relaxed. Sustain the deep breath for about fifteen seconds, let the air out through your mouth and allow the head to fall back slightly, then take another deep breath and continue pushing. The sequence can be followed several times during a contraction. Finally, at the end of the contraction, relax the head, back, and legs, and breathe slowly and deeply. The intervals between contractions are longer during this stage and allow for a period of complete relaxation. Some women experience such a profound state of relaxation that they seem unaware of what is going on around them in the delivery room.

☐ **The Birth**   As you push the baby's head down to the perineum and the vaginal opening begins to dilate widely, you will be able to see the top of the baby's head in the mirror over the delivery table. At this point, your doctor will ask you to stop pushing and begin a series of short little panting exhalations and inhalations through your opened mouth (similar to the panting of a puppy dog). This will give the perineal tissue a chance to stretch slowly. The doctor will support the baby's head to prevent its being delivered too rapidly and will try to stretch the perineum with his fingers to see if he can perform the delivery without an episiotomy (an incision made in the vagina to facilitate the birth; see page 486). If the vaginal tissue will not stretch sufficiently, an episiotomy is made to prevent unnecessary tearing. As you continue panting, the doctor will slowly deliver the baby's head and the anterior (front) shoulder. You will then again be asked to push as the doctor lifts the baby to deliver the posterior shoulder. One long push will help deliver not only the shoulder but the body of the baby. The final push is important because otherwise the doctor might have to pull on the baby's head to complete the delivery, an action which could injure the delicate intracranial nerves.

You can look forward to an extraordinary, joyful sense of release as the baby is finally born. The baby should be handed to you immediately after the birth so you can continue the bonding that began between you and your child long before the delivery.

☐ **The Leboyer Technique of Natural Childbirth**   Dr. Frederick Leboyer* is a French physician whose concept of gentle birth in his book *Birth Without Violence* celebrates the joy of normal birth and protests against unnecessary violence. Instead, a Leboyer birth attempts to recreate the environment inside the womb as closely as possible in the delivery room. Lights are turned down, voices are hushed, the infant is handled gently. The newborn baby is massaged on the mother's stomach and then put in a warm water bath after birth to ease its passage from the intrauterine environment to the outside world. A Leboyer birth teaches respect for the infant by shifting the focus away from the drama of the parents' experience and bringing the infant into a place of central importance in the birth ritual.

The Leboyer concept emerged after years of intensive psychoanalysis in which Dr. Leboyer traced certain persistent anxieties back to the fear he had himself

---

* *Birth Without Violence* (Alfred A. Knopf, 1975).

experienced at birth. Out of this came a new concept of a newborn experience and a belief in infant awareness. "People say—and believe—that a newborn baby feels nothing. *He feels everything!*"

Another formative experience was a visit to India, where he saw traditional births conducted in a quiet manner, with none of the hurry and noise associated with Western hospital births. He also came to believe the influential studies of Konrad Lorenz, the animal behaviorist who showed the effect that "imprinting" has on a young animal's behavior. (Imprinting is by definition the learning process that takes place early in life in social animals.) This only reinforced Leboyer's belief in the importance of the first moments of life to a child's later experiences and personality.

In shifting the focus from the parents to the newborn, Leboyer attacked the methods by which infants are treated on their arrival. His contention is that conventional delivery methods render the transition from intrauterine to extrauterine existence unnecessarily traumatic by abrupt sensory contrasts: bright lights, noise, rough handling. His criticism is extended to such traditional methods of handling the newborn as early clamping of the umbilical cord, routine suctioning, and weighing the infant on a cold scale. Instead, in a Leboyer birth, the baby is placed immediately on the maternal abdomen and massaged gently to stimulate uterine contractions; routine suctioning is avoided; and the clamping of the cord is delayed until it has ceased pulsating. After the separation of the cord, the baby is placed in the water bath. Often the baby responds immediately by opening his or her eyes, relaxing arms and fists, and appearing to gaze around the room.

Leboyer's technique for childbirth thus tries to create a more natural delivery where the child is treated gently after birth. This has begun to affect the delivery of babies throughout the United States. Although very few institutions are following the exact Leboyer technique, many physicians and midwives are beginning to dim the lights during a normal, natural delivery and are trying to eliminate unnecessary noise and bustle. Certainly a gentle approach is a much more natural one and babies appear to do very well without the spanking or the slapping of the feet that were once traditional. But it is useful to remember that these stimulants were used in collaboration with large doses of anesthetics and other medications that made babies so sleepy it was difficult to wake them up after delivery. If very little or no narcotic agents are used, a baby does respond better, has better breathing habits, and does not need to be handled in an ungentle fashion.

☐ **Is the Leboyer Technique Worthwhile?**　In the mid 1970s, a French researcher, Danielle Rapoport, startled psychiatrists by a study which claimed extraordinary benefits from the Leboyer method of birth. Her findings have been largely discredited because they did not take into account the fact that parents who choose Leboyer birth are often better educated than the average couple. But it is true that obstetricians who conduct Leboyer deliveries say there is a remarkable immediate difference in the way the babies respond to their surroundings, and that a Leboyer birth does unite parents and child in an unusually close bond immediately after birth. It is difficult to say how this would affect the future personality of a child, or a child's long-term relationship with the parents, but both could be beneficial. Otherwise clinical observations have failed to substantiate the benefits promised by Leboyer except that women who have planned a Leboyer delivery seem to have shorter labors, perhaps because they are looking forward to the delivery and are anticipating less fear and tension. Differences between the motor skills and general alertness of Leboyer and non-Leboyer babies seem to disappear within a few days of delivery.

☐ *Childbirth with Love*   It is my belief that we should start to think of childbirth in the context of the whole pregnancy, instead of as an event in itself. A successful delivery begins months before the woman enters the labor room. If a woman has had a poor pregnancy, a pregnancy in which she has not taken sufficient care of herself and has not given thought and love to her child, she cannot overcome her neglect by simply doing natural-childbirth exercises in the labor and delivery room, dimming the lights during delivery, and hoping that any damage done during pregnancy will be overcome by avoiding emotional trauma during the birth itself. It is my belief that the outcome is decided long before then. Feelings during pregnancy, nutrition, antenatal care, good health, and anticipation and love for the child before delivery; these in combination with the total process of childbirth education, childbirth techniques, and the understanding of your husband, peers, and family, are essential elements in the delivery of a new child in a loving environment.

A woman whose pregnancy was well cared for, and who has invested time, effort, and energy in the pregnancy, is already well prepared for labor and delivery, although this woman and her husband will benefit considerably from a formal childbirth education class in which they will learn to have limited apprehension about labor and delivery. In my experience, women who have such pregnancies and are completely prepared for labor and delivery, have fewer problems and difficulties than other women. Furthermore, if there is good cooperation between the obstetrician and the patient, and trust in the obstetrician's or midwife's abilities, then a couple will be less fearful of problems and much less fearful of their obstetrician's tricking them into taking unnecessary medications or operative procedures during the birth. Labor and delivery is teamwork; the teamwork of the woman, her husband, the midwife, the physician, and the nurse. This teamwork should be relaxed and honest. It is important for a couple to discuss the labor process with their obstetrician or midwife before the delivery, and if the couple is well educated to all aspects of labor and delivery, including the newer techniques such as fetal monitoring, they will understand normal labor better and be more able to make adjustments if any abnormality should occur. Where there is complete elimination of fear and a partnership between husband and wife in the labor room, a couple can have a wonderful labor and delivery and participate in an exciting birth.

☐ *The Hospital Environment*   I recommend a hospital prepared for a natural approach, with at least one birthing room and modifications in the conventional labor room. Not all couples can use a birthing room because some births require special medical care, but for most couples the birthing room in a hospital is an ideal place to give birth. If anything does go wrong, they have backup emergency facilities available in the same building. A sudden complication can be a very frightening situation, and I have certainly seen cases in which beautiful children were damaged because emergency facilities were not immediately available. Even so, there is no reason why hospitals cannot have a loving, easy, and relaxed atmosphere. There is also no reason why a couple cannot create the atmosphere they desire by dimming the lights or bringing in a tape recorder with music they enjoy. Each person responds differently to labor and delivery, and one couple might want a different type of environment from that of another couple. The aim is to create a peaceful atmosphere so that a woman will be able to concentrate fully on her breathing and the events of the birth.

☐ *Childbirth and the Family* Dick-Read, who had considerable experience with meddling mothers and mothers-in-law in his practice, called such women the "pests of parturition." Implicitly, modern hospitals have also adopted this attitude toward family members other than the husband by rigorously excluding them from the labor floor. Only very recently has this changed as childbirth has become recognized as a family event as well as a mutual experience for the couple. For many women, having their mothers in the labor room with them has provided a strong source of support, perhaps because another woman has a real understanding of labor. Sometimes the relationship is a source of unusual support, or it might be a signal that her mother will accept the newborn.

I once had a patient who was impossible to control in the early stages of labor. Unknown to me, there was some difficulty between her and her husband, and the difficulty went even further because the woman's mother had not completely accepted the fact that she was having a child. Fortunately our hospital, like some others, allows the mother into the labor and delivery rooms, and in this particular case, as in many other instances I have seen, the daughter became more relaxed as her mother stayed with her in the labor room. It was as if at that time she got a signal from her mother—It's going to be okay, we're going to take care of the child, whatever happens to your marriage—that made labor easier. Years ago, the older woman would not have been allowed in with her daughter, but now this has changed. One often sees great benefit from a woman's mother being with her. Sometimes the mother offers even better support than the husband can, although one is not always aware of this initially.

☐ *There Is No Reason to Fear Failure* If labor becomes too difficult during the progress of the birth, you should understand that there are different pain thresholds and it does not mean you are a failure. If you cannot control the pain with breathing techniques, then you should feel completely free to ask for an injection of Phenergan or maybe a small dose of Demerol to take away some of the pain. Most analgesics can still work in harmony with your breathing techniques. When analgesics are not enough to curb the pain and you feel unable to cope in spite of your husband's support, an epidural anesthetic (an injection given in the back to numb the pelvic nerves) could eliminate the fear and the feeling of pain and perhaps give you the relaxation and strength that are important in delivering your child. Women in the past were known to suffer so much in labor that they found it difficult to care for the child. It is important that this does not happen in a modern delivery.

☐ *Birth with Love* The delivery should be done as gently as possible, with dimmed lights and a minimum of noise. Immediately after the birth the baby should gently be rubbed on the back and handed straight to the mother. I do not believe that a baby, as Leboyer suggested, should be placed in a water bath to remind it of the womb because I believe that nature has determined that life for both humans and animals must change from the intrauterine to the extrauterine environment at birth. Instead of the water bath, I believe the mother and child need to be close, with the warmth of their bodies continuing the bonding that was begun inside the womb. If you look closely after such a birth experience you will often see a satisfied smile on the baby's face.

Mammals lick their babies immediately after birth, an instinctive action that stimulates the baby to breathe, and is furthermore, a touching and loving form of bonding. After a human birth, the child should be placed immediately on the mother's abdomen, where warm towels can be used to rub the baby's back. The baby will experience warmth, and the massage will stimulate the baby's natural breathing and the other physiological changes attendant on birth. Both parents can perform the massage. This understanding and gentleness is part of a natural, loving labor and delivery.

Childbirth with love is a birth experience in which each person is completely prepared and fully educated, but each delivery is individual! Every step is done naturally, smoothly, and gently, with time to bond closely after the birth. Labor and delivery will then be pleasurable for the couple and their child will be given a wonderful beginning in life—a start filled with love and hope that should give the child the utmost advantage for his or her lifetime.

27

Labor

Many couples plan the arrival of their baby well in advance. Often they take the due date very seriously, coordinating the relatives' arrival and their other plans with precision—and then becoming upset if something goes wrong. This is understandable, but unrealistic, since you should always bear in mind that the due date your doctor gives you is only an estimated due date. The baby's arrival depends on a number of factors, including the length of the menstrual cycle in the month of conception and exactly when in her cycle a woman conceives. Human beings are born approximately 267 days from the time of conception. Births normally take place a few days before or a few days after the due date. Healthy babies are born two to three weeks before the due date and two to three weeks after. Either variation may in part be genetically determined, depending on each pregnancy.

As the due date approaches, couples who have made careful plans and couples who have been content to let nature take its course are equally caught up in the anticipation of labor. Most women feel that the last weeks of pregnancy seem to go more slowly than the rest of the pregnancy. Other than an increased schedule of visits to the doctor, not much is happening to the pregnancy during the last month, except a considerable increase in weight. Many women feel bloated and cumbersome in the final month. The baby is large enough to exert upward pressure on the stomach and diaphragm and downward pressure on the lower intestines, causing shortness of breath, heartburn, increased desire to urinate and other minor discomforts. Among primiparas the discomfort is usually lessened about two weeks before the birth as the baby's head starts to enter the birth canal, reducing abdominal pressure at least. Lightening, as it is called, occurs later in a multipara, usually just before labor begins. In spite of the physical discomforts of the last stage of pregnancy, you will probably feel an increased sense of excited anticipation because emotionally and physically you are preparing yourself for labor. Often at the end of pregnancy women experience a final spurt of energy—the so-called *nesting instinct*—that drives them to clean the house, prepare the baby's room, and make their final preparations for delivery. A woman is often so wound up in the final weeks of pregnancy that she has difficulty sleeping at night. This sense of excited anticipation is experienced by expectant fathers as well. Participation in childbirth-preparation classes by both parents has resulted in the expectant couple's looking forward to a delivery in which they are finally going to achieve their goal—the birth of their child.

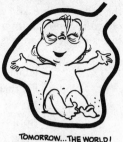

TOMORROW...THE WORLD!

Figure 67: Reproduced by permission from Lester Friedman, Monogram of California, San Francisco, California.

☐ ***The Nesting Instinct***   How prospective parents prepare for their child's birth says much about their personalities and their cultural background. Some couples set up the nursery months ahead of the expected due date, while others wait until the last possible moment, or even until after the baby is born. It is rare to find a woman who does not make some preparation (a complete lack of the nesting instinct is often the sign of a rejected pregnancy), but the amount of preparation in a psychologically healthy pregnancy varies widely.

Among some American ethnic groups the ritual of buying baby clothes and equipment follows a precise and revered tradition. Jewish mothers, for instance, may order the baby's layette and the nursery furniture before the birth, but are not supposed to have them at home until after the baby is born, when the store delivers them to the house. This may be a way to spare the parents unnecessary grief if something goes wrong at the birth. Among ethnic groups that do not honor this custom the expectant parents may use the last few months of pregnancy to set up the baby's room in preparation for the wonderful moment when the baby comes home.

☐ ***When Are Babies Born?***   It is a myth that babies are born at night. Labor frequently starts during the night when the mother is resting and the baby is active (as babies often are at night), triggering labor. But labor that begins at night usually means you will be delivered during the day, since labor lasts anywhere up to twelve hours. (A woman who arrives at the hospital at 3:00 A.M. may not give birth until 10:00 or 11:00 A.M.) According to data collected from a series of births in Germany some years ago, 26 percent of the births occurred between 6:00 A.M. and 12 noon; 22 percent occurred from 12 noon to 6:00 P.M.; 24 percent from 6:00 P.M. to midnight; and 28 percent from 12 midnight to 6:00 A.M. The pattern might be slightly different today, with elective inductions and Cesarean surgery, but births still occur around the clock rather than in a specific time period.

☐ ***Does the Time of Year Make a Difference?***   It is interesting to observe how the birth rate changes throughout the year. An analysis of recent births in the United States by the National Center of Health Statistics has shown that births rise and fall from month to month in a surprisingly predictable pattern. In the following breakdown of American births, 100 represents the mean number of births a month, for a total of 1200 deliveries in a year. The actual number of births in each month is represented by a figure over or under 100.

January	97	July	104
February	100	August	105
March	100	September	108
April	95	October	103
May	93	November	99
June	98	December	100

This demonstrates that a large number of babies are born during the late summer and early fall months. These babies must have been conceived in the fall and early winter months of the preceding year, which suggests that the fall, rather than the summer, is a favorable time for conception. Perhaps the balmy fall weather, when temperatures are moderate and days are often clear and sunny, allows the sperm to survive better than in the heat of summer. A new branch of science called biometeorology, which explores the interaction between weather and health, is trying to come up with scientific explanations for such old beliefs as madness and the moon and the close relationship between sunlight and infertility. The notion that the chances of conception are enhanced by the number of hours of sunshine can clearly be tied in with recent research findings on a hormone called serotonin, which is produced in the brain. High levels of serotonin can apparently decrease the chances of conception by interfering with the brain hormones that control fertility. Sunshine, however, seems to decrease serotonin levels, a phenomenon which has a noticeable effect in northern countries like Lapland, where far more babies are conceived in the long sunny days of summer than the short, sunless days of winter. In the United States serotonin levels must remain relatively high during the hot, humid overcast days of the typical American summer, and probably decrease during the sunny clear days of the fall.

☐   *Delivery and the Full Moon*   The moon was once believed to have a powerful influence on fertility. Even now, the phases of the moon may still have an effect on birth in a modern city. According to two analyses of birth patterns in New York City carried out almost twenty years apart, the lowest number of deliveries seems to take place around the time of the new moon and the highest number just before a full moon. This "lunar effect" could have a biometeorological explanation. Immediately before the full moon, the changes in barometric pressure brought on by the moon's closer proximity to the earth often lead to abrupt shifts in the weather. When this results in low barometric pressure, as it often does, an unusual number of women seem to go into labor, while the opposite phenomenon is seen during periods of high pressure. The tendency to go into labor during bad weather can be explained by the lower pressure outside the uterus affecting the pressure inside the baby's environment, thereby triggering endocrine mechanisms from the baby and beginning labor. Obstetrical units certainly seem to be busier in severe weather conditions—hurricanes, snowstorms, or very rainy days with *low barometric pressure*—than they are on days with high pressure and clear skies.

☐ *Getting Ready for Birth*   As the due date approaches, every expectant woman asks herself, "Will I recognize labor when it begins?"

One of the first signs of the end of pregnancy is the descent of the baby's presenting part, usually the head, into the birth canal. The phenomenon is aptly called *lightening* because the pregnant woman feels less burdened with the shift in the baby's weight. Lightening is nature's way of making sure that the baby is in the correct position for birth. In one sense, this is the first step in the birth of the baby, even though lightening may take place as long as four weeks before a woman in her first pregnancy goes into labor.

Lightening occurs when the uterus shrinks downward and forward, pushing the baby's head into the pelvic canal. This shifts the baby's bulk forward so its weight is resing inside the pelvic bones and not against the surface of the muscles of the uterus. Some women state that they feel the baby drop, a phenomenon that can take place over the space of a few hours; other women only realize that lightening has occurred when they wake up one morning relieved of the abdominal pressure they have been experiencing for the past few weeks. Relief may be localized however, since lightening tends to increase the pressure on the bladder and increases the amount of vaginal discharge.

In a second or third pregnancy, lightening occasionally takes place during the first week or ten days before delivery, but is more likely to occur after labor has already begun. Once the baby has dropped, the uterine weight is resting directly on the large vena cava inferior, the vein that brings the blood back from the legs and pelvis to the heart. It is a good idea to increase the circulation by lying down with your legs elevated at different times during the day to promote the circulation from the legs. Pressure on the vena cava inferior increases the tendency to varicose veins and edema in these final weeks. When you sit down, try to remain slightly tilted to one side to shift the baby's weight away from the abdominal area. Sitting straight with your legs crossed will further decrease the blood flow to the heart and thus decrease the circulation of blood to the baby.

One or two days before delivery, a woman often experiences an increasing number of uterine contractions. These are tiring, and a full-term woman who is about to go into labor often looks tired. Try to rest for as long as two hours during the afternoon in the last weeks before delivery. You are carrying a lot of extra weight and losing energy to the fast-growing baby at this stage of the pregnancy. At night the movements of the baby, which by now have become noticeably more vigorous, often keep a pregnant woman awake.

The fetal movement pattern is another sign of imminent labor. Throughout the last trimester, an alert woman should always keep track of fetal movements; regular movement is a healthy sign (see Chap. 23) but movements tend to lessen at the end of pregnancy. Less movement is usually a sign that labor is about to take place—the baby is more constricted as it engages in the pelvis.

A noticeable lack of fetal movement could also be a sign that the baby is in trouble. A woman must remain alert to the baby's movement pattern and should call her doctor immediately if the baby stops moving for a prolonged period. It could be a warning sign.

☐ *A Checklist Before the Birth Day*   This might be helpful in making your preparations for the hospital stay. Be sure to take a tour of the hospital; find out exactly where the admitting office is and where to go if you need to rush to the delivery floor.

If possible, register in advance at the hospital to avoid waiting in the admitting office. There have been times when a woman was waiting in the office to be admitted and the baby emerged right there.

Make a rehearsal trip to the hospital. Find out how long it takes to drive there and which route is the fastest, any time of the day, even during rush hour.

Find out where to park in the area of the hospital at any time—day or night. If you must park illegally, remember to write a sign saying "At the delivery room" and stick it on the front window of the car; then even if you get a ticket, you can plead not guilty. Also remember to tell the hospital security that you are illegally parked. That will probably prevent your getting a ticket, especially if the car is moved later on.

In the last few days before the due date, be sure you have enough gasoline in the car to make it to the hospital. Don't leave the car empty at night thinking you can get gasoline in the morning, because you may need to rush to the hospital in the middle of the night.

Have the doctor's telephone number easily available and be sure, well before the due date, that you have discussed exactly what you should do in any conceivable eventuality.

Have your suitcase packed with all the necessary equipment before you enter the hospital. This will eliminate the stress of packing at the last minute.

Complete any domestic arrangements in advance so that someone will be available to care for your home or other children when you go into the hospital. When making these arrangements, it is important to remember that you might be in the hospital for up to twenty-four hours before the baby is born.

☐ *Packing Your Suitcase*   About two to three weeks before you expect to deliver, pack a bag or suitcase with the personal items you want to take to the hospital. Some items are routine; others depend on personal preference. Necessary items include: a bathrobe; nightgowns (bring more than one because they become soiled in the hospital); a nursing brassiere; bedroom slippers; a toothbrush and other personal articles. You may also want to bring your own sheets, if the hospital policy permits, and your own pillow or pillows—nothing is more comforting than personal possessions during labor. Another useful item is a bag containing a few biscuits, fruit and several bottles of soda. Although a woman in labor is not usually that hungry and may in any case be receiving fluids intravenously, labor can be hard on the coach, who may not have the hospital cafeteria available to him if labor occurs at night. Also, after the baby is born, you may well be thirsty and will be grateful for something thirst-quenching.

Pack a separate bag with the clothes that you plan to bring the baby home in, or ask a visitor to bring it into the hospital for you. It is better to have this item ready in advance so you will have all the immediate necessities for the baby on hand.

Finally, bring any personal items that you would like to have with you during labor and delivery—pictures of your family, for instance, or a cassette player, or a camera (you must ask your doctor's permission to use a camera in the delivery room). A bottle of champagne or other wine to celebrate the birth is a special item you shouldn't forget. A nurse will usually put the champagne in the delivery floor refrigerator to keep it well chilled until after the delivery.

☐ *False Labor*   Couples who have taken preparation-for-childbirth classes are aware of the need to distinguish false labor from real labor. This is something that worries many women as they look ahead to the baby's delivery. The distinction is not as obscure as it might seem.

Painless intermittent contractions called "Braxton Hicks contractions" occur throughout pregnancy, with increasing frequency toward the end. From time to time, perhaps as frequently as every twenty minutes, the muscles of the uterus tighten and then relax, a sensation that may or may not be evident to you. These uterine contractions exercise the uterine muscles and increase the circulation of maternal blood to the placenta. If you feel your abdomen during a Braxton Hicks contraction you will notice a large firm mass that becomes a softer, indentable mass once the contraction is over. This is the nature of any contraction, including true labor contractions; the difference is that Braxton Hicks contractions occur irregularly, although they may come and go for several hours at a time. Generally they are painless. You may notice them during periods of activity, especially when you get up suddenly from a sitting position or quicken your pace while you are walking. Once you relax, the Braxton Hicks contractions usually subside, unlike true labor contractions, which do not change in intensity as you change your level of activity. True labor pains are persistent and rhythmic. Another difference is that false labor is not accompanied by the other symptoms of early labor: the so-called bloody show or rupture or leakage of the membranes. However, if you are in doubt, call your doctor to discuss your symptoms. Many women find it difficult to distinguish the beginning of true labor and it is better to call your doctor than sit at home worrying.

False labor contractions might continue for weeks before the baby is due, growing stronger and more frequent as labor approaches. They serve a useful function by preparing the uterus for the rigors of true labor.

☐ *The Alcohol Test*   One good old-fashioned home remedy for distinguishing false labor from real labor is the alcohol test. If you sit down with a glass of wine or a cocktail, false labor contractions usually disappear within a few minutes. True labor contractions are unaffected by the relaxant effect of the alcohol. A drink at this time is pleasantly relaxing and will not harm your baby.

☐ *Signs of True Labor*   With the onset of true labor, birth has begun. The first noticeable symptom is often a feeling of discomfort in the lower part of the abdomen, usually described as a menstrual-like pain. Less commonly, it may be felt in the lower back and the legs. Another sign is a characteristic pinkish discharge from the vagina known as the "bloody show." This is caused by the release of the mucous plug from inside the neck of the cervix. A typical "show" is a small quantity of blood, similar in amount to the blood loss at the beginning of a menstrual period, mixed with mucus. Occasionally there is an initial discharge of clear watery material instead of the show, which indicates the imminent rupture of the fetal membranes. The release of the mucous plug is often a sign that labor is on the way, but it can occur a few days before the onset of progressive labor. A third sign that labor is beginning is the rupture of the membrane containing the amniotic fluid, although, once again, this may take place a few days before labor begins, or during labor itself (see below).

At the beginning of the first stage of labor, contractions are usually mild and infrequent. The first contractions last between thirty and sixty seconds and occur irregularly, at intervals of five to twenty minutes. There may or may not be pain at this early stage. Many women do not identify these mild contractions as labor contractions, experiencing only some slight discomfort associated with the abdominal pain or low backache described above. Since each woman has a different labor experience and a different pain threshold, you may recognize the onset of labor earlier or later than other women. (The individual's pain tolerance is a common reason for staying at home until the last moment and then giving birth on the way to the hospital.) Nonetheless, you will usually be able to distinguish a regular pattern of uterine contraction and relaxation from earlier Braxton Hicks contractions. The great majority of women are aware of something much deeper when they go into labor than the occasional contraction, even if the woman has been intensively prepared beforehand through psychoprophylaxis or a Bradley class and is not aware of any really painful sensations. If you are in doubt, always contact your doctor for more information. Sometimes an obstetrician is unable to make a diagnosis from a telephone description and will ask you to go to the hospital for examination. Even if you are not in labor, this will ease your mind, relax you, and help you rest more easily in the intervening days or hours before true labor begins. By getting the rest you need you will have more strength when you do go into labor.

As labor progresses, contractions recur at decreasing intervals and become longer, harder, and increasingly uncomfortable. After the initial period of irregular contractions the uterus begins to contract at regular intervals and the contractions themselves become shorter in duration. Once you experience contractions every ten minutes, your obstetrician should be notified, even though the birth of the baby is usually several hours away. This gives him time to plan ahead and gives you time to make your final preparations at home.

☐ *If the Membranes Rupture*   Spontaneous rupture of the amniotic-fluid sac takes place in 10 to 20 percent of births in the early stage of labor or before labor begins. (I would stress that early rupture is not common to all pregnancies.) The amniotic fluid either gushes out or runs out in a continuous trickle. Sometimes the sac ruptures during the night and soaks through the bed, so it is a good idea to put a plastic sheet under your cotton sheets to avoid damage to the mattress. Fortunately the amount of fluid tends to decrease as the baby approaches or passes the due date. Other women have had the embarrassing experience of the membranes rupturing while they were in the office or out shopping. You will feel safer if you wear a double layer of sanitary pads in the last month. As I have said, a spontaneous rupture is perfectly normal and there is no reason to panic.

Labor usually starts within twelve hours after the membranes have ruptured spontaneously if contractions have not already begun. Unless you are experiencing uterine contractions when the water breaks, a sensible precaution is to lie down and place your hand on your abdomen to see if the baby is moving or not. The most serious problem with spontaneous rupture is the risk of a prolapse of the umbilical cord through the cervix. The cord can become caught between the pelvic bones and the fetal head and strangle the baby. Fetal movement is usually a good sign that the baby is doing well. As soon as you have felt the baby move, call your doctor and inform him of your progress. Most doctors want their patients in the hospital immediately when the amniotic sac ruptures. In that way they can make sure that nothing is wrong and also decrease the chances of infection. In any case, you are likely to go into labor within a few hours if contractions have not already begun. Unfortunately one occasionally sees women who have walked around for days or even weeks without a doctor's supervision and have ended up with such severe amniotic-fluid infections (see Chap. 25) that the baby dies or suffers brain damage. If you do not go into labor almost immediately, and your doctor wants you to stay at home for a prolonged period—more than twenty-four hours—I would certainly recommend that you seek a second opinion from another doctor. In fact, I would suggest you call a perinatologist or an obstetrician specializing in high-risk obstetrics at another medical center than the one at which you are scheduled to give birth. He will probably advise you to go to the hospital immediately for evaluation and possible labor induction.

☐ *What Triggers the Onset of Labor?*   The uterus is a unique organ. It expands over a period of nine months during which it remains almost completely relaxed. It is then suddenly thrown into a frenzy of activity for a few hours, then shrinks back to a fraction of its maximum size in preparation for the next childbirth cycle.

Most pregnancies last the full nine months, but the uterus is capable of contracting at any time if it is given a signal. To prevent this from occurring prematurely, two different types of defense mechanisms are built into the uterus. One involves the special properties of the myometrium, the muscles of the uterine wall; the other a mechanism that prevents all stimuli from reaching the uterus by blocking the nerve impulses and preventing the release of hormonal factors that normally stimulate the uterus into contractions. Exactly how this works is unknown, but the uterus does contain various receptors. Receptors can be compared to keyholes which can be triggered or stimulated only by a specific hormone "key." These receptors are apparently blocked through certain mechanisms and are turned on by other trigger signals.

The muscular walls of the uterus are composed of long, smooth muscle cells built into a network of involuntary muscles. This muscular pattern provides the most efficient conditions for the expulsion of the fetus and the placenta. When a contraction occurs, the entire uterus squeezes, beginning with the upper network of muscle fibers and reaching down to the lower network of fibers. This is the pattern seen during labor. In pregnancy, certain biochemical properties of the myometrium normally block the conducting impulse from one muscle cell to another, thus inhibiting the onset of regular contractions. What happens before or during labor to circumvent this defense mechanism?

It is probably easier to understand the process if one thinks of the onset of labor as a mechanism that can be triggered at any time the defense mechanism is removed. Normally a woman goes to full term, at which point labor occurs. But a spontaneous abortion can take place early in pregnancy, when the mechanism inside the uterus has been damaged in some way and contractions begin. The same is true in a premature labor in which the baby is not yet full-term but a mechanism still triggers labor contractions. This is why it is so important for a woman in a high-risk pregnancy to do all she can to relax the uterus and keep the defense mechanism in the uterus in good condition by resting and avoiding any uterine-stimulating activity.

When conditions inside the uterus are so unfavorable that the fetus begins to suffer, the fetus itself may trigger uterine contractions because the body senses that the baby is suffering and will do better if it is expelled from the uterus. This may well be the phenomenon that occurs during premature labor, when, for instance, oxygenation is reduced and this in turn triggers a mechanism that could lead to contractions. The same might happen at term when the baby has been living inside the uterus for many months and is now too large for its "house"— the uterine environment. Since the placenta no longer provides enough nourishment or oxygen, the baby responds by sending certain hormonal stimuli to the uterus via the placenta, which then triggers labor.

The phenomenon of the fetus triggering labor is one that is seen in many mammals besides humans. Animal studies have also given us a clue to the mechanisms involved in the prevention of uterine contractions before the fetus reaches full term. Among animals the progesterone produced in the placenta throughout pregnancy seems to help prevent the onset of labor, since progesterone appears to block the receptors for oxytocin and prostaglandin, the hormones capable of initiating contractions. Progesterone in animals and in human beings is found to increase steadily throughout pregnancy. We also know that progesterone begins to decrease in the last few weeks of gestation at the time when the placenta has reached its maximum size. In animals, this decrease in progesterone seems to correspond with a rise in estrogen levels in the fetus. The estrogen, in turn, stimulates prostaglandin release, possibly from the placenta; this is perhaps the mechanism that triggers the myometrium to start contractions. At the same time there is a release of oxytocin from the pituitary, which then, in combination with the low level of prostaglandin, starts a series of rhythmic contractions. This pattern is seen in larger mammals such as sheep, and something quite similar appears to happen in the human.

These hormonal changes are part of a complex interaction between the fetus and its environment. In animals an unusual amount of cortisone is secreted from the fetal hypothalamus and the adrenal gland at the inception of labor. When cortisone reaches the placenta it causes an increase in the fetal placental estrogen level and stimulates the release of prostaglandins. Since cortisone is released during stress situations, nature so functions that the fetus signals its distress, and thus begins the process of labor. This is likely to occur when the placenta can no longer support the pregnancy with sufficient nutrition, or some other situation has arisen that stresses the baby.

Stress releases cortisone, and cortisone stimulates estrogen release. Increased estrogen in turn triggers an increase in the number of prostaglandin receptors in the placenta. As prostaglandin begins to increase, it blocks the production of progesterone, making the uterus more sensitive to labor. Uterine sensitivity then increases as the prostaglandin level rises, making the uterus even more sensitive to oxytocin, which is released from the human pituitary in high amounts at that time. Spurts of oxytocin, together with the rise in prostaglandin, will start labor contractions.

Once the first contractions have begun, other factors seem to stimulate labor.

One contraction, for instance, often triggers another as the muscles become tired and need to relax. During this phase of labor, each spurt of oxytocin and prostaglandin causes the contractions to occur rhythmically. At this point, too, the fetal head is pushing against the cervix, which signals the mother's brain to release another spurt of oxytocin. The oxytocin, in combination with the prostaglandins already present, triggers another labor contraction. The combination of small amounts of prostaglandin and oxytocin is therefore enough to begin labor.

As you can see, a variety of fetal "stress" can trigger labor. Premature labor often starts after a urinary tract infection, fever, increased physical activity, sex, malnutrition, or nervous anxiety, and can even be caused by fights between wife and husband. Labor at term is presumably triggered because the baby has outgrown the uterus, and the uterus is "ripe" to be stimulated into labor by any minimal fetal stress factors, such as increased maternal physical activity, sex, fever, anxiety, or diminished fetal nutrition.

☐ *What Happens During Labor*   Labor, put succinctly, is the process whereby the baby, the placenta, the fetal membranes, and the amniotic fluid are expelled from the uterus. The mechanics of labor expel the baby from the uterus in which it has been kept safe for nine months and move it through the birth canal to the outside world. Running through the cervix is a slender canal that connects the neck of the uterus to the vaginal opening. This is the birth canal through which the baby must pass to reach the vulva.

Since this canal is normally impenetrable, by far the longest period of labor is devoted to dilation, or the *first stage of labor*, during which the neck of the uterus is forced open to allow for the expulsion of the baby. During this stage, which can last many hours, uterine contractions gradually push the baby and the amniotic sac downward into the vagina. The first stage ends when the cervix is fully dilated to accommodate the baby's head. The *second stage of labor* is the time from the full dilation of the cervix until the baby is delivered. *The third stage* is the time from the delivery of the baby to the delivery of the placenta—a process that usually takes only a few minutes.

☐ *How Long Does Labor Take?*   The average duration of the first stage of labor in a primigravida is about twelve hours. A multipara, whose labor is always shorter than a primipara's, can expect to labor for about seven hours. These are only averages, however, and individual labors vary greatly. Irregular contractions continue for several hours at the beginning of true labor, and a woman may not be aware of them if she is carrying on with her normal schedule. Labor will then appear much shorter than it really is. It is important not to become frightened when you think about labor—the numbers exist only as a guide. If a woman is tense she will feel labor contractions early on, and make it harder on herself.

The cervix is said to dilate approximately one centimeter an hour, but that is only if one calculates from the beginning to the end of labor. Cervical dilation proceeds very slowly at first and then progresses rapidly when a woman enters the active stage of labor. A woman who has good effacement and dilation can virtually dilate within one to two hours in the active stage. A labor with no disproportion present might only take a few hours, which should make it easier for you to cope successfully.

The average duration of the second stage of labor is fifty minutes in the pri-

mipara and twenty minutes in the multipara. But again, women's experiences
vary greatly, depending on the position of the fetal head, the size of the baby,
and the strength of the contractions. Some women in a first labor find this second stage takes up to one and a half hours or even two hours, but the average is
under an hour. It may take even less time if you are well trained and know how
to push effectively. A second labor sometimes proceeds so quickly in the second
stage that two or three pushes are all that are needed, although most multiparous women take longer. Any woman going into the second stage will find that
the more she knows about labor, the easier the baby's birth will be and the
sooner it will be over.

☐   *Fetal Positions*   The position of the fetus in the uterus before labor
begins is crucial to the course of labor because it determines how labor will proceed and whether a natural labor can be expected or not. About 95 percent of
babies are in the vertex (head first) position by the time labor is ready to begin.
This is the normal, uncomplicated way for a baby to be born. A woman with the
baby in a vertex presentation is more likely to have a natural delivery, if everything else is equal, than a woman whose baby is in another position.

Sometimes the baby presents in the breech position, which means that the
baby's rump presents first instead of the head. Breech presentation occurs in 3 to
4 percent of all deliveries. Breech births are divided into a frank breech in which
the legs are pressed up next to the body or a single or a double footling presentation, in which one foot or both feet extend down into the pelvis. One foot or
both feet, or one or both knees, make it an incomplete breech presentation, different from a frank breech, in which the "breech" or rump of the baby is the
only presenting part. Breech presentation can be distinguished from vertex
presentation by a manual examination in the obstetrician's office or by ultrasonography.

When a baby has settled down into the vertex position it is unlikely to turn
around; definitely not when the fetal head is engaged. Only in a second or third
pregnancy when the amount of fluid is excessive (in a twin pregnancy, for instance) and engagement does not take place until just before delivery might the
baby rotate into another position. Using new techniques, we can now sometimes
relax the uterus and turn the baby before delivery.

A manual examination of the abdomen will determine whether or not the
baby is in the longitudinal or transverse lie. Ninety-nine percent of all babies are
in the longitudinal lie, which means that the baby takes up a vertical position. In
approximately 1 percent of births, the baby is in the transverse or oblique lie, a
position in which the baby lies from side to side or in which the head or breech
has not entered into the pelvic bones. This rarely happens in a first pregnancy; it
is occasionally found in later pregnancies when the uterine muscles are relaxed
and the baby does not engage early into the pelvis. Sometimes labor pushes the
baby into the longitudinal position and a normal delivery can take place. If the
baby gets stuck in the transverse position, the only way to release it is by Cesarean section.

About 85 percent of babies in the vertex position emerge through the birth
canal with their face toward their mother's back. The remaining 15 percent face
front in what is known as the posterior position. In the posterior position the
baby's bony skull is in contact with the mother's spine, creating a sensation of

pressure in the lower back. This will result in "back labor," which is often more difficult and more painful than ordinary labor, although there are ways of relieving the discomfort (see page 405).

The prevalence of vertex or head-first presentation is not totally understood by doctors. One theory suggests that the fetus tries to use the uterine space most economically by choosing a position that fits into the shape of the uterus. A second theory suggests that the head, the heaviest part of the fetus, usually hangs downward in the amniotic fluid and forces the fetus into the vertex position. Indeed, a breech is often seen where some pelvic or uterine abnormality exists and the baby does not adjust well to the shape of the uterus.

Another reason is the construction of the head itself. The fetal head is composed of a group of small bones joined by membranes rather than a solid mass of bone. This makes the head somewhat compressible so it can adapt to the shape of the birth canal, a process that is called *molding*. It is quite common for the baby of a first labor to be born with a so-called "banana head," a head which is molded to a point. This newborn characteristic disappears rapidly—usually within twenty-four hours.

☐ *The Mechanism of Labor*   The mechanism of labor includes the stages of fetal engagement, cervical effacement, and cervical dilation, followed by the birth of the fetal head and the fetal body. The labor mechanism depends somewhat on the position of the baby when labor begins. Since the baby is in the vertex position in 95 percent of labors, the following breakdown of labor will be concerned only with the birth of a baby in the vertex position. In the majority of vertex presentations, the head enters into the pelvis in the transverse, or side position, and in 40 percent of births, the baby is looking to the right when labor begins. Twenty-five percent of babies are facing the other way, to the left, with their back to the right. Another 25 percent face backward toward the mother's back and 10 percent face forward toward the mother's front.

The progress of labor depends on the woman's pelvic structure and the baby's size. A woman with a normal pelvic structure large enough to accommodate her baby is likely to have a normal labor. If there is any pelvic abnormality, a labor dysfunction can occur, a problem that will be discussed later.

There are seven phases that a baby experiences during labor and delivery. They are known as: *engagement, descent, flexion, internal rotation, extension, external rotation,* and *expulsion*. This sequence is basically the same for a first and subsequent pregnancies, although variations do occur at times. The reason for these complicated fetal maneuvers during labor is an anatomical one: the pelvic bones are tilted in such a way that the baby must twist and rotate its way through the pelvis to reach the outside world.

☐ *Engagement*   With engagement, or lightening, the baby's head enters the pelvis. This initial stage of labor usually occurs in the last two to four weeks before delivery in a primapara. A woman who has given birth previously usually experiences engagement just before going into labor. If you are in your second pregnancy and you still feel large, as if you have not really dropped the baby, it is only because the mechanism of labor is somewhat different in the second pregnancy. Once the presenting part has engaged, the baby's weight is resting against the pelvic bones rather than against the muscles of the uterus. The fetal head is now firmly inside the pelvis and has begun to work its way into the bony birth canal (the upper part of the pelvic bone is called the pelvic inlet). In the majority of pregnancies the baby's head enters sideways into the pelvis.

☐ *Descent*   The most important factor in a normal birth is the baby's successful descent through the birth canal. Descent is brought about by uterine contractions, which force the baby into the pelvis via the pressure of the amniotic fluid and push the baby's head farther into the birth canal. This phase begins earlier in the primipara than the multiparous woman. In a woman who has not given birth previously, engagement and descent usually occur before the onset of true labor, whereas a woman who has already given birth will experience engagement and descent during labor itself.

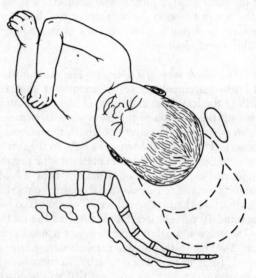

Figure 68: Descent: The baby's head as it enters the pelvic birth canal will position itself sideways to the left or to the right. This descent might begin prior to labor, although full descent occurs only during labor.

☐ *Station of the Presenting Part of the Baby*   The station of the head (an estimation of how far the baby's head has descended) is measured by vaginal or rectal examinations during labor. The doctor performing the internal examination will measure the presenting part and estimate the plane or level it has reached in the pelvis. If the baby's head has not fully entered the inlet of the pelvic bones, it is described as being in a minus station. Once the presenting part is on the level of the spine, the baby is said to be at zero station. At that point, the widest diameter (the biparietal diameter) of the baby's head is just at the level of the pelvic inlet.

A baby who continues to progress down the birth canal and enters into the pelvic bones is in a plus station. The plus one station is a position approximately one-third of the way between the level of the spine and the outlet of the bony part of the pelvis. The plus two station is two-thirds down. The baby then continues to move through the birth canal until the head reaches the perineum, ready to be delivered: in obstetrical language, the plus three station. If your doctor tells you the baby is descending to plus one, that means you should

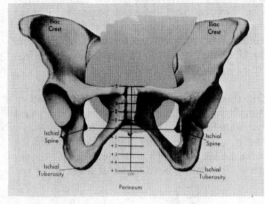

Figure 69: *Stations of Presenting Parts of Emerging Newborn:* A baby's head is illustrated at 0 station as the newborn enters the birth canal at the center of the pelvic bone. When the widest part of the head, called the biparietal diameter, has entered all the way into the pelvic birth canal, vaginal delivery is usually feasible. The leading part of the baby indicates the station. When the biparietal diameter is at the top of the bony birth canal, as seen above, the baby's head is considered to be in the 0 station. For each centimeter that the baby moves through the pelvic birth canal, the stations increase by one: +1 station, +2 station, etc. If the baby is too large and CPD exists, the baby's head will not enter into the pelvis and it will remain at minus level stations.

probably be able to have a natural vaginal delivery, since the presenting part and the pelvis are mutually proportionate. In a labor in which the woman is having difficulties or the baby is disproportionately large for the pelvis, the baby may remain in a minus station position, and would need obstetrical assistance.

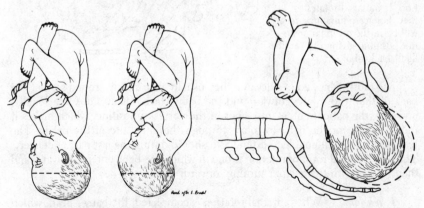

Figure 70: *Flexion:* The flexion of the fetal head during labor occurs as soon as the descending head meets resistance from the cervix. The baby, who initially is looking straight forward (picture at left), will be forced to flex his head and bend his chin to his chest (picture at right).   Figure 71: *Labor:* The baby's head has completely entered the pelvic birth canal and is now ready for internal rotation that allows the labor to continue.

☐ ***Flexion***   As soon as the descended head meets resistance from the cervix or the pelvic wall or floor, flexion occurs, which means that the baby is forced to bend its chin into its chest. This maneuver ensures that the back tip of the baby's head will rotate or turn into the pelvis, and the occiput, the back part (and in this case pointed part) of the head, will be the part that pushes against the cervix and makes it dilate. Studies by Danish researchers have shown that in normal births the baby may even flex the head before it begins to descend through the canal. If flexion does not occur, and the baby extends its head instead, then the presentation becomes what is known as a forehead or a face presentation, where there is a good chance that labor will be arrested and a normal delivery prevented.

☐ ***Internal Rotation***   During this maneuver, the baby turns its head in such a way that the occiput gradually moves from its original position forward toward the pubic bone (although sometimes the baby rotates the other way). This internal rotating movement is also called spinning, and one can indeed see the baby's head spinning into the pelvic canal when a multiparous woman pushes. This spinning motion allows the baby's head to adjust itself inside the pelvic bones.

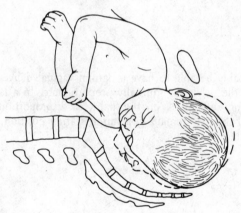

Figure 72: Internal Rotation: During this rotation, the baby's head will move into a position that will allow the head to face backward into the normal occipital anterior position. If the head rotates so that the face points upward, it will be in the occipital posterior position, giving rise to difficult back labor.

Since most babies go in sideways, they usually turn slowly around so that the back of the head rotates forward and the baby's face downward. Occasionally, however, the patient enters into labor in the posterior position, which makes it much harder for the baby to rotate through the curvature of the pelvis. The baby's head is then unable to extend as it should during the last part of delivery. The most natural form of rotation is one in which the baby enters sideways, and then rotates with the occiput turning forward.

☐ ***Extension***   When internal rotation is completed, the baby's head, which until then has been sharply flexed, will begin to extend. The baby's face should now be facing backward as the head enters into the curvature of the sacral bone. From this position the head begins what is known as *extension* in readiness for birth. Extension brings the base of the occiput into direct contact with the under-portion of the pubic bone, thus allowing the head to come down. This

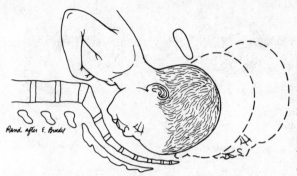

Rand after E. Bradel

Figure 73: Extension:
When the baby's head
is pointed backward, it
will fit perfectly into the
birth canal, making
childbirth easier.

movement enables the baby to pass upward and forward through the opening of the vulva. The top of the baby's scalp then becomes visible as the vulvar opening widens under the pressure of the head.

Before extension can take place the baby must have rotated inside the pelvis so that the head is passing through the narrow space in the pelvic bones. Otherwise delivery cannot occur. For example, a baby in the posterior position cannot extend if it does not rotate spontaneously, even though the woman is fully dilated, pushing, and otherwise ready to give birth. In this case, forceps are applied to rotate the head.

☐ *External Rotation*   Immediately after the birth, the head undergoes another rotation, toward the left side if the occiput was originally directed toward the left, and toward the opposite direction if it was pointed to the other side. The return of the head to its normal position is called the external rotation. The head will rotate to a position corresponding to the position of the fetal body.

☐ *Expulsion*   Almost immediately after the head is born and external rotation is completed, the anterior (front) shoulder appears under the pubic bone and the perineum soon becomes distended to allow delivery of the back, or posterior, shoulder. After the shoulders are free, the rest of the body is quickly delivered into the obstetrician's hands.

☐ *Cervical Effacement*   When labor begins, the baby usually lies curled up inside the uterus in *the fetal position*. Unless the membranes have already broken, it is still protected by the amniotic sac, the fluid-filled balloon enclosed inside the womb. At this point the cervix, or neck, of the womb is thick and uneffaced although some changes in the structure of the cells that make it softer, more pliable, and more susceptible to uterine contractions may occur.

The cervix usually remains firmly closed throughout pregnancy, protecting the fetus and amniotic sac from invasive bacteria. Normally the cervix is long and cylindrical in structure. These are characteristics which alter under the influence of uterine contractions and hormonal interaction during labor, when the cervix gradually becomes conical in shape and becomes part of the wall of the uterus, leaving only one opening between the uterine cavity and the vagina.

First Stage of Labor

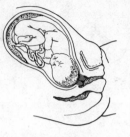 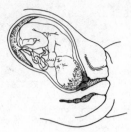

A. Beginning of labor   B. Partial effacement of cervix

Figure 74: Cervical Efface-ment: This picture illustrates cervical changes during the first stage of labor. In figure A, the cervix is long, closed, and uneffaced. In figure B, it is 50 percent effaced. Note that cervical dilatation does not occur until effacement is 100 percent. Figure C illustrates that the cervix is now paper-thin and ready for dilatation. It is now 100 percent effaced, and since it is thin it can easily stretch and begin dilatation. In illustration D, the cervix is completely stretched and fully dilated to accommodate the passage of the baby's head through the cervix.

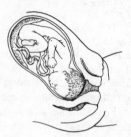

C. Full effacement of cervix   D. End of first stage of labor
   5 cm dilated   Full dilation of cervix

Cervical effacement occurs gradually, often beginning several weeks before the baby is born, and continues up to the end of the first stage of labor. During effacement the cervical tissue becomes progressively softer and shorter and washes away little by little until it virtually disappears. The uneffaced cervix is one and a half inches long. The fully effaced cervix is little more than a thin rim on the edge of the uterine-vaginal junction.

Effacement is necessary before progressive dilatation can occur. A woman might walk around with her cervix one or two centimeters dilated but she will not go into labor until effacement begins. An obstetrician examining a patient just before or just after labor begins is looking, first of all, for progressive cervical effacement. If your cervix has changed and effaced, he might be able to predict how soon labor will begin.

As the cervix effaces, your obstetrician or the hospital staff will estimate its progress in percentages; one can talk about anything from 30 to 80 to 100 percent effacement. A cervix that is 100 percent effaced is paper-thin and ready to dilate or open very quickly. You might begin to dilate slightly several weeks before you deliver, but as long as the cervix has not begun to efface, this dilatation is not only premature but unimportant. Effacement must be initiated before labor can begin.

The early stages of effacement are often painless. Some women go about their normal activities for a couple of days before being admitted to the hospital. Other women go to the hospital in the early stages of labor and still feel no discomfort. You might experience regular uterine contractions, a sign of early labor, without any pain at all. When you do begin to feel discomfort with contractions, this is a sign that the cervix is beginning to stretch, pulling at the nerves. The next stage in the birth process is dilatation, which closely follows progressive cervical effacement.

☐ *Dilatation* Once the cervix is effaced it can begin to dilate, again under the influence of the uterine contractions, or "labor." In fact, the term "labor" was once defined in obstetrical textbooks as "progressive cervical dilatation." Now that we know more about birth than we did a few years ago, labor is believed to begin when cervical effacement is instituted in response to regular uterine contractions, and only then is it followed by dilatation.

Dilatation enables the baby to move gradually down the birth canal and closer to the opening of the cervix. The baby's presenting part, usually the head, and the weight of the fluid in the amniotic sac slowly stretch the cervix through direct pressure. When the uterus contracts, the uterine muscles shorten and pull the upper portion of the uterus downward, pushing the head of the baby deep into the pelvis. As long as the bony pelvis is large enough, the baby moves down the cervical canal in the rotating or spinning motion explained above under *rotation*. As it rotates, the head is pressed downward; this puts pressure on the cervix, which has already undergone effacement and is primed for dilatation. Thus, with each contraction the cervix is slowly stretched and dilated. This cumulative process is slow at first, but with ongoing effacement the cervix is capable of increased stretching and dilatation.

Dilatation may proceed slowly and painlessly at first, but it can also progress rapidly, particularly in a second or third labor, with effective labor contractions. Contractions come closer together as the cervix continues to dilate to its full width. By this time the walls of the uterus have lost their original shape as the uterine muscles contract rhythmically to expel the baby. The nature of this uterine activity is involuntary; it doesn't help to bear down because you have no control over the muscles of the uterus. You can help speed dilatation by remaining as relaxed as possible, although this can be difficult during the active labor stage when the cervix is dilating from five to eight centimeters. Contractions increase in duration and intensity during this active stage. Once the cervix has fully dilated, the second stage of labor, which culminates in birth, is about to begin.

The degree of cervical dilation is expressed in centimeters or fingers. Centimeters are more accurate, since the size of the fingers would depend on the nurse or doctor performing the internal examination. A fully dilated cervix is ten centimeters (approximately four inches) in diameter, wide enough to accommodate the newborn head, with its average biparietal diameter of nine to ten centimeters. Less cervical dilation is required with a premature or small-for-date baby. A doctor who still prefers to estimate cervical dilatation in fingers will talk about five fingers when a woman is ready to begin pushing with a normal full-term baby.

A word of caution: do not begin to push until your doctor tells you the cervix is fully dilated. A woman who starts to push when the cervix is still only partially dilated will push the cervix down with the baby's head, a complication that risks seriously weakening the muscles around the bladder and perhaps causing a bladder prolapse later in life.

☐ *Stripping the Fetal Membrane: One Way to Start Labor*   If labor does not start spontaneously, at or after term, a doctor may try to stimulate labor by a simple procedure known as stripping the membrane, which he can perform during an internal examination. First he slowly inserts a finger into the cervix and gently moves it in between the inner part of the cervix and the fetal membrane, with the membrane still between the baby's head and his fingers. By moving his fingers in small, circular motions, he can often free part of the fetal membrane from its attachment to the uterus. Stripping the membranes in this fashion seems to cause a secretion of labor-inducing hormones, which might in turn trigger labor within twenty-four hours. The mechanism by which it works is thought to be one of two phenomena: either the reflexes will result in the release of oxytocin from the brain or they will cause the production of prostaglandin directly from the fetal membrane. The procedure has been performed for years and is often considered by doctors as a "natural" way to stimulate labor. It is usually not considered dangerous, but it has occasionally been associated with ruptured membranes and subsequent prolapse of the umbilical cord, or heavy vaginal bleeding.

Sexual intercourse is another, even more natural way to stimulate labor, as I have already discussed in Chapter 13. Sperm contain high concentrations of prostaglandins, which can be absorbed from the vagina and trigger labor. If labor does not occur spontaneously within two weeks after the due day, your doctor may consider labor induction by oxytocin infusion (see Chap. 30).

☐ *How Long Can I Stay Home Safely Once Labor Has Begun?*   Couples who take prepared-childbirth courses are usually advised not to call the doctor too early in the labor phase. Sometimes, though, it is difficult for a woman to judge the beginning of labor with confidence since the first contractions are often irregular and only gradually settle into a discernable pattern. Naturally this can be confusing for a woman in her first labor. Also, reactions vary greatly from woman to woman. An inexperienced or anxious woman might put in a call to her doctor immediately she feels Braxton Hicks contractions, while a prepared, confident woman will call only when contractions are well established.

Doctors usually have explicit instructions as to when they should be called. Some doctors like a patient to contact them early on because they can make plans for either a day or night delivery. The doctor will then expect you to call back and give him a progress report within a few hours. A doctor practicing in a group often likes to be called well in advance so he can plan to deliver you himself.

If your obstetrician has examined you a few days previously, he will know whether or not the cervix has begun to efface. This will give him a clearer idea of how quickly labor is likely to progress, and will influence the timing of the move to the hospital; he might suggest waiting until contractions are closer together or he might ask you to come in early if the cervix is effaced and has begun to dilate.

A good general rule is to wait until the contractions build up in intensity before calling the doctor. The first stage of labor is usually long and tends to progress slowly for the first few hours, especially in a first birth. Try not to become too excited early on because you will tire yourself out before you get to the hospital; instead, rest as comfortably as you can at home and continue to monitor the contractions carefully. You should, however, call the doctor immediately if the membranes rupture, as they sometimes do in early labor, whether the loss of the membranes is associated with other signs of labor or not. A doctor usually prefers to see a patient whose membranes have ruptured in the hospital so he can monitor her progress carefully. Very often labor will proceed rapidly when the membranes break, necessitating an immediate move to the hospital.

As long as the membranes are still intact, you can safely delay going to the hospital until contractions get closer together. If the first delivery was a rapid one, you should assume that the next one will be rapid also. If the first delivery was prolonged, your endocrine mechanism might be slow and the second delivery could follow the same pattern—although this is not always true of a second labor.

Another sign of labor progressing is the "show," the mucuslike blood-tinged discharge that is released from the cervical canal. The show, which usually occurs after a group of irregular contractions, tends to speed labor because it frees the cervix, encouraging the onset of good, regular contractions. The show alone does not warrant a doctor's attention, although again, you might call and alert him. If you have no show but you feel labor contractions become more regular and intense, the time to call your doctor depends on the distance you live from the hospital and your previous labor experiences. As long as you can cope with the contractions and make yourself comfortable at home, you might want to wait and then notify your obstetrician when contractions are eight to ten minutes apart. The longer you can comfortably stay at home, the more relaxed you will be and the more easily everything will go. Naturally, if you experience some abnormality—bleeding, or a lack of fetal movement between contractions—you must go to the hospital immediately. Once you are safely there, labor can be monitored with a fetal monitor to make sure that everything is going well. The obstetrician and the hospital staff are equally responsible for the health of the baby and a successful delivery.

☐ **When to Call the Doctor**   Babies are born regardless of the time of day—or night. You may experience the first contractions in the early evening. In this case, call your doctor with your questions before you go to bed rather than calling him in the middle of the night and disturbing him unnecessarily. For many women, labor begins around midnight, which might be tied to increased fetal activity, and contractions continue slowly through the early hours of the morning. Again, there is no reason to call the doctor before labor becomes stronger and more regular. If you think you are definitely in progressive labor, it might be a good idea to call the doctor early enough in the morning to leave the house comfortably before the morning rush hour. Don't hesitate to call your doctor at any time if you experience a warning sign—rupture of the membranes or bleeding; it could be an emergency requiring immediate attention. A safe delivery, your health, and that of the baby, are more important to your obstetrician than a few hours' sleep, which he can always catch up on later.

A couple should never be embarrassed or upset if they call their doctor in the middle of the night to report false labor symptoms, mistakenly thinking the woman is in labor. False labor can easily be confused with progressive labor. Even if you are not really in labor, a conversation with your doctor will reassure you and your partner and give you a clearer idea of how to deal with the symptoms of real labor. He might recommend an alcoholic drink—a vodka and orange juice, for example—to distinguish false labor contractions from real labor, since alcohol will stop false but not real labor. The moment of going into labor is very important in a woman's life, and every sensitive obstetrician should respect his patient's natural concern and very reasonable anxieties.

☐   **How Can I Avoid Being Sent Back Home?**   Before you set off for the hospital, time your contractions. A woman in progressive labor usually experiences regular contractions every five to seven minutes, which are consistently strong enough to cause discomfort. If you go to the hospital at that point in labor, you can be sure that you will not be sent back home. If you have never been in labor before, you cannot be expected to know what labor is like, and you may be confused by false labor contractions or a labor that proceeds irregularly, as some do. Again, women respond differently in the early stage of labor, depending on temperament and experience. If you are in doubt, it is better to call the obstetrician or the birthing center first before setting out for the hospital. An experienced doctor or midwife can usually determine the onset of progressive labor from a patient's description of her symptoms.

In inconclusive cases, I advise my patients to go to the hospital and be checked by a resident doctor or obstetrical nurse rather than stay at home in a state of anxiety. An internal examination will determine the extent of cervical effacement and dilation and put your mind at rest. If you are sent home temporarily, the hospital will often give you a mild sleeping pill such as a Seconal, or a Nembutal—a few hours rest or a good night's relaxed sleep often seem to trigger the onset of real labor. I know how frustrating it is to be sent back home when you are excited about going into labor, but it can be equally frustrating to spend unnecessary time in the hospital waiting room or walking up and down the corridors. Some of the more progressive hospitals have tried to overcome this problem by installing homelike early-labor lounges where patients and their families can talk and watch television in a relaxed, unclinical atmosphere. A woman who suspects she is in labor but has not progressed far enough for formal admission, can spend a few comfortable hours in the labor lounge rather than return straight home and perhaps set out again almost immediately.

An anxious couple should remember that a first birth usually takes at least six hours and generally twelve. The first baby is, therefore, rarely born on the way to the hospital or unexpectedly at home. With a subsequent baby, labor usually progresses much faster, but generally your doctor will have examined you internally before you go into labor and you will have the first labor experience as a guide. In general, don't go to the hospital too early with an uncomplicated labor; wait until you know you are in labor with good progressive contractions before setting out; there is then less chance of being sent back home.

☐   **What Happens When You Go to the Hospital**   If you are planning to deliver the baby in the hospital, your obstetrician will usually call the hospital's labor suite and prepare them for your arrival. If you plan to have your baby in a birthing center, call the birthing center before you set out.

When the contractions are close together, go immediately to the labor floor, where the staff can check your progress. Don't spend time in the admitting office. A major problem is unlikely but it can occur in the early stages of labor—

the placenta could partially separate, causing a decrease in the oxygen supply to the baby, or the umbilical cord could prolapse before the woman reaches the hospital. No time should be lost at the admitting office if labor is progressing rapidly. Your admittance can be formally registered after the nurse on the labor floor has made sure your vital signs are stable and the fetal heartbeat is steady. A first labor is usually quite lengthy, giving your husband plenty of time to go back to park the car properly, register your admission, and get back to act as your coach. Even if it contradicts hospital regulations, don't waste time in the admitting area if you can feel strong contractions. A good reason for both of you to take the hospital tour is to familiarize yourself beforehand with the building entrances and the labor suite, which doors will be open, and where the admitting office is located. Once you are in labor, both of you may be nervous and easily confused by an unfamiliar building.

☐ *The Internal Examination*   When you get to the labor suite, the admitting nurse will monitor the fetal heartbeat and the doctor on duty will check your vital signs—blood pressure, heartbeat, and pulse rate—and perform an internal examination. Internal examinations during labor should be performed under sterile conditions to avoid contamination of the baby. After either washing or spraying the vaginal area, the resident physician will put on sterile gloves and will gently insert one or two fingers into the vagina and feel for the cervix, moving his fingers around the cervix to estimate its length, thickness, dilatation, and amount of cervical effacement. Since full dilation can occur only after the cervix has fully effaced, early labor involves hormonal and endocrine changes occurring inside the cervix in which the cervical tissues soften and become increasingly elastic, so that little by little the cervix thins out, stretches, and finally disappears almost completely. During this ripening process you will experience early labor contractions; then, once the cervix is 100 percent effaced, full cervical dilation accelerates rapidly. If you are told you are 100 percent effaced and four to five centimeters dilated, you have reached an advanced stage of labor, with strong, regular contractions. Always ask the doctor or nurse doing an internal examination to give you an estimate of your progress—it's much easier to use your childbirth techniques effectively if you have a realistic idea of the length of labor.

Next the doctor will examine the pelvic area to determine the presenting part—the head in a vertex delivery or the buttocks in a breech presentation. He will also determine an abnormal position such as a transverse or oblique lie. The great majority of babies enter labor in the vertex or head-down position, but your obstetrician should examine you several times in the final weeks to make sure the baby is not a breech. If any doubt exists as to the baby's position, the obstetrician can order an ultrasound examination before the patient enters the hospital. A breech presentation detected in early labor is usually the result of an oversight by the obstetrician; babies rarely turn in the final stage of pregnancy because there is no room for movement in the birth canal. The only common exception is a twin pregnancy or a pregnancy complicated by hydramnios (see Chaps. 24 and 25). An obstetrician who tries to tell you the baby has turned unexpectedly is probably trying to find an excuse for missing the breech presentation.

Finally, the attending physician will check the position of the presenting part and the degree of engagement in the pelvis. If the head is well engaged in the bony pelvis and turned into the right position, you are likely to have a rapid delivery.

☐   *The Hospital Record*   After the initial examination, the attending nurse usually fills out a labor chart. Your obstetrician will already have sent your prenatal record to the hospital so the obstetrical staff should be aware of any high-risk factors in your pregnancy or any other important information. If high-risk factors do exist, you will need careful monitoring from the time you are admitted. If the staff does not have a patient's prenatal record on hand, it is important for the patient herself to give any vital information to them without waiting for her obstetrician to arrive. It can be irritating to volunteer information or answer questions when you are concentrating on labor, but try to give the staff a good history. The admitting nurse must know whether you have any serious medical problems, are taking any medications, or have a history of allergies.

Once the initial admitting preparations are completed, you are usually given a gown and asked to unpack and make yourself ready. By this time you are considered admitted to the hospital or the birthing center.

☐   *Birthing and Labor Rooms*   Many hospitals now have birthing rooms as well as conventional labor and delivery rooms within the labor suite. An increasing number of them, under pressure from childbirth educators and consumers, have installed or are about to install birthing rooms. Hospitals have made these modifications to stay in business and to satisfy pressure groups within the community who want to see women enjoy a natural childbirth, with medication used only when needed. One of the advantages of using a birthing room is that it is usually staffed by nurses who love their jobs and give expert support to women in labor.

A woman should not use a birthing room if she wants or needs more than the minimum of analgesia or anesthesia. A woman with a low pain threshold who is aware of her need for analgesics or anesthetics during labor can discuss this with her doctor beforehand and arrange to use the conventional labor and delivery facilities. Most major hospitals have several birthing rooms and conventional labor rooms to accommodate their patient's preferences. A high-risk patient is naturally required to use a labor and delivery unit with special monitoring equipment and an anesthesiologist and pediatrician in attendance.

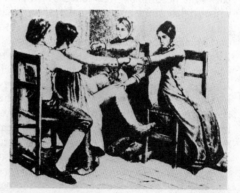

Figure 75: Colonial Birth Scene, Pennsylvania, Nineteenth Century: This picture illustrates a delivery by a midwife in which the woman received assistance and support from the husband, as well as other women. The husband here is being used as a makeshift birthing chair.

Occasionally a hospital makes an error and places a couple in the wrong section of the delivery unit. In this case, don't become unnecessarily upset and allow the mistake to confuse your breathing techniques. Your labor coach is the person who should be responsible for calling the doctor and rectifying the situation. Unless the hospital has only one birthing room, the staff should try to accommodate themselves to your plans and find you the room you would prefer to use during the birth.

☐ *What to Expect Next*   After your doctor has decided to admit you into the hospital, you will probably be faced with a series of standard admitting procedures and tests. These may include the routine prep—shaving of the pubic area, an enema, and an intravenous. Standard procedure in one hospital might not be standard in another hospital. You should discuss the policy of your own doctor and hospital with your obstetrician at least several weeks before you enter labor, if the questions were not raised at an earlier meeting. You will be better prepared and less anxious if you know what to expect. Advance knowledge will help eliminate any possible friction between yourselves and the labor and delivery staff.

☐ *Do I Need to Be Shaved?*   Some years ago, when labor and delivery were assumed to be a major surgical procedure, the routine prep included shaving of the entire pubic area. Routine shaving became controversial after prepared-childbirth teachers questioned the need for it in a normal birth, but it was not until a study conducted by Dr. William Sweeny and co-workers at The New York Hospital-Cornell Medical Center showed no difference in infection rates between shaved and unshaved women that doctors stopped ordering the full "prep" for all patients. Most doctors, including myself, now feel that shaving can safely be restricted to the small area between the vagina and the anus. The reason for this "mini prep" is that it makes it easier to perform a safe and easy episiotomy if this should be required. This minimal prep is favored in many modern hospitals, although I still receive letters from women whose obstetricians or hospitals insist on the full prep. The belief in a completely sterile environment for birth apparently persists, even though babies have been delivered at home for thousands of years without any shaving. In fact, the bacteria a woman normally carries on her skin are usually innocuous—harmful bacteria are those contracted from an alien environment, including the hospital or the doctor's hands.

Once again, this is a subject to discuss with your doctor at an early visit. If the hospital insists on the full prep, you might ask him to relax the rules on your behalf. A mini prep will help eliminate the rare incident of infection in the vaginal area; the full prep is completely unnecessary.

☐ *The Enema—A "Routine" Procedure that Is No Longer Routine*
Twenty years ago, hospitals believed in giving labor patients an enema as part of the standard "prep," or preparation for birth, even though the enema was unpleasant and uncomfortable and increased the fear women had of entering the hospital to give birth. The procedure was not entirely arbitrary, although the practice could have been limited to women who were very constipated. Women tend to become constipated in the last few days of pregnancy as the baby's head

rests on the lower pelvic area and puts pressure on the bowels. In the days before laxatives were added to iron pills this natural tendency to constipation was increased by the pregnant woman's diet. The enema was given to relieve constipation, increase the space in the pelvis, and make delivery easier. Without the enema, the hospital also felt there was a chance of bacteria from the unexpelled stools entering the birth canal and causing infection and other problems. The enema, however, has less of a place today when most pregnant women take proper care of themselves and eat a good, well balanced diet during pregnancy. These changes have led to many hospitals' discontinuing the routine prep for their obstetrical patients.

A sympathetic doctor will usually restrict the routine prep to patients who need it, but hospital staffs vary in their policies. Naturally, if you are somewhat constipated—a fairly normal complaint at the end of pregnancy—then the enema will make you more comfortable and may help trigger labor by increasing the space in the pelvis and allowing the head to press more effectively against the cervix. Otherwise it is unnecessary. I generally discuss this subject with my patients during an antenatal visit or just before they go to the hospital, and I have found no problem in treating each patient individually.

☐ *Do You Really Need an IV?*   Most American hospitals expect their patients to labor with an intravenous (IV), started soon after a woman is admitted to the labor floor. American doctors, unlike their European counterparts, who generally use IVs only in the event of complications, generally favor the IV because a woman who is not allowed to eat or drink during labor runs the risk of dehydration. At least with an IV she will get some fluids, usually a solution of dextrose and water, to counteract the loss of energy and body fluids during a long labor. Another advantage from the doctor's point of view is the ease of giving obstetrical drugs through the open line established by the intravenous. The popularity of epidural anesthesia has also increased the need for the IV. You must have extra intravenous fluids with an epidural to counteract the risk of hypotension, a lowering of the blood pressure, which could in turn decrease the baby's heart rate and damage the brain.

Nonetheless, the idea of giving every laboring woman an IV is possibly an outdated one. The routine intravenous may have been justified years ago when every patient in labor was considered "sick" and confined to bed flat on her back, a position that, as we now realize, prolongs labor unduly. Today, birthing centers do not use IVs and neither do the staff in most of the new hospital birthing rooms. Birthing centers allow women to eat during early labor so that they have enough energy to go through labor without intravenous fluids. A more sensible policy might be to confine the use of IVs to women who are at high risk or who become dehydrated after an unusually long labor, although many hospitals would resist changing their methods at this time. You might want to discuss the routine use of the IV with your doctor before you go into labor. He may or may not be able to relax the normal hospital rules on your behalf.

☐ *May You Eat During Labor?*   Many women going into labor are confused by conflicting opinions on this subject. Most hospitals strictly forbid solid food during labor, given the risk of an anesthetized or heavily sedated woman unconsciously aspirating the contents of her stomach during the delivery. On the other hand, birthing centers or the modern delivery room staff often ask couples to bring food in during the early stages of labor because they do not use IVs and labor can be compromised if a woman becomes dehydrated or hypoglycemic during the delivery.

Labor can be compared with other forms of strenuous physical activity. No athlete would enter a marathon with a large amount of undigested food in her stomach, and neither should a woman going into active labor. Good strong contractions in early labor means you could be at the second stage of labor within a few hours, and pushing on a full stomach can induce an unpleasant bout of nausea and vomiting in the delivery room. At the same time, a woman must avoid dehydration and the risk of becoming acidotic during labor. The body functions better if a woman's energy level is high—another parallel between the athlete who is about to enter a marathon and a woman going into labor. Certainly there can be a reasonable balance between eating and fasting in early labor, even though you must still be careful not to eat once labor begins if you are a high-risk patient who might need surgery, or you anticipate having heavy doses of medication during labor. Naturally, a high-risk or heavily medicated patient will be given an intravenous to prevent dehydration or other problems. Otherwise, a woman who has prepared for a natural delivery with the minimum of drugs can eat a light meal or meals and drink plenty of fluids while she is still at home in early labor. Fluids are preferable to solid food if labor seems to be progressing rapidly (it would be wise to call your doctor first if you are unsure of your progress). A light meal should give you enough energy to get through labor successfully, since most women in progressive labor don't experience hunger until the birth is over. You will usually be allowed crushed ice or water in the labor room, and you might ask your doctor to permit clear liquids like bouillon or tea. And remember, after the baby is born, you should be allowed to drink whatever you want, including a celebratory glass of champagne, as long as you feel well and haven't taken heavy doses of drugs during the delivery.

☐ *Should You Walk Around During Labor?*   Humans are the only mammals that lie down during labor. Other animals move around until it is time for the young to be born, or go through labor in a squatting position. Up until the last century most American women in labor walked around for as long as they could and then sat up, often using a "birthing stool" or an obstetrical chair for the final stages of labor and the birth itself.

Free movement allows the full weight of the baby to press on the cervix and trigger the labor reflex. The force of gravity also pushes the baby down the birth canal, speeding labor and easing discomfort. Studies performed in Guatemala by the eminent obstetrician Dr. Roberto Caldeyro-Barcia concluded that the vertical position shortened the first stage of labor by as much as 25 percent because uterine contractions were considerably more efficient and intense in this position. During the second stage of labor his patients were more comfortable sitting in a special obstetrical chair, rather than lying flat on their backs in the traditional position.

Strictly from a physiological point of view, there is no doubt that you will benefit from walking around during the long first stage of labor while cervical effacement and early dilatation are taking place. Then you might prefer to lie down or sit up when you come to the active phase of labor. As long as you remain at home you can walk around normally, although it is a good idea to relax part of the time because you could tire yourself out before you get to the hospital. You will need all your available energy during the transitional and second stages of labor. Once labor has progressed to the point at which you are more comfortable in bed, the head of the labor bed should be tilted up to allow the weight of the baby to press against the cervix. You can ask your labor coach to help you find the best sitting position by putting pillows between your back and the headrest of the labor bed. One of the disadvantages of electronic monitoring techniques is the physical restriction imposed by the conventional fetal monitor. Certain European hospitals have now introduced an innovative telemetric monitoring device, which gives the patient freedom to move around her room or outside her room while she is still being continuously monitored.

Labor experiences, of course, do vary from woman to woman, and some women are not comfortable walking around during labor. The body's own release of prostaglandin during labor can have some unpleasant side effects; nausea, vomiting, and a low fever are not uncommon in the first stage, and certain women seem to be unusually susceptible to prostaglandin-related discomforts during labor. An overzealous coach can sometimes add to a woman's misery by trying to get her to walk when she would be much more comfortable in bed. A woman with back labor will probably need more rest as well—back labor can be uncomfortable and tiring. One labor can rarely be compared accurately with another, and no one should be subjected to unnecessary stress because her labor is less than "perfect."

☐ *Should the Doctor Rupture the Amniotic Sac?*   Some women enter the hospital after the spontaneous rupture of the fetal membranes at home, but the majority of women enter with the membranes intact. Depending on your obstetrician, the membranes will then either be ruptured artificially or left to rupture spontaneously. Some obstetricians believe in artificially rupturing the membranes as soon as you go into the hospital, the reason being that the rupture causes a release of prostaglandin into the bloodstream. Prostaglandin, in combination with oxytocin naturally released from the pituitary, increases the urgency of the uterine contractions, and labor usually speeds up rapidly about half an hour after the membranes have been ruptured. Other doctors disagree, believing that the membranes are there to protect the baby from undue uterine pressure and should not be ruptured early on. According to Dr. Caldeyro-Barcia, the fluid in the intact membranes protects the baby's head during its descent in the birth canal and helps dilate the cervix. He recommends not rupturing the membranes artificially until birth is just about to take place.

Certainly, if you enter the hospital in good labor, there is no reason to rupture the membranes at an early stage. The membranes usually break spontaneously as the intrauterine pressure increases and the baby's head pushes down against the cervix. Otherwise, if the membranes do not rupture spontaneously, it is often best to rupture them artificially when the cervix is three to four centimeters dilated and the baby's head is well applied to the cervix. By that time the cervix is usually fully effaced and the membranes have performed their role in opening the neck of the womb and effacing the cervix. Once the membranes are ruptured, the uterus is smaller and will work better in speeding up the last part of labor. This, again, is a subject you might like to discuss with your doctor. Another reasonable indication for artificial rupture is a first-stage labor in which the baby has not engaged properly and the membranes are too full of fluid to allow the head to press against the cervix. The doctor would then be justified in rupturing the membrane early on.

Artificial rupture is performed with a small plastic tool with a hook on the end. The doctor inserts his hand into the vagina, slides the device up along his hand and uses the other hand to hook the device into the fetal sac and rip a small hole in the membrane. This can be slightly painful for the mother, but will not harm the baby, since the device touches only the fetal membranes, not the fetal head. Sometimes the membranes are weak enough to rupture during an internal examination without direct assistance.

A procedure known as "stripping the membranes" is sometimes used to stimulate labor in a postdate woman (see above). This is not the same as rupturing the membranes.

☐ *The First Stage of Labor*   The first stage of labor is the time from the onset of true labor up to the full dilation of the cervix. The timing of this stage varies from one woman to another, depending on several factors: how the baby enters into the pelvis; how big the baby is; and how far the cervix has effaced prior to the onset of labor. However, on the average, this first stage takes approximately ten hours the first time a woman gives birth.

This first stage is usually thought of as occurring in three phases. The first is the preliminary phase, or latent phase, in which the contractions last between thirty and forty-five seconds and occur at intervals of five to ten minutes. The cervix usually dilates about two to three centimeters during this phase, which can last up to eight hours, all depending on the timing of the onset of labor. In the next phase, the accelerated phase, contractions usually occur every two to four minutes, and the cervix dilates from three to seven centimeters. Finally, in the transition phase, which can last from one to two hours, contractions usually occur every one to two minutes and last from sixty to ninety seconds. This is the most difficult part of labor—a time when the rapid stretching of the cervix may cause intense discomfort and a woman might need some form of pain relief to see her through the contractions.

It is often difficult to estimate exactly when labor begins. This makes it difficult to time the length of the first stage. However, a general rule is that the cervix dilates at the rate of one centimeter per hour, although naturally this, too, varies among individuals. If you enter the hospital with good regular contractions every three minutes and you are already two centimeters dilated, you should anticipate being in labor for another eight hours until the cervix is fully dilated. You might, of course, be lucky and experience a faster labor, or you might be one of those women who experience some form of dysfunctional labor (see Chap. 30). At least 20 percent of women go through what is known as back labor, in which labor is slowed because the natural forces of labor are impeded by the baby's position, with it entering the birth canal in the posterior position, the face forward instead of backward. Although back labor is frustrating it is easier to cope with if you understand the particular problem of this type of labor (see below).

During the preliminary stage of labor, try to relax as much as you can and make yourself as comfortable as possible. Above all, don't overexcite yourself— be prepared for the length of time it will take to accomplish the birth and try to save your energy for the more taxing transitional stage of labor and the second stage of labor. Since a woman will cope with labor better if she knows what is happening, I like to talk to my patients and give them an honest idea of the progress of cervical dilatation and effacement at frequent intervals during this first stage to make sure they know how well their labor is advancing.

☐ *How Labor Progresses*   Contractions should increase in intensity as the first stage progresses. Initially the cervix is slightly dilated, and contractions are mild to moderate. But toward the end of the first stage (the transitional phase) contractions will be long and intense, with only a short interval between each one. The gradual intensification of the contractions is a sign that labor is progressing normally. Sometimes though, labor will progress up to a certain point and then slow down or stop altogether. A cessation of cervical activity may be a symptom of CPD, cephalo-pelvic disproportion, a complication that might result in a Cesarean (see Chap. 31). It can also be a sign that the uterus is getting "tired." Your doctor may then decide to stimulate the contractions artificially with oxytocic drugs. But normally the mechanism of labor continues to function progressively; natural oxytocin is released through the mechanism of cervical dilation, and the contractions become closer and closer together.

☐ *The Latent Phase*   The pain of labor is associated with dilatation, the opening of the cervix, so there is considerably less discomfort in the preliminary or latent stage of labor than there will be later on, when the cervix dilates from five to ten centimeters. The initial contractions during the latent phase might last from thirty to forty-five seconds and occur every three to four minutes. If you have attended preparation-for-childbirth classes, refer to Chapter 26 for the relaxation and breathing techniques used during early labor.

The preliminary stage is a good time to practice complete muscle relaxation between contractions. Breathe in and out deeply, and try to lose all the tension in your arms and legs by relaxing them completely. Complete relaxation allows more oxygen to reach your muscles so you will have more strength for the next contraction. Additionally, your body's own pain-killer, beta endorphine, will be released and will help to curb the pain (see Chap. 26).

You will find it easier to relax completely between contractions if you can find a comfortable position. Try sitting up in bed with the pillows supporting you from the back, or relax in a side-lying position with a pillow under your knees. Or if you prefer you can walk around between contractions and then stand or squat during the contractions to relieve the pressure on the cervix. Walking around does relieve the monotony of early labor as well as encouraging the baby to move down into the pelvis. If you are already experiencing signs of back labor, kneeling on the bed or the floor, or sitting in the knee-chest position will help take away pressure from the lower back.

Many hospitals use the fetal monitor intermittently during this preliminary stage to make sure that early labor is going well. An obstetrical nurse will put the monitor in place, watch the fetal heartbeat recording for a few minutes, and then disconnect the monitor for a few more minutes, allowing you to walk around freely. Later on in labor the monitor will be reattached to the abdomen and used continuously.

☐ *The Accelerated Phase*   Once the cervix is five centimeters dilated, cervical dilatation accelerates rapidly. Now the uterine contractions recur every two to four minutes and last longer, from forty-five to sixty seconds. The peak of each contraction is higher and more powerful than in the preliminary stage of labor, and you will feel increasing discomfort as dilation progresses. At this point of labor, you will have to concentrate fully on your breathing and relaxation exercises to control the pain. Your coach should time the contractions and count off the seconds as they pass the ten-, twenty-, and thirty-second mark, so you will know how long you have to keep breathing. Then breathe in and out deeply after each contraction is over, making sure you achieve a complete exchange of oxygen and carbon dioxide. Otherwise you might begin to hyperventilate. Contractions occur with increasing rapidity in the accelerated phase, so you must try to focus on each contraction and then conserve your energy between contractions through relaxation and deep breathing.

You may experience some unpleasant side effects of active labor. Because of the increased pressure on the bladder, many women have a continuous desire to urinate (see below). Leg cramps, muscle spasms, and changes in body temperature are also common. Many women become hot and uncomfortable at this stage of labor. Ask your coach to have crushed ice on hand to wet your lips and a damp or wet towel to wipe off your perspiration between contractions. Sometimes the body temperature fluctuates wildly because of sudden changes in the body's vasomotor system (again see below). Your coach might cover you with a blanket if you experience chills or a fit of shaking.

Often a woman in active labor will concentrate so hard on what is happening to her body that she stops communicating with her coach or the other people in the labor room. An understanding coach will quickly learn to interpret facial expressions and hand signals. Sometimes he will see his partner go through periods of agitation or become quite angry or unreasonable. These personality changes are transitory, but they can be upsetting to a man who is trying to help his partner and feels he is being rejected. It is important to remember that a woman in labor may be having difficulty in coping with more than just the contractions, and may find any distraction intensely irritating.

If there are too many noisy people around, close the door. Most labor floors are not peaceful places. You can take a transistor radio or a tape deck into the labor room to help screen out unwanted noise from the staff or the other patients. (You may hear other women screaming during labor because they are unprepared and frightened. Other women make a lot of noise in between contractions because that is one way to relieve tension.) If you feel like moaning or talking loudly, simply ask your coach to shut the door. We never know how we will respond to a stressful situation like labor, and anything that helps relieve tension is valuable.

☐ *Leg Cramps*   Spasms of the legs and calf muscles and the muscles of the foot are a painful nuisance during pregnancy (see Chap. 10). They often occur during delivery also. Cramping in the foot can often be relieved by massage or by walking around. You can also ask your coach to hold your foot and then try to extend your foot as you push against his hand. Another common discomfort is recurrent cramping in the upper part of the leg, but without muscle spasms. The reason probably is the pressure of the head on the nerves, as the nerves in the pelvic area in turn irritate nerves in the back that go down to the skin and the muscles in the leg. This works almost like a reverse acupuncture: whereas acupuncture stimulates an area of the skin which relieves a deep muscle pain, the baby pushes on the large interior nerves, which in turn stimulate the nerves of the skin. The best way to overcome the problem is to change positions or have your coach massage the affected area. Unfortunately, for some women cramping continues throughout labor, because the back of the head rests directly against the spinal nerves. Again, there is no specific treatment, but you can try massage or changing your position. If muscle cramps become so intense that you are extremely uncomfortable, you might need Demerol or some other analgesic to alleviate the pain, or you might decide to accept an epidural. Whatever is necessary to relieve the unpleasant side effects of labor should be done, and there is no reason to feel like a failure if you must accept medication.

Another type of muscle spasm sometimes accompanies an attack of hyperventilation, which is not uncommon during the transitional phase of labor. A woman may find that her hands are clenched into a fist, or her legs become impossible to extend. These spasms are the result of changes in the nerve impulses in the system as the normal balance of carbon dioxide to oxygen is disrupted. Massage will again help relax the muscles and will also alleviate tension, or you can use the paper bag technique (see Chap. 26) to introduce more carbon dioxide into the system. Hyperventilation is another side effect of labor that is more likely to occur as labor intensifies and you become more anxious and tense.

☐ *Bladder Pressure* If you are being given intravenous fluids during labor, the extra fluid will increase your need to urinate. What often happens, though, is that a woman concentrates so hard on her labor that she forgets that her bladder is beginning to fill up. In addition, as the baby moves down, it becomes harder to urinate since the urethra is partly obstructed. If the baby descends, you may feel great pressure on your bladder as the head rotates into the pelvis. It could also be the shoulder of the baby as the head is entering the birth canal that gives you the feeling of pressure. The simplest way to deal with the problem is to try to empty your bladder as often as possible. An empty bladder will also help the baby's head push hard against the cervix to start the Ferguson reflex. Another way to avoid the feeling of discomfort is to change your position; move from one side to another or even try to walk around—whatever you can find to alleviate the pain. If it becomes impossible for you to empty your bladder naturally, you might need to be catheterized.

☐ *If You Become Nauseated* A feeling of nausea in the transitional stage means there is increasing pressure in the pelvic area as the baby's head descends into the pelvis—a sign that labor is well on the way and the end is near.

There is nothing much you can do about the feeling of nausea, although you can try changing your position or your breathing pattern. Antinausea medication is not necessary since the sensation is transitory. If you are in the transitional phase and need Demerol, this medicine will increase your nausea to the point at which you are likely to throw up. Don't worry about it—it might be good to relieve the pressure on your stomach.

☐ ***Don't Forget the Socks During Labor***   During labor, the vasomotor system in the body, the system that regulates the contractions of the small blood vessels, changes in a way that is beneficial to the baby. Blood will therefore be shifted toward the uterus rather than the extremities. The blood vessels will for that reason often be constricted in the feet during labor and delivery, resulting in uncomfortably cold feet, especially during the active and second stages of labor. Since any form of discomfort can make it harder for you to concentrate on your breathing or other prepared-childbirth exercises, most childbirth educators recommend bringing a pair of warm socks in with you for the delivery.

☐ ***Shaking and Chills During Labor***   Shaking and sudden chills are not unusual during labor; again, these are side effects caused by the changing vasomotor nerve system. If your arms and legs become cold, you can ask your labor coach to massage them, or you can ask the nurse to put some warm blankets over you. Sometimes the sensation is one of alternating heat and cold. Women whose labors are induced or stimulated with oxytocin are particularly sensitive to chills and shaking, since oxytocin is known to change the circulation of the blood. Again, your labor coach can massage your arms, your legs, or your back to stimulate the circulation and make you feel warmer.

☐ ***Back Labor***   In a minority of labors, the baby enters into the pelvic inlet in the occiput position, which means that the baby is facing forward with the hardest portion of the fetal skull pressing against the woman's backbone rather than the front of the pelvis. This type of labor usually proceeds more slowly because the natural labor mechanism is altered. The baby's head tends to stay in the posterior position rather than rotate freely in the pelvis, putting great pressure on the nerves within the pelvis. (It can sometimes happen even if the baby is not in the posterior position.) A woman may experience terrible back pain under these circumstances, particularly during each contraction. One way to relieve the pressure is a change in position. If you can walk around, or at least kneel or sit up in the labor bed, you may help trigger the so-called Ferguson reflex, the nerve stimulus from the cervix to the brain which, in turn, triggers release of oxytocin, as the baby's head rests against the cervix. If you cannot sit up, try a side-lying position, with both knees bent and a pillow supporting the upper leg.

Another form of relief is massage. Ask your coach to massage the lumbar spinal area firmly during contractions—the more pressure he can apply, the more relief you will experience (see Chapter 26 on prepared childbirth). Sometimes an ice pack or a heating pad applied to the lower back is helpful. One form of massage now taught in prepared-childbirth classes is *the rubber ball technique*, in which the labor coach continuously rotates two rubber balls or tennis balls between his hands in small circular movements against his partner's lower back. The extra hardness of the rubber balls effectively counteracts the pressure in the lumbar spinal area. Back labor, however, does tend to be longer and more difficult than the average vaginal delivery, and sometimes labor needs to be stimulated by oxytocin to drop the baby's head down and relieve the pressure on the sensitive lumbar nerves.

☐ *The Transitional Phase*   The most active phase of labor is the so-called transitional phase, when the cervix will dilate fully from approximately eight to ten centimeters. Now the uterine contractions are at their maximum intensity, with contractions occurring at thirty- to ninety-second intervals and lasting from sixty to ninety seconds. In this phase of labor each contraction may go through several rather erratic peaks and valleys, instead of rising to a peak and then diminishing. The irregularity of the contractions makes it more difficult to time or "breathe through" each contraction.

The best method is to deal with each contraction at a time. Watch your breathing and use whatever breathing pattern works best for you (the Lamaze breathing exercises are described in Chapter 26). But don't breathe so rapidly that you begin to hyperventilate. If you feel faint or you experience a tingling sensation in your hands and feet, ask your coach to cup his hands or put a paper bag over your nose and mouth. Either will help create a proper exchange of oxygen and carbon dioxide.

As each contraction begins, keep your eyes open and make an intense effort to concentrate on your coach, who will be breathing through the contraction with you. Keep your jaw slack; this will keep you from clenching up your face and increasing tension. Don't be afraid to make noise; moaning is natural and will relieve some of the pain.

As soon as the contraction is finished, relax. You have only a short time between contractions in the transitional stage, so it is very important to relax completely. Your coach should check you carefully for any signs of tension. Keep your legs and arms relaxed; don't clench your hands and fists. Finally, breathe deeply. Slow, deep breathing will prepare your mind and body for the next contraction. When the next one begins, concentrate on it completely. Don't think ahead to the next one, or the next one, or you will lose your concentration and begin to panic. This is important, because once you have lost your concentration you will feel the full pain of the contractions. Your abdominal muscles will then instinctively tighten up and labor will slow down, making the entire transitional phase longer and harder.

Transition often creates a "fog" around a woman, making it difficult to communicate with her. She may say that she "can't go on" or she "wants to quit," or ask for a Cesarean to stop the pain. The coach will find it helps to take his partner's face in his hands and use eye contact as he gives her a firm, verbal order to go on with her breathing techniques. This is a point in labor at which many women become angry or irrational; you may find your partner's touch irritating or you may become angry with anyone who tries to help you. You might also experience some unpleasant physical symptoms, especially just before the end of the transitional phase. Nausea, hiccups, extreme rectal pressure, trembling, chills, perspiration, and even vomiting are not uncommon. (Vomiting is often a good sign, because it usually means a woman is fully dilated and ready to push.)

☐ *Pain Relief in Labor*   Although prepared-childbirth classes usually encourage the minimum of drugs, many trained women find it difficult to control the pain of labor through natural childbirth techniques alone. Each woman, after all, has a different pain threshold and a different perception of pain. A woman whose labor is unexpectedly painful may then face a conflict between her desire to give birth without drugs and her real need for some form of pain relief.

It is important to remember that admitting to pain is *not* a sign of weakness. Women have had children for thousands of years and labor has always been associated with a degree of pain. Even if you are fortunate enough not to require pain medication, you will feel some pain. And for some women, labor is so difficult that they need analgesia or anesthesia to see them through the most painful part of labor. Most childbirth educators talk about obstetrical drugs in their classes because they recognize that many trained women still need medication, even if only some Demerol to take the edge off the pain. (The pros and cons of the different analgesics and anesthetics used in childbirth are discussed later in this chapter.)

There is of course a potential for conflict between a woman who asks for pain relief and a partner who wants his child to have a drug-free birth. I have known women who were pushed by their husbands to continue without medication, but who felt they could not go on any longer without falling apart. If the husband still insists that his child is not going to have drugs, even though his wife is obviously distressed, the father is no longer supporting his wife but demanding what he wants for his child. In that case the husband must understand that she is the one who is suffering, and he should agree to what is in her best interest. Furthermore, acute fetal distress may actually harm the fetus more than the effect of analgesia or anesthesia, according to some new research described later in this chapter.

☐ *"I Can't Do It, Give Me a Cesarean"* Labor for some women is long as well as hard. Sometimes a woman reaches such a low point after hours of labor that she will ask her doctor to do anything, even a Cesarean, to end the pain. By this time the coach too is often exhausted and distraught. I have seen men break down and cry because they don't know how to help their partners out of this crisis point in labor. A doctor is then faced with the choice of operating or seeing the patient through the crisis by some other means.

A number of Cesareans are, in my experience, performed at this critical point of labor because it is easier for everyone involved, and the doctor can go home feeling he has spared his patient unnecessary pain. Unfortunately, however, he may not be acting in the best interests of his patient, since the risks associated with Cesarean section—rates of infection and other serious problems—are much higher than for a woman delivering vaginally. A doctor may properly choose to do a Cesarean if the baby is showing signs of distress, indicated by a specific heart-rate tracing on the monitor (see Chap. 28), or if the patient's progress has been unusually slow (see the section on dysfunctional labor in Chapter 30). Otherwise, the kindest act an obstetrician can perform is to see his patient through the crisis without intervening surgically.

Sometimes the low point of labor is close enough to the end of the transition phase that a woman can get through it with extra encouragement and coaching. But if you cannot cope without medication your doctor may try Demerol or some other form of analgesic to take the edge off the pain. Once the worst of the pain has been curbed, the transitional phase often passes fairly easily. I have had deliveries in which the couple successfully surmounted a crisis with the help of medication and later on felt happy about having a natural delivery. Other women do need regional anesthesia to see them through a difficult labor. The only problem with giving regional anesthesia later in the transitional stage is that the next stage—the pushing stage—is affected. Regional anesthesia numbs all sensation in the abdomen and legs, so you will lose the natural urge to push the baby out. If you are well along in the first stage of labor, you might want to do without the epidural and accept analgesia instead.

☐ *If She Panics*   A woman who loses control of a contraction may have the sensation of drowning as the contraction keeps coming and coming in waves, and she finds it impossible to catch her breath. Once you lose the rhythm of your breathing technique and experience the pain of the contraction it is difficult to regain control because the natural human response to pain is fear. This then is a crucial point in labor because the fear-tension-pain syndrome (see Chap. 26) will only increase with each contraction, making it even more difficult to deal with the next one, and before long a woman may be hyperventilating, or crying, or showing other signs of complete loss of control.

If your partner is beginning to lose control, try squeezing her arm or massaging her back while you verbally encourage her to go on breathing through the contraction. Take a deep breath yourself at the end of the contraction to encourage her to relax and then start breathing through the next contraction with her. You can watch the pattern of the contraction on the fetal monitor and use this to time your breathing. If she is no longer in control of the contractions, make sure to stand up next to her so she realizes that someone is there. The simple act of standing up during a tough moment is probably the most effective action you can take to help your partner regain her control. Then grasp her hand and look straight at her as you encourage her through the next contractions. If you position yourself so your face is about a foot away from hers, she will have no other choice but to pay attention to you. Also massage her hands or her back or touch her face—physical contact is encouraging. Finally, breathe audibly with her through each contraction so she is aware that you are still working along with her.

☐ *The End of the Transitional Phase*   For most women, the transitional phase is unarguably the worst part of labor. Fortunately it is short, averaging only about thirty to forty-five minutes in a first labor. Once the cervix is fully dilated (ten centimeters dilated) it is completely effaced and effectively disappears. Now the baby's head is beginning to move down into the pelvic area. This prompts the nerves in the cervix to transmit messages via the brain to the muscles in the uterus, instituting the pushing reflex. You may experience a premature urge to push even before you are fully dilated. In that event you can begin to bear down slowly *without* pushing. A controlled bearing down without pushing will help the fetal head rotate as it enters the birth canal. If you breathe in and out forcefully, with short, sharp, continuous breaths, you will stop yourself from bearing down and thereby damaging your cervix if you are not yet fully dilated.

With the complete effacement of the cervix, the pain of the contractions decreases considerably because the head has now passed through the cervix, releasing the nerves in the cervical tissues from the direct pressure of the contractions. You will still feel uncomfortable, but it will be a different kind of discomfort from that of the intense uterine contractions you experienced previously.

As soon as you are fully ready to push, a completely different phase of your labor will begin, the second stage of labor. In this second stage, the "pushing phase," different nerve impulses are present and you will find yourself "pushing away" the sensation of pain. And in the second stage you will finally become an active participant in your child's birth.

☐ *The Second Stage of Labor* The second stage of labor begins when the cervix is fully dilated and ends at the time of delivery. The term "pushing phase" has a very good reason behind it: the laboring woman is engaged in pushing the baby out of the birth canal throughout the entire second stage.

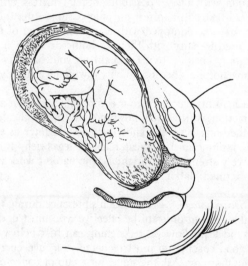

Full dilation of cervix. Beginning of second stage of labor.

Figure 76: Beginning of the Second Stage of Labor: The cervix is fully dilated; it is thin and the head can begin to pass through the cervix. This marks the beginning of the second stage—a woman may now begin pushing. The second stage is from the time of full dilatation until the delivery of the baby.

The length and difficulty of the second phase varies from one woman to another, and from a first labor to a second labor, depending on the strength of the contractions and the position of the baby. The second stage is usually one in which there is some relief from discomfort, and a growing excitement as you reach the final few pushes. It can also be frustrating for those women who find themselves pushing for hours without delivering the baby. No two labors are ever exactly alike, and you may be disappointed if you expect the second stage to progress smoothly and instead encounter some unexpected difficulty. But whatever the circumstances of your delivery (and you may well find the second stage a great relief after the difficult transitional stage) you can prepare by mastering the pushing exercises described in Chapter 26. With preparation and coaching, you will find it much easier to push effectively.

☐ **Pushing**   Preparation and coaching are the key to an easier second-stage labor and a successful birth. There may be discomfort, but with preparation and coaching you will find that pushing the baby out, although very laborious, is exciting and satisfying.

Begin by breathing deeply just before you start pushing with each contraction. This will help increase the oxygen in your body and will fill you with energy. During each contraction you will have a feeling of bearing down that will require great physical exertion. You may feel your face becoming flushed, a normal reaction to physical stress at this stage of labor. An involuntary grunt or groan at the beginning of each contraction is also quite characteristic of second-stage labor.

A woman should be in the best position to encourage the most effective pushing. Some women prefer to lie on their left side, which has advantages because the baby's weight is off the vena cava, allowing more blood through the maternal and the fetal circulation, with a lesser possibility of fetal distress. Other women prefer to sit up with a backrest, or to rest on pillows supporting them from behind. Some hospitals are now equipped with a modern version of the birthing chair that midwives used to carry with them to home deliveries hundreds of years ago. The lithotomy position (lying straight on your back) is no longer encouraged in progressive hospitals because gravity is working against you when you lie down flat.

A supportive coach should help his partner into a comfortable position and assist her during each contraction. With each pushing movement, the legs should be pulled up toward the body, with the knees bent to add force as you push (see Chapter 26 for more information). You can relax the legs briefly as the contraction ends. Pushing is very strenuous; it might be the hardest work you will ever do. This is why it is termed "labor."

☐ **The Coach's Role in the Second Stage**   The coach's presence during this final stage of labor is invaluable. But in order to be effective, you must understand the second stage fully and learn how your coaching can best help your wife. First, in order to be a good coach, you must recharge your own energy, even if it is four o'clock in the morning. Ask the nurse for a cup of coffee or a high-energy snack, splash your face a few times with cold water, and breathe deeply or walk around outside the labor room for few minutes. Then use your renewed energy to help stimulate your wife's courage and fuel her motivation. Many women in their first labor become tired before the pushing phase is completed. A coach, by being there, and realizing what his partner is going through, might well shorten labor by motivating his partner to push harder. Encourage your partner to begin pushing and keep pushing to the end of each contraction, and then help her relax after the contraction is over. Talk to her, breathe with her, and even "push" with her to show her you are sharing the labor with her. Don't ever be afraid of complimenting her when she is pushing as hard as she can.

Try to anticipate your partner's needs. Wipe away the irritating perspiration from her face or body; give her a sip of water or wet her lips with ice chips between contractions. If she is too hot, turn on the air conditioning or direct a fan against her face. If neither is available, use a book or a piece of paper to create a current of air. On the other hand, if she is too cold, wrap a blanket loosely around her.

The best coach has prepared for the birth through classes or reading, but at the same time is naturally sympathetic and supportive toward his partner.

☐ *How Long Is the Second Stage?*   The duration of the second stage can vary from five minutes to two hours, or occasionally three hours. As a rule, the second stage is somewhere between five and thirty minutes in a multipara, while it averages about one hour in a primipara. For some multiparas, the entire second stage is as short as one or two pushes. These variations depend on several factors; first of all, on the strength of the uterine contractions themselves. Contractions may continue strongly throughout the second phase. But it is not unusual for them to begin to taper off as labor progresses. A woman may then continue to push voluntarily, but her labor will inevitably take longer. You might try to stimulate the contractions by sitting up and taking advantage of the force of gravity; even standing up can sometimes be helpful. In an unusually prolonged labor, an intravenous infusion of oxytocin might be needed to strengthen the contractions and make the delivery possible. Even with a normal first labor, you should anticipate a second stage that takes at least an hour, or longer. With a second child, given good uterine contractions and coaching, the second stage can be short and relatively effortless.

Another second-stage factor over which you have no control is the position of the baby as it enters the bony pelvis. The second stage will be shorter and easier if the head is well flexed and fully rotated so it fits into the pelvis. When the baby enters in the posterior position, as it sometimes does, the entire second stage will be longer and more difficult than usual. The size of the baby is also an important factor in second-stage labor. A woman delivering a large baby, especially a woman in her first labor, can expect a harder second stage than a woman delivering a smaller child. There are often very few problems when the pelvis has already been tested by a previous baby, although a very large or poorly positioned baby in a second pregnancy might still prolong labor somewhat. Here a determined woman can sometimes help rotate the baby into the correct position by concentrated, hard pushing.

The one factor over which you do have control is the amount of effort you can exert during this second stage. The muscle contractions of the uterus are involuntary and they may or may not be strong enough to push the baby out unaided. But combined with the laboring woman's voluntary muscles, enough force is usually produced to force the baby down the birth canal and out through the pelvic outlet. An enthusiastic labor coach or an experienced obstetrical nurse or midwife who is really energetic and understands how to get a woman to push will often hasten the second phase by helping the woman through each contraction. When the participants' energy level is lowered, as it often is in a long labor, or a labor that takes place at night, the second stage can be unnecessarily prolonged. I have even seen deliveries in which a Cesarean section was performed because the nursing staff, the obstetrician, and the labor coach did not give a woman the encouragement she needed to push effectively. A second-stage labor can be hard if a woman has little urge to push, or is not coached successfully.

☐ *Is the Second Stage Painful?*   As soon as the second stage begins, you can expect some of the pain you experienced during the transitional stage to disappear. You are now ten centimeters dilated and there are no more nerves left to be stretched. In fact, as you begin to push, you may feel yourself "pushing the pain away" from the area of the cervix. Some women feel an immediate sense of release as they pass into the second stage, often heightened by the excitement of pushing the baby out. At the same time, there is a feeling of pressure in the area of the perineum—pressure which increases as the baby is closer to the moment of birth. This pressure is accompanied with a sense of stretching, sometimes even a burning sensation—particularly if you are delivering a large baby. For some women, this is very painful. Others seem hardly to notice it in the excitement of pushing the baby out. Her experience often seems to be affected by a woman's physical condition. A woman ordered to bed in the last weeks of pregnancy may find the pushing stage difficult because her pelvic muscles have temporarily lost their elasticity. An athletic woman who has been active up until the end of pregnancy will probably find it easier to push through the contractions without becoming tired or discouraged.

☐ *Monitoring the Second Stage*   Most obstetricians consider fetal monitoring an indispensable tool in the second stage of labor and will keep the monitor in place up until the last few minutes when the patient is taken into the delivery room (see Chapter 29 for a further explanation of the timing of delivery). The use of the fetal monitor is only a precaution in most low-risk labors since you can generally expect the second stage to go well; but the heart rate can be affected by cord compression or a sudden oxygen loss. (Again see Chapter 28.) Cord compression is a fairly common complication in the second stage because an umbilical cord caught around the neck or shoulders (this occurs in about 20 percent of pregnancies) will be squeezed as the woman bears down during contractions. Cord compression is not always a matter of concern, but it can result in a pattern of variable deceleration on the fetal monitor. In deliveries in which the monitor shows a persistent pattern of deceleration between contractions, the obstetrician may reposition the mother and give her oxygen by mask to increase the oxygenation within the uterus. If the heart rate continues to decrease, and delivery is still some time away, the obstetrician may decide to take a blood scalp sample to determine the baby's pH balance. A baby in jeopardy may be delivered quickly by forceps or even a Cesarean (see Chap. 31), depending on the position the baby has reached in the birth canal.

☐ *Why Is the Length of the Second Stage Important?*   The baby can be under considerable stress in the second stage because oxygen tension within the uterus is reduced sharply with each contraction. In a healthy pregnancy, the baby is able to withstand this temporary oxygen deprivation by drawing on the oxygen reserves within the placenta. This may, however, become more difficult if the second stage is long or exhausting for the mother, or the baby is in poor condition before labor begins.

One of the advantages of fetal monitoring is that we are now forewarned when a baby is under unusual stress, and can terminate the delivery immediately. Years ago, when monitoring was not available, obstetricians were so concerned about the possible danger of the second stage that they adhered to a principle known as the two-hour second-stage rule, first formulated over a century ago by Dr. Hamilton, a famous British physician. In a paper published in 1861, he stated: "Whenever the cervix has become fully dilated so the ear can be felt, I hold that danger to the child is usually imminent if allowed to remain undelivered much more than two hours." After two hours, Dr. Hamilton and his contemporaries preferred to attempt delivery by forceps rather than wait for nature to take its course.

So frightened were obstetricians of the risks of stillbirth or other damage during the second stage that some of them used forceps (see Chap. 30) as soon as the first stage was over, a procedure which was certainly more dangerous than allowing the second stage to take place naturally. The use of high forceps persisted up to twenty years ago in American delivery rooms, sometimes for social as well as medical reasons. A busy obstetrician who wanted to go home might take a patient to the delivery room, give her general anesthesia, and then apply high forceps to get the baby out, justifying his haste by citing the "dangers" of the second stage. This was one of the abuses that stopped once knowledgeable coaches were allowed into labor rooms.

Now a doctor usually tries to decide what is in the interest of the patient and her baby before acting to terminate the second stage prematurely. In most labors, the baby comes down within a reasonable time, with sustained pushing or oxytocin stimulation. When there is danger, or the patient is exhausted and cannot deliver the baby spontaneously, the delivery might be terminated prematurely with the aid of a low forceps. Occasionally a doctor may even have to resort to a Cesarean at this late stage of the delivery. It is, of course, sad when a woman who has been pushing for an hour to two hours still ends up with a Cesarean, but the lower part of the pelvis is sometimes unusually narrow and neither uterine force nor intravenous oxytocin stimulation are sufficient to push the baby through. At least in a modern delivery, a doctor can be less concerned by the length of a patient's second-stage labor as long as fetal heart rate tracing and fetal blood scalp samplings indicate that the baby is in good condition (see Chap. 28). If any of these reveal serious difficulties, the delivery should be carried out immediately, regardless of the time a woman has spent in labor.

☐ *Does the Urge to Push Differ from Woman to Woman?*   No two labors are alike, and no two women have an equal tolerance of pain. In the same way, the urge to push will vary from one labor to another. This can probably be explained by the position of the head in the pelvis; a head which has rotated properly in the pelvis will exert equal pressure on the cervix, resulting in a more uniform urge to push. The pressure of the head against the cervix seems to stimulate the cervix to send impulses to the brain. This, in turn, will increase the woman's urge to push. On the other hand, in some births the baby remains throughout in the posterior position, and here the urge to push will not be quite as good. Labor can then be expected to take longer and require more concentrated pushing effort.

☐ *Pain Relief During Labor*

Is Labor Painful? The answer is yes, it is never completely pain-free. Labor consists of a series of uterine contractions that become progressively more powerful as time goes on. But the degree of pain a labor patient experiences depends on the individual circumstances of her labor; the size and position of the baby's head, the effectiveness of contractions, and the size of the pelvis are physical factors that are outside a woman's control. Psychological factors also play an important role in labor—including the fear of the unknown.

As long as you are well prepared and have the help of your labor coach during active labor, you may well find you can go through labor without drugs or anesthetics. Avoid medication if you can—a single shot of Demerol could make you so sleepy that you lose your concentration during contractions. And don't let a well-meaning obstetrician force an epidural on you if you can cope without it. It is better for the baby if you have no anesthesia, since the chances of respiratory depression or a forceps or Cesarean birth are smaller with an unanesthetized birth. Even regional anesthesia can have a potentially harmful effect. The more natural the birth, the better it is for the baby. Labor is associated with pain, but the feeling of achievement is extraordinary if you can get through it without medication. On the other hand, if you cannot manage without pain relief, several effective alternatives are open to you. Don't be ashamed if you need medication; some women simply have a low pain threshold or a difficult labor and cannot cope as well as others.

A woman can either take an analgesic or have regional anesthesia. Both of these options are safe when administered properly. But it is important for you and your coach to know the pros and cons of all types of pain-controlling techniques in order to determine which will be best for you and your baby.

Analgesia During Labor Medication given for pain relief during labor and delivery can be divided into two categories: *analgesia* and *anesthesia.*

An analgesic relieves pain without affecting your ability to move around. The most commonly used analgesic is Demerol, a synthetic narcotic that can be given in varying doses. Other analgesics include morphine, fentanyl (Sublimaze), and butorphanol (Stadol). Sedatives such as Valium and Phenergan are not strictly analgesic drugs, but can also be used to relieve pain.

Demerol Demerol is the most commonly used analgesic in the modern American hospital. It will not take away all your pain, but it will take the edge off it. More important, it will help you to relax. Demerol can be given in varying doses (normally 50–100 milligrams), usually in intramuscular form during active labor. Physicians do not like to give Demerol in the early phase of labor since it decreases uterine activity and prolongs labor, nor do they like to administer it just before birth because of the possibility of neonatal depression. After a heavy dose of Demerol, the baby is often lethargic and has difficulty breathing. On the other hand, when Demerol is given during the active stages of labor, it may help speed the uterine contractions by decreasing the amount of adrenaline (a hormone that acts as a cervical constrictor) pumped through your body. Demerol counteracts the constrictive action of adrenaline and actually might speed your labor by simply relaxing the pelvic muscles and allowing the baby's head to descend more rapidly.

The problem with Demerol is that besides relieving pain, it can make you feel nauseated or "high," particularly if the drug is given intravenously in fairly large doses. If you have prepared for labor, a drug like Demerol could make it hard for you to concentrate on your breathing techniques during the really strong contractions. Heavy doses of Demerol given late in the first stage of labor can further have a severely depressive effect in the second stage, when a woman would normally be concentrating on pushing the baby out. A woman who is so "drugged up" she can hardly push will find the second stage unusually difficult and will not enjoy the delivery. Your doctor can minimize the adverse effects of Demerol by administering the drug in small doses. The initial dose can then be repeated as needed. If you need Demerol you can always begin with a small dose and then ask your obstetrician to give you more pain relief as you need it. The normal practice is to administer 50–70 milligrams every three to four hours, but if you want more before the four-hour interval is up, you can ask for it.

What Is the Effect of Demerol on the Baby? All drugs used for pain relief cross the placenta. If you receive Demerol or any other form of analgesia during labor, your labor should be carefully supervised and the effects on the baby monitored by a fetal monitor or frequent auscultation (use of the stethoscope). Demerol and other narcotic drugs tend to produce fetal depression, although effects vary according to the amount of the drug used, and the timing of the administration. It takes from four to five hours for the effects of Demerol to wear off, so if the drug is given one to two hours before birth, there is the chance of high maternal and fetal concentration of Demerol at the time of delivery, and the baby might be sleepy and have temporary breathing problems. Occasionally doctors will see babies who are cyanotic (blue from lack of oxygen) after a heavy concentration of Demerol. The depressing effects of Demerol can, however, often be counteracted by a drug called Narcan (naloxone), which acts as an antagonist to the narcotic drugs. An injection of Narcan, which comes in pediatric doses, can be given quickly after birth to reverse the depressive effects of Demerol. Narcan usually acts rapidly, and the baby will begin to breathe more easily and become pinker and more alert immediately.

The staff should always have an antagonist available in the delivery room or the birthing room. You can even ask the midwife or doctor whether they have Narcan available to give the baby if necessary. Narcan can also be given to the mother just before birth, again to avoid neonatal depression.

Sedatives and Tranquilizers These will not relieve pain, but they will relax you. Sedatives and tranquilizers are not generally used during labor itself. If they are offered during active labor, you might do well to refuse them, since barbiturates can aggravate pain during the active stage, and some barbiturates, such as phenobarbital, can remain in the bloodstream for a long time after birth and have a prolonged depressive effect on the baby. Unlike the case of narcotics, there are no known antidotes to barbiturates or tranquilizers. However, if you go into a hospital in the early stages of labor and are unusually nervous or restless, so nervous that you cannot deal with the contractions, you might be helped by an injection of Phenergan or another tranquilizing drug that will induce a mild sedative effect, enough to cope with early labor. Tranquilizers such as Valium should not be given during active labor because they induce drowsiness and the baby will be lethargic, with poor muscle tone, respiratory depression and an unusually low body temperature postnatally. Barbiturates and tranquilizers generally have a limited use in labor because they are not analgesics and have undesirable side effects; women have told me that tranquilizers during labor have the same effect as "one drink too many." A woman who is confused and uncoordinated is going to have a difficult time breathing through the contractions unless she has an unusually firm coach who can "breathe" with her.

Anesthetics for Pain Relief Anesthetics can also be divided into two categories: general and local anesthetics. The general one most commonly used is *sodium pentothal*. Usually sodium pentothal is given only at the time of delivery and in most cases only for a difficult forceps delivery or a Cesarean birth.

A local or regional anesthesia can be achieved during labor to numb a particular region of the body. Epidurals, caudals, spinals, saddle blocks, or subdural anesthesias are all types of regional anesthesia that leave the patient numb from the waist down. The major disadvantage of this type is the loss of the pushing sensation, the desire to bear down, along with the loss of sensation in the pelvic area. With an epidural or another form of regional anesthesia, a woman will no longer know when she has to push or when she is ready to push. A woman who has attended prepared-childbirth classes will still know how to push, but it might be difficult for her to know when. Here the delivery room staff and her labor coach will be needed to coach her through each contraction.

General anesthesia is rarely considered necessary for a vaginal delivery today, although it was used routinely in the past when doctors believed that birth itself was the most painful part of the delivery. Most women find it tremendously rewarding to be awake for the moment of birth and don't require, or want, general anesthesia. However, in an emergency situation, when the baby is in distress and must be delivered immediately, general anesthesia is often preferred over regional anesthesia because it takes effect very rapidly. Epidurals can be used in elective Cesareans, but the obstetrician will start an epidural only if he feels there is enough time to use regional anesthesia safely.

Finally, a *local anesthetic* such as lidocaine or novocaine is often given to numb the pelvic floor or the perineum—the area between the vagina and the rectum—during an episiotomy. Your doctor will probably administer a local anesthetic in the vaginal area, make a small incision to allow him to deliver the baby without tearing the perineum, and then stitch up the cut while the local anesthetic is still numbing the area.

Inhalation agents: In Europe, a mixture of nitrous oxide and oxygen is used as a light anesthetic called "laughing gas." A few whiffs of this combination anesthetic is often given during active labor and delivery to dull the sensation of pain. Some doctors in the United States like to use an inhalation anesthetic, methoxyfluorane, for the same purpose. This is a reasonably effective form of analgesia, but the patient must be observed carefully. Effects vary from woman to woman: an overpowerful dose can cause excitability—even hysteria—but it works well for some women.

Regional Anesthesia Regional anesthesia results in the elimination of pain in the lower part of the body. Three types are practiced—spinal, epidural, and caudal—although the epidural is by far the most popular of the three in a normal labor.

Spinal Anesthesia Spinal anesthesia is commonly used in Cesarean sections, since it has the advantage of completely numbing the pelvis and legs without the total lack of consciousness experienced with general anesthesia. It is not used as much in vaginal deliveries because a spinal can be administered only during the second stage when most women are reasonably free of discomfort. A spinal administered in the first stage has been known to arrest labor completely. With a spinal, the woman is given a single injection of local anesthetic into the tissues that surround the base of the spinal cord. The injection is effective enough to provide complete pain relief for up to two hours. Its disadvantages in a vaginal delivery include the tendency to severe "spinal" headaches in the postpartum period and the almost routine use of forceps for delivery, since the anesthetic deadens the desire to push for most women. The latter of course is not a factor in Cesarean birth, in which a woman with a spinal anesthetic can remain awake and aware throughout the birth.

Epidural Anesthesia Epidural anesthesia, the most common type of regional anesthesia used in American labor rooms, is achieved by an anesthetic solution injected through the lumbar region of the spine into what is known as the epidural space within the spinal cord. This is the space just before the membrane that separates the spinal fluid. An injection of local anesthetic into the epidural space numbs the nerves that carry sensations of pain to the brain, deadening the sensation of pain in the lower part of the body. To a certain extent it also disrupts motor function.

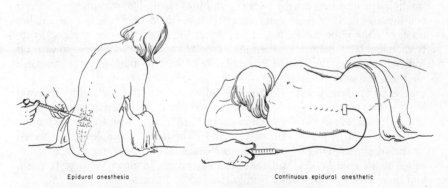

Epidural anesthesia   Continuous epidural anesthetic

Figure 77: Epidural anesthesia: A special epidural needle is inserted in the space between the fourth and fifth lumbar vertebrae, avoiding the spinal fluid itself. The novocaine numbs the nerves in the epidural space. The result is that this type of anesthesia numbs the nerves leading to the uterus and the legs but leaves the respiratory muscles and the other involuntary muscles functioning normally. This is the safest form of labor anesthesia.   *Figure 78: Continuous epidural anesthesia:* After the needle has been inserted into the epidural space, a plastic tube can be threaded through the epidural needle and left in place. This tube is then taped to the woman's back. With continuous epidural anesthesia, the obstetrical anesthesiologist can inject more local anesthetic into the tubing each time the pain-killer wears off without putting the patient through the discomfort of reinserting the needle. A steady concentration of local anesthetic will ensure an almost painless delivery. Additionally, a Cesarean section can be performed under continuous epidural anesthesia.

Before the epidural, the patient is usually given between half a liter and one liter (one full infusion bottle) of Ringer's lactate by intravenous drip. This will increase the total fluid volume and slightly raise the woman's blood pressure. A rise in blood pressure is important because the blood pressure often drops rapidly with the administration of the anesthetic. The epidural is given in a side lying position with the patient's back to the edge of the bed, or with the patient sitting up and arching her back. The anesthesiologist will first prep the site of the anesthesia with an antiseptic solution and mark a point around vertebra number 4 of the lumbar vertebrae. The skin area is numbed with novocaine or Xylocaine and a special epidural needle is pushed through to the epidural space. Once the needle has been guided into the space, a small amount of the anesthetic is given first as a test dose, and the patient's blood pressure is monitored closely for five minutes. A heavy concentration of anesthetic given too rapidly can result in a severe drop in the blood pressure, which will, in turn, decrease the amount of oxygenated blood reaching the baby. If the patient is carefully observed, epidural anesthesia is the safest form of regional anesthesia used today.

After the preliminary test dose is successfully absorbed, an additional 5 milliliters of the anesthetic is injected with the patient lying on her side with her head bent and her knees up toward her chest. The fetal position will ensure that the level of the anesthetic reaches the entire area around the abdomen and legs. If the patient is sitting up the level will be lower, affecting only the area around the vagina.

Often with an epidural anesthesia a plastic catheter is taped to the patient's back to allow the anesthesiologist to administer the pain-killing medication in small, frequent doses, usually forty-five minutes apart. The advantage of using a continuous-injection technique rather than a single injection is that smaller doses of chloroprocaine do not usually affect the blood pressure or cause hypotension and fetal distress. Furthermore, the anesthesia can be allowed to wear off somewhat during the second stage of labor, thereby increasing the woman's alertness and ability to push.

A good epidural anesthetic carefully administered after preloading to avoid hypotension can be extremely helpful to a woman in pain during labor. It effectively eliminates pain in the abdominal area, allowing a woman to concentrate on the labor rather than on the pain of labor. The mind is completely unaffected by the administration of the drug. Second-stage labor, however, can be compromised if the anesthetic is still concentrated enough to affect the urge to push, and there is risk of the baby's being delivered by forceps.

Caudal Anesthesia Some doctors still like to use caudal anesthesia rather than an epidural. This is a form of anesthesia in which the needle is placed deep into the spinal cord, just about one inch from the rectum, and a local anesthetic flows from the needle into the spinal column.

Most anesthesiologists do not like to do caudals because they can be difficult to administer and there is always the risk of puncturing the head when the baby is far down into the pelvis. In addition, the caudal requires a much larger amount of local anesthetic than does the epidural.

Paracervical Block A paracervical block is a form of regional anesthesia in which the anesthesiologist or obstetrician injects novocaine or Xylocaine into the cervical tissue, usually in a circular fashion around the cervix. This numbs the cervical area and reduces the pain of each contraction by numbing the nerves that control the cervix. A paracervical block is a useful form of anesthesia in the active phase of cervical dilation when contractions are unusually intense. Unfortunately, Xylocaine or novocaine is immediately absorbed into the bloodstream, and this quickly affects the baby in turn. The fetal heart rate then goes down, in the same way that it does in an adult who receives any one of these local anesthetics. Most doctors like to protect the baby by monitoring the fetal heart rate continuously on an electric fetal monitor after the mother has received a paracervical block. There is also the risk of the anesthetic's increasing the tonus of the uterus and cutting down the supply of oxygen to the baby. Finally, a paracervical block sometimes upsets the labor pattern by prolonging labor.

What Are the Negative Aspects of Regional Anesthesia? The problem with any form of regional anesthesia is that the entire pelvic area is numb, so you can neither move freely nor feel contractions during the second stage. Regional anesthesia also slows down the uterine contractions, prolonging labor. So, though you will be relatively free of pain, there are negative side effects even with the epidural. Most doctors like to give intravenous oxytocin immediately after an epidural to make sure that labor is not unduly taxing for the mother or baby. Otherwise two to four hours can go by after an epidural when labor stops completely. A forceps delivery is also common after an epidural because the woman's attempts to push are often uncoordinated and spasmodic. The postpartum period will be affected as well, since you will be bedridden for up to twenty-four hours and might have difficulty walking for several days after that. Possible long-term effects include backaches and headaches, infection in the area of the injection, and hematoma.

Epidural anesthesia is the safest form of regional anesthesia for a patient who must have pain relief, but it does have decided disadvantages as well as advantages. This, again, is a subject a couple should discuss between themselves and with their doctor during the pregnancy, whether they have decided on a drug-free delivery or not. The course of labor is not predictable, and neither is a woman's individual tolerance of pain. If you have weighed the pros and cons beforehand, it is easier to make a rapid decision in the labor room when you are under stress. If you are thinking about having an epidural because you feel you will not be able to cope with labor without it, you should discuss the subject with your labor coach and your doctor, bearing in mind that the course of labor will then depend on artificial stimulation and other factors which all have a potential for problems, including the increased chances of a Cesarean section. Once again, however, there is no reason to be ashamed of accepting anesthesia. The positive aspects of safe anesthesia far outweigh the side effects in an otherwise unbearable labor.

What Is the Effect of Regional Anesthesia on the Baby? Some of the anesthetics favored by most anesthesiologists are bupivacaine (Marcaine) and mepivacaine (Carbocaine). Both of them have a low rate of placental transfer and thus have less effect on the newborn's nervous system. Another favorable anesthetic for epidural anesthesia is 2-Chloroprocaine because it is metabolized so quickly in the maternal blood that only an insignificant amount of this drug reaches the fetus. One way to safeguard the baby is to use small doses of either anesthetic and monitor the labor carefully. The major risk of an epidural is usually not the anesthetic used but the possibility of hypotension or prolonged labor, either of which could affect the baby. An epidural should not be used when the baby is very premature, or a woman has severe toxemia or some other serious medical condition that precludes this type of pain relief.

Are There Any Long-Term Effects from Obstetrical Drugs? A few drugs commonly given just before or during labor and delivery, including morphine, Valium, and the barbiturates, are known to have a depressive effect on the baby that can last for weeks. The effects include neonatal depression, delays in weight gain, and a decreased ability to suck. Heavy doses of Demerol can also seriously depress the baby for several days after birth. Otherwise some temporary effects can be expected with all analgesics and anesthetics that enter the newborn's nervous system, even with a moderate dose of drugs or anesthetic; but generally, any slight irritability or depression disappears by the end of the first week.

Very little is known about the long-term effects of analgesics or anesthetics. As far as we know, most obstetrical drugs, when given in controlled doses, have no discernable long-term effects on the child's behavior or learning abilities, but there is always the possibility of some minimal damage which cannot be easily determined. Part of a doctor's responsibility toward his patients is, wherever possible, to avoid drugs during labor or to administer them in only the lowest possible dose. Your doctor should also discuss the known or suspected side effects of analgesia or anesthesia, including the potential effect on the baby, with you before the birth.

Reports you may have read about the prolonged neonatal effects of anesthesia and analgesia during labor do not seem to be as alarming as they might appear. Most researchers have found no differences between the intelligence levels and learning abilities of children whose mothers received anesthesia or analgesia and those who did not, as long as the labor was uncomplicated. Two researchers who did find a long-term effect from obstetrical drugs, Drs. Yvonne Brackbill and Sally Broman, may have come to a different conclusion because they were testing children born in the 1950s and early 1960s, when general anesthesia was almost routine, oxytocin was used indiscriminately, difficult forceps were common, and mothers were given heavy doses of analgesics. A responsible anesthesiologist or obstetrician will not recommend anesthesia unless the patient really needs it, and then only in minimum doses—at least to begin with. Another new factor which should help reduce the ill effects of obstetrical drugs is fetal monitoring, since it allows us to estimate the effect of a drug on the fetal heartbeat immediately.

Anxiety About Labor and Delivery Stress can affect a woman's labor and delivery by elevating the chemical substances known as catecholamines in the blood, which, in turn, can block the release of important hormones such as oxytocin. This is one of the reasons why acute anxiety often leads to prolonged labor. Unrelieved stress can also decrease the amount of blood reaching the uterus and thus deprive the baby of oxygen at a critical time. Severe or prolonged stress could have a very serious effect on fetal circulation. There is also hyperventilation, another side effect of stress, which washes away carbon dioxide from the mother's bloodstream, making her hypotensive and faint—and the baby acidotic. An acidotic baby will produce lactic acid, a substance that causes brain swelling and brain damage.

No one would expect a woman to be completely free of anxiety during labor. A certain amount of stress is natural. The baby, in any case, is protected by the extra oxygen supply available in the placenta and stress would have to be both acute and prolonged before the baby were seriously affected. On the other hand, labor can be difficult or unusually stressful even if a woman is well prepared. Some labors are unexpectedly painful. Others can be unusually prolonged because the baby is in an awkward position or because the contractions themselves are not very efficient. If you experience a painful or prolonged labor, it might be better from the point of view of the baby as well as yourself to accept analgesia or anesthesia, rather than allow yourself to become exhausted or distressed. A state of exhaustion or severe tension could well be more harmful to the baby than the side effects of a controlled dose of Demerol, or an epidural anesthetic.

New research has indicated that excessive pain can have as damaging an effect on the newborn as a heavy dose of obstetrical drugs. A baby may be severely depressed after a painful, unmedicated birth because of the reduction of the uterine blood flow caused by stress. Pain may also prolong the baby's ordeal by encouraging erratic, unproductive contractions. A dose of pain medication might be directly beneficial since it often restores the maternal-uterine blood flow, thus providing the baby with more oxygen, and can regulate the pattern of contractions.

28

Fetal Monitoring

Birth is a stressful time, perhaps one of the most stressful that the individual ever experiences. The baby generally survives it well because nature compensates for the tremendous stress of the uterine contractions by supplying the fetus with a reserve supply of oxygen to draw on during the contractions. At the peak of each contraction, when the normal blood flow through the umbilical cord is briefly decreased, the baby continues to receive oxygen from what is known as the intervillous space—the area of the placenta where maternal and fetal blood interchange. In an uncomplicated pregnancy this reserve oxygen is usually enough to sustain the baby successfully through labor. But when labor is unusually stressful, or the pregnancy is already complicated by an inadequate placenta or poor maternal circulation, a baby may find it difficult to tolerate labor well. Episodes of serious and prolonged deprivation of oxygen could result in fetal brain damage or fetal death. The desire to spare the baby unnecessary stress and avoid brain damage is the reason why doctors try to monitor labor carefully. Unusual heart-rate patterns are often a clue to fetal distress. A distressed baby can be rescued by an emergency Cesarean, or the doctor can take other precautionary measures to safeguard the baby's health.

Techniques of monitoring the fetal heart rate have been known and practiced for over a hundred years, ever since doctors began using the stethoscope to listen to the fetal heartbeat. Electronic fetal monitoring is a recent invention that has come into general use in American hospitals only since the 1970s. The controversy over fetal monitoring therefore is not whether labors should be monitored, but how they should be monitored. Although most doctors agree that high-risk deliveries need the constant surveillance of the electronic fetal monitor, there is still considerable controversy over the role of the electronic fetal monitor in a low-risk birth. Its critics have claimed it unnecessarily increases the Cesarean rate because the information given by the monitor is often inaccurate or confusing; at the same time, more and more labors are being monitored because a very large number of doctors believe that monitors do have a useful function, even in a normal birth. The amount of controversy over this subject makes it an unusually difficult one for a practicing obstetrician and his patients, since many patients feel they don't want or need the monitor, and their doctor may feel that they do.

Two types of monitoring techniques are in common use during labor: *the external monitoring system,* in which an ultrasound device picks up the heartbeat through a device strapped to the abdomen, and *the internal monitoring system,* in which the heartbeat is detected via an electrode placed in the baby's scalp. The internal monitor is the more sensitive of the two but does have disadvantages because of the invasive nature of the technique. A low-risk woman admitted to the hospital is often placed routinely on an external monitor, and will be given an internal monitor only if a serious abnormality develops or the external monitor is incapable of achieving an accurate record of contractions.

A low-risk labor can be monitored quite successfully by a nurse or a doctor listening to the fetal heart rate with a fetoscope at ten- to fifteen-minute intervals. The advantage of electronic fetal monitoring is its continuous record of the heart rate and its ability to monitor the fetal heart during the repetitive stress of contractions. It is difficult for the fetoscope to pick up the heart-rate pattern accurately during contractions because the sounds become very weak. This means that the electronic monitor can detect such common problems as cord compression, which are often missed by the fetoscope. There are many situations in which the first sign of a problem appears on the fetal monitor and the doctor can then intervene in time. Intervention does not have to be Cesarean section, since much new knowledge has been obtained as doctors understand fetal heart-rate monitoring techniques better and have learned to interpret the information more accurately.

☐ ***External and Internal Monitoring Techniques***   *The external fetal monitoring device* consists of a fetal monitoring unit and two transducers, which are secured by belts on the abdomen—one usually placed just above the pubic hair line and the other just below the navel. The lower transducer monitors the fetal heart rate, which is continuously recorded on the fetal monitoring paper passing through the unit, while the second transducer picks up the frequency and duration of the uterine contractions. The external fetal heart-rate device uses ultrasound (see Chap. 23) to detect changes in the moving values of the fetal heart.

Unlike an electrocardiogram (ECG) the Doppler ultrasound unit does not provide a precise recording of each heartbeat but gives a more generalized picture of the fetal heart rate. The uterine contractions are picked up by a "finger" inside the transducer pressing onto the abdomen and recording its movement upward as the uterus goes into a contraction. The duration of each contraction is recorded as a curve on the fetal monitoring paper and you or your coach can anticipate the next contraction by studying the activity of the fetal contraction signals.

External monitoring is safe and useful, but it does have disadvantages. Although it provides a continuous record of the heart rate, the ultrasound signal is intermittently interrupted as the baby moves around during labor. The strength

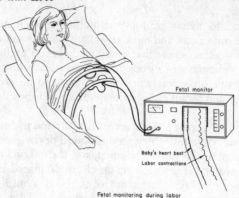

Fetal monitor

Baby's heart beat
Labor contractions

Fetal monitoring during labor

Figure 79: The external fetal monitor: The monitor records the fetal heartbeat by means of the Doppler fetal heart transducer strapped around the upper section of the mother's abdomen. The fetal heart rate is then traced continuously on the strip of fetal monitoring paper fed through the machine. A pressure transducer attached to the lower abdomen records the duration of the uterine contractions. Fetal monitoring, used properly, has helped decrease brain damage because the unit will alert the staff to a potential problem long before it becomes serious enough to injure the fetus.

of the signals varies from monitor to monitor, but there is a tendency to distortion in all external monitors because of the relative weakness of the signals. While the monitor picks up the heart rate, it usually does not give beat-to-beat variations, except with two modern fetal monitoring systems. Another disadvantage is that many external monitors work best when the patient is in the supine position, a position known to prolong labor because it decreases the pressure on the cervix. Some hospitals try to overcome the problem by placing the patient in a semisitting position supported by pillows or a backrest, or have the patient walk or stand near the bed during early labor. With this in mind, new forms of fetal monitoring are now being developed that allow a woman to move freely or assume any position she finds comfortable during labor.

Internal monitoring, or what is known as direct monitoring, gives a more precise record of the fetal heartbeat and the uterine contractions. The internal monitor is either inserted after the membranes have ruptured, or the membranes are ruptured to insert a catheter into the uterus. The fetal heart rate is transmitted via a small electrode attached to the baby's scalp.

Internal monitoring is more accurate than external monitoring because it records each heartbeat separately and interprets the exact strength of the uterine pressure as well as the duration of the contractions. The latter feature can be used to good advantage during intense periods of labor when you can follow a contraction through its peak and then begin to relax as it diminishes in intensity. The capacity to measure internal pressure is a great advantage during labor induction and stimulation with oxytocin, since the doctor can watch the effect of the oxytocin on the uterus. These special features make the internal monitor far more useful than the external monitor in a high-risk labor. The two major disadvantages with internal monitoring are the need to rupture the amniotic sac to insert the internal devices in the uterus and the increased risk of infection for mother and baby. The baby's scalp is usually cleansed with an antiseptic solution after birth to reduce the chances of infection at the site of the electrode.

☐ *Who Needs Electronic Fetal Monitoring?* Electronic fetal monitoring is recommended in any labor in which the patient has a preexisting medical condition such as diabetes or hypertension or has developed complications during pregnancy, such as preeclampsia or a postterm pregnancy. Monitoring should always be used when women with a high-risk factor go into labor. Electronic monitoring is invaluable in a high-risk labor because the baby is already under stress before encountering the additional stress of labor.

The situation is different with a low-risk patient. Here, as I have already said, most labors go well. But a serious problem can occur even during an apparently low-risk labor, a complication that cannot be predicted before labor begins. Labor may slow down unexpectedly, the second stage may be unusually prolonged, or the patient may need oxytocics to augment insufficient labor contractions. With such conditions, fetal monitoring is a must. Perhaps one in every ten labors develops some abnormal factor that requires careful surveillance from the staff and the use of the fetal monitor. Electronic monitoring is also recommended if the patient needs an epidural or some other form of conduction anesthesia or a paracervical block, because these forms of anesthetics can affect the woman's blood pressure and therefore the fetal heart rate. This still leaves a large number of women who theoretically should not need electronic fetal monitoring at all, *except* for the small but ever present risk of unexpected fetal distress. Unfortunately it is not possible to predict who will develop fetal distress, and this is one of the reasons why doctors prefer to screen all their patients with an external fetal monitor.

While unexpected fetal distress may have many causes, one of the most common is cord compression as the umbilical cord becomes tangled around the baby's neck or arm during the delivery. With each contraction the cord tightens and the blood flow from the placenta is reduced, stressing the baby and reducing its oxygen supply. The fetal heart rate then develops a pattern known as variable deceleration, in which the heartbeat is slow to return to its normal rate after the cord pressure has been released. Late deceleration (see page 466) is another potentially alarming pattern, which is caused by decreased oxygen passage through the placenta. These are both fetal heart-rate patterns that the electronic fetal monitor can pick up far more quickly than the stethoscope—allowing the doctor time to protect the baby by measures that do not necessarily include a Cesarean section. In fact, the fetal monitor can often prevent a Cesarean because the doctor can detect fetal distress early enough to correct it. Often fetal distress is treated effectively by placing the patient on her side and giving her oxygen, which in turn will reach the baby and improve its condition. Fetal distress might also, in the case of a labor induction, be caused by too much oxytocin, resulting in too strong contractions. This can be corrected by stopping the oxytocin infusion. Before electronic fetal monitoring, such problems were either difficult to detect or resulted in such alarm that the woman was rushed into the delivery room for an immediate Cesarean section. (Complications such as cord compression can lead to brain damage if fetal distress is allowed to continue throughout labor.) Other, more subtle changes in the fetal heart rate that may be missed by traditional methods can be detected through electronic fetal monitoring.

☐ *Does Monitoring Increase the Cesarean Rate?* We have all heard the argument that fetal monitoring increases the Cesarean rate. Some critics say that the introduction of monitoring into a hospital can increase that hospital's Cesarean rate by as much as 25 percent. But while it may be true that doctors faced with an unfamiliar technology made many mistakes in the first years of fetal monitoring, this is no longer the case in hospitals with experienced obstetrical staffs. A few years ago, when a doctor saw a suspicious heart-rate tracing, his first reaction was often to rush the woman into an emergency Cesarean. Now he will usually wait, watch the monitor and the patient carefully and perhaps try a change in the woman's position or give oxygen inhalation. Many of these transient problems correct themselves and fortunately don't need further intervention. In general, the large medical centers where fetal monitoring has been used for years are performing far fewer unnecessary Cesareans than a few years ago, although the smallest hospitals that have just acquired fetal monitoring units may still be experiencing a high Cesarean rate. In any case, the relatively high Cesarean rate throughout the United States is the result of other factors besides the monitoring. Many difficult labors that used to be ended by oxytocins and forceps, potentially damaging the baby, are now delivered by Cesarean section. Doctors nowadays would rather do a Cesarean than risk brain damage to the baby. We know more now too about the effects of prolonged stress during labor, and are less willing to let a woman labor on for hours than doctors were in the past.

☐ *How Can Fetal Monitoring Be Combined with Natural Childbirth?*   It would be unfair to say that the electronic fetal monitor has not had an effect on the labor experience. Many women understandably dislike the idea of being hooked up to a machine for hours, afraid to move in case a transducer becomes accidentally dislodged. This has been partly overcome by developing longer cords on the newer types of monitors to allow the patient to get out of bed and move around during labor. One way to minimize the time spent in bed is to put the monitor in place for about ten to fifteen minutes when the patient is admitted in relatively early labor and then disconnect the monitor and have the patient walk freely around until the contractions become stronger. (The entire labor, however, must be monitored if the heart rate looks suspicious early on.) This is one way to combine the advantages of monitoring with free movement and a more natural labor. Later on, as labor gets stronger, the fetal heart rate should be monitored continuously, even in a low-risk labor, because that is when problems can occur. One advantage that the prepared couple certainly has over the unprepared couple is a familiarity with the principles of fetal monitoring. The monitor might look frightening to an unprepared woman, but a prepared couple who understands the function of the fetal monitor often finds the experience reassuring rather than alarming.

☐ *What Do Fetal Heart-Rate Tracings Mean?*   The heart rate is the tracing found on the upper portion of the fetal monitoring paper. Unlike the lower tracing showing the rise and fall of each labor contraction, the heart rate is usually more or less stable in a healthy fetus just as it is in the healthy adult, although there is a small difference between each fetal (as well as adult) heartbeat. The amount of variability is recorded on the monitoring paper by the needle moving up and down. The base-line heart rate in a normal fetus during labor is between 120 and 160 beats a minute, about twice that of the healthy adult.

The slight variations you will see on the monitor from moment to moment are not only normal, but an indication that the baby is in good health and responding well to labor. If the heart rate flattens and this beat-to-beat variability is lost, it could mean that the baby is beginning to experience hypoxia, a slight decrease in the oxygen supply, which could be dangerous. The fetal heart rate also tends to flatten after a woman has been given Demerol or some other drug during labor or delivery, since drugs tend to depress the maternal nervous system and therefore the fetal nervous system as well. As you and your labor coach watch the monitor, look for a good variability pattern and alert the staff if you see an absence of beat-to-beat variability.

Of more concern is the speed of the heart rate. If the heart rate shows a *persistent* pattern of fast heartbeats, *tachycardia,* (more than 160 beats a minute), or a slow heartbeat, *bradycardia,* (fewer than 120 beats a minute), the obstetrician needs to find the cause. One will often notice a short period of tachycardia as the baby responds to sudden stress, but this does not suggest serious distress. Prolonged tachycardia is rare, and is often the result of elevated maternal temperature caused by an infection. A more common cause for concern is bradycardia, since a depressed heart rate means the baby is not receiving enough oxygen, and a bradycardiac condition that cannot be counteracted by placing the patient on her side or giving her oxygen means an immediate delivery by forceps or a Cesarean.

Another phenomenon to watch for is the response of the fetal heart rate to each uterine contraction. The heart rate should remain reasonably steady during each contraction, indicating a steady supply of oxygen throughout the contraction. But you should not expect to see the heart rate remain in a completely straight line; a healthy fetus will have a normal heart-rate variation of about three to five cycles per minute. These slight fluctuations are a sign that the baby is receiving adequate oxygenation. Occasionally you might see a more pronounced drop in the heart rate that will last only a few seconds. One such deceleration is usually quite insignificant; it could be caused by the baby's movements, which frequently disturb the heart-rate monitor and falsely indicate a drop in the baby's heart rate. If, on the other hand, you see a persistent pattern of heart-rate decelerations, it could be an early warning sign.

There are three major types of decelerations that occur so frequently that they have been classified as *early, late* and *variable* decelerations, depending on their relationship to the uterine contractions. It is important for you as parents to understand how to interpret monitoring patterns because you will better be able to appreciate your doctor's response to any warning signals and cooperate with his management in an emergency.

☐ *Early Deceleration* There may be periodic heart rate changes that do not indicate fetal distress. A pattern known as *early deceleration* sometimes develops in which the heart rate decreases during a contraction and then returns to normal as the contraction disappears. This pattern, which is not a danger sign, occurs as the baby's head is compressed or squeezed during the contraction, temporarily affecting the nervous system and therefore the heart rate. Early deceleration is not dangerous because the heart rate goes back up again immediately when the contraction is over. In fact, some head compression is inevitable during labor since the uterus is putting tremendous pressure on the baby's head.

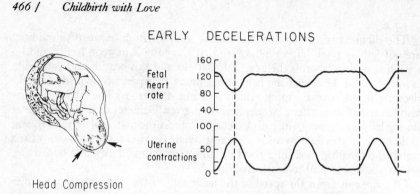

Head Compression

Figure 80: Early decelerations of the fetal heart rate occur when pressure is exerted on the fetal head. One will see the fetal heart rate drop at the peak of the uterine contraction when more pressure than usual is exerted on the fetal head. The deceleration disappears with the end of the contraction. An early deceleration is not a dangerous pattern and requires no intervention.

The reason there is no danger with early deceleration is that the baby's oxygen level remains basically steady.

☐ **Late Deceleration**   Late deceleration is potentially alarming. A late deceleration is one in which the heart rate begins to decrease a few seconds after each uterine contraction has begun, indicating that the contracting uterus is squeezing the placenta and decreasing the oxygen supply to the baby. If the baby continues to suffer oxygen loss, brain damage can occur because of the inadequate supply of oxygen in the fetal circulation. Typically, a pattern of late deceleration will begin with a decrease in the heart rate *after* each contraction has begun, a deceleration that will continue throughout the contraction, recovering only when the uterus is completely relaxed between contractions. The rate of recovery will be slow. While one or two abnormal tracings may not be significant, a late deceleration pattern that repeats itself time after time could indicate severe distress. Persistent late deceleration is often accompanied by a relaxation of the fetal sphincter muscles, spilling stool, or meconium, into the amniotic fluid. The appearance of this meconium-stained fluid through the vagina can be serious, particularly if the meconium is very *thick:* a heavy show of meconium could indicate that the fetal brain has already been damaged. Second, the baby might aspirate the meconium during labor, endangering the lungs. Pneumonitis or pneumothorax, collapse of the baby's lungs, is not an uncommon complication of the newborn after a heavy show of meconium.

A pattern of late deceleration should be reported to the labor-floor staff immediately. Usually the nurse will move you onto your side to relieve the pressure on the large vein, the inferior vena cava, which immediately increases the amount of blood returning to your heart and into the fetal circulation. At the same time the nurse may give you oxygen by face mask to increase the supply of oxygen to the placenta. If you are being given oxytocin, the pump or drip will be turned off to decrease fetal stress. When the late deceleration pattern persists, despite these conservative measures, your obstetrician must make a further decision: should he proceed with an emergency Cesarean section or should he wait and evaluate the fetal condition further with fetal scalp blood sampling? (See below.)

LATE DECELERATIONS

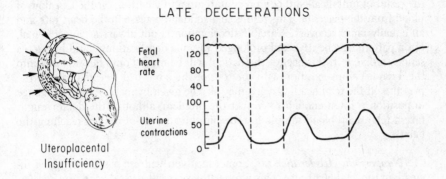

Uteroplacental
Insufficiency

Figure 81: Late decelerations are caused by uteroplacental insufficiency, a condition in which the placenta begins to malfunction because it is not receiving enough blood to guarantee the fetal oxygen supply. During a late deceleration the fetal heart rate drops significantly during the uterine contraction and then recovers after the contraction is over. A late deceleration might be difficult to detect by the untrained eye. The one illustrated here represents a textbook case with a clear repeated decrease in the heart rate with each uterine contraction and a slow recovery after the contraction is finished. This is a dangerous pattern that should be evaluated further with fetal scalp blood-sampling to analyze the fetal pH values. A low pH level would argue the need for an emergency delivery.

VARIABLE DECELERATIONS

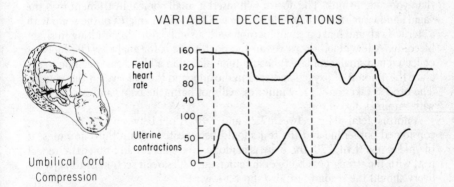

Umbilical Cord
Compression

Figure 82: Variable decelerations are fetal heart-rate decelerations occurring at any time that is not related to the uterine contractions. The compression of the umbilical cord is often the cause of the characteristic pattern illustrated here. One can see that variable decelerations often take a U or a V form as a sudden drop occurs in the heart rate, to be followed by an equally rapid recovery. The temporary effects of cord compression are usually counteracted by placing the mother on her side and giving oxygen by mask. Only if the pattern persists will the doctor proceed to other techniques, such as fetal blood-sampling and, possibly, an emergency delivery.

☐ **Variable Deceleration**   In *variable deceleration,* the heart rate drops suddenly, not necessarily during a uterine contraction, and then recovers rapidly, a pattern that will show up in a U-like or V-like tracing. Variable deceleration is the result of umbilical-cord compression temporarily cutting off the free flow of blood from the placenta. This results in a sudden decrease in the heart rate and an equally rapid recovery. Variable deceleration is not always a danger signal, but a pattern of repetitive and prolonged variable decelerations could become a serious problem. If this occurs, the patient will be moved onto her side and into the Trendelenburg position with the foot of the labor bed elevated to take the pressure off the fetal head. Oxygen may also be given by mask. A simple change in position is often enough to correct the problem, although the doctor might take a fetal scalp blood sample to estimate the amount of oxygen reaching the baby.

☐ **Nonperiodic Acceleration**   Sometimes you will see a sudden, quick increase in the fetal heart rate. This is a healthy sign called *fetal heart-rate acceleration.* The flurry of activity is associated with fetal movement and shows that the baby is responding well to labor and is not depressed. The fetal heartbeat, like an adult's, increases with physical activity, thus supplying the body with extra oxygen. An increased fetal heart rate in response to fetal movement is, therefore, an indication that the baby's nervous system is working correctly.

☐ **Fetal Scalp Blood Sampling**   When the fetal heart rate is persistently abnormal, a doctor should take a fetal blood sample to evaluate fetal condition more accurately, rather than proceeding to an immediate Cesarean section. The fetal blood sample is used to estimate the baby's acid/alkali balance; an important piece of information, because an overly acidotic baby can become brain damaged (see pages 458–59). Obtaining a fetal blood sample is simpler and safer than you might think. The doctor will insert a small conical instrument into the vagina and visualize the baby's head. He will then clean an area of the scalp with a sterile swab and make a small incision with a small knife tip, resulting in slight bleeding. A few blood drops are all the doctor needs for analysis. The blood is collected in a small capillary tube and then placed in a blood-gas machine to analyze the amount of oxygen and carbon dioxide, and the pH level of the sample. The process takes only a few minutes, will not harm the baby, and is associated with minimal discomfort.

A normal fetal pH is between 7.25 and 7.40. A pH between 7.20 and 7.25 is considered borderline and the test should be repeated within thirty minutes. If the pH is less than 7.20, the baby is acidotic; this calls for an immediate repeat test, with the strong possibility of an emergency Cesarean section or forceps delivery should the second test also show a low pH.

Fetal blood sampling used in association with fetal heart-rate monitoring has saved numerous babies from unnecessary Cesarean sections after the acid-base state was found to be normal, despite a pattern of heart rate deceleration. Certain obstetricians are skilled in the method of fetal scalp blood sampling. On the other hand, quite a few have as yet no knowledge of the technique. Unfortunately, a doctor who does not use acid-base blood sampling may not know enough about fetal monitoring to prevent an unnecessary Cesarean. You should ask your doctor how he would handle fetal distress; if his answer simply is "A Cesarean," you would probably do well to look for another obstetrician.

A new electronic device has recently been developed to read continuous pH measurement through a small electrode placed inside the regular scalp electrode attached to the fetal monitor. A doctor can use this new technology to analyze fetal pH in association with fetal heart-rate abnormalities. This type of advanced monitoring technique will mean less surgical intervention in future deliveries and a quicker detection of babies at risk—not only fewer Cesarean, but fewer babies born with birth-related brain damage.

29

The Birth

The culmination of the nine months of pregnancy is at hand when a woman approaches the end of the second stage. Until this point, labor has been only the forerunner of the most important event in your pregnancy—the birth itself.

The first and second stages of labor might seem endless to the expectant parents. The birth itself will take only a few minutes. It may take no more than thirty seconds from the time the head is visible in the birth canal until the moment the baby is born, although the normal duration for this stage is two or three minutes. Since the birth happens so rapidly, the mechanism of birth should be looked at as a distinct phase of labor. When a couple is taken into the delivery room they should understand what is going to happen in order for them to participate fully in and to enjoy the birth.

Each birth is, of course, a unique event, even for an obstetrician who has been present at hundreds of them. It never fails to thrill me to deliver a child and feel the new life in my hands. Women often tell me that giving birth immediately erases negative memories of difficulties during labor.

☐ *Where Should the Baby Be Born?* Most American hospitals still have separate labor and delivery rooms, which means that you are likely to labor in the labor room and then be taken "down" to the delivery room where you are ready to deliver.

☐ *Giving Birth in a Delivery Room* A delivery room looks virtually like a standard operating room, with an anesthesia machine, oxygen tanks, and a large table on which the patient lies or sits during the delivery. The staff and the labor coach wear caps, gowns, and masks.

Delivery-room tables are made so that the lower portion of the table slides

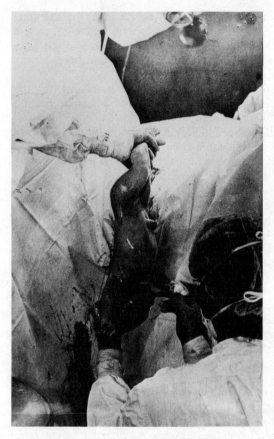

Figure 83: Birth Yesterday: A typical birth picture taken less than ten years ago. The patient is placed in stirrups under the strong overhead lights of the delivery room. The baby has just been delivered and is being held upside down to stimulate breathing, a position that most obstetricians no longer favor because of the risk of hip dislocation. A nurse or an intern, or in this case the obstetrician, is suctioning the baby's mouth to remove any excessive mucus. A few minutes after this picture was taken the baby was separated from his mother and sent up to the newborn nursery for the next twenty-four hours, a routine procedure that meant the mother had no time to bond with her baby. This harsh approach to birth has been generally eliminated in most, though not all, modern hospitals.

under the upper portion. The patient is then positioned with her feet in stirrups so that she is resting at the edge of the table. Most delivery tables are equipped with handles, metal hand-pieces, or bars, which can be used to apply pressure during the pushing stage. The delivery area is usually illuminated by a large overhead surgical light, and a mirror is often attached to provide the patient with a view of the baby's birth.

In most hospitals the patient is asked to put her legs in stirrups. A few doctors, unfortunately, still strap the patient's legs to the table, a procedure that dates from the time when women were given high doses of Demerol plus scopolamine as an analgesic during labor. Scopolamine, also called the "truth serum," has such disturbing side effects that its use has been virtually discontinued in the modern hospital. Women under the influence of scopolamine were so restless and disoriented that involuntary movements were a problem, and the only way to control the patient was to strap her legs down during the delivery. Although most hospitals no longer favor scopolamine, some still insist on strapping women down, for reasons that have more to do with tradition than necessity.

Since the practice is both uncomfortable and humiliating, you should include delivery-room procedures among your list of questions before you look at a particular hospital. Arrange to have an early tour of the hospital, and when the staff shows you the labor room, find out whether the hospital insists on strapping down or not. Some progressive hospitals have even discontinued the routine use of the stirrups and will allow a woman to deliver with her feet flat on the table. This is a less humiliating position than the traditional one, and gives you the freedom that is important for a natural delivery.

Other standard equipment in the delivery room includes an incubator for the baby and a table for infant resuscitation with an overhead infra-red heating lamp and suctioning equipment. Emergency oxygen is available should it be necessary. The delivery room is well equipped to deal with emergencies, but has little warmth or friendliness about it, although a couple can still experience a wonderful birth in one if the staff is sympathetic and the hospital has modified its old-fashioned standards sufficiently for the modern birthing couple.

☐ *From the Labor Room to Delivery Room: What Is the Procedure?*   In most hospitals a primapara is moved from the labor room to the delivery room just before the baby is born. The second stage of a first labor often lasts longer than an hour. Even two hours is common. During this time period, the attending doctor usually performs several vaginal examinations to ascertain the position of the baby's head in the birth canal. A doctor can usually tell the birth is imminent once the top part of the baby's skull can be seen between the open lips of the vagina, the moment known as crowning. The move to the delivery room is usually made when birth is likely to take place within five to ten minutes. In a second or subsequent labor, the second stage is usually quite short. Here again, the doctor will perform a vaginal examination with a sterile glove to make sure that the head is rotating into the pelvic area. Sometimes in a second birth the head will rotate extremely rapidly, and the second stage can be as short as five minutes. The vaginal examination will also give an idea of how well the baby's body is entering the pelvis. When the woman is delivering a large child with large shoulders, it is not enough just for the head to move down into the pelvis, but the cervix has to stretch over the shoulders as well, requiring energetic pushing from the woman herself. The second stage can take even longer if the shoulders are very large. Again, that is a factor the doctor must bear in mind in timing the move into the delivery room. Actually, you may feel the head crowning all the way down to the pelvic outlet as you push, but between contractions the baby will move far back inside you again as the cervix pulls the shoulders back in. You will then have to push harder to get the shoulders delivered. Finally, when your obstetrician assumes you are ready to deliver within one or two pushes, he will give the signal to move you into the delivery room.

☐ *What Is the Advantage of Staying in the Labor Room?*   Most hospitals today prefer that the patient remain in the labor room until just before giving birth. This enables the staff to keep the fetal monitor in place as long as possible. A number of things can go wrong at the end of labor, as the baby is being pushed all the way down the birth canal. The umbilical cord, from which the baby receives its only source of oxygen, may be stretched or constricted, reducing the blood entering the fetal circulation. A late deceleration (see p. 466) in the heart rate is much more frequent in the second stage of labor than the first, and this possibility alone would call for careful monitoring for as long as possible in the second stage.

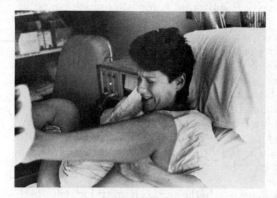

Figure 84: Second Stage of Labor: Pushing; Brenda is sitting up and pulling her legs toward her to increase the effectiveness of the contractions. Brenda was able to deliver her baby spontaneously in the birthing bed in which she is seen. The fetal monitor in the background was used intermittently during labor to make sure that the fetal heart rate was responding normally.

The risks are greater at this point in labor since oxygen tension is normally somewhat lower during the second stage. The baby usually has a built-in mechanism within the placenta that can withstand this oxygen loss, but not for a prolonged time. That is why, if the heart rate does remain down, oxygen tension does too, which means that the baby can become acidotic. A significant drop in pH is often a danger sign, because the acidotic baby produces lactic acid, a substance that causes brain swelling, and hence brain damage. Again, this is unusual in the low-risk birth, but the possibility of acidosis makes fetal monitoring an important part of the management of the second stage of labor.

One way for you to increase the oxygen reaching the baby is to breathe deeply in between pushes to increase the oxygen in your own circulation. If the heart rate decelerates for several seconds, your obstetrician might prefer to turn you on your side rather than have you labor in a flat or semisitting position.

As long as pushing proceeds normally and the baby is moving satisfactorily into the birth canal, the second stage can continue peacefully. If the fetal heart rate is normal, and your blood pressure is normal, then you will be moved to the delivery room at the very last moment before the birth of the baby. On the other hand, if something does go wrong, you must expect to be moved there immediately. On occasion, when the heart rate goes down and stays down, your doctor might give you emergency oxygen by face mask in the labor room rather than take you straight to the delivery room. The face mask and oxygen supply are usually available right above the labor bed. Once the extra oxygen has entered your circulation, the baby will benefit from the higher concentration of oxygen in your bloodstream. This extra oxygen can be vital in an emergency because it may prevent brain damage. If the heart rate remains depressed in spite of the oxygen, you will be taken to the delivery room and delivered immediately, either by forceps or Cesarean section, depending on the position of the baby in the birth canal.

☐ *The Importance of the Labor Coach* Because problems can occur unexpectedly in the last few minutes before birth, the progress of labor is exciting, but also worrisome for the obstetrician, who knows that there could come a time when a decision must be made very quickly. The end of labor is all the more arduous since the baby, who is pushing downward during most of the second stage, must suddenly, at the very end of labor, push slightly upward through the upward configuration of the pelvis. Consequently, the latter phase can be exhausting and difficult for a woman pushing to get the baby out, as well as nerve-racking for the obstetrician and the labor coach. It is very easy to give up at the end of the pushing phase when you are tired, exhausted, and unable to push further, although you cannot possibly stop at this point because the baby is still trapped inside the pelvis. Here your labor coach can be very important; his encouragement may help you through the last few pushes, even though you feel you are at the point of exhaustion. It may seem as if the birth is never going to happen, but in fact you are only a few minutes away from the moment you have both been looking forward to for so long—the baby's arrival. Because the obstetrician, the labor coach, and the nurses are so nervous in these tense final minutes, everyone is all the more excited when the birth finally takes place.

☐ *Moving into the Delivery Room*   In the average hospital the staff wheels the labor bed into the delivery room. Moving onto the table itself can be difficult, although the nurses will adjust the delivery table to the level of your labor bed to make the maneuver easier for you. At this point of labor a woman is usually tired and won't feel like making any extra physical effort.

The best way to move over to the delivery table is to turn around or sit on your side and slide over. Try to do this as quickly as possible, between contractions. Once you are finally on the delivery table, your coach should help you get into a comfortable position by placing pillows behind your back and making sure that the backrest is adjusted so you are sitting up at a 30- to 60-degree angle. In this position gravity will assist you as you push. Ideally the delivery table will be adjusted in such a way that the stirrups are lowered and you are half sitting rather than lying on your back—the traditional lithotomy position is not the way a modern birth should take place, since it fights the natural forces of gravity. I would also ask your doctor not to put you in stirrups, unless you are having a forceps delivery. Sitting up, you will see the baby being born and you will find it easier to control the delivery. As your coach is helping you into a comfortable position on the delivery table, your obstetrician will usually be scrubbing and gowning up for the delivery.

☐ *Why Is a Delivery Room Necessary?*   Many women want to know why they must be moved from the labor room to the delivery room when the experience of moving at this crucial point of labor is so uncomfortable. Why can't a woman simply deliver in the same bed she used during labor? Many hospitals and clinics throughout the world are indeed encouraging women to do so, using a modern labor bed. In other hospitals or clinics, the patient simply delivers in an ordinary hospital bed. There are certain situations, however, when an obstetrician will find it simpler to deliver a woman on a conventional delivery table. For example, it is easier to deliver a large baby if the woman has her legs apart with her feet resting in a stirrup heel rest. Also, an obstetrician will need room to apply forceps in a forceps delivery, although forceps can be used in a labor room equipped with the modern type of labor bed with an adjustable end.

If something should go wrong, your obstetrician will use the quickest method to get the baby delivered. Because of complications, a delivery room is still necessary in the modern hospital, although fewer women will probably use it in the

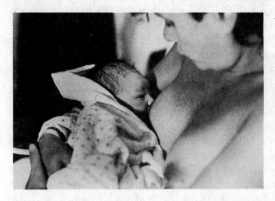

Figure 85: Brenda and her son Adam are together within just a few minutes of his birth, which took place five minutes after the previous photograph was taken. While still in the birthing room, Brenda was able to breast-feed her son and continue the bonding that began between them long before birth. A relaxed and happy Adam was born without drugs into a quiet, peaceful atmosphere.

future. The delivery room is not the ideal environment for a woman who is delivering with the minimum of drugs and the support of her labor coach. Many hospitals are belatedly installing birthing rooms, which, among their other advantages, allow a woman to labor and deliver in the same, comfortable environment. Other hospitals are permitting patients to deliver in an ordinary labor room. Obstetricians have found that many of their patients prefer to remain in the same bed throughout labor and delivery, although a labor room is not nearly as pleasant as a birthing room when energy and imagination have been put into its design.

☐ *Just Before the Birth* Just before the birth you will be pushing very hard and you may well begin to feel exhausted. There may be pain, although the pain will be different from that you experienced during the transitional stage. Experiences at this stage of labor vary from woman to woman. Some women feel very little discomfort while others experience pressure—a feeling of distention in the vaginal area that can be painful. Naturally, during a first pregnancy this discomfort is more pronounced, and a sensation of tearing and burning is not uncommon as you feel the baby pushing through the vagina.

Pushing at this late stage can seem extraordinarily hard. Then, suddenly, the baby will rotate inside the pelvis and move down quickly as it enters the extension phase from the flexion phase. At this point some women feel some relief from pressure together with a tremendous urge to continue pushing because the baby is almost ready to be born. This can be a difficult moment if you need to be moved to a delivery room for the birth. Naturally, if you are in a birthing room, you can continue with only one or two more controlled pushes and the birth will be over. In the traditional hospital, the patient is asked to stop pushing while she is being moved into the delivery room. If the urge to push is becoming unbearable, try a pattern of short quick pants. Panting can be done effectively by putting your head back and breathing in and out rapidly.

As soon as you get onto the delivery table, get yourself into an upright position. Don't, as I have already said, put your feet in the stirrups if it is a natural delivery. If there is a rest for your knees you can place them in the knee rests on the delivery table; if you are in a birthing bed you can either rest your legs on the edge of the bed or put your heels into the edges of the stirrups, which act as heel supporters. Meanwhile your coach should place pillows underneath your back to elevate your position; the same holds true of a birthing-bed delivery. If you are sitting up you can see the baby being born and you have better control over the birth process. You will then feel pressure and a sense of tension as the baby is finally ready to make its appearance. Some women find this very painful, while others feel that these last few pushes are associated with a great sense of relief.

☐ *The Delivery*   As the head descends farther down into the birth canal, the perineum, the area around the vulva, begins to bulge noticeably, and the skin becomes stretched and tense. With the further progression of the second stage, the perineum bulges more and more with each contraction, and the vulva begins to form a distinct circular opening around the top of the head (crowning). The head usually disappears back into the birth canal with the end of each contraction as the bulky shoulders push the baby back up again. Once the head has gone through the cervix, the shoulders are the next sizable part of the baby that must be pushed through the cervical canal. That may take some time if the baby is large, and you need to continue your pushing after the head has crowned. You will also feel a sensation that is one of relief when the shoulders have gone through. (You will know the shoulders have passed through the cervix when the baby's head stays down and remains on the perineum after each contraction.) Once the shoulders are free of the cervix, the last part of the delivery will be much easier.

As the head becomes increasingly visible, the vulva is stretched further and further apart, and a small circle of vulval tissue will form around the baby's head. The baby's head is now completely pushed down the birth canal, and it will appear almost as if the area between the vagina and the rectum has disappeared as the perineum stretches around the top of the baby's head. The reason

CROWNING

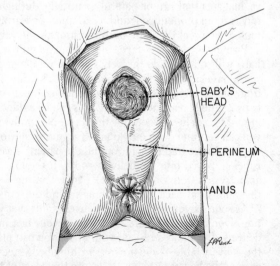

Figure 86: Crowning: The vulval tissue is stretched tightly over the top of the baby's head, forming a small protrusion that resembles a crown circling the head of the baby. An episiotomy is usually made at this time if the obstetrician feels that the baby's head is too large to pass through the vulva without tearing.

DELIVERY OF HEAD

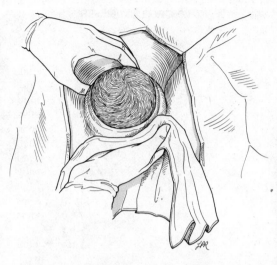

Figure 87: As the head emerges further, the doctor supports it with his left hand to prevent its being pushed out too rapidly while he slowly lifts the baby's head with his right hand. The towel is kept between the anus and the vulval opening to avoid contaminating the vulva and the baby.

this is called crowning is that it looks as if the baby's head is surrounded by a crown of thin, paperlike skin (see Figs. 86 and 87). The skin is usually thinner in the back area of the perineum than in the front. The changes in the perineum allow the head to move through the vaginal opening, but at the same time there is the risk of ripping the vagina and vulva and tearing the skin on both sides of the rectum and the bladder if a woman pushes too hard. At this crucial point, complete control is necessary. You should watch your doctor very carefully and follow his directions on when to push and when to desist from pushing, if necessary using short panting breaths to control the pushing urge.

With each contraction more and more of the baby's head now becomes visible. In between contractions, a doctor who is trying to avoid an episiotomy will put a finger in the lower portion of the perineum and stretch it gently from side to side—massaging the perineum, as it is called. In a multiparous woman (a woman who previously has given birth) in whom the vaginal tissues have already been stretched, this massage can often open and stretch the paper-thin skin of the perineum sufficiently to allow a gentle delivery without an episiotomy or any substantial tearing.

By now the doctor will be resting his left hand on the baby's head. He can then keep the birth under control should you push suddenly or uncontrollably. With his other hand, he will take a towel and then put the hand underneath the rectum, between the edge of the sacral bone and the rectum (see Fig. 87). The towel will prevent the stool from contaminating his gloves. Then, by pushing his hand in and upward, he will be able to feel the baby's chin through the perineum, while the other hand gently supports the head to prevent it being delivered too fast.

The baby, at this point, is still looking downward. Once the doctor has palpated the area underneath the baby's head and found the chin, he will lift the

CONTROLLED DELIVERY

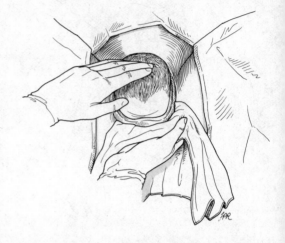

Figure 88: More and more of the head is becoming visible as the doctor continues to ease the head through the vulval opening. A slow, controlled delivery allows the delicate tissues around the vulva time to stretch spontaneously, without ripping. Otherwise, there will be damage to the perineal area that may be difficult to repair.

chin up and slowly lift the baby forward with one hand underneath and the other hand still supporting the top of the baby's head (see Fig. 88). This must be done slowly and gently to give the tissues around the vagina a chance to stretch naturally, without rupturing, as the baby's head is born. This maneuver is called the Ritgen maneuver, after the physician who originally described it. The Ritgen maneuver allows the doctor to control the delivery of the head, and also encourages the extension of the head in a natural way (see Fig. 89). By watching the perineal area carefully at this delicate moment, your doctor may be able to make the delivery without an episiotomy. If he feels he cannot do so without tearing, he will choose to do the episiotomy before the head is delivered. The episiotomy can be made with a small cut in the area between the vagina and the rectum (the midline episiotomy) or out to the side of the rectum (a mediolateral episiotomy) to give more space for the shoulders, the widest dimension of the body. The head is often born between two contractions and as slowly as possible. During the delivery you will be asked to pant quickly with short, quick breaths to help overcome the urge to push. Finally, you will see the widest diameter of the head emerge through the perineum, and within a few seconds the entire head will be born (see Fig. 90). After the birth of the head is completed, the head will rotate to the left or right side to align itself with the rest of the body.

Immediately after the birth of the head, the doctor will usually open the baby's mouth gently with one finger, insert a small syringe, and suction out the mucus. Excess mucus should always be suctioned out of the mouth before the baby takes its first breath to make sure that no meconium or blood-mixed fluid is aspirated into the lungs. By this time the baby may have already opened its eyes and the obstetrician can judge its condition by its alertness and skin color; a healthy baby will mean an unhurried, smooth completion of the delivery. It is fascinating to see the baby's eyes open and look up, perhaps surprised by the

COMPLETION OF DELIVERY OF HEAD

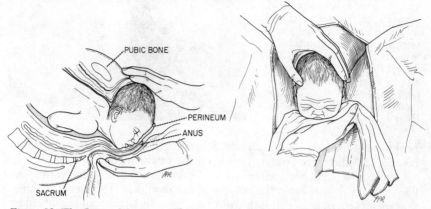

Figure 89: The Ritgen Maneuver: This maneuver allows the obstetrician to control a spontaneous delivery. One hand is placed underneath the rectum (the towel is used as a protection against contamination); the doctor then reaches for the chin and slowly lifts the baby's head while he uses the other hand to steady the head and avoid an overrapid delivery.   *Figure 90:* Still using the Ritgen maneuver, the obstetrician now slowly lifts the baby's chin and finally delivers the head. He then pushes the perineum backward to make sure that the chin is free. At this point the obstetrician can see the face well enough to judge the baby's reflexes and make some preliminary judgment of the baby's condition.

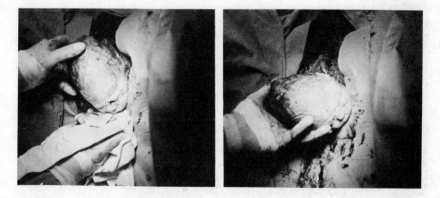

Figures 91 and 92: External Rotation: Immediately after the head is born it will rotate itself to the right or to the left to align itself with the rest of the body. In this instance the baby's head has just been born, supported by the hands of the doctor. The slight protrusion of the baby's head is called "molding."

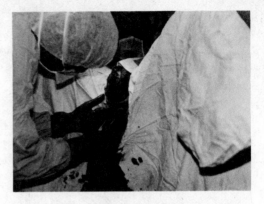

Figure 93: Aspiration of the Baby's Mouth: Immediately after the head is born, the doctor will open the mouth with his fingers and then insert a small syringe. It is important to aspirate excess mucus from the baby's mouth before he takes his first breath, when he might aspirate some blood-stained mucus, damaging the lungs.

brightness of the room. A sympathetic delivery with low lighting does appear to ease the transition into extrauterine life for the newborn child.

Now that the head has been delivered, the doctor will gently feel for the position of the body and begin the delivery of the shoulders. This can be a rather delicate maneuver, especially if the baby has unusually large shoulders. Shoulder distortion is a difficult problem for an obstetrician and is one of the reasons that some doctors are wary of birthing-room deliveries, in which the woman is positioned at the end of a birthing bed, making it difficult to push the baby's head far enough down to deliver the shoulders without harming the child. It does not usually present a serious problem for the experienced obstetrician, and I have personally delivered babies of nine and a half pounds in a birthing bed without the use of forceps or any other manipulation. If a doctor cannot deliver the shoulders easily, he might put the patient on a bedpan to allow him more room to manipulate the shoulders.

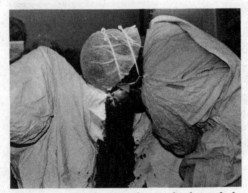

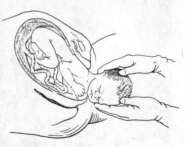

Head is completely delivered and now turned to the side, immediately before delivery of shoulders.

Figure 94a: This drawing shows a birth just before the delivery of the shoulders. The anterior (front) shoulder is underneath the pubic bone, so the doctor will next proceed to pull the head downward to deliver the front shoulder. Sometimes shoulder distortion occurs with a very large baby, a complication that can make this maneuver the most difficult part of the delivery.   *Figure 94b: Delivery of the Posterior Shoulder:* After the anterior shoulder is born, the posterior (back) shoulder is delivered by lifting the baby forward as the mother pushes through the next contraction. Here you can see the posterior shoulder being delivered. Again, careful manipulation by the obstetrician will avoid tearing.

In most cases, the shoulders appear at the vulva just after the external rotation of the head. Again, you will feel a tremendous urge to push. At this point you should put all of your pushing efforts into completing the delivery while the doctor places one hand on each side of the baby's head and pulls the baby downward to deliver the front shoulder. At the same time the obstetrical nurse or midwife may exert pressure on the abdomen just above the pubic bone to help press the shoulders down underneath the pubic bone and out through the vaginal opening.

As soon as the anterior (front) shoulder appears through the upper part of the vulva, the doctor will begin to lift the baby upward to deliver the posterior shoulder. Here again, continue to push. After the anterior shoulder is delivered, the posterior shoulder will usually appear fairly promptly, as will the remainder of the baby's body. If there is a good collaboration between your doctor and you, he will ask you to push very hard for the shoulders, and then when the body is ready to be born he will ask you to push again to free the baby completely from the birth canal. As you push, he will gently position his hands to help the baby as the body is delivered. The rest of the body is usually delivered easily and painlessly, with one small push. This is not surprising, if you remember that the

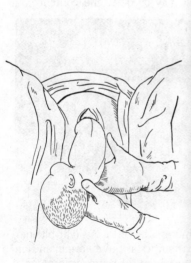

Delivery of the baby

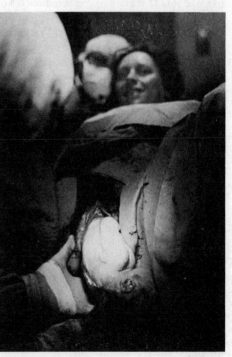

Figure 95: After the shoulders are born the rest of the body will be delivered quickly and easily since the trunk is usually narrower than the head and the shoulders. The woman is asked to push and the doctor gently supports the baby as the body is born.   *Figure 96: Completion of the Birth:* Here the baby's body is being delivered as the doctor gently supports the baby with his hand. The mother can control this final stage of the delivery—a stage that takes only a few seconds. This photograph shows the completion of a natural, drug-free delivery.

head is the widest part, followed by the shoulders and the relatively slender body. If the baby does not deliver easily, the obstetrician may push with his hand next to the shoulder and gently pull with the other hand underneath the baby's armpit. At the same time, the attending nurse may put her hand on your abdomen and help guide or push the baby down. In a natural delivery you will see the baby immediately, either as he or she is delivered into the doctor's arms, or onto the birthing bed.

Immediately after the birth, there is usually a gush of amniotic fluid often mixed with blood. This is the fluid that was trapped above the baby's body and did not escape when the membranes initially ruptured.

After the head is born, but before the shoulders emerge, the obstetrician will usually feel for the umbilical cord. Occasionally this will be wrapped tightly around the baby's neck and the doctor might have to clamp and cut the cord rapidly to prevent its tightening around the neck and strangling the baby. Otherwise the doctor will deliver the baby and cut the cord after the delivery is completed.

☐   ***The Baby***   As the body is born, the doctor will again suction the mouth to make sure that all the fluid is removed from the upper trachea before the baby takes its first full breath. By this point the baby should begin to breathe. A healthy baby may or may not cry. We may have been taught that a healthy baby must cry immediately after delivery, but this is a misconception. A baby born in a gentle manner into a friendly, quiet environment and allowed skin-to-skin contact with the mother immediately after birth may be quiet and content, and need not cry.

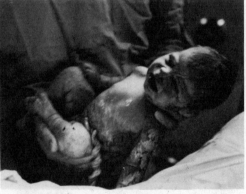

Figure 97: A healthy newborn baby immediately after delivery. The baby looks happy and peaceful after this natural birth. Note how the umbilical cord is still attached even though the baby is breathing on his own.

A healthy baby is pink at birth or a few minutes after birth. A slight blueness immediately after birth, particularly of the extremities, is quite normal and understandable, if you consider that the baby comes from the warm atmosphere of the uterus and birth canal into an environment at normal room temperature or below. The baby's circulation can be stimulated by a gentle massage with warm towels while it is lying on the mother's abdomen. The massage acts as a stimulus to the baby's circulation and breathing in the same way that a cat or dog uses her tongue to stimulate her young after birth.

As long as the baby is breathing well and has good color (see the section on the Apgar Score later in this chapter) he or she should be handed to the mother

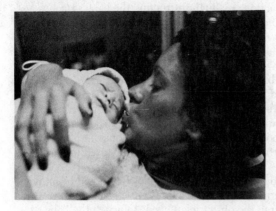

Figure 98: I Love You: A few seconds after birth, a happy mother is holding her beautiful son Rory. Muki and Peter had the opportunity of bonding immediately with their newborn.

immediately after birth. This is an important moment for you—be sure to tell your doctor you want to hold the baby immediately and have skin-to-skin contact. As you hold the baby, massage the trunk with the palm of your hands, talk to him or her, and observe the baby's breathing and color as the baby responds to the warmth of your skin and touch. Once the umbilical cord is cut, your arms and your body are the baby's new lifeline. Even if you have a forceps delivery or a Cesarean birth, it is important for the baby to bond with you immediately. Only if there is some initial difficulty in breathing should the nurses attend to the baby first before giving it to you, and even if it needs assistance and oxygen, there is usually no reason why you cannot hold it yourself within a few minutes. I would favor immediate bonding with the parents in all births, whenever possible. It is an important moment when the cord has been cut, severing the former connection between mother and child. The baby needs warmth and bodily contact immediately after birth; the Leboyer water bath is, I think, a poor substitute for maternal warmth, because the baby has been in "water" for nine months and must now adjust to an extrauterine life surrounded by air. Bonding, begun in the uterus, should be continued after birth in the loving arms of the parents.

As the baby is handed to you, the obstetrician will initially clamp the umbilical cord with a metal clamp to prevent any further exchange of blood between the placenta and the newborn. The umbilical cord is then cut with scissors. The

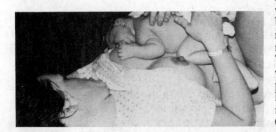

Figure 99: Postpartum Bonding: A baby needs warmth and body contact after birth. Hold the baby close to you; skin-to-skin contact or a warm blanket will help maintain the infant's body temperature. Breast-feeding can begin as soon as mother and baby are ready. The photograph records a wonderful moment for these parents: Rosemary had just delivered her third baby naturally after two previous Cesarean sections.

obstetrician will be ready to suction any fluid obstructing the baby's trachea and the staff can give oxygen if the child is not breathing well. Sometimes a baby needs a little extra oxygen to get the lungs started properly. Sometimes, but only sometimes, does it need a small slap underneath the palms of the feet to stimulate breathing, usually if Demerol or other analgesics have been given as a painkiller. Years ago the newborn baby was held up by the feet and slapped firmly on the rump to dislodge any fluid remaining in the lungs. This was not only an unnecessarily violent and unnatural practice, but a potentially dangerous one as well. According to Dr. Edmund Crelin, an anatomy professor at Yale Medical School, this tradition was responsible for dislocated hips in one out of every four hundred newborn babies. Fortunately the technique is rarely used in American hospitals today and one hopes it is no longer used anywhere.

Narcan (naloxone), an antidote to Demerol (see Chap. 19) should be immediately available in injectable form to reverse the depressant effects of drugs. With a forceps delivery or an epidural, the obstetrician needs to watch the baby's respiration carefully, and in general closely supervise the first minutes after birth.

If a difficult birth is anticipated, or if the baby's heartbeat drops before delivery (fetal distress), the birth must take place in a delivery room, where adequate resuscitation equipment is available. A pediatrician is often called to the delivery room before the birth to make sure that the proper assistance is at hand immediately.

☐ **Cutting the Umbilical Cord**   The umbilical cord can be cut either immediately after the birth or a few minutes after delivery, depending on the preference of the obstetrician. In some primitive societies the cord is never tied or cut until after the delivery of the placenta. In general, most physicians clamp the cord with a metal clamp immediately after birth. Certain doctors do prefer to allow the cord to continue pulsating for a few minutes after birth before clamping and cutting. Four to five minutes after delivery, spasms in the umbilical cord will naturally cut off the placental blood supply.

The preference for early clamping and cutting is based on the belief that neither early nor late cutting has any influence on the child's later development, and early clamping avoids the possibility of increased neonatal jaundice. The cord continues to supply blood to the baby for several minutes after birth, and this extra blood, added to the postnatal blood, may be deleterious. A baby is born with a relatively higher blood count than it will have in extrauterine life to compensate for the lower oxygen level in the uterus. Immediately after birth, the excess number of red blood cells is destroyed in a natural process that brings the blood count down to a normal level. Otherwise there is a risk of neonatal jaundice, since the baby's liver may not be quite mature enough to metabolize the extra blood.

Often the doctor hands the scissors to the father, who will be the one to cut the cord. This can be a very exciting moment, and I have known fathers to keep the surgical scissors they used to cut their child's cord as a memento of their part of the delivery. The umbilical cord is subsequently clamped with a plastic clamp and cut a few inches from the navel. The tying of the cord has nothing to do with an "inner" or "outer" navel—that is all determined by a baby's genes, since the umbilical cord will eventually shrink and fall off a few days after the birth.

After the cord is cut, it should be checked to see if it contains the normal two arteries and one vein. A sample of umbilical cord blood is usually sent to the laboratory to check the baby's blood count, blood type, and general status.

☐ *Delivery of the Placenta—The Third Stage of Labor*   The third stage of labor is the time from the delivery of the child to the delivery of the placenta. This can take anywhere from a few minutes to thirty minutes, although the average is in the area of ten to fifteen minutes.

Once the umbilical cord is clamped, the doctor usually awaits the spontaneous separation of the placenta. This is caused by contractions of the uterine muscles. These contractions cut down the blood supply to the placenta, and the placenta usually begins to separate at its middle portion. This is slowly followed by the separation of its margin. In fact, the placenta is almost turned inside out by the time it is delivered.

Just before delivery of the placenta, the umbilical cord is usually left alone, although some physicians unclamp the cord and let it bleed to aid the separation of the placenta and the ease of its delivery. What is important to understand is that the delivery is not complete until the placenta is delivered; and it is essential that it be delivered intact and with care. Otherwise there can be excessive postpartum bleeding.

During the delivery of the placenta, the obstetrician should place one hand on the abdomen and rotate it in small, circular movements to stimulate the release of any remaining prostaglandins inside the uterus. These prostaglandins will make the uterus contract more thoroughly and thus hasten the expulsion of the placenta. At this point the doctor can easily deliver the placenta by pushing with one hand on the abdomen and at the same time pulling gently on the umbilical cord with the other.

As the placenta is delivered, it will usually be turned inside out so that the first section delivered will be its fetal side, the area in which the amniotic fluid and the baby had rested during gestation. The other part of the placenta, called the maternal side, the area where the placenta had been implanted into the uterus, is distinguished by its vascularity and irregularity. As soon as the placenta is delivered, the doctor will examine it to make sure it is delivered *in toto*, and

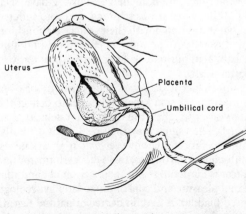

Uterus

Placenta

Umbilical cord

Spontaneous delivery of the placenta

Figure 100: The End of the Third Stage of Labor: The placenta is seen shedding itself from the lining of the uterus as the doctor gently massages the outside of the abdomen to help the uterus begin to contract. The mother will be asked to push at the same time. A slight cramping sensation is experienced as the placenta is delivered.

will then hand it to another doctor or leave it on the delivery table for a later, thorough examination. The doctor should keep one hand on the abdomen and continue to perform circular movements to push the uterus down. This maneuver can be slightly painful for the patient, but it is important in keeping the uterus contracted and diminishing the risk of bleeding. No sutures can be put inside the uterus, so when it contracts, the contractions help constrict the blood vessels inside it and eliminate bleeding.

The same purpose is achieved by the injection of oxytocin favored by many hospitals immediately after the delivery of the placenta. The injection is given intravenously or intramuscularly, or else by what is known as *half and half*—half intravenously and half intramuscularly. The oxytocin will reach the uterus quickly and cause it to contract. Whether you are given oxytocin or not, the doctor should continue the uterine massage for a few minutes after the delivery of the placenta and may then ask you or your labor coach to continue the massage intermittently for one to two hours after the birth. Through this cutting down on postpartum bleeding, your blood count will remain higher and you will have less tendency toward anemia. If your blood count is high, you will heal faster and you will be less susceptible to postpartum depression and other problems.

If the bleeding cannot be controlled after the delivery of the placenta, the obstetrician may elect to give you an intravenous or intramuscular injection of ergotrate or methergine. These oxytocic drugs are also uterine contracting agents. A serious bout of postpartum bleeding might require a blood transfusion. Prolonged bleeding can lead to a D&C in the postpartum period and, on rare occasions, has resulted in hysterectomy.

The patient will usually stay in the labor and delivery area for about two to three hours after the birth to allow time for careful observation by the staff. It takes a few hours to make sure that no major postpartum problems will occur.

☐ *The Episiotomy—Is It Necessary?*   A calm, controlled delivery performed by a skillful obstetrician might prevent vaginal tearing, particularly in a woman who has already borne a child. However, in a first delivery, an episiotomy is often called for to prevent excessive laceration in the relatively inelastic vaginal area—tearing that can sometimes result in nerve injury. I have seen women who did not have an episiotomy when it was required, and who suffered such damage of the vaginal area that it interfered with their sexual relationships. Given the risk of serious damage, it is better to perform an episiotomy in doubtful cases rather than deliver the baby without one, as long as the episiotomy itself is performed by a skillful obstetrician.

The advantage of the episiotomy is that it decreases the possibility of overstretching and lacerating the perineal muscles and makes it easier to deliver the baby's head. In addition, it is often easier to repair the vagina after delivery if an episiotomy has been performed first. The vagina may then heal more naturally, with less postpartum pain. A routine episiotomy, however, is not always necessary, especially in a second or subsequent birth. Doctors who perform routine episiotomies argue that a jagged tear is harder to repair than a clean cut and that any tearing will interfere with sexual pleasure and contribute to later gynecological problems, including a prolapsed bladder. A certain degree of natural tearing can, however, be repaired successfully and may not cause later problems. An

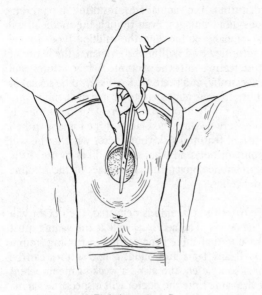

Episiotomy

Figure 101: Episiotomy: First, the area of the perineum is anesthetized with a local anesthetic. Second, the cut is made through the perineum at a time when the perineal tissues are almost paper-thin. Here the obstetrician is making a median (midline) episiotomy. This type of episiotomy usually causes less pain and heals faster than the mediolateral episiotomy.

episiotomy has never been proven to benefit the baby either, even though it makes the delivery easier. Quite the opposite: the squeezing of the baby's chest through the intact perineum may serve a function by helping expel mucus from the lungs.

Despite contradictory opinions on the subject, an episiotomy is routinely performed in most hospital births in the United States, depending on where the doctor received his training. European midwives often conduct their deliveries without an episiotomy, although their patients do experience more tearing.

There are two types of episiotomies: the midline or median episiotomy, and the mediolateral episiotomy.

The midline or median episiotomy is a straight cut between the lower portion of the vagina toward the rectum. This is often considered the better procedure of the two, since the cut is made in an area of less vascularity—resulting in less bleeding—and there are fewer nerves in the area, and therefore less pain afterward. The midline episiotomy also heals faster, because there is less fatty tissue and the cut therefore is easier to suture after birth. The disadvantage is that a very large baby may be too large for a midline episiotomy, causing a third- or fourth-degree laceration—a tearing through the anal sphincter, the muscles around the rectum. A fourth-degree laceration may tear into the anus itself.

The mediolateral episiotomy is cut from the bottom of the vagina into the side of the anus. This type of episiotomy will cut into the fatty tissues but avoids the sphincter muscles. The advantage of this type of cut is that any tearing will penetrate the fatty tissues but not the sphincter muscles or the rectum. However, the mediolateral episiotomy is harder to repair than the median episiotomy and does not always heal as well because it is cut into the fatty tissues, which can easily become infected. Since this type of episiotomy usually heals more slowly, the patient is likely to have a harder time moving around after the birth, and there is a greater chance of its disturbing the vaginal area, resulting in pain during intercourse. These are serious disadvantages, even though the mediolateral episiotomy accommodates a larger baby better than the midline type. In my opinion, a midline episiotomy performed by a skillful obstetrician is the better of the two, even if it does result in tearing into the rectum. A few sutures will usually repair any rectal tears successfully, and there are less likely to be sexual or other problems later on. More obstetricians now seem to be aware of the advantages of the midline episiotomy—even with a forceps delivery. (An episiotomy is always necessary with a forceps delivery because the blades of the forceps stretch the vulval area and add to the risk of tearing.) Ask your doctor whether he will be performing a routine episiotomy or not, and what type he likes to use. If he says mediolateral, question his preference, given the advantages of the midline episiotomy in most, if not all, deliveries.

☐ *Suturing the Episiotomy*   After the placenta is delivered, the doctor will usually inspect the vagina and the cervix. The cervix as well as the vagina must be looked over carefully to make sure that there is no tearing or ripping from a large baby or a forceps delivery. If any tears are found, a few sutures can be placed in the cervix to help it heal completely and avoid a weak or incompetent cervix in future pregnancies. At the same time the doctor will inspect the vagina to make sure there is no tear in its upper portion. No major lacerations should result from a carefully controlled delivery.

In a forceps delivery there is a chance of the forceps tearing into the vagina and increasing the need for more extensive surgical repair. Occasionally the forceps will rupture a blood vessel and produce very heavy bleeding. In this case, the woman's obstetrician will need other doctors to help him retract the vagina to assure proper suturing. In a few of these cases, patients have bled so profusely postpartum that a blood transfusion became necessary. Generally, however, a thorough obstetrician will be able to locate any tears and deal with them easily by suturing meticulously. Most obstetricians now use chromic catgut sutures, which are self-absorbent, and which heal faster and with less pain than the old-fashioned type.

The repair of the episiotomy itself is next. If the cut was of the midline type it is usually easy to repair. With a small episiotomy, one running suture is all that is necessary to secure the vagina, although it is important that the transverse perineum muscles which hold the vagina together are carefully sutured from side to side to build up good support in the vaginal tissue. The muscles surrounding the vagina will then remain tight, preventing a prolapse at some future time, which could interfere with your sexual relationship. A careful suturing is also associated with fewer immediate problems. The suture should be placed subcuticularly—immediately under the skin tissue so that no suture is visible from the outside. This ensures a minimal scar and much less nerve damage or pain in the postpartum period. With careful suturing, a controlled midline episiotomy usually heals quickly with little discomfort and little loss of sensitivity and sexual pleasure in the future. A mediolateral episiotomy, as I have already explained, may be associated with more immediate pain and a slower recovery time because it is cut through the fatty tissue. Even if tearing does penetrate into the rectum, as it may do with the midline episiotomy, a competent physician can carefully suture the rectum together and repair the sphincter muscles, the muscles that surround the rectum. As long as the sutures are placed correctly, a properly repaired tear will not result in any future problems with bowel movements or a woman's sexual function. Nor does it lead to hemorrhoids, which often develop during pregnancy through pressure on the veins in the rectum, and have nothing to do with the type of episiotomy used during the delivery. A thorough, competent physician will probably elect to do a midline episiotomy and can usually repair it with few harmful effects to your future sexual or childbearing functions.

The episiotomy is usually sutured under a local anesthetic (lidocaine or Xylocaine) if you did not have epidural anesthesia during the delivery.

☐ *Care of the Episiotomy*   It is normal to experience pain and swelling after the episiotomy, although the discomfort can be alleviated by an ice pack placed on the affected area. Keeping an ice pack in place for a few hours will ease the swelling and make the transition easier. Other effective methods of relief are sitz baths or a lidocaine spray applied to the area of the episiotomy. Your doctor will usually leave a prescription for pain-killers to be taken for the first few days. Prescriptions vary from hospital to hospital, depending on physician preference. Caution is of course required if you are breast-feeding since the baby will get some of the medication through the breast milk, and you might prefer to forgo medication altogether, or at least ask for the minimum dose.

☐ *Why Do Women Have Chills After the Birth?*   Many women experience a sudden attack of chills after the delivery of the placenta. This is often unpleasant as well as unexpected. Some doctors feel it is a natural side effect caused by the postpartum blood loss but it is more likely to be a reaction to the oxytocin injection given after the delivery of the placenta, since a woman can bleed very little and still experience symptoms of shock. Pitocin (synthetic oxytocin) is known to have a side effect on the temperature-regulating center in the brain. If you suddenly experience chills or a fit of shivering, ask for some warm blankets; the sensation usually disappears within a few minutes and your body temperature will stabilize again.

☐ *How Will the Baby Look After Birth?*   At birth, the baby will usually be covered with a substance called *vernix caseosa*, which has been described as cheesy and white, or as greasy and yellow. This substance protects the skin of the baby from the liquid environment inside the uterus. The vernix is sometimes washed off during the delivery but is usually not fully removed until the baby is given a bath in the nursery. The vernix has a function during birth as well as before birth, since it enables the baby to slip more easily through the vagina.

The newborn's skin is thin, and you may see the veins more clearly than you would in an adult. The body, in particular the back, may be covered with fine downy hairs called *lanugo* hair, which will disappear in the first month of life. Some blood from the delivery may also be present on the normal newborn's skin.

The skin color changes somewhat after delivery. While the trunk may be pink, the hands and feet are usually bluish because the blood circulation is slower in reaching the extremities—especially in a cold room. Small white spots called *milia* are often apparent on the nose, cheeks, and chin, caused by distended sebaceous cysts. Other distinctive marks, light red areas on the back of the neck or the bridge of the nose, are caused by clusters of tiny blood vessels. Most of these birthmarks will fade with time. Many black or Asian babies are born with what are known as Mongolian spots, which look like black or blue bruises on the back or bottom. These may take longer to fade, although they too usually disappear by the time the child is older. It is interesting that black, Asian, and Mediterranean babies are born relatively light-skinned—skin pigmentation does not appear until several days after birth.

Usually the face and eyelids are puffy and reddish after birth because of the pressure of passing through the vagina. Interestingly, no tears will appear for the first few weeks.

The unusual appearance of many newborn's heads, the "banana head," is something that concerns many parents but is normal and transient. The banana shape occurs because the fetal head is soft and malleable enough to conform to the shape of the pelvic bones and becomes elongated or swollen as it passes through the birth canal. Any swelling will usually disappear within a day or two of birth and so will the strange banana shape of the head. Neither is a reflection of the child's later intelligence level.

☐ *Evaluation and Care of the Newborn*   First the baby is quickly checked to make sure it is healthy and has ten fingers, ten toes, and a generally normal appearance. If any abnormality is immediately apparent, the obstetrician will call on a pediatrician or a neonatologist to examine the baby. Otherwise the obstetrician will evaluate the baby's condition himself, following a series of routine procedures. Immediately after the birth, the obstetrician will again aspirate the excess mucus from the mouth and then make sure that the baby is breathing. If the baby is blue or not breathing satisfactorily, the doctor will clamp and cut the umbilical cord and move the baby to a resuscitation table, where the anesthesiologist or pediatrician will begin emergency resuscitation. The baby must be encouraged to breathe on his own: up until that point a newborn has received all his oxygen through the umbilical cord, and breathing air is still a foreign experience that will exert great stress physiologically as the blood begins to pass through the lungs. If the baby's breathing is depressed by Demerol, or he has some other difficulty, he may not be able to adjust immediately to his new environment. The obstetrician's job is to evaluate the newborn's capacity to hold his own without help. As long as the baby is pink and breathing well, showing a good adjustment to the extrauterine environment, he can be safely handed to the parents within a minute or two of birth. The obstetrician might briefly use a stethoscope or feel with his fingers to check the heartbeat, but otherwise there is no reason to separate an apparently healthy child from his parents. The newborn was once put in a warmed crib to maintain body temperature after the delivery, but skin contact with the mother on the delivery table will usually keep the baby sufficiently warm as well as increase intimacy between parent and child. Most delivery rooms are equipped with an overhead heater, or the baby can be loosely covered with a towel or blanket on the delivery table.

If there is a moment of concern after birth, immediate action will be taken to remove mucus and amniotic fluid from the stomach and the trachea and begin oxygenation. Sometimes a newborn will begin to breathe on his own only after he is given a few breaths of oxygen. If the baby is depressed by the effects of Demerol or some other analgesics, he may also require an antidote such as Narcan to reverse the effects of the drug. In a birth in which you have had an epidural during the delivery and required forceps for delivery, the baby is usually unaffected by the method of delivery and can be handed to the parents immediately. Only if forceps have been used in a case of fetal distress—a decreased heart rate and therefore lower oxygenation—may the baby need resuscitation or oxygenation before he is ready to breathe on his own. Parents are naturally concerned if forceps have been used, but no harm should result if a forceps delivery is undertaken carefully (see Chap. 30).

☐ *The Apgar Score*   The Apgar Score, a rating system that indicates the condition of the newborn, is given at one minute, at five minutes and occasionally at ten minutes after birth. Dr. Virginia Apgar, a celebrated pediatrician at Columbia Presbyterian Hospital in New York, was the first doctor to realize the importance of a uniform scoring system so that obstetricians and pediatricians throughout the world would have a standard way of determining the newborn's condition in the crucial minutes after birth. Immediately after birth, a baby may go through a characteristic series of reactions similar to those of an adult recovering from anesthesia—grunting, respiratory movements, fast or slow heart rate, and color changes. Following the initial shock of birth, the baby usually begins to adjust—a physiological change that is evaluated by the two Apgar Scores.

APGAR SCORE

SIGN	0	1	2
Heart rate	absent	slow (below 100)	Over 100
Respiratory effort	absent	weak cry; hypoventilation	good effort; strong cry
Muscle tone	limp	some flexion of extremities	active motion: extremities well flexed
Reflex irritability (response to stimulation) of skin of feet	no response	some motion (grimace)	crying and active
Color	Blue, pale	body pink; extremities blue	completely pink

The Apgar Score evaluates five crucial determinants of the baby's condition: heart rate, respiratory capacity, muscle tone, reflexes, and skin color. An Apgar Score of 2 in each category means that the baby has a normal heart rate, normal respiration, is active and alert, cries vigorously when stimulated, and is completely pink. If the baby is generally healthy with good breathing, a steady heart rate, and strong muscle tone he will usually get an overall Apgar Score of 9 at one minute after birth. The baby must be completely pink to get the full Apgar Score of 10, and that is rare because it usually takes a little time for the oxygen to reach the skin tissues in the extremities.

The next evaluation is made five minutes after birth. The five-minute Apgar Score is the more significant of the two because many babies are born with some initial breathing difficulties and require resuscitation or a shot of Narcan before they can breathe well on their own. Again, the breathing, muscle tone, reflexes, heart rate, and color are evaluated separately. Most normal babies will receive a 9 or 10 at five minutes; but a score of 7 or higher is not associated with future learning disabilities or behavioral abnormalities.

In one large-scale study, the Collaborative Perinatal Project, in which several large hospitals went through their labor and delivery records and then evaluated the babies one year and five years later, babies with different Apgar Scores were followed to estimate the connection between the Apgar Score and neurological damage later on in life. This study found that most babies with a score of 7 or higher *at five minutes* were doing well and had no neurological impairment. It was the babies with lower five-minute Apgar Scores who were more likely to be impaired. Even this is only a gross estimate, because the real test comes when a child enters school. An obstetrician naturally likes to see a baby with an Apgar score of 9 at one minute and 10 at five minutes—average scores for a healthy child—but there is no need to worry about the future of the baby if the scores are several points lower. Many, many babies have immediate difficulties and then overcome them quickly. The newborn is also surprisingly resilient and adaptable; a child with a poor Apgar Score often does well within a few weeks after birth.

A ten-minute Apgar Score is occasionally given, but this is of real importance only if the baby is sick at birth and requires resuscitation.

If a baby is delivered under completely natural circumstances without analgesics or anesthesia, it will usually have good Apgar Scores and be much bouncier and healthier at birth than the baby of a medicated mother. Another healthy sign after birth is urination and erection of the penis in a boy.

☐ *The Birth Weight*   Babies were once routinely weighed in the delivery room so the birth weight could be entered immediately on the hospital record. Today most babies are not weighed until they arrive at the hospital nursery— half an hour or more after birth. The change has come about because hospital staffs are more concerned with the baby's temperature stabilizing after birth than an immediate record of the birth weight. Delivery rooms are deliberately kept at a low temperature to discourage infection; and this, together with the cold surface of the metal scales, can make it more difficult for the baby to retain body warmth after delivery. Obstetricians and pediatricians, in any case, no longer regard the baby's initial weight as the most significant indicator of the baby's condition. As long as your child is thriving—breathing well and doing well—the exact weight is not important, unless he is very small or considered premature. Later, after bonding, when the baby is warm and comfortable, the pediatric nurse will weigh the baby and give you the birth weight. The baby's length and head circumference will be measured at the same time.

The average birth weight of a healthy child in the United States is slightly higher than seven pounds; at least a half pound heavier than the average birth-weight only one decade ago. Babies are larger now partly because of better pre-natal nutrition. It is not uncommon for a woman to give birth to a baby of eight pounds or more, depending on genetic factors and her pregnancy care.

☐ *Silver Nitrate Eyedrops—Are They Really Necessary?*   According to Board of Health requirements in almost every state, precautions must be taken against gonorrhea-induced blindness after every birth. The baby of an infected mother can pick up the gonorrhea as it passes through the birth canal. This is a rare occurrence in newborns since the chance of gonorrhea is extremely slim in a woman who is living in a caring relationship—but the law is still on the books in most states, except Massachusetts. Many hospitals use the traditional 1 percent solution of silver nitrate in each eye—an unpleasant procedure, since silver nitrate is highly irritating and will blur the baby's vision for several hours. The parents then cannot fully bond with their baby after birth, since eye-to-eye contact is lost. Another disadvantage of silver nitrate is that newborns often develop a chemical-induced conjunctivitis, which can last for several days after birth.

Many hospitals are now beginning to favor other forms of antibiotics that are less irritating, such as 1 percent tetracycline ophthalmic ointment. This will still interfere with the baby's vision, but to a lesser degree. An injection of 50,000 units of penicillin is another alternative to silver nitrate. Bonding is then not af-fected, but the injection can be painful and the chance of penicillin allergy could be another problem. If your hospital favors drops or ointments, you should ask the pediatric nurse to wait for an hour or so after the birth before treating the baby. You will then have a chance to be close to the baby immedi-ately after birth. Drops placed two hours after birth are as effective as they would be two hours earlier. Never allow the nurse to use silver nitrate.

☐ *Vitamin K Injections*   By law the baby should also receive a 1.25 milli-gram injection of vitamin K immediately after birth. This is a sensible require-ment since a baby has an insufficient supply of vitamin K naturally for several days after birth and is therefore vulnerable to internal bleeding. It takes a few days for the baby's gastrointestinal tract to produce enough intestinal flora to form vitamin K. Some doctors and midwives, concerned with the baby's sensitiv-ity at birth, now give vitamin K orally—a practice that may be routine in the future.

☐ *Footprints*   A footprint of the baby as well as a fingerprint of the mother is by law a part of the baby's records. This is for identification purposes should there be any temporary confusion in the nursery—though a mother who takes the "wrong" baby home may exist in fiction but is very rare in reality. When the nurse takes the footprint, you can ask her to give you a copy for your own files and for the baby's scrapbook. The baby's I.D. bracelet, with your name and hos-pital number on it, can be added to your collection later.

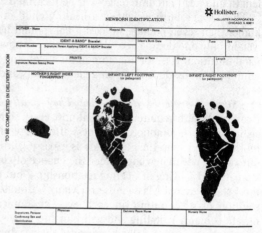

Figure 102: *Delivery Room Identification Chart:* Immediately after the baby is born his footprints will be recorded on a newborn identification chart. Note, too, the print of the mother's right index finger. Such marks guarantee correct identification in the rare event of a mixup in the nursery.

☐ *Birth Certificate*   By law a birth certificate must be filled out within twenty-four hours of the birth. Most doctors fill out and sign a preliminary form immediately after the delivery, and the hospital's administrative office will then combine this data with the information they already have on file about the parents. Any complications during pregnancy and delivery, the time of delivery, and the baby's Apgar Scores are placed on record by the attending obstetrician at the time of birth.

☐ *Photographing the Birth*   The birth of their baby is an event many couples want to record for posterity. Some couples prefer not to photograph the delivery per se but like to take photographs immediately after the birth. Any pictures will be exciting for the child as he or she grows up.

Remember, the use of camera equipment in the delivery room must be approved by your doctor, and no flash attachment should be used, since the flash can hurt the baby's eyes and might be dangerous if there is oxygen in the room.

☐ *Champagne—for the Birth Day*   If you are lucky enough to have a delivery without Demerol or an epidural anesthesia, you can celebrate your child's arrival with an ad hoc picnic after the birth. The birthing room staff will usually allow the labor coach to bring in a bottle of champagne or other wine, and you can either bring or order out food for yourself, your husband, and the doctor and nurses to celebrate this special birth day. After a successful delivery, everyone can relax, discuss the events of the birth, and toast a happy life for the newcomer.

☐ *The Recovery Room*   A postpartum patient will usually stay in the recovery room for two to three hours after the delivery. This is necessary because the uterus must contract in the first few hours to prevent excessive postpartum bleeding. The recovery room nurse will check your vital signs at regular intervals and massage your abdomen to help firm up the uterus. You will also be encouraged to empty your bladder at the first opportunity, since the uterus will tend to bleed more if the bladder is distended. Emptying your bladder can be difficult at the beginning if the skin around the urethra is swollen and irritated after the episiotomy. You might need to be catheterized the first or second time you pass urine until the swelling around the urethra has disappeared.

After two hours, as long as the uterus is well contracted, there is only minimal bleeding, and you have no trouble urinating, you will be moved to your room on the postpartum floor. The staff will continue to watch your progress carefully for several days. If you should develop problems such as increased bleeding, you must alert the nursing staff and be seen by your doctor. The doctor will examine your uterus to make sure it is well contracted and inspect the vagina to rule out any laceration that needs to be resutured. He might also prescribe ergotrate or methergine tablets, 0.2 milligram, every four hours for one to two days to help contract the uterus and stop the bleeding. A woman commonly experiences more bleeding in the first two or three days after birth because the milk let-down reflex is not yet established (see Chapter 32 on breast-feeding). The baby's sucking releases oxytocin from the pituitary gland which in turn contracts the uterus, but in the first two or three days the baby is not sucking enough to release sufficient oxytocin. You can expect the uterus to heal quickly once breast-feeding is well established.

☐ *Bonding* Bonding is defined as the growth of attachment between two human beings. It is crucial to human survival because without it no parent would be willing to make the sacrifices necessary to taking care of an infant or bringing up a child. Neither is it one-sided: a child's growing attachment to the parents only strengthens their attachment to their child.

Writers and researchers who have studied bonding believe it begins very early, in the first moments after birth, when subtle, almost imperceptible interchanges occur that hasten the growth of attachment. When Drs. John Kennell and Marshall Klaus, pediatricians at Case Western University in Cleveland, began observing maternal infant bonding in the 1950s, they discovered that a woman given her baby for the first time will usually follow an instinctive pattern—touching the face with her fingertips, massaging the trunk, caressing and stroking the baby and trying to establish eye-to-eye contact. (Fathers, too, repeat this sequence when they first hold their babies). The baby is alert and responsive in the first hour or so after birth and will respond in his own way to the excitement of his parents. This complementary behavior encourages immediate and close contact between parent and child.

The special quality of the first hour after birth has caused it to be termed a "sensitive period" in the growth of human attachment, similar to that seen among animals who engage in characteristic behavior immediately after giving birth. At the same time, researchers on bonding in humans have emphasized that, unlike animals, who may permanently reject the offspring taken away from them immediately after birth, humans can bond with their babies at other times after the first "sensitive period." Because a parent misses, or is deprived of early bonding, it does not mean that the sequence of attachment is permanently disrupted; adoptive parents may, for instance, be as attached to their children as natural parents. However, traditional hospital practices, which separate mother and baby immediately after birth and for several days thereafter, do make it difficult for new parents to establish bonding early on, and *may*, in some cases, permanently affect the relationship with the child. Isolating the newborn in a nursery away from his parents, at a time when he needs their physical closeness, seems not only unnecessary but cruel.

The newborn is physically helpless, but he comes into the world with a remarkable array of social and sensory skills. A baby will discriminate visually at birth. He is also capable of following a moving object at a twelve- to fifteen-inch distance. In the quiet, alert state, characteristic of the first hour of life, the baby will open his eyes and focus intensely on a chosen object, preferably the human face. The human eye is fascinating to newborns, perhaps because of its brilliance and mobility. The mother recipro-

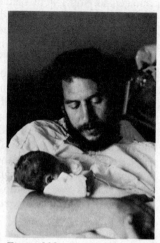

Figure 103

cates, placing the newborn about a foot away in the face-to-face position where he can see her best, and engaging in prolonged mutual gazing (behavior that is also seen in adults who are in love). The newborn's hearing, too, is already sufficiently acute that he will turn his head to follow the sound of the human voice. Mothers, again instinctively, use an unusually high-pitched voice in talking to their babies; the higher resonances are apparently more attractive to the newborn than the lower pitch of the typical male voice, although the newborn has been observed to follow both his parents' voices in the delivery room (this finding is among the new pre- and postnatal research to be found in Chapter 14). As the mother speaks, the baby will respond by moving rhythmically—often moving a foot or raising an eyebrow as she pauses or accents a syllable. Like social smiling, which does not develop until a few weeks later, these behaviors seem to quicken the parents' interest in their baby, thus increasing their desire to protect and care for him. "You can't love a dishrag," is the way Klaus and Kennell have summarized the reciprocal nature of early attachment.

☐ ***Bonding in the Hospital***   Ten minutes of bonding in the delivery room followed by separation of mother and baby is not long enough for you and your child to establish effectual early bonding. An extended period of time—at least thirty minutes—should be made available to you after the birth. If you are not using a birthing room, ask the staff to place you in a private recovery area where you can be undisturbed with the baby, or at least get the nurse to draw the curtains around the delivery bed once your obstetrician has finished any necessary suturing of the episiotomy.

You can ask for the baby as soon as the delivery is completed, or you can wait a few moments until you feel ready to hold the baby. Many women need a few minutes to "catch their breath" before they are ready for the next important step. The father should, in this case, hold the baby until the mother is ready. If the baby's temperature has stabilized he can be dried off and handed to you unwrapped. The natural way to maintain the infant's body heat is skin to skin contact, although the labor or delivery bed may come equipped with an overhead radiant-heat warmer.

If you plan to breast-feed, you can begin immediately by placing the baby close to your breast and allowing him to root for the nipple. Most newborns will take to the breast, first nuzzling or licking the nipple. There will not be much milk this early on, but if you massage the breast gently with your

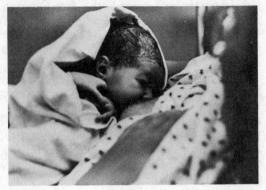

Figure 104

hand a few times and squeeze the nipple into the baby's mouth, this will be enough to encourage the baby to continue to suck. Most babies delivered under minimal anesthesia will begin breast-feeding almost immediately. Hold the baby close and rub him gently up and down to stimulate his blood circulation and let him feel the warmth of your hands and skin. A newborn who feels warm and secure will remain quiet and content. Talk to him: the voices he heard from inside the uterus are already familiar and will help soothe and reassure him.

Be sure to allow yourself time for both of you to touch and fondle the baby. Communication and touch hasten the father's as well as the mother's bonding with the baby. When a man feels close to his child from the beginning—the child he had a part in creating—it can influence his attitude to his child later in life. Many men who have also experienced a traditional delivery, one in which there was no period of bonding after birth, have told me that being there with the baby eased the stresses of the first month home and may have permanently affected their relationship with a particular child. This has been borne out by research linking the father's behavior later on to the time spent with the baby in the first three days of life.

As long as the baby is warm and breathing well there is no reason not to stay together for an extended time, at least thirty minutes. After thirty to forty minutes the baby and the mother will often fall into a deep sleep. The child will be taken to the newborn nursery for a few hours, while you are taken to your hospital room. Most hospitals, even those with rooming in, feel the baby needs to go to the nursery for a period of observation because problems can occur in the first twenty-four hours of life as the baby is learning to breathe on his own. Also, after the excitement of the birth, you may be too tired to watch the baby yourself. If you are in a hospital with rooming in, the baby can be placed in your room after the initial period of observation, and some hospitals will allow the father to sleep in with you, increasing the contact with the baby in these first, important days. New parents who have rooming in or modified rooming in are usually less anxious when they go home than parents who have been forced to leave their babies with the hospital staff.

☐ *Postpartum Bonding*   Postpartum bonding is possible whether you deliver in a birthing room or in a delivery room; whether you have a natural delivery or a forceps or Cesarean birth. Many Cesarean deliveries are now performed under spinal anesthesia, which allows the parents time with the baby after the birth is over. A baby delivered by Cesarean is not necessarily a baby that needs special care, although the staff may observe the baby more closely in the recovery period.

☐ *If You Cannot Bond Immediately*   Bonding may begin with birth, but it also continues for the days, weeks, and months to come. Parents who are not allowed to bond immediately after birth can still be loving, successful parents. Although the research on bonding has stressed the importance of establishing early, effectual ties, ongoing opportunities for attachment continue throughout the life of any relationship. One researcher believes that some mothers fall in love with their children even before birth; while some feel a powerful attachment in the first week after birth, and still others bond successfully only once the baby is several weeks old or even older. Early bonding, in any case, will not always counteract the stresses of parenthood. Even so, if hospitals generally were to change their philosophy of care, all parents and newborns would benefit from a more humane approach to birth, and the effects might be felt long after the children and parents had left the hospital.

☐ *The Biorhythm of the Newborn Baby*   The baby may remain in the quiet, alert state for about an hour after birth, the optimum time for bonding, and will then fall into a deep sleep lasting three or four hours. Similar sleeping-waking cycles recur in the next few days, although the baby may be restless and cry more on the second and third day after birth. The period of restlessness is a natural one because he must adapt to extrauterine life and readjust his biorhythms. Continual contact with his mother will help him establish his new biorhythmic cycle. After the third day a baby whose mother is physically close to him will usually cry less and be more alert when his mother holds him. Even if he is not in the quiet, alert state, he will become attentive when he sees and hears his mother. By the eighth day he may respond at least 50 percent of the time to his mother's holding him—about double his capability on the second day of life. Alertness increases as a child grows older, and by six to eight weeks social smiling usually begins.

30

Complicated Births

Couples who attend childbirth-preparation classes usually have a good understanding of a natural delivery. But they may not be so knowledgeable about such common complications as prolonged labor, abnormal presentations, or forceps deliveries. This is unfortunate because today, when more older women are having first babies and more couples want to participate fully in their pregnancies and deliveries, they should know that birth is not always a smooth and easy process. They should also try not to be unduly upset if something does go wrong at their own delivery. Too many couples who have unexpectedly difficult births blame themselves for the last-minute Cesarean or the need to resort to anesthesia, only because they had not realized that a high percentage of deliveries can be *expected* to encounter problems. It may be easier for a doctor or a childbirth instructor to imply that every couple will have a normal delivery, but a couple will be *less* afraid to face the possibility of a complication during labor if they understand potential complications, and the way in which they should be handled. They may indeed find the information reassuring rather than frightening. Of course, a couple must educate themselves as far as is possible, must ask questions, and must not be afraid to discuss possible complications with their obstetrician or their childbirth instructor. By knowing what to anticipate, it becomes much easier for a couple to cope with a complication and much easier to understand why the complication has occurred.

☐ *Understanding Childbirth*   The two previous chapters explain in some detail how labor is initiated, and how the various stages of labor progress in an uncomplicated vertex delivery. An understanding of the progression of natural labor is essential to an understanding of the complications of labor.

You might be under the impression that your delivery will be an uncomplicated one if your pregnancy has gone smoothly and your baby is lying in the correct position (the vertex, or head-first, position). But this is a misconception.

Not all vertex deliveries are uncomplicated. First of all, a patient might rupture her fetal membranes before labor contractions begin (premature rupture of the membranes—PROM). In that event, labor never progresses quite as smoothly as it would otherwise. A woman with PROM might not go into labor for several hours, and when she does go into labor, her labor is often longer, or needs to be stimulated by intravenous administration of oxytocin. Often the baby in these circumstances enters the birth canal in the so-called posterior position, in which the head faces forward in its passage through the bony pelvis—a position that prolongs labor and often makes it harder (as explained in Chapter 27).

Another complication may occur when the fetal head fails to enter the pelvis in the weeks before delivery. In a first birth, though not in subsequent births, the head usually engages itself with the bony part of the pelvis two to four weeks before labor begins. Then as time goes on the Braxton Hicks contractions slowly push the head far into the pelvis, into the right position for labor. Simultaneously the cervix changes, or becomes effaced, in readiness for labor. If these changes take place in the proper sequence, it may well be an easy, normal delivery. Your obstetrician can even tell you whether to expect an easy or a difficult birth from the position of the head in the pelvis and the degree of cervical effacement.

In most first labors the head will engage in readiness for an uncomplicated delivery. Sometimes, however, the head fails to engage because the head is very large, the pelvis is unusually small, or the baby is in the wrong position for birth. You might then be facing dystocia—or difficult birth—and your labor might be unusually hard and long. A birth complicated by dystocia will often need stimulation with synthetic oxytocin (Pitocin) to achieve a vaginal delivery. Even with oxytocin stimulation, a vaginal delivery might be accomplished only with the aid of forceps or a vacuum extractor. And if dystocia is not managed properly, you might be forced into an unnecessary Cesarean delivery. Since management of dystocia is a controversial subject, it will be discussed both in this chapter and in the next chapter, on Cesarean birth.

Each labor is different, and a variation in labor patterns is to be expected among individual women. Some women, therefore, experience a natural but prolonged labor. But if labor is unusually prolonged, an obstetrician will probably decide to stimulate the contractions with oxytocin rather than allow labor to continue for many hours without relief.

Another complication occurs when a woman fails to go into labor at term. There is then the risk of postmaturity, a potentially dangerous condition which is explained in Chapter 25. A postdate or postmature pregnancy can be induced artificially by oxytocin infusion—another controversial subject that is discussed in this chapter.

So far I have discussed only vertex deliveries, either easy, natural ones, or those in which complications can occur. I haven't even mentioned breeches. Unfortunately a small but sizable percentage of all deliveries do end up in a breech delivery, which puts these births in a different category from vertex deliveries. Today many obstetricians in private practice don't give a woman with a breech presentation the chance to deliver vaginally, even if the breech is a relatively uncomplicated one. The result is that some breeches unnecessarily end up in a Cesarean birth. If you do experience a breech presentation, you would be wise to discuss your delivery plans carefully with your doctor several weeks be-

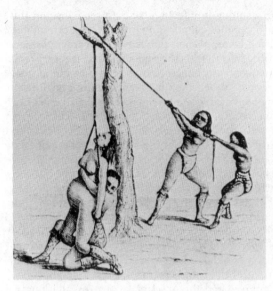

Figure 105: Although most labors proceed naturally, all cultures have devised methods of dealing with complicated deliveries. This picture depicts a difficult birth among the Coyotero Apache Indians. A rope has been tied around the woman's chest just beneath her arms and the other end thrown over the stump limb of a nearby tree. The two men have pulled the patient up until her feet barely touch the ground. The midwife is exerting pressure with tightly wrapped arms just above the abdomen to encourage the baby's descent.

fore you go into labor (see below) and perhaps seek a second opinion if you are doubtful about his approach or his competence.

The term "complicated birth" might sound frightening to most people, but it should not alarm you unnecessarily. A competent obstetrician can guide you through a difficult birth and help make the delivery as joyful a moment as that of any natural birth. If you and your partner have educated yourselves as to your specific problem it will help alleviate fear, and allow you to participate more actively in the birth itself. A so-called difficult birth will then be transformed into an experience you will remember with happiness.

☐ **Management of PROM—Premature Rupture of the Membranes**   The term PROM, or premature rupture of the membranes, is generally used when a woman enters the hospital with rupture of the membranes before the onset of labor. This occurs in about 12 percent of all pregnancies and is somewhat more frequent among women who give birth prematurely before the thirty-sixth week of gestation.

Premature rupture has many possible causes, although the exact reason can often only be guessed at. One explanation is that, if the cervix is slightly dilated before labor occurs, bacteria could enter from the vagina and into the fetal membranes. A local inflammatory reaction will then result in weakening of the membranes. Any weak spot in the membranes is vulnerable to leakage or rupture as the baby moves; this causes the membranes to leak amniotic fluid or rupture completely. A rupture sometimes takes place in their lower portion, around the cervix, although the weakened area occasionally is higher up in the uterus. If a "high" leak occurs the leakage of fluid will go on for several days.

In a woman at full term, rupture of the membranes often leads to spontaneous onset of contractions, presenting no problem. But if labor does not occur spontaneously, there is the risk of infection both pre- and postpartum. Once the protective membranes are gone, bacteria already in the vagina could enter and contaminate the amniotic sac, resulting in infections of both the baby and the uterus and placenta as well as the amniotic fluid. A uterine infection can induce severe problems and fever during labor, placing the baby in jeopardy; postpartum infection with endometritis, infection of the endometrium, is also likely.

Another problem with a spontaneous premature rupture is that the normal progress of labor is often disrupted. When the membranes rupture before the onset of labor contractions, the fetal head often becomes wedged at the neck of the uterus, and the natural mechanism of labor is slowed down. Then, once labor begins, the uterine contractions will often take much longer than usual to push the baby through the birth canal. Flexion of the head often does not take place naturally with a case of PROM, and the baby will remain in the posterior position with the head facing forward throughout the labor. In other words, you should be aware that things will not always go smoothly when the membranes rupture before labor begins. This is a common complication you must familiarize yourself with, since it occurs in more than 12 percent of all births.

☐ *When Does Labor Begin After PROM?*   The interval between the rupture of the membranes and the onset of labor is less than 24 hours in 80 percent of women who are at or near term. If the baby is premature, less than 36 weeks, the time period between the rupture and the onset of labor is usually longer.

Rupture of membranes at or near term will result in spontaneous labor within 6 hours in 30 percent of cases; within 12 hours in 50 percent of patients; and in 80 percent within 24 hours after PROM. Ninety to 95 percent of women go into labor spontaneously within 48 hours of ruptured membranes.

Because of the infection possibilities associated with PROM, each hospital has a standard procedure for dealing with the problem, including a period of observation before inducing labor artificially. A woman whose membranes have ruptured is usually asked to come into the hospital and is then placed immediately on a fetal monitor to watch for the onset of labor. Frequent internal examinations should be avoided. Each time a doctor or resident performs a vaginal examination there is the risk of introducing bacteria into the amniotic sac. I would even advise you to contact your obstetrician by phone before permitting a hospital doctor or resident to examine you. Often spontaneous labor will occur quickly. That is the best that can happen under these circumstances because the chance of the baby's rotating into the correct position is greatly enhanced. You are then likely to enjoy a normal, spontaneous delivery. Otherwise, if labor does not occur normally, there is a higher possibility of problems.

☐ *What Happens if Labor Does Not Start Spontaneously?*   If labor does not begin within a certain time frame, the chance of an infection entering from the vagina into the uterus increases. For this reason, most hospitals begin intravenous oxytocin stimulation after twelve hours if there is no sign of spontaneous labor. Each hospital has its own policy when it comes to PROM. Some hospitals start inducing labor as little as six hours after PROM because their statistics show a higher infection rate after this period, while others will wait twenty-four hours or longer because they feel the risks are not all that high.

The oxytocin infusion is usually started in very low doses with an infusion pump, and slowly increased if necessary. Meanwhile the fetal heartbeat will be monitored continuously to make sure that the baby is not under too much stress.

With proper care, labor stimulated by oxytocin infusion should not be dangerous.

Induced labor is usually harder and stronger than spontaneous labor. This is unfortunate, but one has to balance the problem of infection against waiting for a labor to begin spontaneously. PROM is one of the labor complications that can be handled very well in a modern hospital, but it does call for careful observation and, sometimes, intervention.

☐ *PROM in Premature Births* With a premature labor, rupture commonly precedes the onset of contractions by several days, and in this case the doctor will often wait, observing the patient before deciding if delivery is necessary. (See Chapter 25, on premature labor.) The delay is designed to give the fetal lungs a chance to mature. Chapter 25 contains further information on the management of ruptured membranes in cases of prematurity.

☐ *Should Antibiotics Be Given with Ruptured Membranes?* A woman with ruptured membranes who enters into spontaneous labor usually does not need antibiotics. But if there is any sign of infection, the doctor will take a culture from the baby and the placenta after the birth. He might then start the patient on antibiotic treatment immediately, or he might wait a few days until the culture comes back. One of the advantages of taking a routine culture is that the baby too can be treated in the event of an infection. When the onset of labor is unduly prolonged, or an infection is suspected because the patient has developed a fever or because a blood count shows a proliferation of white blood cells, the doctor might prescribe an antibiotic such as penicillin, which is safe for use in pregnancy if the patient doesn't have penicillin allergy. Penicillin will cut the risk of infection for the baby as well as the mother, but the pediatrician should still take a culture after the birth and treat the baby if necessary. Fortunately the amniotic fluid is usually bacteriostatic—that is, it possesses an ability to fight infection spontaneously—so even if the uterus is infected, the baby will often escape.

☐ *Chorioamnionitis—Infection of the Amniotic Sac* Most hospitals will, as I have said, induce a woman's labor no later than twelve hours after the membranes have ruptured to avoid chorioamnionitis, infection of the amniotic sac. Even mild contractions can result in bacteria's invading the amniotic fluid and moving into the amniotic sac. Chorioamnionitis may also occur before the membranes rupture (see Chap. 25). Bacteria may, even with intact membranes, ascend from the vagina, penetrate the fetal membranes, and cause inflammation of the amniotic sac. The first symptom of infection is a fever that occurs before the onset of labor. The doctor must then decide whether the fever is due to a virus infection, a urinary-tract infection (which are fairly common in pregnancy; see Chapter 24), or to chorioamnionitis or even some other infection. If the obstetrician judges the source of the infection to be chorioamnionitis, he will bring the patient into the hospital, monitor the labor, and then begin induction of labor if the baby is at term. When the baby is still premature, the doctor may choose instead to treat the patient with high doses of antibiotics. As a precautionary measure, he should also perform ultrasonography and amniocentesis to collect a specimen of the amniotic fluid for laboratory culture to check the effect of the chosen antibiotic. Chorioamnionitis must always be promptly treated since it can cause high fever and prolonged healing and other difficulties postpartum, as well as potentially endangering the baby. Many babies, even term babies, who are affected by amniotic-fluid infections need special care, including intravenous feeding and heavy doses of antibiotics. Antibiotic therapy in itself poses problems: although we have powerful antibiotics available today, some of them are relatively new, and the obstetrician should be cautious in prescribing them for the unborn or the newborn. A careful pediatrician-neonatologist will take blood cultures, urine cultures, and skin cultures to make sure that the prescribed antibiotics are best for the baby. A mother affected by chorioamnionitis will also be treated with high doses of antibiotics after the birth. Sometimes only one type of antibiotic is needed, but at other times triple antibiotic therapy—a combination of three powerful antibiotics—is required to provide the right therapy for a particular kind of bacteria.

Chorioamnionitis, as you can see, is a serious problem; it requires careful diagnosis and an understanding of the new antibiotic therapy. Some complex research has gone into these new antibiotics, but not all doctors are familiar with the latest findings in this area. If you have a fever postpartum that does not respond within a few days to the antibiotics prescribed by your doctor, you might want to call in a consultant. A prolonged infection after birth will delay healing and may even irreparably damage the uterus and Fallopian tubes, causing infertility in the future.

☐ *Dystocia—Difficult Labor*   "Dystocia" is a Greek word meaning "difficult labor." Medically, it can be defined as a cessation of the normal progress of labor due to an abnormality in the mechanism of labor. Dystocia is an old problem in obstetrics, especially in first labors (it used to be said that a woman who had one baby successfully could bear other children without difficulty). The incidence of dystocia seems to have increased in recent years, perhaps because women giving birth to their first child are generally older than they were in the past, so the uterine tissues may not be as elastic as those of a younger woman. Today, too, babies are larger than in the past; so births are more likely to end in a CPD—cephalo-pelvic disproportion—which means that the cephal, the head of the baby, is in disproportion with the pelvis. (In simple terms, the mother's pelvis is too small for the baby to be born naturally.)

Basically, three reasons for dystocia exist. *First*, the uterine contractions may not be strong enough to push the baby through the bony part of the birth canal. Weakness of uterine contractions is known as *uterine dysfunction* or *uterine inertia*. The *second reason* for dystocia is an abnormal fetal presentation, such as a breech presentation or a transverse or oblique lie. The *third reason* is a disproportion between the size of the baby as compared to the size or configuration of the birth canal. Often a case of CPD is termed a relative CPD, since some babies do not enter properly into the pelvic bones but are otherwise not disproportionate to the birth canal. In that case, dystocia may lead to a Cesarean section in a first birth, but it does not mean that any future children must be born by this method.

☐ *Inadequate Labor—Uterine Dysfunction*   A pattern of ineffective labor contractions, or uterine dysfunction, as it is termed by the obstetrician, has always been one of the most serious problems in obstetrics. Dystocia throughout history resulted in innumerable stillbirths and fatal damage to women whose birth attendants ripped them apart in attempting to deliver the child.

A spontaneous labor follows a fairly predictable pattern. Approximate timing of normal cervical dilatation begins with a latent phase of several hours during which the cervix becomes effaced, but dilates only slightly. This latent phase is followed by an active phase of accelerated labor in which the cervix dilates rather rapidly, and, more important, progressively. The normal timing of these stages of labor has been plotted on a curve known as a *Friedman Curve,* after the obstetrician Dr. Emanuel Friedman of Boston, who devised it from his analysis of a large number of women in labor. With first labor, according to the Friedman Curve, the cervix usually dilates slowly, up to three centimeters, for eight to nine hours, then dilates very rapidly in the two to three hours of the active phase (see figure). If any significant deviation in the pattern of normal cervical dilatation exists, an obstetrician should be alerted to the possibility of uterine dysfunction, or an unsuspected cephalo-pelvic disproportion. The obstetrician must then decide whether the irregularity is indeed caused by uterine dysfunction, which means that the uterine contractions are not strong enough, or is the result of a cephalo-pelvic disproportion.

Generally, if the progress of labor does not follow the Friedman Curve, the obstetrician will begin intravenous injections of oxytocin in very small doses to stimulate labor (see below). The infusion should be given in combination with fetal monitoring to make sure that the baby's heart rate remains normal—a sign that the baby is receiving enough oxygen during contractions. As long as the proper precautions are observed, the administration of oxytocin is the recommended way to speed up labor and to test the capacity of the woman's pelvis. Increased uterine contractions will often make the baby enter the pelvis and rotate normally through the birth canal, so given time, oxytocin stimulation may well avoid the need for a forceps delivery or a Cesarean section.

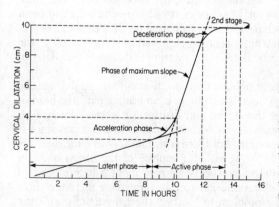

Figure 106: The Friedman Curve: This is the type of chart used in many hospitals to compare a woman's progress in labor against the normal labor pattern. The average labor curve, known as the *Friedman curve,* charts the slow cervical dilatation (eight to ten hours) in a first birth. There initially is a relatively flat pattern followed by the acceleration phase (three to four hours) in which dilatation occurs rapidly and the curve becomes considerably steeper. If a woman's pattern of dilatation is distinctly slower than that indicated on the curve she might need intravenous oxytocin to bring on more effective contractions.

Uterine dysfunction sometimes appears with prematurely ruptured membranes; it seems that if the membranes are ruptured over a prolonged period, the uterine muscles can become infected and are therefore weaker than usual. Many other reasons exist for insufficient labor contractions: with an older woman, for instance, the uterus often does not seem to respond as it would in a younger woman, or sometimes the baby is a large one, and greater force than usual is required to push it through the pelvis. Whenever a woman fails to dilate normally, her doctor should consider the possibility of uterine dysfunction and, in the absence of certain contraindications, try stimulating labor with oxytocin. The oxytocin infusion will establish whether labor has stopped because uterine contractions are insufficient, or will rule out uterine inertia as the cause of the arrested labor.

Oxytocin stimulation should be attempted only if the baby is in the longitudinal position, which means either the vertex position or what is known as a frank breech. Oxytocin is ineffective and harmful if the baby is in the transverse or oblique lie.

☐ *Secondary Arrest of Labor* Obstetricians sometimes talk about "secondary arrest of labor." Secondary arrest is basically the same as *uterine dysfunction.* In other words, labor progresses normally until a certain point and then stops. A doctor may interpret secondary arrest as a case of CPD, but we know that this is not always so. Sometimes labor will stop because the baby is too large to enter the birth canal, but sometimes the problem is that the baby does not enter in the right position, thus disrupting the normal stimulation mechanism from the cervix to the brain. Other causes seem to be premature rupture of the membranes or some weakness of the uterus itself. Thus, if labor stops at some point, the obstetrician is not required to resort immediately to a Cesarean section, except perhaps in the case of a very large baby. Even then, before doing a section, an obstetrician might do well to get a second opinion.

☐ *Dystocia Caused by an Abnormal Presentation or Position of the Fetus* In approximately 95 percent of all births the baby will settle down in the vertex or head-first position. In about 1 percent of births, the baby will be in the transverse, or oblique, lie, and in about 3 to 4 percent of births, the baby will be in the breech presentation. Breech presentation will often result in dystocia, particularly if it is a compound presentation in which a foot or a leg as well as the buttocks are the presenting parts. Breech presentation is discussed fully later in the chapter.

With a baby in a transverse or oblique position, the only way to manage the birth is by Cesarean section. A lie in which there is no leading part, the head or the buttocks, pressing against the cervix, will disrupt the normal mechanism of labor. Under these circumstances oxytocin stimulation is dangerous since it will increase the uterine contractions, but there is still no way to force the baby through the vagina without inflicting either a rupture of the uterus or brain damage to the child. An obstetrician who is worried about a baby's position can scan the abdomen with ultrasound and get an immediate picture of how the baby is lying. If there is a problem in locating the baby exactly with the sonogram, one flat-plate abdominal X-ray will give an accurate picture of the baby's position. Following the results of the sonogram or X-ray, an obstetrician will go straight to a Cesarean if the baby is shown to be in the transverse lie.

Abnormal positions can also occur in the vertex presentation if the baby's head has not rotated itself correctly into the pelvis and the occiput, or back part of the head, faces toward the mother's spine. The occiput posterior position causes what is known as back labor, which often leads to dystocia because the natural labor force is lessened by the lack of rotation. This kind of dystocia can often be overcome by intravenous oxytocin augmentation. With increased uterine activity, the baby will usually slowly rotate into the occiput anterior position, in which the baby will be looking backward rather than forward at the time of delivery.

☐   *Abnormality of the Pelvis*   If the pelvis does not have an anatomically normal bone structure, delivery can be difficult. There may be genetic reasons why the pelvis is abnormal, or there might be damage from an accident or a childhood illness. Indication of the pelvic size can be gathered from a woman's height—a taller woman usually has a larger pelvis than a shorter woman—through a patient's obstetrical history, and through manual measurement by the obstetrician. From the first routine visits, an obstetrician should be able to get an impression of the size of the patient's pelvis by manually palpating the pelvic bone structure and estimating the pelvic size. The important measurement is the *diagonal conjugate*, the distance from the undersurface of the pubic bone in front to the top of the sacrum (the posterior bony wall of the lower part of the spine). If this measurement is five inches or longer, one can almost be certain that the upper part of the pelvis, the so-called pelvic inlet, is of adequate size. The obstetrician will at the same time palpate the abdomen and pelvis to discover the general shape and contour of the bony pelvis. He should also try to determine whether the lower part of the pelvis (the pelvic outlet) is of adequate size for a natural birth.

☐   *Contracted Pelvis*   A contracted pelvis (one that is too small for normal childbirth) can be inherited or might be the result of malnutrition or poor hygiene during the years of growth. One reason for a contracted pelvis that was common in the past was *rickets*—a bone disease that ravaged American and European children one hundred years ago. When a girl has rickets, the bones are weakened and the pelvic bones flatten out in a way that makes later childbearing difficult. Rickets still exists in parts of the world where the diet is severely lacking in calcium and vitamins A and D, and children are deprived of ultraviolet sunlight by crowded city conditions. Although the disease is rarely seen in the United States today, just a few years ago, about 2 percent of American white women and 15 percent of black women had contractions of the pelvis that were the legacy of a childhood attack of rickets.

☐   *Pelvic Distortions Caused by Fracture*   Occasionally a pelvic fracture is so damaging that it permanently changes the configuration of the pelvis. Any pregnant woman who has had a severe accident in which the pelvis was fractured or broken, is advised to have an X-ray of the pelvis to make sure there is enough space in the pelvis to deliver. Other than this, indications for X-ray pelvimetry are very few.

☐   *X-rays During Labor—Pelvimetry*   Why would a woman need an X-ray during labor? The answer is that she probably doesn't but her doctor might recommend X-ray pelvimetry—a specialized form of X-ray capable of delineating the pelvic area—if he suspects a breech delivery or a cephalo-pelvic disproportion. Obstetricians who still favor X-rays are generally older men who were trained in pelvimetry techniques when they were residents. Don't, however, agree to measurement by pelvimetry unless the information cannot be achieved by any other means. X-ray pelvimetry exposes the fetus to a significant amount of radiation. An ultrasound examination will usually detect an abnormal presentation and, as far as we know, will achieve the same result with far less danger to the fetus (see the section on breech later in this chapter). Pelvimetry will delineate the proportions of the pelvis in a suspected case of cephalo-pelvic disproportion, but a woman's doctor will inevitably detect an inadequate pelvis once labor stops because the fetal head is not descending properly.

The FDA has recommended that pelvimetry be used *only* in the few instances in which they believe pelvimetry to be specifically indicated—in, for example, a case of congenital deformity of the pelvis. If your doctor insists on ordering pelvimetry, at least ask him to explain why he thinks the X-ray will be beneficial. If possible, try to get a second opinion by calling in another doctor on the staff or by contacting the nearest university hospital and asking to speak to a physician on the perinatal team.

☐   *Dystocia Due to Cephalo-Pelvic Disproportion*   Dystocia caused by CPD is the most important single reason for the recent rapid rise in Cesarean section rates in American hospitals. Cephalo-pelvic disproportion has several possible origins. Occasionally the pelvic structure is abnormal. The pelvis may be so small that it is inadequate for even a normal-sized baby. Sometimes the baby is simply a large baby. Many cases of CPD, however, are cases of *relative* disproportion, in which the dystocia results from the abnormal way in which the baby's head enters the pelvis. For example, a persistent posterior position might prevent a perfect fit between the head and the pelvic bone structure. Labor will then fail to progress and the doctor might be forced to resort to a Cesarean to prevent brain damage to the baby. Another common cause of CPD is what is known as soft-tissue distortion, from abnormalities of the tissues rather than of the bony part of the pelvis. This may be the problem in a labor in which, in spite of good, strong contractions, the cervix fails to dilate or does not dilate at a rate equivalent to the Friedman Curve (see picture). The complication can be handled without the doctor's necessarily resorting to a Cesarean.

Tension is sometimes a cause of dystocia. If a woman is unusually tense, she will instinctively tighten her pelvic muscles and thus prevent the fetal head from pushing hard enough against the cervix to open it. Analgesia or an epidural anesthesia will sometimes relax the pelvic muscles enough to turn a potential dystocia into a natural delivery. Occasionally an athletic woman with well developed abdominal muscles finds it so difficult to relax her muscles that the delivery becomes almost impossible to achieve naturally.

Uterine abnormalities or fibroid tumors can also cause dystocia. For example, a large fibroid tumor could obstruct the birth canal (see Chap. 24) and would slow down or stop the baby's birth progress.

☐ **Management of Dystocia**   Observation and careful evaluation are needed in a case of dystocia. Pelvic configuration, can, as I have already mentioned, be evaluated without the use of X-ray pelvimetry, but the doctor must rule out another cause of dystocia—an abnormal lie—before he turns to the use of oxytocin. Once he has decided that the cause of the dystocia is inadequate uterine contractions, he can begin uterine stimulation with the oxytocin and watch its effects on the contractions. He must, of course, give an adequate amount of oxytocin, and at the same time monitor its effect on the baby with care. Electronic fetal monitoring is important in such instances to monitor both the fetal heart rate and the uterine contractions. After a proper period of observation, the doctor can usually determine whether a vaginal delivery is possible or not. Sometimes, though, the use of oxytocin may stimulate good uterine activity but labor still fails to progress, because the pain from the stimulated labor is so strong that the woman instinctively tightens her pelvic muscles and impedes the baby's descent. In a case of this kind, an epidural anesthesia is often the best solution: relaxation of the pelvic muscles under the epidural may increase the chances of a vaginal delivery without harming the baby.

A woman whose labor is complicated by dystocia may be able to push the baby down through the birth canal but not through the pelvic outlet to complete the delivery. The baby may also be very large, or there may be a tight fit between the head and the pelvis. In cases of dystocia in which the pelvis is adequate but the woman is unable to push the baby out by her own efforts, the obstetrician can choose a forceps delivery (see below). If, on the other hand, the presenting part fails to enter the pelvis and the doctor diagnoses a case of true CPD, he can elect to perform a Cesarean section; but only after he has consulted with another obstetrician on the staff and only after he has documented the uterine contractions for several hours to evaluate his patient's progress against the Friedman Curve.

☐ **Nipple Stimulation for Arrested Labor**   We talk about arrested labor when labor is progressing very slowly, or the uterine contractions become less frequent as time goes on. The reasons for this are varied. The baby's head may not be pressing sufficiently against the cervix to trigger new waves of contractions, or the uterine muscle fibers may be showing signs of fatigue, etc. It is often suggested, at this point, that the woman walk or change positions in order to increase the pressure of the baby against the cervix and stimulate uterine activity. If dystocia is diagnosed, a doctor might also suggest intravenous oxytocin augmentation to help the labor progress.

A natural alternative to drugs is gentle nipple stimulation. Stimulating the nipple by slightly twisting and pulling it between the fingers of the woman or her mate, triggers the so-called milk ejection reflex, normally initiated by the suckling infant. As part of this reflex, nerve stimulation is sent to the hypothalamus, causing it to release the hormone oxytocin to the pituitary, and from there into the bloodstream. Nipple stimulation thus results in a surge of oxytocin, which might be enough to stimulate uterine contractions. Since oxytocin will also stimulate the breast tissue, the woman may feel slight contraction pain in the breast itself and possibly see colostrum secreted from the nipple.

Every woman in labor should familiarize herself with this nipple-stimulation technique, since it is an excellent, natural means of aiding the birth process.

☐ **Elective Induction of Labor—Is It Safe?**   A few years ago, American and European hospitals routinely used oxytocic drugs (Pitocin), to start labor artificially in full term, uncomplicated pregnancies, a procedure still favored in some countries. Unfortunately the practice of inducing women for reasons of *convenience* resulted in a higher rate of prematurity and unnecessary cases of brain damage. Doctors did not have or were not using modern techniques to estimate gestational age (see Chap. 23), and simply admitted women into the hospital on the assumption they were "ready" to give birth. A statement like "You're big enough—let's induce you" was commonplace in the American obstetrician's office of the 1950s and 1960s. This careless attitude toward elective induction led to the delivery of thousands of premature babies whose gestational age had not been estimated correctly.

Oxytocin, which is a powerful drug, was often overprescribed or improperly supervised during the induction, with serious results. Too much oxytocin induces a state called hypertonus, in which the uterus goes into unusually prolonged, violent, spastic contractions. When hypertonus occurs, the oxygen supply in the uterus is reduced considerably, in turn reducing the oxygen supply to the fetal brain; the baby's heart rate then goes down and fetal brain damage can result. Among multipara, hypertonus carries the additional risk of rupture of the uterus, which, on a number of occasions, led to the woman's losing the baby and her life.

In view of these unnecessary risks, the government outlawed elective inductions in 1977, while still permitting induction for medical reasons (see below). At the same time, stricter rules were put into effect governing the use of synthetic oxytocins, including the requirement that patients receiving intravenous oxytocin must be under continuous observation by a doctor or obstetrical nurse. Consequently, oxytocin should be given only in small initial doses, gradually increased until the contractions reach the intensity of *normal* labor.

☐ **Medically Indicated Labor Inductions**   Labor induction may still be indicated for *medical* reasons in cases in which the pregnancy has some unusual complicating factor. For example, a woman who passes her due date by more than two weeks may be suffering from postmaturity, a dangerous condition in which the placenta begins to disintegrate. A postmature woman will need, first, nonstress testing and possibly labor induction. A nonstress test that is judged nonreactive (see Chap. 23) can be followed by an oxytocin challenge test, and labor started artificially if the second test also reveals abnormalities. Here an induction could save the baby's life.

Labor induction is also called for in pregnancies complicated by diabetes, in which labor often fails to occur at term, or toxemic pregnancies, in which the mother's elevated blood pressure and renal failure endanger her and her baby. Any high-risk condition in which the baby could be endangered by its continued intrauterine existence would call for testing and possible labor induction. Legitimate instances therefore exist in which a doctor might consider inducing labor, although you are certainly within your rights as a patient to discuss the matter thoroughly before giving your consent to such a procedure.

A responsible doctor should be aware of the negative side of labor induction: the risk of uterine hypertonus and uterine rupture, and the other serious problems associated with poorly conducted inductions. On the other hand, labor does not occur normally in all pregnancies, and instances do exist of a doctor's being justified in inducing labor to assure a healthy outcome. If your doctor can give convincing reasons for inducing labor, don't fight his decision; there are good reasons for inducing labor, even today.

☐ *How Is Labor Induction Performed?*   A labor induction is always carried out in the hospital. The patient is either admitted the night before and induced early in the morning, or the induction takes place on the day of admission. In Britain, the patient is usually admitted the day before and given a prostaglandin suppository or gel overnight to induce mild contractions and prime the cervix. This method is not used in the United States as yet, but preliminary studies on prostaglandin labor induction have found it to be useful in cases in which induction is normally difficult. The induction patient in an American hospital is placed in bed, given an IV, and attached to a fetal monitor to make sure that the fetal heart rate remains normal during the induction. This precaution is particularly important after a positive nonstress test or oxytocin challenge test. Labor is then induced with Pitocin (oxytocin) infused intravenously through a device known as a constant infusion pump, a means by which oxytocin can be started in very low doses and increased as needed. Pitocin is a powerful drug and should always be administered cautiously. By using an infusion pump rather than an oxytocin drip, the physician can observe the patient carefully and slowly increase the infusion until labor contractions are well established. If contractions become too intense at any point, the pump can be turned down. In this way, a careful, skillful physician who observes the proper precautions can induce labor without unduly stressing either mother or child. A woman induced for medical reasons is considered a high-risk patient, and will be allowed to labor only in a conventional labor and delivery suite, not a birthing room or birthing center.

After labor has begun and the patient is three to four centimeters dilated, the attending obstetrician might rupture the fetal membranes in the hope of stimulating spontaneous labor contractions. Once the patient is producing her own oxytocin the pump can be turned off and the woman allowed to labor on her own. When the patient is supervised carefully, labor begun by synthetic oxytocin often ends in a natural, vaginal delivery.

One fact to bear in mind with oxytocin induction is the increased intensity of the uterine contractions. Labor is always stronger and more painful with an induction, although that can be controlled if the doctor modifies the infusion rate. You may need an epidural with an induced labor, something you and your labor coach should bear in mind as you enter labor.

☐ *Is There a Connection Between Oxytocin Stimulation and Brain Damage?*
A few years ago a woman successfully sued her obstetrician on behalf of her son, who was born with severe brain damage after an elective delivery induced by oxytocin. This was the case that prompted the FDA to change its regulations governing the use of oxytocin, resulting in a ban on elective inductions and modifications in the way oxytocin stimulation is used during deliveries. In the 1950s and 1960s oxytocin was usually given continuously by intravenous drip, so it was difficult for a doctor to estimate just how much oxytocin a patient was receiving. *Hypertonus*—uterine overstimulation—occurred all too often in consequence. Since uterine relaxation is necessary to allow for an exchange of oxygen to the

placenta, prolonged uterine hypertonus deprives the baby of oxygen and can result in serious brain damage. Nowadays an obstetrician who uses a fetal heart-rate monitor can detect a persistent pattern of fetal bradycardia (a heart rate that drops to a low level without recovering) early on and stop or slow down the oxytocin infusion in good time. If necessary he will also give the mother oxygen by mask to enhance the oxygen supply to the baby. The safety of the procedure is increased by the modern preference for an infusion pump; with a pump rather than a drip one can safely achieve regular contractions with good uterine relaxation in between. And as long as the heart rate remains normal, we know that the baby is receiving enough oxygenation to protect him from brain damage. If the proper precautions are taken during labor induction or stimulation, the chance of brain damage is virtually nonexistent.

☐ *Oxytocin Augmentation in Arrested Labor*   If labor slows down or stops (secondary arrest), intravenous oxytocin augmentation is usually given to speed up the contractions. An infusion often results in vaginal delivery within a few hours. Otherwise, if the head does not move further down into the pelvis after an hour or two of good, strong contractions, the doctor will presume that no further progress can be expected and a Cesarean section is probably needed to deliver the baby. Sometimes an unsuspected case of cephalo-pelvic disproportion is discovered at this relatively late stage of labor, more commonly in a woman who has already had children. Often the problem is some unexpected labor dysfunction that holds up progress even though the woman is having good contractions. In either case, the doctor's decision to proceed with a Cesarean section is a reasonable one. A labor that goes on for hours without progress or relief in spite of adequate uterine contractions, can be safely concluded only by a Cesarean. One must keep in mind that a long, hard labor subjects the baby's head to hours of battering against the unyielding bones inside the pelvis. The result may be intracranial hemorrhage and permanent brain damage.

☐ *Oxytocin Stimulation During Epidural Anesthesia*   When a woman is given an epidural anesthetic (see the section on anesthesia in Chapter 27) the pain disappears completely but so does the stimulus of labor. Although contractions reappear after a short interval, they are less effective than before and labor is often prolonged. Many obstetricians like to give the patient an oxytocin infusion with the epidural to avoid prolonging labor and stressing the baby unduly.

☐ *Oxytocin Augmentation and Irregular Contractions*   Oxytocin stimulation or augmentation is favored during labor in other specific situations, although, again, the drug should be used only under careful supervision. For example, a woman with weak or irregular contractions may benefit from a carefully measured and controlled infusion of oxytocin. The extra oxytocin is often sufficient to regulate or stimulate labor enough to save the patient from a Cesarean section.

☐ *Neonatal Jaundice and Oxytocin Infusion*   Newborn babies have an increased tendency to neonatal jaundice after the use of pitocin to induce or stimulate labor. This may be the result of pitocin's effect on the newborn's liver or liver enzymes, or it may be caused by a hematoma, a small collection of blood underneath the fetal skin caused by strong prolonged labor. These hematomas can break down after delivery and increase the circulating blood to the point at which the liver is unable to metabolize it properly. The baby then becomes jaundiced as the bilirubin (the breakdown product of red blood cells) enters into the bloodstream. A slight degree of neonatal jaundice is common and is not dangerous, but there is a possibility of brain damage if the degree of jaundice becomes acute. Some researchers feel that there are no increased incidents of newborn jaundice after oxytocin stimulation. Others believe there is a direct effect and most women who have received oxytocin for a long time during labor can expect their baby to become jaundiced.

A baby who shows signs of increasing jaundice that does not regress spontaneously is best placed naked under ultraviolet light for one to several days in the neonatal nursery (see Chap. 33). This light will hasten the more rapid breakdown of the bilirubin.

☐ *Forceps Delivery*   Forceps still have their place in a modern delivery, even though the nature of the forceps delivery has changed and Cesareans have replaced forceps in many births. Today a responsible obstetrician will no longer attempt what is known as a high midforceps delivery, a difficult delivery in which he must place the forceps far up into the pelvis, but will do a Cesarean instead. But forceps are still routinely used to complete a delivery when the baby has reached the last portion of the birth canal but his mother is either too exhausted to push or needs help in pushing him out. Especially with the increase in epidurals, a low forceps delivery can be expected in many births because the anesthesia decreases the woman's urge to push. Unfortunately, the modern obstetrician may not be as well trained as his predecessors in handling forceps deliveries because many training hospitals have encouraged their residents to rely on a Cesarean any time a baby is not delivered normally. This is not good obstetrics; we must have a balance between Cesareans and forceps deliveries to protect patients from unnecessary Cesareans, and give the best and safest of care to both the child and the mother.

☐ *What Are Forceps?*   The word "forceps" is Latin and means "a pair of tongs." The word is supposed to be derived from the Latin words *formus* (hot) and *capere* (to take). The modern obstetrical forceps consist of two crossing branches, each composed of a blade, a handle, a shaft, and a lock. The blade is designed to rest behind the baby's ears, so when forceps are applied correctly no undue pressure should be put on the fetal brain. Once the blades are in place the lock is used to secure the blades in place. The obstetrician completes the delivery by applying force to the handle and guiding the child out of the pelvis.

☐ *Types of Forceps Delivery*   Forceps deliveries are classified according to the position of the head at the time the forceps are applied.

A *low forceps* operation is a delivery in which the forceps are applied after the fetal head has reached far down into the pelvis, past the pelvic inlet.

A *midforceps* operation is a delivery in which the forceps are applied before the widest diameter of the head has passed through the pelvic inlet.

A *high forceps* operation is one in which the forceps are applied before the fetal head has completely engaged in the bony pelvis.

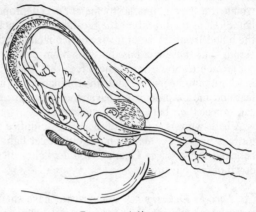

Figure 107: If a woman is having difficulty delivering spontaneously a doctor may decide to use forceps to complete the delivery. The blades are placed on each side of the baby's head and the doctor then gently applies pressure to pull the baby out. Forceps used properly are safe and often avoid the need to resort to a Cesarean section in the final minutes of labor.

Forceps delivery

☐ *When Is a Forceps Delivery Justified?*   The obstetrical forceps are nothing more than a mechanical extension of the human hand. Like the obstetrician's hand, it is used to complete a delivery or to rotate the head in a difficult delivery. There are a variety of forceps available, but most obstetricians work with one or two types which they prefer or with which they are most familiar— the Simpson forceps and the DeLee forceps are those commonly used in the low forceps deliveries of primiparous patients.

Termination of labor by forceps can be done very simply, and without serious risks, if it is performed carefully by a trained obstetrician. Indications for a forceps delivery are: a case of eclampsia or severe toxemia in which a woman is not allowed to push; a case of heart disease in which the pushing stage would be dangerous for the patient; other acute medical problems that would make it difficult for the patient to push; separation of the placenta; cases of infection in which the uterine contractions are ineffectual; prolapse of the cord; and shock and bleeding. Forceps are commonly used in dystocia cases when the patient needs assistance in pushing the baby through the last section of the birth canal. They are also used where there is a prolonged second stage but the baby is small enough to pass through the pelvis.

☐ *Contraindications to a Forceps Delivery*   Contraindications are: evidence of a cephalo-pelvic disproportion; an unengaged head (the danger of high forceps delivery is discussed below); face presentations in which the chin is stuck in the hollow of the sacrum; and the presence of a soft-tissue abnormality, including a fibroid tumor or tumors obstructing the birth canal.

Most obstetricians would regard any situation that required high or midforceps as in itself a contraindication to the use of forceps. The risks of serious trauma to the vagina and bladder and the possible neurological damage to the baby preclude the use of forceps in a high or high midforceps delivery.

☐ *How Does the Obstetrician Use Forceps?*   Correct placement of forceps is important. Improper placement might cause nerve-system damage or lifetime scarring for the baby. The obstetrician should first carefully examine the patient internally to ascertain the exact position of the baby. If he is unable to feel the head, a forceps delivery is potentially dangerous and should not be attempted. Each blade is inserted separately; the doctor holds the handle in one hand while he gently inserts two fingers inside, between the vaginal wall and the baby's head. He then slides one blade of the forceps in between his fingers and lines it up next to the baby's head. His assistant will hold the handle of the forceps as the obstetrician inserts the first blade. The second blade is placed in the same fashion. The doctor then palpates the vagina to make sure the forceps are resting correctly against the skull. If the blades are in the right position, he will lock them in place and ask the woman to push hard with the next contraction. As she pushes, the doctor will coordinate his pulling with her pushing and slowly pull the baby down by exerting traction on the handle of the forceps. During this maneuver he can rotate the baby if necessary. When the baby is about to be delivered, he will put his hand underneath the chin and perform the Ritgen maneuver to achieve a slow, controlled delivery. Once the head is delivered, he will gently take off the forceps and finish up the delivery as if it were a spontaneous vaginal birth.

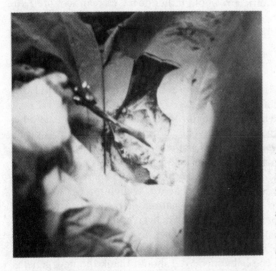

Figure 108: Here one can see the forceps in place. The vulva is "crowning" as the head is slowly and gently delivered. Forceps are removed as soon as the head is fully born. The remainder of the delivery is performed in the same fashion as in a natural birth.

Since the forceps are used for only a few minutes, the baby can usually be handed to the parents immediately after the delivery. There may be some marks or bruises, but they usually disappear within five to six days after birth. In the hands of an unqualified physician, of course, there are dangers: a blade placed incorrectly so that it cuts into the skin and nerves might result in scarring, facial paralysis, or permanent brain damage.

□ *Low Forceps* A delivery that requires low forceps is one in which the baby has passed through the pelvic plane, but the mother is unable to push the baby through the last part of the birth canal due to uterine inertia or fatigue. A low forceps delivery is a safe way to deliver a baby as long as the obstetrician follows the precautions I have just described. And there is no reason for a couple to be frightened or upset if their obstetrician must use forceps. Even an apparently uncomplicated birth can end in low forceps because an unexpected problem has arisen during the delivery.

☐   *Midforceps*   The term "midforceps" includes what are known as low midforceps and high midforceps deliveries. In a low midforceps delivery, the obstetrician will be delivering a baby positioned in the midportion of the bony pelvis. Here a skillful obstetrician will be able to put the forceps in place, and then rotate and deliver the baby with no problem. Other obstetricians would prefer to do a Cesarean at this point rather than risk using forceps; this is particularly true of younger doctors who have not much experience in doing forceps deliveries. In fact, the degree of your doctor's skill might determine the outcome of your delivery.

☐   *High Midforceps*   A high midforceps operation is potentially dangerous because an obstetrician can easily misjudge the position of the baby's head up in the pelvis and place the blades of the forceps incorrectly. The resultant pulling and tugging could cause permanent scarring or brain damage. Understandably, therefore, most obstetricians would rather do a Cesarean section than risk a high midforceps delivery. There are exceptional circumstances, however; the heart rate may, for instance, decrease so rapidly that there is no time for an emergency Cesarean, so the obstetrician is forced into a high midforceps delivery.

☐   *High Forceps*   When the obstetrician uses high forceps, he must put the forceps in place before the fetal head has engaged itself into the pelvis. He certainly will not be sure that the blades of the forceps are correctly in place, and he must exert tremendous pressure to pull the baby out. Both circumstances place the baby in danger. In addition, an obstetrician who is trying to rush through a delivery may be tempted to place the blades before the cervix is completely dilated; he will then run the risk of ripping the woman's vagina apart so badly that she will need vaginal reconstruction later on. The use of high forceps was often abused before childbirth educators encouraged natural deliveries, because most women were put to sleep before they entered the delivery room. It was easy then for the obstetrician, even a respected one, to butcher his patients by terminating the delivery prematurely. I even saw one delivery in which the forceps blade severed the umbilical cord and the baby died. We should thank the new generation of childbirth professionals who have brought more humane attitudes into the delivery room.

☐   *Forceps vs Cesarean*   By the best obstetrical standards, forceps should be used only when the procedure is safe for both mother and child. If there is any doubt about its safety, a responsible doctor would prefer to do an emergency Cesarean. Unfortunately the change in policy has had an effect on the Cesarean section rate, which has increased considerably as the use of forceps has declined. (This is often forgotten when the subject of forceps comes up in a childbirth class or in a doctor's office.) In the future, perhaps, we need to balance the risks and the benefits of Cesarean and forceps deliveries more carefully than we do now.

☐ *Vacuum Extraction*   The vacuum extractor was introduced as an alternative to the obstetrical forceps in Sweden in the mid-1950s. The device consists of a metal cup that is closely applied to the top of the fetal head. A controlled amount of negative pressure is then created inside the cup by a vacuum pump, which provides just enough pressure to fix the cup firmly in place without damaging the head. Once a vacuum has been created, the obstetrician will pull the chain connected to the cup to bring the baby out. The maneuver is usually carried out as the mother pushes. This allows the doctor to use the force of the uterine contractions as well as that of the vacuum extractor.

The vacuum extractor has become increasingly popular in the last ten years and is now used in many hospitals in the United States as well as around the world. It presents many advantages over forceps. Forceps often cause laceration in the vaginal area. They also occupy substantial space in the vagina, so there is a great advantage in using the vacuum extractor when there is a tight fit between the head and pelvis.

The main disadvantage of the vacuum extractor is the likelihood of lacerations and hematoma in the scalp area and the possibility of neonatal jaundice when the hematoma breaks down, just as there would be after any traumatic delivery. However, any hematoma or swelling usually disappears promptly after a vacuum extraction delivery, normally within twenty-four to forty-eight hours. There are no reports of brain damage, and most obstetricians are confident of the safety of the vacuum extractor since one can apply only a certain amount of pressure to the head. The cup will come off if the obstetrician pulls too hard.

☐ *Breech Births*   Although 3 to 4 percent may not seem like a very large percentage of the total births in the United States, the figure represents thousands of women every year who experience a breech delivery. If you are one of them, you will need to weigh your options very carefully. Most breech babies used to be delivered vaginally, but for a number of reasons the modern obstetrician usually favors a Cesarean in any case of breech, even a relatively uncomplicated one. As I will explain later, this may not always be in the best interests of the patient. Be prepared to question your obstetrician closely before consenting to a Cesarean or a vaginal delivery. Also be prepared to seek a second opinion or even change obstetricians if you are not satisfied with your obstetrician's approach.

☐ *What Is a Breech Presentation?*   There are three types of this presentation: the *frank*, the *full*, and the *footling* breech presentation. The frank breech presentation is the most common. Here the thighs are folded up next to the abdomen with the calves straight up so that the baby's toes touch his shoulder, and the buttocks reach down in the pelvis. This is a difficult position for an adult, but not for a tiny baby whose joints are still loose and flexible. A full breech presentation is one in which the baby has his legs up alongside the body, with the knees bent, almost in a lotus position. A full breech is rare. In a footling breech, one or both feet or one or both knees are positioned straight down in the lower portion of the birth canal, as though the baby were in a semistanding position. A footling breech is also known as an incomplete breech presentation.

☐ *Diagnosis of Breech Presentation*   When an obstetrician palpates the abdomen he will usually be able to locate an irregular soft mass, the outline of the buttocks, in the upper portion of the uterus and the hard round mass of the head in the lower portion of the uterus. Quite the opposite pertains in a breech presentation; the hard fetal head occupies the fundus, or top part of the uterus, while the back, the buttocks, and the legs point downward toward the pelvis. A skillful obstetrician can often diagnose a breech presentation during pregnancy, but unfortunately not all obstetricians are sufficiently experienced to pick up a breech by palpation; the result is that patients do enter into labor with unsuspected breech presentations.

In modern obstetrics a much surer way to diagnose a breech is by ultrasonography (see Chap. 23). The ultrasound examination will not only pick up a breech but will usually distinguish between a frank breech and a footling breech. In doubtful cases the position can be verified by one flat-plate X-ray of the abdomen, which invariably gives a clear picture of the baby's presentation.

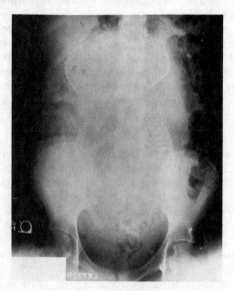

Figure 109: An X-ray of a Baby in the Breech Presentation: This pelvimetric X-ray confirms that the baby is in the frank breech position. Many frank breech babies can be delivered without a Cesarean.

Finally, a vaginal examination, just before labor begins, will often detect a breech. If the cervix is slightly dilated the doctor may actually feel the hard mass of the head through the fetal membranes as he makes his internal examination. This method is not foolproof, however; there have been cases in which an inexperienced doctor has mistaken the buttocks for the head and discovered his mistake only when the patient was well along in labor.

Difficulties often arise in twin gestations, where one baby is commonly in the vertex position and the other in the breech presentation. Here ultrasonography is recommended to detect the position of each twin. Sometimes the second baby in a twin presentation of this type will turn around into the vertex presentation during labor itself, which of course makes delivery considerably easier.

☐ *What to Do When a Breech Presentation Is Diagnosed*   When a breech presentation is detected by an ultrasound or a manual examination in the seventh or eighth month, the situation is less problematic if the patient is in a second or third pregnancy. After one or two pregnancies, the uterus is roomier so there is a good chance that the baby will still be able to kick its way around into a vertex presentation. This could happen right up to birth. In a first pregnancy the uterine space is restricted and the baby tends to settle down in the bony pelvis earlier than in a subsequent pregnancy. The baby is then unable to move freely once the presenting part is engaged. The time to try disengaging a breech yourself is the seventh or early eighth month when the fetus can still turn around within its plentiful supply of amniotic fluid.

An easy, natural method to turn a breech presentation is to adopt what is known as the *Trendelenburg* position by elevating the foot end of the bed or putting a stack of books under the foot end of the mattress so the feet and pelvic area are higher than the head. As you shift your weight, the baby is pushed up, away from the bony pelvis, and this should release the presenting part, the breech, from its position in the pelvis. If you sleep on your side in the Trendelenburg position, the baby has space to kick around during the night and may turn itself into the vertex presentation. (Nighttime is a period of intense activity for many babies because the blood sugar produced by the final meal of the day reaches the fetal circulation a few hours later and will trigger increased fetal movements.) This simple change in position is often enough to turn the baby into the vertex presentation—in fact, you may feel the baby's weight shift as the head moves down into the pelvis. After the baby has turned you can go back to your normal sleeping position to keep the baby in the vertex presentation.

☐ *A New Method of Turning Breech Presentation*   A doctor can now turn a breech presentation by using a technique known as external fetal version. External manual version was done frequently in the past, although many babies stubbornly resumed the breech position within a few days after version. Then external version fell out of favor when serious hazards were associated with the procedure, including the risk of turning the baby too violently and disturbing the placenta or twisting the umbilical cord around the baby's neck during the maneuver. Obstetricians generally have not done versions since the 1960s.

Recently some leading obstetrical institutions throughout the country have begun to use a new method combining ultrasound with the new uterine relaxant drug, ritodrine (Yutopar), and the traditional external version technique. The woman is admitted into the hospital, given an intravenous infusion, and placed on a fetal heart-rate monitor. Ritodrine is then given intravenously for fifteen to twenty minutes. Once the uterus is fully relaxed, an obstetrical specialist carefully pushes the baby around with his hand on the outside of the abdomen. (Turning is very simple when the uterus is relaxed.) Ultrasonography is used throughout the version to make sure that the cord is free and the placenta is undisturbed. After the maneuver is completed, the patient is observed in the hospital for an hour or two until the ritodrine has metabolized and has been excreted from the body, and the uterus is back to its normal shape. The baby will remain in the vertex position because the slightly contracted uterus will prevent it from turning back into a breech presentation. A child can then be expected to stay in the vertex position until full-term labor begins.

Since this is a new technique, a patient with a breech presentation can ask her doctor to do the procedure himself or refer her to a specialist, a perinatologist, at a local university medical center, where they have the facilities to perform the

version. You might avoid an unnecessary Cesarean by taking advantage of this
new perinatal method.

☐ **Term Breech Deliveries**   Breech delivery at term (thirty-six to forty-two
weeks of gestation) would depend on the type of breech involved. A woman who
enters the hospital with a frank breech presentation should be allowed a trial of
labor, unless there is some special complication. A patient with a footling
breech, on the other hand, should be delivered by Cesarean section: the legs in a
footling breech often get in the way of normal rotation, so the doctor risks frac-
turing the extremities or damaging the nervous system during vaginal delivery.
    Most breeches present in the frank breech position. These women should be
able to deliver vaginally as long as the baby descends satisfactorily and the cervix
continues to dilate. Progress can usually be expected if the leading part, the buttocks, is fully engaged in the bony pelvis and pressed against the cervix. As long
as the labor meets these criteria, there should be no serious difficulties and a
woman should be allowed to deliver vaginally. Naturally, her obstetrician must
be skillful, must be aware of how to manage a breech delivery, and must have
assistants available.

☐ **Premature Labor and Breech**   Twenty to 30 percent of pregnancies with
breech presentations begin prematurely, usually with a premature rupture of the
membranes. The reason for this high incidence of premature rupture is unclear,
but it may be explained by the fact that the fetal kicking seems to be more damaging to the fetal membranes than the pressure of the fetal head. Because a very
premature baby is fragile, vaginal premature breech deliveries have been found
to have a high risk of fetal damage, including cerebral palsy and damage to the
nerves in the arms and shoulders. A Cesarean section is probably the safest and
smoothest way to deliver a premature breech baby between twenty-eight and
thirty-six weeks of gestation. Once the breech baby reaches term or is close to
term, he is usually strong enough to allow for at least the option of a vaginal delivery.

☐ **The Mechanism of Labor in a Breech Presentation**   The mechanism of
labor is somewhat different in a breech from what it is in a vertex. The anterior
hip of the baby is often tilted to one side or another and will therefore descend
more rapidly than the posterior. The rotation of the breech usually takes place
inside the pelvis; after rotation, the baby continues to descend to the perineum,
with legs and feet following the breech in a frank breech presentation. Then,
once the presenting part, the breech, has passed through the vagina, a slight external rotation takes place with the back turning forward. Immediately after the
shoulder is delivered, the head is usually delivered by using a special extraction
maneuver (see below).

☐ **Is X-Ray Pelvimetry Necessary in Breech Deliveries?**   Although it is
rarely used today, X-ray pelvimetry is still suggested as a preliminary procedure
before attempting the vaginal breech delivery of a woman in labor with her first
child (primipara) because it is important to establish the configuration of a
woman's pelvis. During a breech delivery, unlike the normal vertex delivery, the
first part to be delivered is the buttocks, which are narrower than the head and

will usually slip out easily. The last part to be delivered is the head, and here the obstetrician may encounter problems because a large head is easily trapped in the birth canal and would require extraordinary maneuvers to dislodge. The obstetrician will, therefore, order a pelvic X-ray of a primipara to have a clear idea of the pelvic configuration and to make sure that the baby's head is well flexed. He must not attempt a vaginal delivery in the absence of adequate flexion. If, on the other hand, a breech baby is apparently too large to deliver vaginally, or the patient has been in labor for a while with no sign of descent, the doctor will assume that the pelvis is too small or the baby too large and will proceed to a Cesarean section. If a woman has given birth previously (multiparous) an X-ray of the pelvis—pelvimetry—is not necessary since the pelvis has already been tested during the previous birth or births. Only if the obstetrician suspects dystocia in a multiparous woman in labor with a breech is a pelvimetry probably necessary. The doctor should then explain why he is ordering the X-ray.

☐ *Vaginal Delivery of the Breech Baby*   No doctor, as I will explain later, should attempt to deliver anything but a frank breech vaginally, and then only under certain circumstances. Once a vaginal delivery has been decided on, you can still expect the labor and delivery to be somewhat different from the normal vertex delivery. Even the speed of delivery is different. Very often labor will last longer; a labor complicated by breech averages about nine hours for a primipara and six hours for a multipara. But labor may go very quickly, at least in certain cases of breech. It is important for the obstetrician to examine his patient at repeated intervals to make sure that the presenting part, the buttocks, is pressing down on the cervix, because only then can the cervix be expected to dilate successfully and expedite labor. There are more unsuccessful vaginal deliveries with the frank breech presentation just because the breech does not always fit well into the pelvis.

Once the birth reaches the second stage, a woman with a frank breech must push much harder than usual because her doctor will not be able to use forceps to help her deliver. Training and concentration are therefore even more important in a vaginal breech delivery than in a vertex delivery. The presenting part, the breech, will be pushed out first. (The doctor will perform a midline or mediolateral episiotomy to make sure there is enough space for the baby's head.) After the breech is born, the mother will be asked to continue pushing as hard as she can; any pulling by the doctor at this critical point may result in damage to the nerves. The attending obstetrician usually likes to see the mother push the baby out spontaneously as far as the level of the navel; he will then take over the delivery, supporting the baby and gently delivering the legs. With a frank breech, he will usually bend one of the baby's knees and deliver the first leg and then the other leg. Next he will pull the baby downward and rotate the body to slowly deliver the anterior arm, bending the arm out gently because it can be damaged rather easily. He will then carefully rotate the baby 180 degrees by placing a hand on both sides of the chest and pulling downward. This maneuver will usually help deliver the other arm, if it is not delivered spontaneously. (When the doctor delivers the shoulders he usually places a hot, wet towel between his hands and the baby's slippery body because it makes it easier for him to manipulate and deliver the shoulders.)

After the shoulders are delivered the doctor inserts one hand into the vagina

522 /   *Childbirth with Love*

and will try to place one finger into the baby's mouth. He will then let the baby rest over one arm, placing the other hand over the baby's shoulder while the mother is asked to continue pushing. A gentle maneuver of this kind will usually deliver the baby vaginally without trauma. If the head is difficult to deliver the obstetrician will put special forceps, the so-called Piper's forceps, underneath the baby so the baby is resting on the forceps as the head is delivered. But most skilled obstetricians can deliver a breech just by the technique I have just described, the technique known as the Mauriceau-Smellie-Veit maneuver.

A vaginal breech delivery is a challenge, but a skillful doctor can usually manage the delivery without any long-lasting effect on the baby.

☐ *How Does the Breech Baby Appear After Birth?*   Because of the difference in the mechanism of delivery, a vaginally delivered breech baby will have a rather different appearance, immediately after birth, from a baby born head first. Most newborns have, at least temporarily, the characteristic elongated head known colloquially as a "banana head." The head has this strange appearance because it has been molded in the descent through the pelvis. In a breech birth, the buttocks take the place of the head, so the buttocks aften suffer temporarily from hematomas, bruises, and swelling. The head, on the other hand, is often more rounded than usual; and because it has rested up against the top of the uterus, the fundus, during the pregnancy, it will be flat on the top rather than elongated. The shape of any newborn's head, of course, changes in the first twenty-four to forty-eight hours of extrauterine life, when it begins to take on the appearance it will have later in life. This is true of both vertex and breech babies.

Many breech babies have temporary hip or joint problems after delivery. This is hardly surprising, since the breech baby has spent months in the womb sitting with his legs bent up next to the body—a position that impedes normal fetal movement and proper muscle development. Any congenital weakness of the hips or joints can be cured completely by prompt treatment after birth. Special orthopedic braces are usually recommended for a few months to keep the legs in the right position and to encourage the rebuilding of the hip joints. I know that parents find this remedial measure difficult initially, but it will avoid problems later on when the child learns to walk. Otherwise, breech babies born at term or near term are generally healthy. As long as the delivery goes smoothly and the Apgar Scores are satisfactory, a breech baby can bond with the parents immediately after birth and will respond to care like any other healthy newborn.

☐ *What Are the Risks of a Vaginal Delivery in a Breech Presentation?*   A breech presentation is always associated with more complications than a vertex presentation. To begin with, the fetal membranes often rupture prematurely, precipitating labor weeks before term. Second, there is more fluid in the amniotic sac because the head does not obstruct the pelvis as it does in a vertex presentation; consequently there is a risk of the umbilical cord's prolapsing. Third, labor itself is often more difficult than usual because the presenting part does not always fit as it should into the pelvis. Finally, it is important to realize that an obstetrician, particularly an inexperienced one, can run into difficulties during a vaginal breech delivery. Breech babies have been known to sustain serious traumas including hypoxia (decreased oxygen level) and injuries to the head, neck, and arms, during a mismanaged breech delivery. Out of fear of malpractice suits, among other reasons, many doctors prefer to section all their breech patients rather than allow a woman with an apparently uncomplicated breech to go into labor naturally. And certainly, some of the follow-up studies of vaginally delivered breech infants would seem to endorse the almost universal Cesareans of breech babies. One long-term study, for instance, was undertaken in Indianapolis, where a group of breech babies from one hospital was followed for nine years after birth. Of the babies who were delivered vaginally, the study found that 25 percent needed to repeat one school year, a startling contrast with the group delivered by Cesarean, none of whom were held back through the early school years. Another study from France concluded that breech babies delivered by Cesarean section did significantly better during the neonatal period than those delivered vaginally.

Studies such as these may, however, not be the final word on the subject of breech deliveries. Disturbed by the risk of Cesarean delivery to the mother— maternal mortality is about five times higher among Cesarean-sectioned women than among those delivered vaginally—doctors in the larger university medical centers are now going back to delivering *certain* cases of breech vaginally. While they continue to recommend a Cesarean section if the mother has a small pelvis, if the baby is large—eight and a half pounds or more—or the breech is an incomplete or footling breech, they are delivering babies in the frank breech position vaginally, as long as the labor continues to progress smoothly. A vaginal delivery may present a slightly higher risk of damage to the nerves in the arms, but this condition usually disappears within a few days when the swelling goes down. Otherwise such deliveries usually go well. Here, of course, I am talking about a breech delivery managed by an experienced obstetrician. The problem is that many obstetricians, especially younger ones trained outside the large medical centers, have never been taught the technique of the vaginal breech delivery, and a well-meaning but inexperienced doctor could endanger a baby or a mother by attempting to deliver a breech vaginally. This situation makes it important for a couple with a diagnosed breech presentation to question their obstetrician closely. If he does not appear competent to deliver the baby vaginally, but no other obstetrician is available, you would probably do better to ask for a Cesarean rather than subject yourself to a hazardous vaginal delivery. The risk of birth injury, including that of cerebral palsy, is too serious to allow for any doubts about your obstetrician's skill. But if you are fortunate enough to have an experienced obstetrician, you and your doctor can make a decision based on the individual circumstances of your pregnancy. Of course, he must protect both his patients—you and the baby—but the baby may do just as well with a vaginal delivery.

☐ *Emergency Delivery* Each birth is different; and so is a woman's experience from one birth to another. Some deliveries take a long time, some go very fast. It all depends on the baby's size relative to the mother's pelvis and on the way in which the baby enters the pelvis. If for some reason or other labor begins very rapidly and the cervix is already effaced and dilated, birth can progress so rapidly that, for instance, a woman might wake up in the middle of the night already in the active stage of labor and fail to make it to the hospital in time. An unexpected delivery at home or on the way to the hospital is comparatively uncommon, but every expectant couple should still know how to deal with an emergency childbirth, just in case it should happen to them.

☐ *If You Feel That the Birth Is Imminent . . .*   As soon as you experience definite signs of labor, call your doctor and tell him or his answering service what is happening. If the doctor is not available and does not return your call immediately, don't wait for him to call back but give his service the message that you are on the way to the hospital. Then rush to the hospital. If on the other hand you feel that the baby's birth is imminent, don't try to get to the hospital because you probably will not get there in time. Call your doctor, inform him of the emergency, and then try to get help. If you must, you can manage an emergency childbirth on your own, but the presence of your partner or a trusted neighbor or friend will not only reassure you but will mean that help is on hand if something should go wrong.

You really do not need any special equipment for an emergency delivery. The kettle of boiling water is a myth. All you need to do is to keep calm. A birth that is progressing rapidly is usually an easy one. Indeed, if all births were only that simple, we would hardly need doctors, or at least, many fewer doctors than we have now.

☐ *Delivering the Baby*   First, empty your bladder. Second, sit down and lean your back against a solid object with your legs slightly apart and your knees spread as wide as possible. Don't lie down—you will lose the force of gravity if you do and you won't be able to see what is happening.

As you would with a delivery in the hospital, don't begin to push when you feel the initial urge to do so. That first urge to push often occurs before the cervix is completely dilated. If you begin to push too early on, you run the risk of ripping the cervix and causing bleeding that cannot be stopped without medical assistance. Wait instead until the urge to push is so irresistible that you feel you *must* push, using your breathing techniques meanwhile to control the delivery.

Once you no longer feel you can refrain from pushing, begin to push with each contraction, bearing down steadily with the contractions and taking a deep breath to help you as you push. Remember to exhale quickly and take in another breath in between contractions. Try to achieve a complete exchange of oxygen and carbon dioxide, because otherwise you might begin to hyperventilate and make yourself dizzy and frightened. It is important to bear down as hard as you can with each contraction because you will shorten the delivery by hard pushing and will, at the same time, relieve any sensation of pain or discomfort. In between contractions, relax your pushing position and rest.

When you feel a burning or a stretching sensation, stop pushing temporarily. This is usually a sign of "crowning." If you keep pushing as the head is crowning you can rip the perineum so badly that stitches would be necessary to close it. Instead, take short, rapid breaths to suppress the pushing urge. As you see more of the baby's head appear with each contraction, hold your hands against the head to prevent it from emerging too rapidly. The head will probably be rotating in the normal position, facing your backbone. After the head emerges, the baby will rotate so he faces frontways. Lift the head gently as he does so to prevent vaginal tearing. Once the head is born, be sure to squeeze one finger inside the mouth and move it around gently to dislodge any mucus. Next, feel for the position of the umbilical cord. Sometimes the cord will be wrapped around the neck. If so, you can usually slip it gently over the head and release the neck. Don't pull—too much pressure may rupture the cord. Finally, begin to push with the next contractions and slowly guide the body of the baby out. If you keep sitting in an upright position, the anterior shoulder will be delivered easily. Once the first shoulder is out, support the baby and slowly lift him forward and upward to deliver the back shoulder and the rest of the body. There is no danger of dropping the baby if you are sitting upright on a bed or the floor, although the body will be slippery, with its coating of vernix. Remember to lift the baby slightly forward and upward; this is a good way to prevent tearing the vagina. Once the shoulders have been born, the rest of the baby will follow easily and all you need to do to complete the birth is to lift the baby and pull slightly as the trunk and legs are born.

As soon as the birth is completed, you should protect the baby's body temperature by drying the skin with a blanket or towel. Keep rubbing the baby gently to make sure that he is warm. A healthy child will appear vigorous and alert or will cry. (It would be wise to check once again that there is no mucus obstructing the trachea or clogging the mouth and nose.)

A minute or so after birth, the umbilical cord will stop pulsating, and your partner can tie two pieces of cord or string a few inches apart around the umbilical cord and then cut through the section with ordinary scissors. Neither the string nor the scissors have to be sterile, because the cord will fall off naturally. If you are alone, complete the delivery and leave the baby between your legs, watching to make sure he is breathing well. You will feel another urge to push within a few minutes when the placenta is delivered; it is best to wait until the placenta is delivered to tie the cord.

When, a few minutes after the birth, you feel the next urge to bear down, do so. At the same time, put one hand on your abdomen just above the uterus, where you will feel the hard ball of the placenta. Gently press down with the palm of your hand on the uterus with each contraction to help push the placenta out. Little by little the uterus will contract and deliver the placenta. Don't pull on the umbilical cord, since you might rip it, but keep pushing and the placenta will come out easily. Finally, a little gentle pressure on the cord and the placenta will come out in its entirety. If it sheds off easily, it's usually intact. For safety, have the placenta examined by a doctor or midwife. Afterward, continue to massage the uterus or ask your partner to massage it for you, since continuous massage will release the hormones in the uterus that keep it contracted and help prevent postpartum hemorrhaging. Breast-feeding the baby immediately after birth will also release oxytocin and help firm up the uterus and cut down on postpartum bleeding.

☐ *Should You Go to the Hospital if You Have an Emergency Home Delivery?*
It is a wise precaution to go to the hospital as soon as you can after an emergency home delivery. There the baby will be examined by a pediatrician and you will be checked to make sure no serious tearing has occurred. Also, in case of any unexpected postpartum complications, you and the baby will be in safer surroundings than at home. An uncomplicated birth is rarely followed by postpartum complications, but it is better to have professional care close at hand for a few days after the birth.

31

Cesarean Birth

□ *Whatever Happened to "Natural" Childbirth?*   The average childbirth couple enter the hospital expecting a natural birth. They have already prepared for a vaginal delivery through books and childbirth classes and they look forward to participating in the birth of their child. What no one, including their doctor or their childbirth educator, may have told them is that they face an almost one-in-six chance of having a Cesarean birth instead of the natural delivery they have spent months preparing for. This means that the mother will not only go through a surgical procedure instead of giving birth vaginally, but in many hospitals she will be separated from her husband, isolated from the baby for up to twenty-four hours after the delivery, and will face a longer and more painful postpartum period than a woman whose baby is delivered vaginally. With the Cesarean rate at an unprecedented high level, and still rising, no wonder so many people are asking the question: Whatever happened to natural childbirth?

□ *Why Are There So Many Cesareans?*   For years a Cesarean delivery was resorted to only when the life of the mother or the baby was in jeopardy. In the early 1960s Cesarean deliveries were still only 5 percent of American births. Then in the 1970s, the Cesarean rate rose dramatically, until by 1980 the national Cesarean rate was 15 percent, making delivery by Cesarean the tenth most common surgical procedure in the nation. The rate is now close to 17 percent and some obstetricians have predicted a Cesarean-section rate of 25–30 percent in the near future, if the present trend continues. Already the section rate in some American hospitals is so high that one out of every three obstetrical patients is delivered surgically instead of vaginally. It is not surprising that the American obstetrician has been accused of "grabbing the knife" instead of making a serious attempt to achieve a vaginal birth.

The section rate has risen for a number of reasons, several of which have to do with some long-term trends in obstetrical care. First of all, the operation itself is much safer than it was in the past. With improvements in surgical techniques and the introduction of potent antibiotics, it has become much more acceptable for the obstetrician to make the decision to operate. At the same time, he faces new pressures to deliver a healthy baby. With couples having fewer children, there is more concern for the individual pregnancy. While doctors once did difficult vaginal deliveries, using dangerous high forceps to pull the baby out in a case of cephalo-pelvic disproportion, or trying to manipulate a baby in a complicated breech birth, a modern obstetrician will usually choose to deliver the baby surgically. This change has undoubtedly saved lives and has prevented birth-related brain damage for thousands of children. But it is a trend that is also dangerous because women have died during Cesareans or have suffered serious postpartum complications.

The introduction of sophisticated new medical technologies has also affected the Cesarean rate. A baby subject to acute stress during labor is delivered by Cesarean section to prevent death or brain damage. In the past, doctors and nurses used the fetoscope, an obstetrical stethoscope, to monitor the fetal heartbeat. Now that American hospitals have fetal monitors, a doctor can detect signs of fetal distress early on and act accordingly to protect the baby. Consequently, the number of sections performed for fetal distress has gone up in the last few years. Critics of electronic fetal monitoring claim this to be the chief cause of the increased Cesarean rate. They point to cases in which doctors, faced with an unfamiliar machine, have misinterpreted heart-rate tracings and rushed their patients into the operating room. But as doctors become more familiar with fetal monitors (see Chap. 28), the number of Cesareans for reasons of fetal distress can be expected to decrease. And an even newer technique, fetal scalp blood sampling, can now be used to back up the monitor's findings if an obstetrician feels a Cesarean may be necessary. Doctors have made deliveries safer by using Cesareans, but they have also chosen to do Cesareans in births in which the baby could be delivered vaginally. This trend is responsible for thousands of Cesareans each year. The two most common indications for a Cesarean today are dystocia, or lack of progress in labor, and the repeat Cesarean. A repeat Cesarean is one performed because a woman's previous pregnancy ended in a Cesarean.

Dystocia accounts for about 30 percent of all Cesarean births. Sometimes

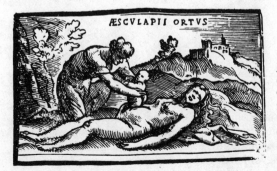

Figure 110: Birth of Asklepios (Asclepius): Apollo, the Sun God, is removing the baby from his mother, the wood nymph, Coronis. The wood cut is from the 1549 edition of Alessandro Benedetti's *De Re Medica.*

labor fails to progress because the baby is too large for the pelvis (a cephalo-pelvic disproportion). Then the baby must be delivered abdominally. But many cases of dystocia are cases of prolonged labor that could be managed vaginally by a careful obstetrician (see below). Instead, many women are now given Cesareans as soon as labor has ceased to progress, or sometimes even before real dystocia has been verified.

Medical-legal issues have played a part in the sudden popularity of Cesareans. As parents have become more sophisticated and more demanding, obstetricians are increasingly reluctant to take risks that might lead to litigation. Obstetricians have found that if they let nature take its course, as in a case of dystocia or breech, they run a serious risk of a lawsuit if the vaginal delivery results in a baby with problems. Consequently, the obstetrician may rush his patient into the operating room at the first sign of fetal distress or dysfunctional labor. Many obstetricians are afraid to perform a simple forceps delivery or an uncomplicated vaginal breech delivery because they might be held liable for electing not to do a Cesarean.

□ *Why Should We Be Concerned About the Rise in Cesarean Births?*
Many of the Cesareans performed each year are undoubtedly justified by the circumstances of the delivery (see below for a breakdown of the indications for Cesarean birth). But in deciding to do a Cesarean, the benefits to the baby must be weighed against the potential risks for the mother. Maternal mortality is low for all births, but there is still a two to four times greater chance of a woman's dying after a Cesarean than after a vaginal birth. The risk of major complications, including infection, is much higher with a Cesarean. The hospital stay is longer, the financial cost is greater, and increasingly women are aware of the psychological costs as well. If the Cesarean rate reaches 25–30 percent, that means that one out of every four women giving birth will face the risks of a major surgical procedure and subsequent complications.

□ *Reasons for Increases in Cesarean Sections*   Years ago, a Cesarean was performed only to save the life of the mother or the fetus. Today the four most common reasons for a Cesarean section are as follows:

INDICATIONS	PERCENT OF ALL CESAREANS DONE FOR THIS INDICATION	PERCENT RESPONSIBLE FOR THE INCREASE IN CESAREAN BIRTH RATE
Dystocia	31%	30%
Repeat Cesarean section	31%	25–30%
Breech presentation	12%	10–15%
Fetal distress	5%	10–15%

You can see from this breakdown that the two major indications responsible for the recent increase in Cesarean births are dystocia (or dysfunctional labor, see Chap. 30) and repeat Cesareans. Together these two indications account for 60 percent of the recent increase in Cesarean births. Obstetricians who feel that the Cesarean rate is too high favor looking at dystocia cases more carefully (see below) in an effort to reverse the trend. Dystocia often occurs in a first pregnancy, so the number of repeat Cesareans would also be reduced if fewer women were C-sectioned because of dysfunctional labor.

☐ **When Is a Cesarean Birth Really Necessary?**   Certain *obstetrical emergencies* indicate the need for an immediate Cesarean. The most common emergencies are a placenta previa (the placenta is partially or wholly blocking the birth canal); an abruptio placentae (the placenta partially or completely detaches itself from the uterine wall); prolapse of the umbilical cord; a severe hemorrhage; and cases of fetal distress in which the fetal heart rate drops to below eighty beats per minute and does not recover, or when the fetal heart-rate pattern indicates that the fetus is at jeopardy. A suspected case of fetal distress should be verified by a fetal scalp blood sample before a Cesarean is done. This will aid in preventing unnecessary C sections for this indication (see Chap. 28).

A *maternal illness* may also necessitate a Cesarean. The baby of a diabetic mother is often delivered abdominally (see Chap. 24), especially if the baby is large. Maternal hypertension or severe toxemia might call for a Cesarean to avoid the maternal stress of a long labor. Active vaginal herpes and intrauterine infection might also call for a C birth. Finally, if a woman has had a previous pelvic fracture or has a congenitally abnormal pelvis, a Cesarean will be the safest mode of delivery.

Breech deliveries: The premature breech baby is at special risk in a vaginal delivery. Premature breech babies delivered vaginally often suffer traumatic birth injuries because the head, which at this time is much larger than the body, is trapped by the unripe cervix. These tiny babies stand a better chance of survival if they are delivered by Cesarean (see below). Term breeches with the baby in the complete or footling breech position (see Chap. 30) are considered high-risk and are also best delivered by a Cesarean. Babies in the frank breech position, the easiest position to deliver vaginally, are often delivered by Cesarean if the baby is very large, but surgical delivery may not be necessary in every case of a frank breech. Vaginal delivery of more breech births would help reverse the trend toward Cesarean births. If your baby is in the breech position you should discuss the delivery plans with your doctor well in advance (see Chap. 30).

☐ **Cephalo-Pelvic Disproportion (CPD)**   In a case of CPD the baby's head is too large to negotiate its way through the bony pelvis, either because of its size or because of the configuration of the pelvis itself. A CPD is usually diagnosed when the cervix ceases to dilate in the active phase of labor. A doctor may occasionally take an X-ray of the pelvis to confirm the disproportion between the head and the pelvis and then deliver the baby abdominally if the bony pelvis is absolutely too small for the baby's head.

☐ **Dystocia**   Dystocia is medically defined as a cessation of the normal progress of labor due to an abnormality in the mechanism of labor. It is often just referred to as lack of progress (see Chap. 30).

An unnecessarily high number of dystocia cases end in Cesareans because obstetricians rush through deliveries and are not willing to wait for labor to take its own time. Dysfunctions of labor can often be managed by simple means: by helping the patient relax, changing the patient's position, encouraging her to walk around, or giving increased intravenous fluids. If these simple remedies do not encourage a good progression of labor, the doctor can monitor the strength of the contractions with an internal monitor (see Chap. 28) and give the patient intravenous oxytocin to help speed the contractions. Once oxytocin infusion has been tried and failed, a doctor may elect to perform a Cesarean. You should realize, though, that in the absence of fetal distress, your doctor has plenty of time to allow for a real trial of labor. He should not rush into a Cesarean until the evidence of real dystocia is clear to him, and to you and your husband.

☐ *Repeat Cesarean Section*   A repeat Cesarean is considered necessary if a woman has had a previous classical Cesarean (see below) or if the indication that led to the previous Cesarean section is present in the subsequent pregnancy. Otherwise, this is a controversial subject that is treated more fully later in the chapter.

☐ *How Cesarean-Section Rates Vary*   Statistics from various hospitals have evidenced a great difference in the incidence of Cesarean section from one hospital to another. In New York City, for instance, the North Central Bronx Hospital in the Bronx has a Cesarean rate of only 9.2 percent, the city's lowest, while New York University Hospital, on the other hand, has a Cesarean rate of 26 percent. Of course, some large university hospitals, which have a much higher population of high-risk patients, can be expected to have a higher Cesarean rate than a hospital, such as North Central Bronx, in which the population has a relatively high birth rate and women come to the hospital for their second or third child. However, the C section rate in hospitals that serve middle class families is also surprisingly high; one hospital on Staten Island (New York City) reports that a Cesarean section is performed on over one-third of its obstetrical patients.

The National Institutes of Health has strongly urged hospitals to review their section rates, case by case, to help bring the Cesarean-section rate in the United States under control. It is important for you as the consumer to know the section rate in your hospital. Some hospitals have shown a steady rate, while others have had a rapid increase in recent years, a sign that the obstetrical division may not be exercising the proper control. You might want to bear this in mind when you make your choice of an obstetrician or a hospital.

☐ *How to Avoid an Unnecessary Cesarean*   A low rate of Cesarean birth in a hospital does not necessarily guarantee careful decision-making, but a couple choosing an obstetrician or a hospital should ask some basic questions at the initial interview. The choice of a particular obstetrician might mean the difference between a vaginal or a Cesarean birth.

Consider asking the obstetrician the following question: Does the hospital with which he is affiliated demand a second opinion before a Cesarean birth can be performed? One good example is a public hospital in New York, the Municipal Hospital, which has a much lower Cesarean-section rate than most private hospitals. The reason is that two doctors must share the decision to perform a Cesarean.

A second question concerns what is known as the "repeat Cesarean." Will the obstetrician allow women with a previous Cesarean section to deliver vaginally if the next delivery is without complications? A number of the larger medical centers are now encouraging women to attempt a vaginal delivery the second time around; another reason why the Cesarean section rate is lower in certain hospitals than in others.

Also ask your obstetrician whether the hospital uses fetal scalp blood sampling techniques (described fully in Chapter 28). By using fetal blood-sampling, an obstetrician can determine whether a suspicious fetal heart-rate pattern on the fetal monitor means the oxygen level is decreasing or fetal acidity is increasing. If either problem is occurring, the obstetrician will do a Cesarean section to protect the baby's health. Fetal blood-sampling used in conjunction with fetal monitoring may also avoid unnecessary Cesareans, since the additional test will confirm or disprove a suspicious heart-rate pattern. Not all hospitals have fetal blood-sampling techniques available, so a couple might want to consider booking a hospital in their locality that offers the new technique.

☐ *Does Cesarean Section Depend on Maternal Age?*   Recent statistics from the United States do show a connection between maternal age and the Cesarean-section rate. Presently, 17 percent of births in the United States end in Cesarean section; for very young women, under the age of twenty, the rate is 14.5 percent. This increases to 15.8 percent for women between twenty and twenty-four, and to 16.7 percent for women between the ages of twenty-five and twenty-nine. By the time a woman is between thirty-five and thirty-nine, there is a 20 percent chance of her undergoing a Cesarean, and for women over forty, the highest percentage of all—21.2 percent.

☐ *The History of Cesarean Section*   The technique of delivering the unborn child by an incision of the abdominal wall has been known since prehistoric times. Cave paintings in Africa show the operation being performed by shamans. Greek mythology includes numerous stories of abdominal births. The sun god Apollo, for instance, was said to have removed his unborn son Asklepios from the abdomen of his beloved Coronis, whom Apollo had ordered killed because of her infidelity. Among Eastern religions, both Brahma and Buddha were said to have emerged from the abdomens of their mothers.

The "Cesarean section" dates back to an early Roman law that directed that a child should be removed from the uterus of any woman dying in late pregnancy (Muma Pompilus—a law that was known initially as the *lex regia.* The law persisted under later rulers, and acquired the name *lex Caesarea* under the rule of the Caesars. There is no evidence that Julius Caesar, born about 100 B.C., was delivered abdominally, nor, contrary to common belief, was the procedure named after him).

The first documented Cesarean section on a living patient was performed on April 21, 1610, by Jeremias Trautmann of Saxony. The mother lived twenty days after the operation, before dying from complications. The technique was first described in a treatise on gynecology in 1663, and became more popular after that time, although it could be used only in an extreme emergency. In those early days the babies were sometimes saved but the mothers inevitably died of hemorrhage and infection. The first successful Cesarean section—that is, the first section in which both mother and child lived—was performed by a Dr. Knowles of Birmingham, England, in 1836. Women generally failed to survive the operation because the uterus was not closed after surgery, exposing the mother to massive infection and invariably death.

Then, in 1882, a German physician, Dr. Max Sanger, published a thesis on Cesarean section that called attention to the importance of sewing the uterine incision firmly together after the baby was born. Careful suturing was to increase considerably the chances of a woman's surviving the operation. Another improvement was the introduction of the low-cervical Cesarean section, first described in 1907, instead of the customary classic one. Not only have surgical techniques improved, but a greater emphasis has been placed on asepsis—the prevention of bacterial contamination. Both have added immeasurably to the safety of the operation.

☐ **The Cesarean Operation**　　A Cesarean section is defined as the delivery of an infant through an incision in the abdominal and uterine walls. The word "Cesarean" was derived sometime in the Middle Ages from the Latin verb *caedere* meaning "to cut." The word "section" is derived from the Latin verb *secare*, which also means "to cut." The term "Cesarean section" is, therefore, a tautology.

There are two types of the operation: the low-segment section, which is also referred to as a "low flap" or low-cervical Cesarean section, and the classical Cesarean section.

A low-segment uterine incision is an incision made inside the uterus after the bladder is freed from its firm attachment to the lower portion of the uterus. The surgeon then pushes the bladder out of the way down into the pelvis and makes an incision into the area of the uterus previously covered by the bladder. After the baby has been delivered, the uterus is sutured together, and the bladder flap pushed over the incision to make it stronger. There is then less chance of rupture in a future delivery, and fewer immediate complications as the incision heals.

With a classical Cesarean section, the type favored some years ago, the incision inside the uterus is made vertically. Consequently, the scar is not covered by the bladder flap after the operation; this means that the uterine incision is relatively weak, since it is cut vertically through the muscle wall of the uterus. A vertical incision may be followed by some immediate problems, such as infection and the weakness of the uterine wall, and problems in subsequent pregnancies because of the risk of rupture with this type of incision. The latter is the reason why a woman who has had a classical Cesarean section cannot attempt a vaginal delivery in a subsequent pregnancy. A woman won't know which form of incision has been made within the uterus just by looking at the scar on her abdomen.

☐ **The "Bikini" Incision Versus the Up-Down Incision**　　The abdomen is entered through a skin incision. Two types exist. The most popular, known as the bikini incision, is made transversely across the lower part of the abdomen just below the pubic hairline. Since the pubic hair will grow back over the incision, the scar will be almost invisible later on. This type of cut is also called a Pfannenstiel incision (named after a German physician of that name) or a "smiling" incision. The other type, the midline or the up-down incision is made vertically from the navel to the pubic hairline. This used to be the most common form of abdominal incision but it is less favored nowadays because it leaves an obvious scar.

Most obstetricians use the bikini cut in all types of Cesareans. Sometimes the old-fashioned up-down incision is recommended if there is a real emergency, such as a case of fetal distress, because a surgeon can enter the abdomen faster with a vertical cut. But a decision is often made because of a doctor's particular training or skill. Many obstetricians can enter the abdomen as fast (or even faster) using the bikini cut as the up-down incision. I personally prefer the Pfannenstiel incision since it heals better and only rarely results in the development of a hernia. If you are scheduled for a Cesarean section, ask your doctor what type of incision he plans to perform. If your doctor does not know about the "bikini" incision, give yourself time to look for a doctor who can perform any type of abdominal incision.

☐ *Preparation for Cesarean Birth*   A nurse will prepare you for the operation. Preoperative medication may be given to dry the secretions in your mouth and the upper airway. This is usually atropine. With atropine, there will be less chance of your coughing or aspirating fluid after the surgery. The lower part of the abdomen is washed and shaved to remove any hair around the line of the incision. Next a catheter is placed into the bladder before the surgery to keep it empty since the bladder is located next to the area where the Cesarean will be performed. The catheter will usually be kept in for twenty-four hours after surgery because you may not feel like getting up to go to the bathroom right away; some obstetricians, though, remove the catheter right after surgery. An intravenous infusion is also started that permits the anesthesiologist and the obstetrician to give you medication through the open intravenous line. Finally, a blood sample should be obtained so that your blood can be typed and cross-matched in the case of an emergency blood transfusion.

You will then be taken to the operating room, where a decision will have to be made by the obstetrician and the anesthesiologist as to general or epidural anesthesia. The pros and cons of both types of anesthesia will be discussed below.

The speed at which these preparations will take place depends on the circumstances of the Cesarean. If it is being performed for a reason such as dystocia, there will be time to ask questions while the preoperative procedures are being completed. But in the case of fetal distress, the baby must be delivered within a few minutes. The preliminaries will then be rushed through, and you might have very little chance to ask questions. I would advise asking your obstetrician important questions in a routine office visit. Because so many women do give birth by Cesarean, it would be wise to find out what type of incision he will perform and what type of anesthesia would be used in an emergency Cesarean.

☐ *What Type of Anesthesia Is Best for a Cesarean Birth?*   Two types of anesthesia are currently used for Cesarean birth: epidural anesthesia and general anesthesia. In the past the majority of hospitals preferred to use general anesthesia; the patient was put to sleep quickly, the abdominal muscles were completely relaxed so that the delivery was usually completed easily. General anesthesia has the added advantage of taking effect quickly—an important factor in an emergency Cesarean. It also ensures a pain-free birth. However, the situation has changed now that anesthesiology is more sophisticated and there is more emphasis on childbirth education. Many women prefer a form of anesthesia that allows them to stay awake during the operation; and many anesthesiologists favor epidural anesthesia over general anesthesia because the baby is less depressed with it. Most hospitals now use epidurals except in an emergency in which the patient must be put to sleep in a hurry to deliver the baby as quickly as possible. An additional advantage with the epidural is the extra time it allows the obstetrician during the operation. With general anesthesia, the baby must be delivered within a few minutes of the anesthesia's taking effect, otherwise the baby may be unconscious by the time he is born.

☐ *Epidural Anesthesia*   It often takes ten to thirty minutes for the epidural to take effect. Consequently it should be used only when you are expecting what is known as a prepared Cesarean section—one that can be anticipated at least thirty minutes in advance of surgery either because of dystocia, a repeated Cesarean section, or because of some other problem that allows time for preparation. The epidural cannot be used in a case of fetal distress because it does not take effect quickly enough, unless you are already in labor with an epidural. This is, of course, one of the advantages of epidural anesthesia during an apparently normal labor; the same anesthetic can be used for a Cesarean birth.

The technique of administering epidural anesthesia has already been described in Chapter 27. While from a medical point of view there are advantages and disadvantages to this type of anesthesia, there is no doubt that the epidural is by far the preferred form of anesthesia for a woman who wants to be awake and aware during and after the birth. And with an epidural, an increasing number of hospitals will allow your partner to share the birth with you. Another advantage of epidural anesthesia is that the local anesthetic used during an epidural does not have the same paralyzing effect on the baby as general anesthesia. The anesthetic might be transferred across the placenta, but the chances of severe depression are far less with epidural than with general anesthesia.

The epidural is difficult to administer and must be supervised by an anesthesiologist. If you are giving birth in a good-sized hospital, the chances are that a skilled anesthesia staff will be available around the clock. A small suburban or rural hospital may not be able to provide an anesthesiologist at short notice who can administer an epidural. If you need to have a repeat Cesarean, look for an obstetrician with admitting privileges in a larger hospital where epidural anesthesia is routinely performed. Ask also whether the hospital will allow your husband to be present during the birth, and whether the institution will allow both of you to bond with the baby after the birth. Try making your plans well in advance, or at least in time to change to another doctor if you are not pleased with his hospital's policy.

☐ *General Anesthesia*   With general anesthesia the patient is taken into a delivery room where the entire obstetrical team, the anesthesiologist, the obstetrician, the assistant obstetrician, and the surgical nurses, are standing by in readiness for the procedure. The abdomen is completely shaved and draped. Once the preparations are completed, the anesthesiologist will introduce sodium pentathol into the patient's IV. Within a few seconds the patient will be asleep;

the anesthesiologist then usually gives a combination of nitrous oxide and pure oxygen to maintain the anesthesia.

The operation itself follows the normal sequence: an incision is made into the abdomen to open up the peritoneal cavity; the doctor then visualizes the uterus and makes his incision in it to deliver the baby. It takes no longer than five to ten minutes from the abdominal incision until the birth of the baby. Finally the doctor sews up the uterus while the patient is still completely anesthetized.

A Cesarean section done under general anesthesia is not a difficult operation. Nonetheless, more complications can be expected because the patient is unconscious and her respiration must be artificially maintained. If by mistake the patient does not get enough oxygen, brain damage or even death can occur. With epidural anesthesia, on the other hand, the patient is breathing on her own so the chance of complications is less.

☐ *Performing the Cesarean*   The doctor will first make an incision into the abdomen (either a low bikini incision or an up-down incision, depending on the circumstances I have discussed previously). After the incision has been made, the doctor will free the surface of the facia (fibrous membrane covering the muscles) and cut it with a pair of surgical scissors. Next he will isolate the muscles of the abdomen and spread them apart. The muscles are *not* cut. He will then reach into the area of the peritoneum, which he will incise with scissors. By then the abdomen will be exposed and the obstetrician will be able to see the bowel and the uterus. The uterus is the next organ to come into view because it is pushed up to the front by the baby. Once the uterus has been visualized, the doctor must determine its exact position; retractors will be inserted to insure continued visualization. The peritoneum covering the uterus will next be surgically incised and the bladder pushed downward, exposing the lower segment of the uterus. This is very thin during labor. The doctor will subsequently make as small an incision in the lower segment of the uterus as possible. If this is to be a classical Cesarean section, the incision will be made vertically in the uterus. During this operation the doctor will cut from up to down into the front wall of the uterus. The physician will next put his hand into the organ and feel for the baby's head. The delivery will be made as he lifts up the baby's head with one hand and pushes on its bottom with the other to pull the baby up through the abdominal incision.

A Cesarean delivery thus follows the pattern of a normal delivery inasmuch as the head is generally delivered first, and the shoulders and the rest of the body follow. In the case of a breech presentation, the buttocks or legs are delivered first. Once the baby is born, the mouth is suctioned with a syringe, and the umbilical cord is clamped and cut. The pediatric staff, who should be standing by in the operating room, will then take over the baby's care. Most hospitals require that a pediatrician be immediately available if resuscitation or some other emergency care becomes necessary—a wise precaution.

After the baby is born, the obstetrician will put his hand into the uterus to locate the placenta, which he will free from the uterine wall and deliver. Immediately after the placenta is delivered, the anesthesiologist will inject oxytocin into the patient's IV to help contract the uterus. The doctor will then inspect the uterus to be sure there is no laceration or any other abnormality, and to be

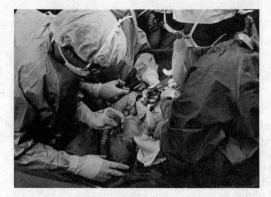

Figure 111: Cesarean Birth:
The mother has received a
local anesthetic and is awake
during the birth. The baby is
delivered within a few minutes
of the anesthetic's taking effect. This healthy infant is
being examined by the doctor
to check his skin color and
muscle tone. Later on the parents will be able to bond with
their baby even though it was
a Cesarean birth.

sure that the entire placenta has been removed. When that is done, he will close
the uterus with two layers of sutures to secure it firmly enough for any other
pregnancy and birth. After the uterine wall has been closed, the bladder flap,
which had been pushed down prior to the incision, will be lifted and placed over
the incision, then closed with sutures. (With the up-down uterine incision, there
is no bladder flap, so the incision will be more prone to rupture.) Once the
uterus is closed, the doctor will clean the abdomen, perhaps washing it with a
saline solution, and will close the anterior peritoneum with catgut sutures. Then
the fascia will be closed with strong dissolving sutures; sturdy sutures are used
since the fascia is the most important layer in the closing up of the abdomen.
The final layers of muscle and skin will then be secured and stitched together.
You can see from the complexity of the procedure that the type of incision
made in the abdomen is not related to the type of incision made inside the
uterus.

The baby should be examined by a pediatrician immediately after the delivery. Unless he is having difficulty breathing, events immediately after the birth
follow the sequence of a vaginal birth, including the recording of the one- and
five-minute Apgar Scores. If you are awake and your husband is with you, both
of you will see the baby immediately and your husband may be able to hold him
for a few minutes. A husband who has not been allowed into the delivery room
will be shown the baby as soon after the birth as possible. Although the pediatric
staff used to take the baby away to the nursery almost immediately after a Cesarean, most hospitals now allow the baby to stay in the delivery room to give the
parents time to bond with the newborn.

☐ *Bonding After a Cesarean*   In a hospital that encourages bonding after a
Cesarean birth, the baby will be put in a heated bassinet or under a heating
panel until the surgical team has completed the procedure. This usually takes
about fifty minutes, during which time your husband can begin to familiarize
himself with the baby. Then both of you and the baby will be united in the recovery room where you should be able to bond with the baby for fifteen to
twenty minutes or longer, depending on the hospital. With an epidural you
should feel well enough to hold the baby and begin breast-feeding immediately

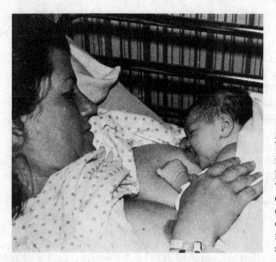

Figure 112: Rosemary is breast-feeding her baby after a natural delivery following two previous Cesarean' births. A woman who has had a previous Cesarean or Cesareans can often give birth spontaneously even though many doctors still insist on a repeat Cesarean for such patients.

just as you would after a vaginal delivery. If you had general anesthesia, you might be too groggy to hold the baby for very long, but even a few private minutes with the baby will give both of you great happiness.

Some hospitals have not yet relaxed their rules to allow bonding after a Cesarean birth. If your hospital rigidly adheres to the old policy of separating parents and babies almost immediately after birth, you should think of choosing another hospital next time around.

☐ **Breast-Feeding After a Cesarean**   There is no reason not to breast-feed immediately after a Cesarean birth. With a modern Cesarean you can expect very few complications and you can also expect to recover fairly quickly. Even if you are not able to take solid food for a day or so, the extra fluids will encourage the milk let-down. Although the first two days after a Cesarean birth can be difficult, the full breast milk supply will usually come in three days or so after the birth, and after that there is usually no problem with breast-feeding.

Another advantage of the bikini cut is that it will allow you to hold the baby with less discomfort than the old-fashioned up-down incision. Try lying on your side when you breast-feed, with the baby lying on a pillow next to you. This position will minimize the pain of the incision.

The only contraindication to breast-feeding after a Cesarean is a heavy dose of antibiotic therapy, which may be prescribed by your doctor as a protection against infection. Although many antibiotics, such as ampicillin and penicillin, are reasonably safe for the breast-feeding mother (see Chap. 32), certain antibiotics, such as sulfa and the modern broad-spectrum antibiotics, are not recommended in conjunction with breast-feeding. However, most antibiotic therapy can be stopped within a few days after the birth. Meanwhile you can use a breast pump to keep the milk reflex going, and then start to breast-feed once you are off the medication.

Most women find that breast-feeding the baby often gives them a more positive attitude toward the birth and even helps the body heal faster. And since you can expect to recover fully within three to four weeks of birth (a much shorter recovery period than women experienced years ago), you should be able to continue breast-feeding successfully once you get back home.

☐ *What Are the Risks Associated with Cesarean Section?*   A baby delivered by Cesarean section is spared the trauma of a vaginal birth. But for the mother, a Cesarean is a potentially dangerous operation. Nationally the mortality rate associated with Cesarean section is about two to four times that of a vaginal delivery. The two major life-threatening risks with a Cesarean are anesthesia-induced complications and pulmonary embolism (blood clots in the lungs) after the operation.

Major complications such as infection and hemorrhage also occur almost twice as often after a Cesarean section as they do after a vaginal delivery. The post-Cesarean patient often develops a urinary-tract infection, a wound infection, or endometritis, an infection of the uterine lining. Major infections will prolong the time spent in the hospital and delay a full recovery when the patient gets home.

The decision to perform a Cesarean section is a serious one. The operation is not an "easy" way to deliver the baby quickly, it is major surgery with all the attendant complications of any major surgery. A doctor who rushes a woman into surgery without exploring the other options is not acting in the best interest of the patient.

☐ *Reducing Postoperative Complications*   One of the remaining major complications of modern obstetrics is infection after a Cesarean birth. Most post-Cesarean infections are wound infections or uterine infections.

The risk of infection is higher if a patient has been placed on an internal fetal monitor or has been in labor for several hours before the Cesarean, because both circumstances encourage the entry of bacteria through the dilated cervix and up into the uterus.

Many doctors give their patients intravenous doses of antibiotics followed by oral antibiotics in the postpartum period. Even if there is no sign of infection, antibiotics given as preventive medicine will cut down postpartum complications and promote healing. This has been proven in several studies. Your obstetrician will know how to prescribe an antibiotic that is safe for the breast-feeding mother. Penicillin, ampicillin or cefazolin sodium is often used after a Cesarean birth.

The first symptom of infection is usually fever, an elevated temperature of 100 degrees or more. A postpartum patient who develops a fever should be evaluated immediately and have cultures taken from the vagina, the uterus, and the urine to determine the reasons for the infection. If the tests reveal a serious postpartum infection, the patient should be treated with potent broad-spectrum antibiotics. Several antibiotics might need to be given in combination. If the infection appears very serious and your obstetrician is not familiar with the modern type of antibiotics, an infection specialist should be called in.

☐ *Once a Cesarean, Always a Cesarean?*   Following a Cesarean delivery, most women who subsequently give birth undergo what is known as a repeat Cesarean section. This practice, which is at least eighty years old, was popularized by the famous saying "Once a Cesarean, always a Cesarean," made back in 1912 by a Dr. Edwin Cragin of New York City. At the time, Dr. Cragin and his fellow obstetricians were probably right in insisting on the repeat Cesarean, since doctors then routinely performed the classical Cesarean section, which had a high incidence of rupture in a subsequent vaginal delivery. But what is surprising is that many obstetricians still support that old rule "Once a Cesarean, always a Cesarean" even though many studies have found that a vaginal delivery after a previous Cesarean birth is reasonably safe. Contemporary obstetricians now use the low-flap uterine incision, which is much stronger than the classical incision because it is cut through the collagen tissue, not through the muscles of the uterus. A rupture is still possible with the low-flap abdominal incision but the risk of rupture is less than with the classical type of incision (see below).

Since the repeat Cesarean, like any type of the operation, carries the risk of postoperative complication such as infection or even death for the mother, many consumer activists and doctors are beginning to believe that the repeat Cesarean is open to question. Several recent studies indeed confirm that a vaginal delivery after an uncomplicated low-segment Cesarean is safe for most women. Pregnant women with previous Cesareans should therefore look for open-minded physicians who are familiar with vaginal deliveries after a previous C birth. If women are persistent, doctors will have to change their policies!

☐ *What Is a Trial of Labor?* Instead of automatically scheduling a repeat Cesarean for a patient whose previous pregnancy ended with a surgical delivery, a doctor can decide whether or not the patient's history warrants a trial of labor. "A trial of labor" means that a woman is allowed to go through a spontaneous labor until she delivers vaginally or the circumstances indicate that she must have another Cesarean. Several conditions, however, must be met before the doctor and patient can decide on a trial of labor.

The first and most important is the type of uterine incision performed during the previous Cesarean. Women who have undergone a classical Cesarean cannot attempt a vaginal delivery because of the high risk of uterine rupture. The incidence of uterine rupture with a vertical incision varies between 1.5 percent to 4 percent in a subsequent trial of labor.

Women whose previous Cesarean was of the low-segment type may be candidates for a trial of labor. The incidence of rupture with an uncomplicated low-segment incision is very low: from .25 percent to 1.5 percent. A healthy woman whose previous abdominal surgery left her with an uncomplicated low-segment incision could therefore attempt a trial of labor although other factors must be taken into consideration as well. These are:

(a) A woman must be fully informed of the risks and benefits of a trial of labor and must understand that the trial of labor can be terminated at her doctor's discretion. Only highly motivated women are suitable candidates for a trial of labor after a previous C birth.

(b) The complication that led to the first Cesarean must be not present in the subsequent pregnancy. For instance, a woman whose previous baby was too large for her pelvis should not be allowed a trial of labor if the baby of the subsequent pregnancy is as large as or larger than the first. However, the circumstances of the subsequent pregnancy are often different, especially if a woman experienced a problem such as dysfunctional labor in the earlier pregnancy.

(c) There must be no additional reasons for a Cesarean in the subsequent pregnancy. A new complication would terminate the trial of labor immediately.

(d) The fetus must be a singleton, weighing less than 8.8 pounds, who is lying in the vertex position.

(e) The patient must be clearly informed of the risks and benefits of a vaginal delivery and told that a repeat Cesarean might be necessary in the case of complications.

(f) The patient must be monitored closely through labor; a physician or a nurse must watch her continuously to detect abnormal pain or changes in the vital signs that might indicate the onset of uterine rupture.

(g) The delivery-room staff must be prepared to do an immediate Cesarean section should a crisis arise. The woman's blood must be typed and cross-matched, and surgical equipment must be readily available.

☐ *What About Anesthesia with a Repeat Cesarean?*   Epidural anesthesia is not given during a trial of labor because the anesthesia will mask any specific pain that could be a precursor of uterine rupture. Demerol or some other analgesia can be given instead to relieve the pain.

☐ *What Are the Chances of Avoiding a Repeat Cesarean?*   From the present studies it seems there is better than a 50 percent chance of avoiding a repeat Cesarean. In one study of almost five thousand women, 68 percent of the women were allowed to enter labor. The rest were excluded because of complications in the current pregnancy. Sixty-seven percent of these women went on to have a normal vaginal delivery, while the others developed complications during the labor that necessitated a repeat Cesarean.

☐ *Will Your Doctor Agree to a Trial of Labor?*   Many doctors still routinely recommend a repeat Cesarean. But a number of doctors have accepted patients who want to attempt a vaginal delivery, with the understanding that a trial of labor does not guarantee a vaginal delivery. I believe that a woman who is fully informed and wants to attempt a vaginal delivery should be given the opportunity to do so, if the circumstances permit. The patient motivation is of course very important. Some women would rather not incur the risks or the uncertainty of a trial of labor and opt for a repeat Cesarean instead. No physician should pressure a woman into attempting a vaginal delivery when she is uncertain or fearful of the possible consequences.

Your obstetrician's circumstances may also influence his policy on repeat Cesareans. It may be impossible for an obstetrician in private practice to spend twenty-four hours or more monitoring the labor of one patient. Your first choice for a doctor is probably an obstetrician associated with a large medical center where an obstetrical staff is constantly at hand. A university hospital will also have blood bank facilities and a full range of emergency services.

☐ *Postoperative Care*   During the immediate postoperative period, you will usually be kept in bed for a period of six to eight hours. After that you will be encouraged to move around. If you have had general anesthesia you will be asked to get up and sit in a chair, since early mobility will help prevent complications, particularly blood clots (see Chap. 24) or pneumonia. If you have had an epidural, you might be kept in bed longer, but you can still change your position and breathe deeply to clear your lungs. The first few times out of bed, you should be accompanied by a nurse or someone in your family since you might feel faint.

The Foley catheter is usually kept in for twelve to twenty-four hours. If the Cesarean was performed during the night, it is usually taken out the next day, but it is good to keep it overnight so your sleep is not disturbed. The following day when the catheter is removed you should be able to move around on your own.

Intravenous fluids are usually continued for a few days after the Cesarean, depending on the hospital and your obstetrician. Fluids by mouth are usually allowed on the first day after the delivery, and you will be advanced to a regular diet within two or three days. A hospital will not put you on a regular diet immediately since your stomach is likely to be upset and you will vomit if you are given solid food too early. Many hospitals remove the intravenous feeding within twenty-four to forty-eight hours after a Cesarean section and encourage you to drink plenty of fluids. It doesn't matter what you eat initially; just drink enough fluids to prevent dehydration. You should also keep taking your prenatal vitamins after the birth. I always tell my patients to take two prenatal vitamins as soon as they begin to eat, after both a vaginal and an abdominal birth, to help the body heal more quickly. Extra vitamin C in particular will help you heal faster, since vitamin C both encourages womb healing and helps the body's retention of iron. You should continue to take vitamin C and prenatal vitamins for several weeks after you get home. If you are breast-feeding you need to continue the vitamins until you stop nursing the baby.

☐ *The Emotional Effect of Cesarean Birth*   Many women feel like a failure after a Cesarean birth. As more parents take childbirth classes in the hope of participating more fully in their children's births, parents whose births have not matched their plans or expectations often experience a deep sense of disappointment. A new mother may be jealous of other women who have given birth "successfully"; she may be angry or depressed; she may blame herself for her "loss of control" over the birth. The sense of failure may be particularly strong in a woman who has been able to control her life successfully in the past. Unfortunately, couples who have enthusiastically prepared for "an awake and aware" birth are often those who feel the disappointment most keenly. These feelings can persist for many weeks, or even months. Some Cesarean mothers find it difficult to establish breast-feeding, or are more ambivalent about caring for their newborns. This may be the result of a hospital's policy that routinely separates Cesarean mothers and children in the first twenty-four hours after birth.

Not all parents have such negative responses to a Cesarean birth. But you should be prepared for conflicting feelings if you do experience a Cesarean, particularly an emergency one. It is natural to feel a sense of inadequacy or failure, but you should remember that the decision to perform a Cesarean is purely a medical one. It has nothing to do with how well you were prepared for your baby's arrival or how well you dealt with labor and delivery.

The circumstances of her Cesarean can be expected to affect a woman's emotions in the postpartum period. Women have said they found it easier to cope with the aftermath of a Cesarean if they were fully informed at the time of the operation and understood why a vaginal birth would be impossible. If a woman and her husband feel their doctor honestly attempted to see them through a vaginal delivery, and resorted to a Cesarean only to safeguard the baby's health, they are likely to feel less guilty themselves about the Cesarean. If, on the other hand, a woman feels her doctor made a hasty decision or pushed her into an unnecessary Cesarean, she may not only hate her doctor but feel angry at herself because she was deprived of the experience of a natural birth.

If you do need counseling and help after a Cesarean birth, there are several organizations that will give you information or put you in touch with a support group in your area. Write to:

C-Sec Inc., Patricia Erikson, Membership, 23 Cedar Street, Cambridge, MA 02140

Cesarean Birth Association, 133–29 122 Street, South Ozone Park, NY 11420

Cesarean Birth Booklet, Westchester Chapter ASPO, Box 123, Scarsborough, Briarcliff Manor, NY 10510 (send $2.50 by mail).

There may also be local support groups you can contact.

32

The Joy of Breast-Feeding

Breast-feeding was once as natural to human beings as it is to other mammals that know no other way to feed their young. For centuries, breast-feeding was the only way a child could be fed, and breast milk knew no competition; it was as normal a source of nutrition for a baby as bread or meat was for an adult. Without nursing, the newborn had no hope of survival. Furthermore, breast-feeding fostered the closest possible contact between the mother and her child—a natural means of continuing the nurturing relationship after the umbilical cord was severed.

Until the nineteenth century all children were breast-fed unless death or abandonment made artificial feeding a necessity. Babies "reared by hand" rarely survived because feeding methods other than nursing were still primitive and unhygienic. Women who could not, or chose not to breast-feed, hired lactating women to nurse the baby for them. This surrogate mother, the wet nurse, occupied a prestigious position in the family and often played a significant role in the life of the child. For centuries the breast-feeding woman was a universally regarded symbol of a woman's devotion toward her child, and a powerful expression of femininity; one of the most popular themes of medieval and Renaissance painters was that of the Virgin offering her breast to the infant Jesus. In both art and literature, breast-feeding was always considered a central event in the life of the family.

It was not until the Industrial Revolution, when women left their homes and entered factories, that there was a need for widespread artificial feeding. Even after the baby bottle was generally available at the end of the nineteenth century, women who were able to feed their children themselves preferred to do so because bottles were unhygienic and it was impossible to store fresh milk successfully without refrigeration. Only among poor American and European fami-

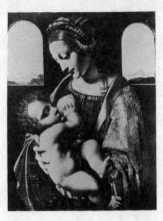

Figure 113: Breast-Feeding the Infant Jesus: The Virgin in this fifteenth-century Italian picture is wearing a typical maternity garment of the fifteenth and sixteenth centuries, which can be opened and closed for nursing. This detail indicates how naturally nursing was viewed at the time. The painting is from the workshop of Leonardo da Vinci; his pupil Ambrogio de Predis painted it between 1485 and 1490. The work is now in the Hermitage Museum in Leningrad.

lies did the bottle have any popularity until just before the Second World War, when bottle feeding suddenly became fashionable among middle-class women. The general introduction of bottle feeding has been called the biggest change in feeding practices since the invention of cooking. The idea that bottle feeding was a modern, scientific way to feed babies became accepted so quickly that the majority of American women abandoned breast-feeding and turned to the bottle instead. By the early 1960s, only 18 percent of American women bothered to establish breast-feeding, and many of them stopped nursing soon after leaving the hospital.

☐ ***The Rediscovery of Breast-Feeding***   In the past few years there has been an increasing interest in breast-feeding as natural childbirth methods have gained popularity and new evidence has emerged on the superiority of breast milk over formula feeding. Rates of breast-feeding have doubled in the last ten years, suggesting that women are not only convinced that breast milk is better but are ready to take the time and energy needed to breast-feed.

The breast-versus-bottle controversy is one that has been going on since the 1940s. Two decades ago, few doctors and pediatricians advocated breast-feeding because they felt it meant difficulties for the mother and incessant telephone calls to the doctor. Given the medical profession's confidence in formula feeding, it seemed easier for all involved to encourage a woman to bottle-feed. Now, influenced by the new research studies emphasizing the unique health benefits of breast-feeding, a subject that will be discussed later in this chapter, physicians as well as mothers are again beginning to appreciate its importance. Unfortunately, it is still only better-educated women who seem to favor the breast over the bottle: 48 percent of women in one study who breast-fed had at least twelve years of education, while only 24 percent of the babies born to the women with less than twelve years' schooling were breast-fed. I hope that one day every pregnant woman in our society will know enough about breast-feeding to help her make an informed decision about the way she feeds her child.

In clinics and hospitals where physicians as well as childbirth educators and maternity staff sponsor breast-feeding, up to 80 percent of women are now choosing to breast-feed. Most of these babies are still breast-fed for only a few weeks and then switched to formula. This provides the baby with some valuable immunity to disease but it does not give the baby the full health benefits of prolonged nursing. Nonetheless, the first few weeks are the time when the baby needs the superior nutrition and the immunological factors in breast milk, which cannot be duplicated by formula. A woman should not be afraid to nurse because she can nurse for only a short time, although ideally a child should be breast-fed for three months or longer.

Every woman should at least attempt to breast-feed, other than in very exceptional cases. At least 95 percent of American women are physically able to breast-feed successfully and the reasons that they do not are psychological, usually the result of anxiety, fear, or negative feelings about breast-feeding among family, friends, or physicians.

☐ *Myths About Breast-Feeding*   A number of persistent myths have encouraged women not to breast-feed. "You won't have enough milk" is one of them. This negative attitude is the result of ignorance about the mechanics of breast-feeding. Usually every woman has the ability to produce a good supply of milk if she knows what to do or is given help by a knowledgeable relative or a professional. Once the milk supply is well established, a woman should have no problem feeding her child.

A second, equally destructive myth is that breast-feeding is tiring. A surprising number of women believe that it is more exhausting than bottle-feeding, even though there is no special preparation involved with breast-feeding as there is with bottle-feeding. The breast-fed baby does require more attention at the beginning than the bottle-fed child, but once breast-feeding is well established, mother and baby usually develop a rhythm that allows four to six hours between feeds; enough time for a reasonable night's sleep. The fact that some breast-feeding women are harried and exhausted has more to do with the sudden responsibility of a young child than breast-feeding per se.

"Breast-feeding hurts." Many women are deterred from breast-feeding because they believe it is painful. Again, this is not necessarily true. The initial period of engorgement is sometimes uncomfortable but it passes in a few days, and once the milk flow is well established a woman usually enjoys nursing. If there is pain, it is because the let-down reflex is hindered by insufficient rest, anxiety, or some other surmountable problem. Problems with sore or cracked nipples are lessened if you learn to toughen them before you begin nursing, a simple process which is described later in this chapter.

Finally, there is the belief that "breast-feeding spoils the figure." This is perhaps the most pervasive myth of all. Our culture is one that sees the breasts as objects of eroticism rather than a source of nourishment, so it is not surprising that women won't risk losing their youthful appearance or that many men still prefer their partners not to breast-feed. The truth is that breast-feeding does not ruin the figure. Breast shape changes with the first pregnancy whether the woman breast-feeds or not, but the degree to which the breast tissue becomes softer during pregnancy is determined by other factors as well, including heredity and age. A woman who decides to breast-feed need only buy a good nursing bra that gives her breasts full support to avoid the exaggerated stretching falsely associated with nursing. Nursing may even improve a woman's physical appearance because the extra fat built up around the hips and waist during pregnancy disappears gradually during lactation.

☐ **Why Is Breast-Feeding Important?** Breast-feeding might well help your infant to a better life. There is good evidence that breast-fed babies have fewer serious illnesses, especially gastrointestinal and respiratory illnesses, than bottle-fed babies, and this immunity to certain diseases seems to persist even after a baby has been weaned to the bottle. According to some recent research, mother's milk may naturally protect a child against obesity, promote brain development, and guard against serious adult disorders such as heart disease. It is of course more economical and convenient, and, depending on the parents, usually more emotionally satisfying for mother, father, and baby than formula feeding. A woman who is breast-feeding can take pride in using a natural resource rather than a substitution.

The contents of breast milk meet the specific needs of the human infant. In certain vital ways it is quite different from cow's milk, goat's milk, or any other source of infant nutrition. It also contains antibodies and sensitized white blood cells that provide the infant with a natural immunity to a large number of infections and may, possibly, protect babies against the development of food allergies in later life. Mother's milk apparently contains antibodies to virtually all strains of infectious organisms a newborn is exposed to. The natural protection offered by mother's milk is so powerful that even babies nursed as little as one month gain some resistance to disease, although the advantages are greater the longer the baby is nursed. One researcher who compared formula-fed and breast-fed babies found one-third fewer serious illnesses among the breast-fed group in the first year, while the formula-fed children were fifteen times more likely to experience a respiratory infection and two and a half times more likely to suffer vomiting and diarrhea. The bottle-fed babies were nine times more likely to be admitted to the hospital before their first birthdays than the breast-fed babies. In one British study, the sudden infant death syndrome was far more common among bottle-fed babies than breast-fed babies.

☐ **Cow's Milk Is for Calves** Infant formulas have generally been based on the constituents of cow's milk, in the belief that cow's milk is as beneficial for the baby as human milk. In recent years this assumption has been seriously questioned. There are significant differences between human and cow's milk that were not appreciated in the days when obstetricians and pediatricians encouraged formulas rather than breast-feeding. Human milk is considerably lower in protein than cow's milk, a fact that might appear to favor cow's milk unless one compares the special needs of calves and human infants. A calf, which becomes independent of its mother after the first few months, requires a food that increases growth rapidly and encourages muscle mass. The human infant, on the other hand, is dependent on its mother for a number of years. Muscle, therefore, is less important than the development of the central nervous system and a gradual increase in weight through a steady supply of small amounts of protein. The rapid weight gain and large body size that we think of as healthy may in fact be an undesirable side effect of universal bottle feeding, since the bottle-fed child continues to require large amounts of protein in later life, with the risk of obesity, heart disease, and breast and colon cancer in middle age.

Not only does human milk contain four times less protein than cow's milk but the constituents of the proteins themselves are quite different. Easily digestible proteins abound in human milk, while cow's milk consists mostly of casein, which is much harder for the baby to digest and increases the tendency to constipation and hard stools among bottle-fed babies. Breast milk also naturally contains high amounts of the amino acid cystine, and low amounts of another amino acid, phenylalanine. Phenylalanine is relatively high in cow's milk, another disadvantage of formula feeding, because large amounts are metabolized slowly by the human infant. Another important amino acid is taurine, a substance which seems to promote nerve development and may stimulate the growth of the human brain. This is found in relatively high amounts in breast milk but not in cow's milk.

One of the reasons why breast-fed babies seem to have fewer digestive problems than bottle-fed babies is that the lipids in human milk, which contain over 40 percent of its calories, are highly absorbent. The fats in human milk are also quite different from the fats in cow's milk or formula since they are, perhaps surprisingly, unusually high in cholesterol. The long-term function of this is unknown, but it may be that the high serum cholesterol concentration in human milk stimulates enzymes that allow the individual to fight off high cholesterol levels later in life. More immediately, they help to protect the infant from infectious organisms in the immature gut, which might otherwise cause gastrointestinal problems. Potential problems from the high cholesterol content of human milk are undoubtedly mitigated because breast milk lipids are generally polyunsaturated fatty acids rather than the saturated animal fats found in cow's milk.

Another advantage of human milk is its superior vitamin and mineral content. Cow's milk is a poor source of vitamins C and E, copper, and iron, although commercial formulas are generally fortified with extra vitamins and minerals. The iron content of human milk is relatively low by the standard of other foods but it is virtually completely absorbable, removing the need for supplementary iron during the breast-feeding period.

Given this new evidence on the health benefits of breast milk, it is not surprising that the American Academy of Pediatrics believes that breast milk is "the best food for every newborn human infant." If the baby cannot be breast-fed, a woman and her pediatrician should select a formula that as much as possible imitates human milk.

☐　*How Breast Milk Protects the Newborn*　Breast milk protects the infant from several sources of major infection. The newborn emerges from the nine months of gestation with certain natural protections against infection already inherited from its mother across the placenta. These are the antibodies known as type IgG, which give the fetus and the newborn months of protection from bacterial and viral diseases to which the mother herself is immune. Another important group of antibodies, those known as IgA, can however be supplied only through human milk, and those the baby receives during the breast-feeding period. These are the antibodies that protect the otherwise vulnerable newborn from coli bacteria and other microorganisms in the intestinal walls. Interestingly, colostrum, the "first" milk, is even higher in bacteria-fighting substances than ordinary breast milk. Between one million and three million macrophage cells, which have the ability to absorb bacteria, viruses, and fungi are secreted daily in breast milk, providing the infant with defenses against respiratory illnesses, bacterial diarrhea, and allergy-triggering substances. Breast-fed babies from families with severe allergies have fewer allergic reactions in later life than bottle-fed siblings. Breast milk may also act to protect the infant by stimulating its immature antibody system early in life.

☐ *Breast Milk and Brain Development*   Breast milk promotes brain development in the period immediately after birth when the brain is still immature. This is another reason why formulas containing a higher protein content than breast milk may not be good for the newborn, especially the premature newborn. A high protein content encourages the build-up of blood tyrosine levels, which seems to foster certain learning disorders later in life. Among one group of prematures fed formula, learning disabilities were far more common than among a similar group who were breast-fed. Breast milk also contains taurine, an important amino acid in the development of the newborn brain. Again, these are factors that encourage breast-feeding rather than formula feeding.

☐ *Bonding and Breast-Feeding*   Breast-feeding is a natural continuation of the bonding begun before a baby is born. A breast-feeding baby not only hears the reassuring sound of the mother's heartbeat but enjoys intimate contact with the mother through touch, warmth (the breasts become warmer during nursing), smell (newborns have an acute sense of smell and can distinguish their mothers from other women within a few days of birth), and eye contact. When the baby cries the mother picks him up; at the same time the blood flow increases to the breasts, encouraging the flow of milk. Each of these stimuli reinforces the close relationship between the newborn and the mother, and continues to reinforce it throughout the nursing period. Interestingly, prolactin, the hormone responsible for the milk flow, is a "love" hormone in birds, encouraging the female to take care of the nest and nestlings. The natural increase in prolactin just before the baby nurses may be nature's way of fostering attachment between human mothers and their babies. No wonder that women who enjoy breast-feeding often talk about a special intimacy during the nursing period and look back on nursing as one of the most satisfying experiences of their lives.

The long-term effect on breast-fed babies is difficult to estimate, although they are generally more peaceful and contented, have less colic, and sleep more quietly than bottle-fed babies. Early experiences, including feeding, do undoubtedly influence later behavior, but exactly how is unknown. Certainly anything that fosters the relationship between mother and child must increase a child's sense of security and self-confidence later on.

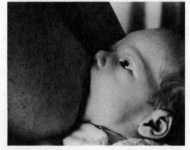

Figure 114

Breast-feeding can, and should, begin either directly after the delivery or within a few hours after birth. Before hospitals routinely separated mothers and babies after birth, the baby was always put to the breast immediately and encouraged to nurse. This firmly established the mother-child relationship within a few minutes of birth, following the behavioral pattern seen in animals. There are not only biological reasons for early nursing but psychological advantages as well. In the first few hours after birth the baby is unusually alert and responsive to both parents, making it an optimal time for bonding and beginning nursing. Parents who are given the opportunity to bond with their babies in the first twelve hours after delivery are, according to two celebrated researchers on bonding, Drs. Marshall Klaus and John Kennell, more likely to show affectionate behavior several months later than parents denied early contact. A baby who is breast-fed in the "sensitive period" is also more likely to be breast-fed several months later than a baby who begins nursing after the sensitive period is over.

In their famous book *Maternal-Infant Bonding*, Klaus and Kennell made no distinction in the matter of bonding between the breast-feeding mother and the nonbreast-feeding mother who bonds early with her baby. However, they talk about the more intimate involvement of the breast-feeding pair as compared to the bottle-feeding pair. It is my own observation, however, that breast-fed babies seem much closer to their mothers and appear to be more adjusted later in life than bottle-fed children. I would certainly advise all mothers to try to breast-feed their babies even if it is for only a short time. The initial bonding associated with nursing can be of great importance in a mother's later relationship with her child.

☐ **Sexual Feelings During Nursing**   Breast-feeding does seem to heighten sexual pleasure. The uterus contracts with the release of oxytocin from the brain during nursing periods; these contractions are often experienced as a deep, warm, pleasurable feeling similar to that experienced during orgasm. Interestingly, even though nursing mothers generally do not ovulate for several months after the birth, which would normally inhibit sexual pleasure, women who breast-feed seem to have a greater desire for sexual relations than women who do not breast-feed. Masters and Johnson, who originally made this observation, also interviewed women who were so disturbed by this aspect of breast-feeding that they gave it up, feeling it was somehow "perverted." Women have nursed daughters but not sons for the same reason. Again, these are women who are not confident sexually or are worried about their sexual relations with their partner. Breast-feeding should be viewed as something as natural—and as enjoyable—as a loving sexual relationship.

☐ **Why Don't More Women Breast-Feed?**   One of the biggest factors in choosing or not choosing to breast-feed is a woman's attitude toward her body. If she and her mate regard the breasts solely as sex objects, it can be very difficult to breast-feed without feelings of shame or embarrassment. A number of women who try nursing quickly give it up because they associate it with a sexual act or they find it physically pleasurable and therefore threatening. When a woman cannot accept nursing as part of the biological role of motherhood, it is almost impossible for her to nurse successfully, even if she understands the health advantages of breast-feeding. The habit of regarding bodily secretions as "unclean" is also difficult to overcome for some women. It is not unusual to hear a woman refer to breast-feeding as "icky." These cultural attitudes to nursing can be expected to change, although slowly, as women become more at ease with themselves physically. Change would come more quickly if nursing were accepted as a normal part of life, as it is in non-Western countries, instead of expecting the breast-feeding mother to retire modestly into her bedroom when she has to feed the baby. If we saw more women breast-feeding at work or in public places, the breasts would soon stop being purely a sex object, and far more women would be encouraged to breast-feed.

☐ *Preparation for Breast-Feeding*   Every woman should at least attempt to breast-feed. One good way to diminish anxieties about breast-feeding is to understand how breast-feeding works.

☐ *Anatomy of the Breast*   The breast is mostly built of fatty tissues, smooth-muscle tissues, and glands, and is held against the chest with the pectoral muscles. The milk-production mechanism in the breast exists from the time of puberty but is dormant unless a woman is pregnant. It is made up of the milk glands, tiny glands which secrete the milk and then release it into the milk ducts when it is needed. Stimulation is provided by the hormone prolactin, which is produced by the pituitary gland. The prolactin level increases slowly during pregnancy and then increases rapidly immediately before and after delivery. Under the influence of the pituitary hormone, milk production is increased in the milk glands, and the milk is then led through a network of milk ducts, all of which are surrounded by the fine smooth muscles which, through contraction, lead the milk out toward the larger ducts in the area of the areola and nipple. If the stimulation is very strong, milk can spray out or drip out rapidly.

ANATOMY OF THE BREAST

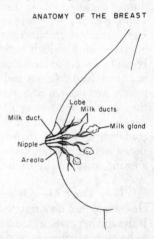

Lobe
Milk ducts
Milk duct
Milk gland
Nipple
Areola

Figure 115: Fifteen to twenty milk ducts are clustered just behind the areolar tissue, each one receiving milk from the corresponding milk gland in the breast. Each duct leads to the main duct that passes the milk through the nipple.

The central portion where the ducts collect is the nipple. When the baby begins to suck, the nerves around the nipple and areola send messages to the brain to release the precursor of the hormone oxytocin from the hypothalamus. Oxytocin is then directed to the pituitary, from which it is led into the bloodstream and carried to the breast again. Here it acts on the small, smooth muscles, which begin to contract and push the milk toward the nipple. The release of oxytocin occurs not only when the baby stimulates the nipple but when the breast is touched or stimulated manually. During lovemaking, for instance, milk is often excreted spontaneously. Oxytocin can also be released mentally when a mother hears her baby cry. In each case, oxytocin release stimulates the *milk reflex.* Although every woman who has a normal hormonal system will develop milk glands during pregnancy, some form of stimulation is always needed in order to begin and maintain the milk reflex. Without suckling or other stimulation, milk production will cease. Beginning and maintaining this "let-down" mechanism is the key to successful breast-feeding.

☐ ***Does Breast Size Make Any Difference?***   The size of the breasts is no indication of how much milk a breast can produce. Women with small breasts have been known to produce quantities of milk, while women with large breasts might produce considerably less. The size of your breasts should not have any bearing on whether or not you decide to breast-feed. As a normal, healthy woman you should certainly be able to breast-feed successfully.

☐ ***Breast Asymmetry***   It is not unusual for one breast to be larger than the other. Anatomical structures are often asymmetrical; a man, for instance, has a larger testicle on one side than the other. Differences in breast size sometimes

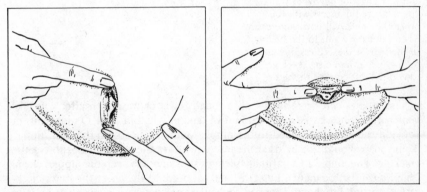

Figure 116: Hoffman's Exercise: This exercise is particularly good for inverted nipples. Even if your nipples are not inverted, you can use the exercise during pregnancy to help prepare for breast feeding.

become more prominent with pregnancy, but the larger breast does not produce more milk than the other; it is just a physiological change and should not worry you or prevent you from breast-feeding.

☐ ***Inverted Nipples***   Nipples come in different shapes and sizes. Some nipples are prominent, others are flat until stimulated; others are inverted, with the center of the nipple pulled inward. An inverted nipple is usually the result of some adhesion in the breast tissue that occurred during breast development. Flat nipples are often confused with inverted nipples, but a completely inverted nipple is rare and can readily be distinguished because it is folded inside the skin. If you are among the few women who have inverted nipples, a special exercise called Hoffman's exercise can be used to prepare for breast-feeding. This exercise consists of placing the forefinger and thumb on the edge of the areola, pressing them into the breast, and then stretching the skin from side to side. Skin adhesions at the base of the nipple will then be slowly stretched out and the nipple released. Do this several times a day for a few months before the birth. It is not too late to begin Hoffman's exercise immediately after delivery.

☐ *Preparing the Breasts for Breast-Feeding*   Nipples are often unduly sensitive when a woman begins breast-feeding because Western culture encourages bras and other soft clothing that discourage exposure to friction or the air. Women with fair skins are often unusually susceptible to the problem of sore nipples. You can begin to prepare for breast-feeding one or two months before the birth by toughening the nipples and performing breast exercises designed to stimulate the milk flow.

Figure 117: Finger Exercise: If you roll each nipple between your fingers just prior to breast-feeding you will stimulate the milk-ejection reflex. Roll the nipple between the thumb and first finger of one hand while you massage the breast with the other. The milk will flow more easily when the baby is put to the breast, so the baby will exert less pressure on the nipples as he sucks—a good way to prevent cracked nipples.

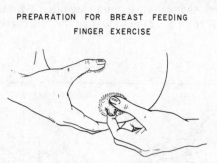

PREPARATION FOR BREAST FEEDING
FINGER EXERCISE

The nipples can be rubbed with a rough towel or washcloth after you take your bath or shower. A small amount of lanolin, vitamin A or D ointment, or baby oil can then be applied to the nipples and areola to keep the skin supple. Toilet soap should not be used because it will dry the skin and possibly cause cracking. The nipple area naturally secretes substances to keep the nipples clean. Nipples can be toughened by occasional exposure to the air or the outer clothing. A nursing bra, bought toward the end of pregnancy, is convenient because you can open the center flap and expose the nipples while still supporting the breasts.

Breast exercises are not essential to good nursing, but they are useful. These can be done alone, or in combination with your partner, who might enjoy stimulating the breasts orally and manually. A gentle sucking simulates the suction of the baby and helps to encourage the let-down reflex essential to good breast-feeding.

Simple nipple-rolling exercises should be done once or twice a day. Place the nipple between your finger and thumb and pull it out firmly enough so you feel it, but not enough so it hurts. As you draw the nipple forward, hold it there for a few seconds and then roll it between your fingers for a minute or two. Your husband can do this for you. Then rub lanolin or some other ointment into the areola and onto the side of the nipples. *Note:* Don't be tempted to stimulate the breast to such a degree that you excrete colostrum before the birth. This could trigger release of the hormone oxytocin, which might stimulate premature labor. There is no particular benefit to encouraging the secretion of colostrum before the birth.

☐ *Prenatal Advice for Women Who Want to Breast-Feed*   Professional help for women who want to breast-feed is unfortunately still rather unreliable. Some hospitals are not interested in breast-feeding or their staffs are too busy to help mothers establish nursing. It would be wise to take a breast-feeding class through the La Leche League or your natural-childbirth instructor to make sure you have a good initial preparation for breast-feeding. One essential step is to make sure your obstetrician, midwife, or the staff in the maternity ward know you want to breast-feed. This information should be clearly understood, since certain hospitals still give routine injections or medications to dry up milk after delivery. Also make sure the nursery staff and your pediatrician know you want to breast-feed the baby whenever he or she is hungry. This will prevent the nursery nurses from giving a supplementary bottle rather than bringing the baby in for feedings that do not conform to the normal schedule. (A hospital with twenty-four-hour rooming in is always the first choice for a nursing mother.) You should establish nursing early—the colostrum may look less nutritious than bottled formula, but it is ideally suited to the needs of the very young baby.

Immediately after the birth, hold the baby to your breasts to help establish the sucking reflex. Early on, the sucking reflex is well established and the breast is easy to grasp. Later, as the breast fills up with milk it becomes full and hard, and sucking is more difficult for the baby and more uncomfortable for the mother. Additionally, the loss of the first feed denies the baby the valuable colostrum, the nutritious fluid that provides protein and early antibody protection. Once the baby has experienced sucking in the delivery room or soon after delivery, he or she will have no difficulty in establishing nursing a day or two later when the full supply of milk comes in.

☐ *Factors Influencing the Ability to Nurse a Baby*   As I have already mentioned, the size of the breasts is no indication of your ability to produce milk. The breasts change during pregnancy, whatever their original shape or density, and a small breast has the same number of milk glands as a larger breast. To some extent, breast-feeding does depend on the amount of chemical stimulation released by your hormones, a factor that is not under your control. Nonetheless, these hormones are related to those present in pregnancy and delivery, and even women who have premature babies produce milk. This natural supply of milk can be stimulated to breast-feed the child successfully.

One important element in successful breast-feeding is an adequate, well balanced diet. Try to resist the desire to lose all your weight in the immediate postpartum period; hormonal changes continue to occur in the weeks after birth, and the body must be in a healthy condition. The remaining weight is designed to sustain you through the early nursing period and will then be shed naturally. The body stores about two to four pounds of extra fat during pregnancy as an energy supply for lactation, which provides about two hundred extra calories a day for the first one hundred days of nursing. In all, a lactating mother should increase the calorie content of her diet by about five hundred calories over the pregnancy period during the first three months of breast-feeding and increase her protein intake by about twenty grams. Other requirements—calcium, minerals, and vitamins—remain much the same as they do during pregnancy, although you need extra vitamin C, A, and the B's during lactation. In general, a woman's diet affects a woman's milk less than you would think. A poorly nourished woman will still produce good quality milk, although it will be lower in certain amino acids than the well nourished woman's. The main sufferer is the woman herself, since nature acts to protect the baby at the expense of the mother.

Fluids are important. A nursing woman needs at least three quarts of fluids a day. This may consist of anything you like to drink, not just milk. Although large amounts of alcohol are harmful to the baby, a light cocktail or a glass of wine might even help you to relax before a feeding and stimulate the milk flow.

The body is consuming extra energy in producing enough milk for the baby and in meeting the demands of feedings around the clock. A short nap in the middle of the day and extra rest at all times will help provide the body with a

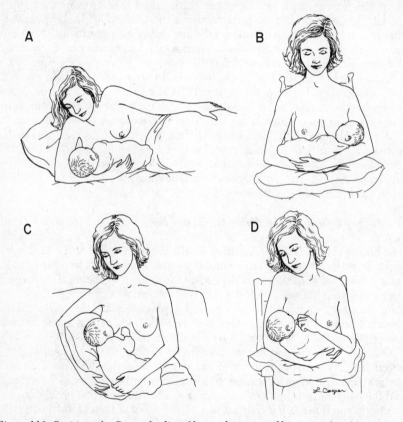

Figure 118: Positions for Breast-feeding: If you place yourself in a comfortable position for breast-feeding you will avoid unnecessary stress. You might find that lying on your side with your arm around the baby is the most comfortable (A). Another possible position is to sit up and cradle the baby resting on a pillow (B). If you have had a Cesarean birth you might find position A to be comfortable, or you might want to put one or two pillows on one side and rest the baby on the pillows with your arms around him (C). Many women feel the most comfortable sitting in a chair with an arm rest. Place pillows or blankets on your lap to help support the baby and then place the baby at the breast. You can continue to hold the baby for long periods of time without tiring yourself.

good balance in the first few weeks at home. Exhaustion, unfortunately, is a common reason for switching to bottle feeding, even though breast-feeding is not really more tiring than bottle feeding.

Emotional relaxation is an important, and underestimated, factor in breast-feeding. Milk secretion is, to a certain degree, influenced by the mother's emotional state, since the action of the hypothalamus is affected when the mother is tense and upset. Milk production ceases only on rare occasions, but a mother who is tense is more likely to experience difficulty than a calmer woman. It is always a good idea to prepare yourself beforehand and have confidence in your abilities to breast-feed before you begin. I have frequently seen an emotional upset or state of tension diminish the flow of milk temporarily and the woman become frustrated because the baby was not taking the breast well enough or seemed dissatisfied after a feeding. As soon as the woman calmed down, the full flow returned.

One way to decrease anxiety is to relax as you sit down to nurse, using your prenatal relaxation breathing exercises to decrease physical tension. Breathe slowly and calmly and relax your face, shoulder and leg muscles as you begin to nurse. A glass of wine is helpful for some women, or you might like to play a favorite piece of music. Nursing is an experience to be savored; don't try to combine it with other activities or rush through it—satisfaction and pleasure come with calm, concentrated nursing. One of the pleasant side effects of nursing is the emotional tranquillity breast-feeding mothers usually experience once nursing is well established. Again, this is undoubtedly a natural occurence that protects mothers and babies in the important nursing period. The mood cycle during lactation is more even because ovulation and menstruation, with their hormonal variations, are suppressed for the first few months.

Be confident: as long as you are relaxed you will be able to breast-feed.

☐ **The First Feed** Ideally a baby will have the first feed immediately after birth and then again six hours later. During this first day, nursing time should be kept short to prevent your nipples from becoming sore. If you have had anesthesia the baby, too, may appear sleepy and uninterested at first until he or she has become adjusted to life outside the womb. There is no reason to be concerned; the baby is born with enough energy reserves to survive well without nourishment for the first few hours. Babies normally lose about 10 percent of their initial birth weight in the first few days of life without any detrimental effect because the newborn has a natural store of extra fluid in the body tissues. By the second or third breast-feeding the baby usually seems more alert and interested in nursing.

Feedings are best given on demand when the baby is hungry. The traditional four-hour schedule followed in the hospital is not conducive to breast-feeding. Breast-fed babies usually like to nurse at least once every three hours at the beginning. Instead of waiting for a scheduled feed, ask the nurse to bring the baby to you when he or she seems restless and ready to nurse. A crying baby should be brought in to you and *not* given a supplementary bottle in the nursery. Supplementary bottles at this early stage are a good way to make a child lose interest in breast-feeding. This does not preclude the bottle of glucose water given after each breast-feeding in the first few days to increase the baby's fluid intake. Once your milk has come in, the glucose water can be safely discontinued.

Initial periods of nursing should be kept short, not longer than five minutes on each breast on the first day. If the baby sucks too long, tender nipples can become damaged and cracked. One way to avoid sore nipples is to make sure the baby grasps the *whole nipple and most of the areola* to encourage proper suction and does not pull on the nipple as he or she is taken from the breast. Generally any temporary soreness that does appear in the first few days disappears naturally as you continue to nurse, but any area of redness or tenderness should be examined by a nurse, who can supply you with a nipple shield, a gauze shield placed over the breast that discourages the baby from sucking right on the tender nipples.

When you begin to nurse, make yourself comfortable in bed or sit down in a low chair that gives support to your arms. If you have had an episiotomy, the most comfortable position is usually a side-lying one with the baby lying on the bed next to you. Then hold the baby close to your breast so that its cheek touches the nipple and stimulates the let-down reflex. Babies will generally move the head from side to side to find the nipple (the rooting reflex); this encourages the nipple to become erect and makes it easier to grasp. If your baby does not grasp the nipple spontaneously, you can guide it into his or her mouth. You can tell whether or not the baby is sucking successfully by the up and down pressure of the jaw on the areola area, a motion which encourages the milk ducts to release their stored milk and triggers the reflexes that cause milk production. A baby biting down on the nipple rather than the whole areola will cause a painful sensation which can be prevented by removing the baby from the breast and beginning again with the correct nursing technique. The baby can be removed gently from the breast by pressing the breast away from the corner of the mouth with your forefinger to break the suction, and then slipping your finger into his or her mouth.

It is a good idea to use both breasts at one feeding session since emptying each breast helps to prevent clogging of the milk ducts. You can start with five minutes on each side and then gradually increase the length of each feed to twenty or thirty minutes, encouraging the baby to empty the first breast in the first ten minutes or so when he or she is really hungry, and then changing to the second breast for the rest of the feed. Then begin the next feed with the breast used last in the previous feed.

Help the baby bring up air before you offer the second breast and after nursing is completed; burping will release any trapped gas from the stomach. Breast-fed babies tend to take in less air than bottle-fed babies but burping is still part of the feeding routine, a fact that a patient of mine, who insisted on leaving the hospital a few hours after the birth, failed to understand. Her baby did well for about twenty-four hours and then almost died when he aspirated with the build-up of gas in the lungs. The mother had never realized that burping was important.

By the third or fourth day the full milk supply is beginning to come in and by the end of the second week breast-feeding will be well established. You should expect to feed the baby not less often than five times a day, with extra nursing time during periods of rapid growth (see page 561).

☐ *Approximate Nursing Times*   On the first day the baby should be nursed for approximately five minutes on both breasts. By the third day the time can be lengthened to ten minutes on each breast; the fourth day, fifteen minutes; and the fifth, fifteen to twenty minutes. Sometimes a baby will go on sucking after he or she is full because the sensation is enjoyable; this time should be limited in the first few days, as otherwise your nipples will become cracked or sore.

☐ *What Is the Difference Between Colostrum and Mature Milk?* Colostrum is the thick yellowish fluid secreted before birth and in the first days after delivery. It is rich in protein, and contains more minerals and less carbohydrate and fat than mature human milk. The antibody protection it offers is ever superior to that of the mature milk. Colostrum continues to be secreted during the first four weeks of nursing while the mature milk is coming in. Mature milk has a thinner consistency than colostrum, and a whitish-bluish appearance, rather like that of skimmed cow's milk.

☐ *Engorgement* Engorgement is the swelling of the breasts that accompanies the second stage of milk production when the mature milk begins to come in the second or third day after birth. The breasts often become full, hard, and tender, making nursing difficult. Increased vascularity in the breast tissues and increased blood flow in the veins as well as the extra milk contribute to the characteristic symptoms. Engorgement can be temporarily upsetting and painful but it will not prevent you from continuing to breast-feed successfully; quite the contrary, there will be plenty of milk once proper lactation is established.

Engorgement may affect the areola area or the body of the breast or both areas at once. With an engorged areola, the baby is unable to grasp anything but the nipple. This makes nursing extremely painful for the mother and frustrating for the infant, since the milk ducts are not being stimulated. The best way to overcome this is to gently press out a small quantity of milk from each breast, using the technique described below ("Hand Expression of Milk"). Once the milk has been stimulated manually, the baby can be put to the breast. Compressing the areola between two fingers as you induce the baby to nurse will make the breast easier to grasp. As soon as the baby begins to nurse vigorously, the milk flow will return.

When the body of the breast is engorged, the breasts may become uncomfortably tense and warm to the touch. If this occurs, the first step is to wear a nursing bra that gives the breasts support. This should be worn day and night until the period of engorgement is over. The best way to release the milk flow is to stimulate the breasts during a warm shower or to place a warm towel directly on the breasts. The heat and massage act as signals to the pituitary, which in turn releases the oxytocin that stimulates the milk let-down. Once the breasts have been stimulated manually, the baby is usually capable of releasing the rest of the milk through suction. Any remaining milk should be hand-expressed after the feeding is over, since complete drainage of the milk ducts is the key to preventing engorgement. A hand pump or electric breast pump might be needed for a few days to keep the milk flowing freely. As soon as the milk let-down is fully established, through whatever means, you should have no further difficulty with engorgement. One of the advantages of starting breast-feeding soon after delivery is that women who do so experience less engorgement than the average breast-feeding mother.

☐ *Hand Expression of Milk*   Expressing milk through massage is similar to the natural suction of the baby and should be learned by every woman who plans to breast-feed. The best teacher is a sympathetic nurse or another breast-feeding woman. You can familiarize yourself with the techniques before the birth, but as I have already mentioned, it is unwise to begin hand-expressing colostrum during pregnancy because it may stimulate premature labor. Before you begin, wash your hands thoroughly and rub lanolin or skin cream into the palms of your hands. Then support the left breast with your left hand (most women find it easier to express the left breast with their right hand and vice versa) and squeeze the milk reservoir area behind the areola with your right hand, placing the tips of the thumb and first finger or middle finger on the opposite sides of the areola, just on the outer edge of the areola area. Press the thumb into the breast and then squeeze the finger and thumb together, repeating the motion at short rhythmic intervals. The pressure must be firm to express the first drops of milk, but after that the milk will come in more easily. Remember not to allow

Figure 119: Manual Exercise: Every breast-feeding woman should learn how to express milk from the breasts manually. Manual expression after a feed will help make sure that the breast is empty. It is a particularly important technique in the days before the milk flow is established, since it will help prevent breast engorgement. The breast must be massaged gently from the outer portion to the center in order to stimulate the breast glands and encourage the milk to enter the nipples. Once the milk appears you can begin to express the milk to make sure that the first drops are flowing freely. After this the baby will find it easier to take to the breast.

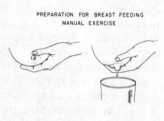

PREPARATION FOR BREAST FEEDING
MANUAL EXERCISE

the fingers to slide over the skin of the areola or to touch the nipple itself—pressure should be used only in the area behind the nipple to avoid hurting the tender areas of the breast. Once the milk is flowing you can move the thumb and finger around to the other side of the areola to make sure that all the milk glands are emptied. Extra milk can be collected in a jar and used for feeding of premature infants or stored in the refrigerator. Hand expression can be tiring at first, but the hands become stronger with practice and you will soon learn to massage the breasts efficiently. This technique is useful in the first week when you are establishing nursing; it is not one that is used much in the normal course of breast-feeding unless you want to store bottles of breast milk while you are away from the baby for a few hours.

☐ *Should a Breast Pump Be Used?*   There is nothing wrong with using a breast pump if you have a hard time expressing milk by hand. Most hospitals have hand breast pumps available. Ask the nurses on the labor floor to help you locate a hand or electric pump when breast-feeding is difficult during the first week.

A hand-held pump is placed around the nipple and the balloon section pressed to create a vacuum. This encourages the milk to flow into a container positioned underneath the pump (see Fig. 120). You might at the same time massage the milk ducts and the upper portion of the breasts to help let the milk down. The milk can then be collected to feed the baby temporarily while you establish nursing, or you can feed the baby yourself once the breast pump has relieved the initial engorgement. Encourage the baby to feed directly from the breast if you can; a baby who regularly drinks breast milk from a bottle might not want the extra work of sucking from the breast itself.

HAND BREAST PUMP

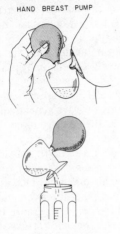

Figure 120: Breast Pump: A hand-held or electrical breast pump can be useful in the first few days if you find it difficult to establish the milk flow. Massage the breast gently first or press a hot towel to the breast to stimulate the milk ducts. Then place the breast pump over the nipple. At first the bow syringe is pushed in so that a vacuum occurs. After this the milk will flow into the attached flask. The use of the pump will expel milk more quickly than by hand expression and is invaluable if the mother wants to store breast milk in bottles while she is away from the baby for a few hours. Women who have their babies in the premature nursery can produce milk even though the baby is not ready to feed from the breast itself. Another use of the breast pump is to help evacuate unwanted milk if breast engorgement has occurred.

The Engell electrical breast pump is even more efficient than the hand-held type in relieving engorgement, as long as it is used with care. You can ask the nursing station to supply you with an Engell pump, or you can rent one from a medical supply store for a few days when you get home. Avoid the old-fashioned type of electric breast pump; they are dangerous and resemble instruments of torture! Both hand and electric breast pumps are helpful to women who have initial difficulties in establishing the let-down reflex and there is nothing to be ashamed of in using one. They are also invaluable when the baby is premature. A woman can use a breast pump to express a regular supply of milk for the baby as well as keeping her milk reflex going until the baby is mature enough to suck directly from the breasts. It requires persistence to feed a premature baby yourself, but many women have done so successfully.

☐ *Can You Store Your Milk?* While mothers and babies can often travel together or enjoy other normal activities without being separated, a woman who needs to be away from home does not have to resort to formula feeding. Breast milk can be expressed by hand or breast pump and stored in a sterile bottle in the refrigerator or freezer. Studies show that human milk can be safely stored in a deep-freeze unit for about three years, in a large freezer unit for up to four months, and the small freezer compartment of a standard refrigerator for about two weeks. In other words, a woman can go to work or even be away for a considerable period of time and still feed the baby with her own milk.

Breast milk's storage qualities have encouraged unpaid volunteers to donate extra breast milk to babies who are sick or who cannot tolerate formula. A voluntary organization of mothers called *Milk for Life* has provided hundreds of gallons of human milk for children whose mothers are unable to feed their sick babies themselves or whose babies are allergic to formula.

☐ *Breast-Feeding After a Cesarean*   There is no reason not to breast-feed after a Cesarean. Breast-feeding can not only be initiated successfully, it is as desirable after a Cesarean as it is after a vaginal birth. The production of milk is not usually affected by the procedure because the milk let-down reflex is dependent not on the method of delivery but on the release of hormones after the birth of the placenta. In other words, a Cesarean birth makes no difference in the natural sequence of events. The only problem is that a woman may not feel alert enough to nurse in the first day or so after anesthesia.

Even with a Cesarean, a woman should ideally begin nursing immediately. As long as you are given regional anesthesia, you can breast-feed the baby in the delivery room and take it with you into the recovery room—if you and your doctor agree. (Some hospitals still insist on keeping the baby in a special-care unit under observation for a period of time after birth.) If you have general anesthesia, most hospitals keep the baby in an incubator in the delivery room but let you hold the baby when you are awake to encourage bonding after delivery. When mother and baby are separated for a longer period after birth, milk can be expressed by hand until the baby is ready to begin feeding. Women who are given a prophylactic antibiotic after a Cesarean might sometimes face difficulties, since the antibiotic will cross into the milk. It is important for you and your obstetrician to discuss breast-feeding in advance of the delivery because he can prescribe, for example, penicillin or ampicillin, which are safe for use during breast-feeding.

Breast-feeding after a Cesarean can be uncomfortable at first because the incision often makes it difficult to sit up in bed comfortably. Usually this can be overcome with the cooperation of the nursing staff. Ask the nurse to help you turn over after you have finished nursing on the first side. A side-lying position with the baby next to you in the bed is easiest in the beginning. Later on you can get out of bed and nurse the baby in a chair. The more you move around, the faster your body will heal and the more optimistic you will feel about handling breast-feeding successfully. If you and the baby are separated, try to massage your breasts regularly; even though you cannot shower you can use a hot towel and lanolin or some other cream to help stimulate the flow of milk. A hand or electric pump is useful in encouraging the let-down reflex.

A Cesarean birth today is usually without complications serious enough to inhibit nursing.

☐ *Breast-Feeding the Premature Infant*   A small-for-date or premature baby is often benefited by breast milk. A baby who is large enough to suck can do so directly from the breast. A baby who is very premature may have to be fed intravenously at first but can be fed breast milk from the bottle or breast with increasing maturity. As long as a woman establishes the let-down reflex with manual stimulation or a breast pump, she will be able to continue expressing milk for weeks or even months until she can feed the baby herself. I would first recommend a close association with the doctors and staff in the premature nursery since methods of feeding prematures vary from hospital to hospital. Some neonatologists favor breast milk for the tiny premature, and some favor a special formula to promote faster growth. If you can provide milk for the baby yourself, the staff can use the breast milk to feed the baby through a stomach tube. And even if the baby can't use the breast milk at first, you can continue to express milk and establish nursing later. In either case, breast milk will be much better for the child than formula feeding because of its immunological and nutritional advantages. Providing the baby with a source of sustenance is also a valuable way to establish bonding in the premature nursery where normal interaction between mother and child is sometimes difficult. Feeding a premature baby does take persistence, but many mothers have been able to breast-feed successfully at home even after a baby has stayed in the premature nursery for two or three months.

☐ *Not Enough Milk* More women stop nursing because they feel their milk supply is inadequate than for any other reason. Very often they are deterred by the initial period of engorgement, and give up nursing before the let-down reflex has been properly established. Sometimes the problem is a strict feeding regimen in the hospital, when the baby wakes up long before the next feed and is exhausted with crying by the time the scheduled feed takes place. Unless the staff is sympathetic to breast-feeding, a woman in difficulty is often encouraged to put her baby on the bottle because it does not seem to be doing well on the breast. Tension, insecurity, lack of sleep, postnatal depression also contribute by inhibiting the free flow of milk in the crucial first days after birth. There is no doubt that many women do not lactate as well in the hospital as they would if they were at home, and this is a great pity because the mother's confidence has been destroyed before she has had a chance to establish nursing. Remember, too, a baby normally loses weight in the first days after birth and it does not mean you should give up nursing. Once the milk supply is well established, weight gain is usually rapid.

When a woman gets home, lack of sleep, postnatal depression, insecurity or lack of support from family members can temporarily affect the milk supply. In order to relax and enjoy breast-feeding it is necessary to simplify your domestic life and spend as much time with the baby as possible. Tiredness is a problem for any new mother, whether she is breast-feeding or not. Try to rest during the day in between feeds for as long as the baby continues to keep you up at night. Don't hesitate to call on professional or other help if you need it; there are bound to be uncertainties at first.

A difficult period is often encountered ten to fourteen days after birth when the baby may seem dissatisfied after a feeding, especially during the afternoon and evening. This is what is known as a "hunger age," a period when the baby is growing quickly and develops an increased appetite. Unfortunately some women give up nursing at this point, thinking their milk supply is inadequate. All you need to do is nurse more frequently for a few days until the milk supply increases to meet the demand. Other "hunger ages" often occur at six weeks and then again at three months. At other times, the baby might not appear as hungry, and again, this is normal. As long as the baby is gaining weight, urinating frequently, and sleeping between feedings, you can be sure he or she is getting enough milk.

☐ *Too Much Milk* Just as some women seem to be able to produce milk more readily than others, some women feel they produce too much. An over-bountiful supply of milk can be gratifying but it can also be embarrassing. To reduce the first flow, which can be overwhelming for a young baby, douche the breasts with cold water just before feeding or express some milk before putting

562 /   *Childbirth with Love*

the baby to the breast. Eventually when you persist with nursing, the milk flow will adjust itself to the baby's demands.

If you secrete milk between feeds and during the night, use breast pads or absorbent material inside the nursing bra. A sudden flow of milk between feedings can be unobtrusively dealt with by folding your arms across your breasts and pressing down firmly on your nipples with the palms of your hands. Leakage of breast milk during intercourse, an embarrassing problem for some women, might be lessened by making love after a feed. Most breast-feeding women encounter this phenomenon when the breasts are stimulated during lovemaking, but it can also happen as a result of the release of oxytocin during intercourse. This may continue for up to one year after the birth.

It is important to remember that an apparent oversupply of milk does not affect its quality.

☐ *Where to Turn for Help*   Women who have had the support of the staff during their stay in the hospital or birthing center may worry about what to do or where to turn for help when they get home and are suddenly on their own with the baby. The first source of support is family members, friends, or neighbors who are knowledgeable about breast-feeding. Although older relatives may have bottle-fed, there are young friends and relatives who might have nursed and will be sympathetic to your problems. Try to be open enough to look for help from any supportive person. Professional help, of course, should be available as well. The obstetrician and pediatrician you choose should not only approve of breast-feeding, but have the time and understanding to help you overcome the minor difficulties that every woman experiences in the first few weeks. Don't be ashamed to get help if you do encounter problems; most "lactation crises" can be dealt with successfully. Some women unfortunately give up nursing early because there is no one to help them.

One outstanding source of support is La Leche League (*leche* means "milk" in Spanish), an international organization established in 1956. The purpose of La Leche is to promote breast-feeding by helping mothers become successful breast-feeders. La Leche members, women who have breast-fed or interested professionals, form a local network that provides telephone assistance to nursing mothers. If you are interested in becoming a member or would like to talk to other breast-feeding women, contact your local La Leche League chapter either before or after delivery. You can find the chapter in your area by writing to: La Leche League, International, 9616 Minneapolis Avenue, Franklin Park, Illinois 60131. The telephone number is 312-455-7730.

☐ *How Long Should You Breast-Feed?*   The longer you can breast-feed the better. Ideally a baby should be breast-fed for six months to a year, but, as I have already said, a woman who can manage to breast-feed for only a few weeks is immeasurably benefiting her baby. If you know you can only breast-feed for a limited time, try to continue for at least the first three months before switching to formula. This will give the baby the full benefit of the early nursing period. It may be possible to combine breast and bottle feeding by leaving a bottle of formula with a baby sitter and feeding the baby yourself when you get home. Such an arrangement makes it possible for a working mother both to work and nurse at the same time.

Of course each woman's life is different, but unless there is some compelling reason for giving up breast-feeding early on, I would encourage a woman to continue nursing her baby for as long as possible. It is one of those experiences a woman may never have a chance to enjoy again.

☐ *Mothering the Mother*   "Mothering the mother" is an accepted practice in non-Western cultures in which a new mother is formally assisted by her female relatives in the weeks after the birth of her child. This is part of a cultural tradition in which the young woman's transition to motherhood is as highly regarded as the adjustment of the infant to extrauterine life. Given the ambivalence about becoming a mother in our society and the lack of support from family members, who are often hundreds of miles away from their daughters and sons, it is not really surprising that an equivalent tradition is rarely found in America. Instead, new mothers are expected to fend for themselves after they get back from the hospital. No wonder that some women become anxious and find breast-feeding too difficult to continue beyond the first week or so.

One writer on nursing, Dana Raphael, has suggested that every breast-feeding woman try to enlist the help of a doula in the first weeks home. *Doula* is the Greek word for a friend or relative who helps the mother establish herself at home after a birth. A sympathetic doula can usually see the mother through the initial cycle of panic that inexperienced women often experience when they get home. A calm mother will help the baby nurse peacefully and sleep well between feedings, reinforcing the mother's confidence in her abilities to nurse.

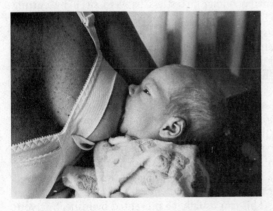

Figure 121a: Breast-feeding: An expression of contented satisfaction is seen on the baby's face as she breast-feeds. Breast-feeding brings mother and child together in a unique and special relationship. A special nursing bra is useful because a woman can breast-feed her baby wherever she might be. Pads can be placed inside each cup to avoid leakage between feedings.

There is no reason why the father cannot fill the doula's role. He can provide encouragement and physical assistance in the first weeks home, even if he is home only a part of the time. A relaxing massage or a quiet evening together are often enough to encourage the let-down reflex. One important function of the doula is to prevent the mother from becoming discouraged by negative "advice" from friends and other relatives who are unfriendly to breast-feeding. Here a supportive husband can be invaluable.

☐ *Social Drugs During Breast-Feeding*   Heavy smoking inhibits the let-down reflex and decreases the quantity of breast milk. The effects of small quantities of nicotine in milk are unknown, but this does not mean it is harmless. If you cannot give up smoking, at least cut down and avoid smoking during feeding periods, so the baby is not exposed directly to cigarette smoke or hot ash from burning cigarettes.

Marijuana is fat-soluble and enters human milk. A few babies have reportedly become drowsy after their mothers smoked marijuana. A more serious problem is the possibility of marijuana interfering with brain cell development in the sensitive period of infancy. Common sense dictates that smoking anything should be kept to a minimum during lactation just as it would during pregnancy. Most substances, including social drugs, that the mother eats, drinks, or smokes go into breast milk and might affect the baby.

Breast-feeding and large amounts of alcohol are not a good combination. Children have developed severe endocrine disorders with heavy concentrations of alcohol; in one instance the baby became obese, showed high levels of cortisone in the blood, and developed a moon-shaped face—symptoms of Cushing syndrome. There is no problem with an occasional glass of wine or beer or a cocktail, and many breast-feeding experts recommend the occasional glass of wine before a feed to help stimulate the let-down reflex.

☐ *Can You Drink Coffee or Eat Cabbage if You Are Nursing?*   A hyperactive baby who sleeps poorly may be getting a hefty dose of caffeine from an accumulation of tea, coffee, and cola drinks. A mother who drinks more than six to eight cups of any beverage containing caffeine a day is probably overstimulating the baby, who is likely to sleep only short periods of time and be unusually alert during waking hours. You can encourage a restless baby to sleep by cutting down on your caffeine intake.

Other foods that upset nursing vary from baby to baby. Cabbage, broccoli, beans, or onions sometimes cause a slight stomach upset or colic, but there is no reason to avoid a specific food unless you notice an effect on the baby. The same is true of chocolate, which is harmless in small quantities.

☐ *Breast Problems: Breast Abscess and Mastitis*   Mastitis and breast abscesses are relatively common among breast-feeding women. A breast infection usually begins when one of the breast ducts become clogged. Milk remains blocked behind the clogged area, and bacteria then move into the nipple through the breast duct and infect the area. The classic sign of a breast abscess is an inflamed, tender lump on the breast. If the clogged area is not relieved promptly, the breast can become increasingly inflamed, with the whole breast becoming swollen and tender. This can usually be prevented by inspecting your breasts carefully every day for signs of breast inflammation and using hand massage or a breast pump to express any milk left in the breast after a feeding. As soon as the obstruction is removed, the infection will disappear. An untreated breast infection can result in mastitis—symptoms of which include painful, swollen breasts, chills, headache, and a high fever. In severe cases, the skin can break and ulceration or an abscess appear on the breast area. Contact your doctor as soon as you experience symptoms of mastitis. He should prescribe pain relievers and antibiotics to treat the condition as well as suggesting hot compresses and hand massage or a breast pump to empty the breasts completely. Continue breast-feeding as you would normally. Many antibiotics are safe for use during breast-feeding, including penicillin, ampicillin, or erythromycin, although ampicillin is associated with diarrhea. Nursing can be continued safely as long as the infection is the nonepidemic form of mastitis; in fact it should be encouraged to avoid engorgement and other problems. The infectious organism is not excreted in the milk, so the baby is not affected. By contrast, a rarer, more severe form of mastitis is epidemic mastitis, a staphylococcus infection transmitted in hospital nurseries. If a milk culture shows the presence of staphylococci, the mother must stop breast-feeding and be treated promptly with antibiotics.

Breast infections during nursing can be prevented by toughening the nipples and avoiding drying agents, including soaps.

☐ *Vaginitis During Breast-Feeding* Soreness and irritation of the vagina are commonly experienced during breast-feeding, although the subject of vaginitis is rarely discussed in a breast-feeding preparation class. A breast-feeding woman's estrogen level is low, and the vagina may become atrophic. It then lacks its normal protective mechanism and invites the growth of yeastlike organisms. Antiyeast creams or suppositories are helpful; so is Mycolog cream applied to the outer portion of the vaginal lips to decrease irritation and soreness.

Vaginitis is so common during breast-feeding that no woman should be surprised if it occurs. Fortunately it is easy to treat. Another problem is the pain some women encounter during sexual intercourse, again because breast-feeding lowers the estrogen level. K-Y jelly applied to the opening of the vagina will make intercourse easier.

☐ *Breast-Feeding and Contraception* Breast-feeding stimulates the release of the brain hormone prolactin, which in turn suppresses the production of estrogen in the ovaries. This is one of the reasons a woman's estrogen level is lower and the vagina becomes dryer. At the same time, ovulation generally ceases during breast-feeding. Protection is usually complete for the first three months after delivery but nursing mothers are advised to use some form of contraception because ovulation does occasionally occur even before menstruation has been reestablished. As a general rule, as long as a woman does not experience bleeding, she is usually not fertile. After menstruation returns, often at about the fourth to sixth month, breast-feeding may still offer some protection, but it is highly unreliable.

The best form of contraception during breast-feeding is the barrier method. It might be better to use foams or condoms in the beginning because the vagina tends to heal slowly with the low estrogen level. Then you can switch to a diaphragm as the vagina becomes healthier. The use of birth control pills is not encouraged because the hormones may enter the milk or affect the milk supply. This is of particular concern with high-estrogen combination pills; the high doses of estrogen could inhibit lactation. Low estrogen combined or progesterone-only contraceptives do not affect breast-feeding once it is established, but there is still a chance of the hormones' entering the milk. Risks with low combination pills, or better yet, progesterone-only pills, are probably minimal, but it would be better to avoid them altogether if you have a choice.

☐ *Drugs and Breast-Feeding* The amount of any drug excreted into breast milk varies greatly from drug to drug, although with any drug, including over-the-counter preparations, a woman should be aware of the potential risks involved in taking medications during lactation. In general, drugs that are fat-soluble tend to concentrate in the milk more readily than drugs that are water-soluble. (This phenomenon is reversed in the first few days of nursing, when water-soluble drugs enter the colostrum easily). Weakly alkaline drugs are also excreted more readily than weakly acidic drugs.

The best way for a nursing mother to protect her baby is to remember that most drugs, taken in large enough quantities, will concentrate in breast milk, and drugs are to be avoided in lactation just as they are during pregnancy. If your doctor decides you do need a specific drug, he should ask himself whether the drug he prescribes for you is one that could be given safely to the baby. An example of a drug that cannot be given safely to infants is lithium. Phenobarbital, on the other hand, can be given in small dosages to infants; so can antibiotics such as penicillin. With a tranquilizer such as phenobarbital, the question then is whether enough is reaching the baby to cause symptoms of respiratory depression. One way to minimize the effect on the baby is to take a prescription drug immediately after a nursing period to give the drug time to metabolize and leave the body. If you are taking medication, try to watch for unusual symptoms such as a change in sleeping habits and call your pediatrician and internist to discuss anything that disturbs you.

Among nonprescription drugs, large doses of aspirin are known to enter breast milk with a possible alteration of platelet function in the baby. No studies have been made on the concentration of Tylenol in breast milk. In general as little is known of the effect of nonprescription drugs during lactation as is known in pregnancy; which means you should be just as cautious during nursing as you were during pregnancy. Don't stop nursing, however, because you have taken an over-the-counter drug or need to take a prescription drug. A few drugs are definitely contraindicated, but a single dose of a nonprescription drug is unlikely to harm the baby, and many prescription drugs can be used with reasonable safety during breast-feeding. Sometimes a prescription can be changed to a safer drug.

☐ *Environmental Pollution and Breast-Feeding*   The nursing mother, like everyone else, is exposed to environmental pollution. The two environmental substances that have caused most concern are DDT and the polychlorinated biphenyls, PCB and PBB. DDT has been banned in the United States since 1970, but it was a persistent enough compound to be stored in human fat over a long period of time and has appeared in human milk as recently as 1977. This is alarming, but concentrations vary greatly from woman to woman and in any case residual concentrations are found in cow's milk as well as breast milk. The polychlorinated biphenyls are a group of industrial chemicals that have been widely used in the electrical industry. In the 1970s waste products containing PCBs were found to have contaminated lakes and rivers in the central United States, causing heavy concentrations in fresh-water fish. Individuals who eat contaminated fish, drink contaminated water, or come into contact with PCBs at work, store PCBs, which persist in body fat over a long period of time.

Since lipids in breast milk are made up from the body's storage of fat, not from the fat eaten during the time of milk production, the nursing baby is thus exposed to the effects of the chemical. Effects of moderate exposure are virtually unknown, although very high levels of PCB infestation do have immediate and long-term detrimental effects. Generally, a woman who is not aware of any concentrated exposure to PCBs is encouraged to go on breast-feeding, avoiding only a sudden weight loss, which could release the chemical from fat stores. It is possible to have your milk tested, but the testing procedure takes so long—at least six weeks—that the American Academy of Pediatrics recommends it only when a woman is aware of a heavy occupational or environmental exposure. For the average woman, the risk of the baby's ingesting more than a small amount of PCBs or PBBs is small.

Other substances that cause concern are pesticides such as dieldrin or chlordane. Environmental exposure to these substances has been linked to birth defects. Don't use garden chemicals while you are nursing, and have your milk tested if you are aware of heavy exposure to agricultural sprays.

☐ *Fibrocystic Breast Disease and Breast-Feeding*   Fibrocystic breast disease is a benign condition in which a cyst or cysts develop in different areas of the breasts. One out of every five women suffers from fibrocystic breast disease at some point in her life; more often than not this happens in the teens, thirties, and forties. New research reveals that it is not a precancerous condition; but it is caused by hormonal imbalance resulting in changes in breast tissue when the tissues thicken and become cystic and painful. The condition gets worse with the ingestion of large amounts of caffeine. A woman with a painful case of fibrocystic breast disease can now be treated successfully with an oral medication: Danocrine, an antihormone that has been approved for this use by the FDA.

If you are troubled by fibrocystic breast disease, breast-feeding is encouraged rather than contraindicated because the breast tissues are stimulated during nursing as the breast is used for its natural purpose. The function of childbirth in deterring or curing fibrocystic breast disease is confirmed by the fact that women who postpone childbearing are more likely to suffer from it than women who have children at an early age. When you have a tendency to fibrocystic breast disease, try to breast-feed for as long a time as possible, cut down on your caffeine intake, and then seek help if the condition becomes worse after you stop breast-feeding. Remember, there is effective medication available if the condition does not disappear after nursing.

☐ *Does Breast-Feeding Prevent Cancer?*   Breast-feeding may help prevent cancer, but there are other factors involved. The risk of breast cancer seems to increase when a woman has no children or a first child after the age of thirty. Women whose first child is born when they are under eighteen have about one-third the risk of developing cancer in comparison with a woman whose first child is born when she is over thirty-five. The first full-term pregnancy seems to have some effect on the breast tissue that makes it less susceptible to neoplasms. Some people feel that breast-feeding offers additional protection by prolonging the time of absent menstruation and hormonal fluctuation; others think that breast-feeding per se is a relatively unimportant factor compared with pregnancy itself. Interestingly, though, in cultures in which women traditionally use only one breast to feed their babies, there does seem to be a higher incidence of cancer in the unsuckled breast.

☐ *If You Decide to Bottle-Feed*   You may have decided to bottle-feed because you feel it is impossible for you to breast-feed successfully, or you have bottle-fed your other children and don't want to change your routine. You could be planning an early return to work, or you might need to travel, or there might be some other personal factor that makes long-term breast-feeding impossible. Sometimes the thought of breast-feeding is unattractive because of the potential problems associated with it, or some women simply find the process itself unappealing. These are understandable reasons. However, by changing your plans and breast-feeding for the first few weeks, the baby would at least get the important antibodies present in breast milk but absent in formula. A short period of breast-feeding gives several months of protection until the immature immune system is further developed. Then if you don't want to continue breast-feeding after the first few weeks you can switch to formula.

Although no formula can match breast milk's value, there are some good formulas available that will provide excellent nutrition for the rest of the first year. Companies that make formulas have changed their products in recent years in an attempt to approximate the composition of breast milk rather than cow's milk, and several formulas are on the market that provide a reasonable balance of protein, carbohydrates, fats, and minerals. Your pediatrician will help you choose the best brand for your baby. It is important to use formula in the first year rather than powdered milk or fresh milk. Cow's milk is relatively indigestible; the extra protein may overload the baby's kidneys; it is high in sodium and relatively low in essential minerals and vitamins. Whether breast-fed or bottle-fed, your baby should not be started on cow's milk until well into its second year.

Babies differ in their tolerance of different formulas. Excessive gas, constipation, or other signs of intestinal discomfort should be discussed with your pediatrician, who may recommend trying another type of formula. Very occasionally a baby is sensitive to the proteins in milk and will need a special soy-based formula.

If you do turn to formula feeding, you can still feed the baby on demand, and encourage physical contact during feeding by holding the baby so he or she can see your face and feel your warmth. A formula-fed baby may not get breast milk but he or she isn't therefore deprived of parental attention or affection. Mothers who bottle-feed their babies can be just as loving parents as breast-feeding mothers; not that professionals would encourage bottle feeding, but it is important for a woman not to carry guilt feelings about the way she cares for her children.

☐ *How to Stop Milk Production—Estrogen Injections and Parlodel*   Until recently, women who chose not to breast-feed were given estrogen injections immediately after the birth to prevent the milk supply from coming in. After adverse reports about the effects of estrogens, particularly DES, this routine has been halted. Many physicians now prefer not to give medication but instead recommend tight bras to stop lactation gradually. The problem is that many women suffer from painfully engorged breasts, symptoms which often persist for as long as a week or two despite treatment with ice packs or analgesics. *This is unnecessary.* Recent studies on the action of prolactin, the hormone that produces breast milk, have yielded a new drug that has recently been approved by the FDA under the name Parlodel. This drug contains a hormone known as bromocryptine mesulate rather than the traditional estrogen hormone and is a safe way to block the elevated level of prolactin in the postpartum period.

Recommended doses of Parlodel are one 2.5-milligram tablet taken three times a day with meals while you are in the hospital. You should start the regimen as soon as you decide not to breast-feed. After you have been on the initial dose of Parlodel for three or four days you can cut down to two tablets a day and stay on that dosage for about two to three weeks. Breast engorgement is thus avoided, and the absence of unnecessary pain will help you heal better after the birth and take good care of your child.

Note: Parlodel is so new that your obstetrician might not be aware of it yet. If he does not discuss it with you, ask him to prescribe it yourself once you have decided not to breast-feed. At least you can be sure of feeling better after the birth when you make this important and sensitive decision.

☐ *Weaning* Whether the baby is breast-fed or bottle-fed, don't rush into introducing solid foods too early. The immature digestive system and the swallowing mechanism are not well suited to solids in the first months of life. Wait until the baby is at least four to six months old before introducing an iron-fortified baby cereal into the child's diet. The tradition of starting solid foods early, popular in the mid-1960s, is no longer favored because early weaning is unnecessary and encourages overfeeding and obesity.

There is no reason to give up breast-feeding once the baby begins on solid food. As long as the baby receives extra iron from another source besides breast milk, breast milk remains a nutritionally complete food for the rest of the first year. If you are planning a return to work or a full work schedule, you can continue to breast-feed night and morning and rely on formula or expressed breast milk during the day. Older babies continue to enjoy being breast-fed, especially if you have been away part of the day. Some American women are now continuing to breast-feed well into the second year. The baby by this time is receiving nutrition from a number of other sources, but the emotional closeness of nursing is still pleasurable for mother and child.

Whenever you decide to wean, do it gradually. Abrupt weaning is traumatic for both the mother and the baby. By eliminating one feed at a time, giving the baby formula from a cup or bottle instead, your milk supply will decrease gradually until the breasts cease to produce milk. Sudden weaning can be done, but the breasts often become engorged and remain uncomfortable for several days. Sometimes a hastily weaned older baby is reluctant to use a bottle for the first few days and will accept only solids.

33

Postpartum: What to Expect After the Birth

Now you have finally delivered the child whose arrival you have awaited for so long. The excitement of giving birth is sometimes so intense that you may not believe the baby is really here, or is really yours.

Once you pass through those first euphoric moments after the birth, you will probably find yourself experiencing a multitude of emotions. In this respect the postpartum period is as rewarding and as difficult a time as pregnancy itself. One common sensation is relief. Fears about childbirth, which even well-prepared women experience, have been eliminated, and you should have a wonderful feeling of accomplishment. Regardless of whether the birth went as you imagined, you have achieved your goal, you have your baby, you are now a mother. Women sometimes say this is the first time in their lives that they have something of their own; something that no one can ever take away from them. This new responsibility is exciting, and a little frightening. No wonder many postpartum women experience a temporary sense of disequilibrium; the reality of a woman's becoming a mother is so incredible that no one can really predict how she will react until the baby is born.

Both parents commonly go through a period of uncertainty as they face the responsibilities of parenthood for the first time. You know you love the baby, yet you are afraid; afraid of the future, afraid that you will not be a good parent. What will this child do to your life? Will it make the family stronger? Or will it create tension that drives you and your partner apart? It may help to remember that parenthood is as much a learned as an instinctive skill. Plan to discuss your feelings and concerns with your partner, with other family members, and with your friends. As the time passes, you will find your confidence growing and you will begin to experience the joy of motherhood.

Despite the excitement and the emotional conflicts of the postpartum period, a woman may feel slightly "let down" after the baby is born. It is hard to have a positive feeling about caring for the child because many babies are sleepy and unresponsive in the first few days. This let-down feeling is intensified by traditional nursery arrangements that separate mothers and babies except at feeding times. Perhaps, too, it is only human to look back with regret at the high expectations you had about childbirth and motherhood. Sometimes anticipation is more pleasurable than reality, or it may seem that way initially.

You can expect the first weeks postpartum to be a confusing if not a difficult time. So many things are happening; so many decisions must be made; so much must be done. Facing the changes in your life will be easier if you know what to expect and have an understanding of the complex physiological and emotional changes all postpartum women experience. A new mother who is tired after a long labor or is still recuperating from a difficult birth may not realize that her feelings of weakness, or even anger at the demands suddenly put on her are completely natural. Instead of suppressing your feelings, as some women do because they feel guilty or inadequate, ask for help. Support is essential. You always need your family and friends, but one time in your life you surely need them is after a birth. Fatigue is normal after childbirth, but the less fatigued you are, the more you can concentrate on building your inner strength. Furthermore, it will be easier for you to take care of the baby once you feel more confident about yourself. If you don't plan to have professional help, ask your mother or your mother-in-law or a close relative or friend for assistance. You will need that help in the first weeks after you get home.

☐ **Your Body**   You may be disappointed when you find that your body has not changed much in the immediate postpartum period. Even though you have delivered the baby and the placenta and "dropped" almost twelve pounds, you can expect your weight to be almost the same after the birth as it was just before the birth. One reason is that the body's composition has changed because of pregnancy and is now loaded with excess fluid. Another is that the circulation and hormonal balance are temporarily altered after a birth. These changes encourage edema, especially in the legs, which often become almost twice their normal size immediately postpartum.

Anemia is another common postpartum complaint, caused by the loss of blood during and after the delivery. People who are anemic often experience edema of the feet and face. Watch your diet, eat food rich in iron and vitamins, and continue to take your prenatal vitamin supplement after the birth. I encourage my patients to double their normal prenatal supplement during the postpartum weeks to restore the nutrients lost during the childbirth. An extra iron supplement is also important for at least a month after the birth. If you can rebuild your strength quickly you will find it much easier to take care of the baby, as well as deal with the postpartum blues. After a few days the extra fluid will begin to disappear little by little as the body regains its normal balance and strength. As you lose the extra fluid you will see your weight begin to decrease as well.

Be prepared for your abdomen to look rather flabby for a time after the birth. You must understand that the uterus develops a thick wall of muscles over the nine months of pregnancy and those muscles do not disappear overnight. However, the uterus is an amazing organ; within a week or so the muscles begin to degenerate and the uterus will shrink down to its normal size, smaller than a pear. Nonetheless, the extra muscles and fatty tissue will be around for some time after birth, so you cannot expect to see a change immediately. I tell my patients not to worry about the extra weight because they need to rebuild their physical stamina first before they can go on a diet. As long as you eat well and get plenty of rest you will see your body change, little by little, as the weight goes down and you go back to your normal shape. Women who breast-feed often find this takes place quickly because the body naturally draws on the excess fat stored during pregnancy to provide the extra energy needed for lactation. Concentrate on good nutrition while you are breast-feeding; a lactating woman needs even more calories each day than a woman who is pregnant. Dieting can be dangerous while you are breast-feeding because the breakdown of the carbohydrates in the body might increase ketone concentration, which in turn may poison the milk.

☐ *The Episiotomy*   You will feel some pain from the stitches in the first few days and notice some swelling. Both are normal although unpleasant. Treat the area locally with a medicated spray or ointment or try soaking the episiotomy in a sitz bath. The episiotomy will begin to heal up once the swelling goes away a few days later. Remember, though, it takes several weeks for the torn tissues to restore themselves.

I would not recommend resuming sexual intercourse until after the first postnatal check-up three to six weeks postpartum, when your doctor can make sure the episiotomy has healed completely. If you have intercourse too early on you might tear the fragile tissue. Be particularly cautious when you are breast-feeding because the breast-feeding woman has a lower estrogen level than normal and the tissues consequently take a longer time to heal, making early intercourse painful and occasionally damaging.

Anything unusual about the episiotomy should be reported to your doctor immediately. An infection will heal faster when it is treated early, before it damages the tissue or even leads to an abscess.

A few women find intercourse is still painful a year after their episiotomy. This is why the episiotomy should be avoided, if possible. If one must be performed, a midline or median episiotomy is preferred (see Chap. 29).

☐ *Lactating Breasts*   Whether a woman is breast-feeding or not, she needs to wear a support bra or a good maternity bra until her breasts return to their normal size. If your breasts become painful, put ice packs on them to reduce the swelling, and keep them bound with a bra night and day. A woman who has decided not to breast-feed can ask her doctor to prescribe bromocryptine or another medication to stop lactation and avoid painful breast engorgement. Any abnormality, infection, or pain should be reported to your doctor immediately, since it could be the beginning of a breast abscess and would need medical attention right away.

Many women find that they continue to lactate for a year or a year and a half after they have stopped nursing. This is a quite normal phenomenon. Sometimes a sudden gush of milk will occur during lovemaking because the oxytocin, stimulated by intercourse, enters the bloodstream and stimulates mammary muscles around the milk ducts. You may find this embarrassing or annoying, but it is in no way abnormal and is even enjoyable for some couples.

☐ **Constipation**   Before you leave the hospital, the bowel function should be fairly regular. Constipation is a common complaint in the postpartum period. It is only to be expected. With all the extra weight in the last few weeks of pregnancy, the extended uterus tends to press down on the bowels, and the bowels lose their normal sensitivity. Then after the birth, you may be afraid to push too hard because you don't want the episiotomy to hurt or rip apart. A good way to deal with the problem naturally is to eat a diet including extra salads or bran, prune juice, and plenty of other fluids. If diet alone does not help regulate the system and the problem persists, a bowel softener such as milk of magnesia or Colace twice daily is safe for the breast-feeding mother. You must remember one thing: the episiotomy stitches will not break, although it might hurt to put pressure on them initially. If the natural approach does not work, the best alternative is to use an enema to avoid a prolonged problem with constipation.

☐ **Difficulty Urinating**   Normal urination is sometimes difficult immediately after the baby is born or in the first few days postpartum. After childbirth the urethra is often stretched to such a degree that normal muscle control is lost. A few women lose complete muscle control for weeks or even several months postpartum, depending often on whether they have delivered a large child, or are breast-feeding. As I have mentioned in Chapter 32, breast-feeding depresses your estrogen production, and estrogen, the female hormone, is an essential factor in the speed with which the vaginal tissue heals. I would suggest practicing the Kegel exercise twenty or thirty times a day, beginning a few days postpartum, to begin to retone the vaginal muscles so that they become firm and tight again (see below). Strong vaginal muscles will help establish full control over urination.

If you find urination difficult after the delivery, the doctor might decide to insert a catheter temporarily into the bladder. Women who have had difficult deliveries or an epidural are particularly prone to this problem. After a day or two, the system usually returns to normal. You shouldn't be catheterized for too long, because this may introduce an infection into the bladder.

The desire to urinate increases between the second and fifth day after delivery as the body begins to rid itself of the extra water accumulated in the tissues during pregnancy. From then on, the bladder can be expected to function normally.

☐ **The Lochia—How Long Does It Last?**   Uterine bleeding is often fairly heavy in the first couple of days, particularly after a long labor. The lochia, the postpartum discharge, is bright red following delivery and becomes brown as the uterus goes back to its normal size. The amount of discharge gradually decreases; at first you may find yourself changing sanitary pads about twice a day, then after a while you will notice some occasional spotting. Finally the vaginal discharge will stop completely. Some bleeding is quite normal for as long as four to six weeks after a delivery, although many women find the bleeding stops in about twenty-one days.

Uterine contractions continue through the postpartum period. Women who breast-feed notice them more because the uterus will contract as oxytocin is released into the bloodstream each time the baby sucks on the nipple (the milk-ejecting reflex). A sharp contraction of the uterus during breast-feeding will often expel a small blood clot together with the lochia. You may experience this for several weeks postpartum, but it is not harmful.

After you go home, take it easy for the first few weeks even if you do feel energetic enough to follow your normal schedule. After childbirth the uterus is almost like an open sore that needs time to heal, and overexerting yourself can bring on a sudden increase in bleeding. Any abnormal bleeding should be reported to your doctor immediately. He might prescribe methergine or ergotrate to hasten the uterine contractions and thus slow down the bleeding. Or your problem might be some retained placental tissue, which may require minor surgery, a dilatation and curettage, to remove it from the uterus. Otherwise the uterus will continue to bleed, or might become infected.

Occasionally a woman experiences what is known as a *postpartum hemorrhage* several weeks after the birth. Don't be afraid to call your doctor if at any time you experience increased discharge or heavy bleeding. On occasion a postpartum hemorrhage can be very severe and blood transfusions might be necessary in addition to surgery to control the bleeding and replace the blood loss. A postpartum hemorrhage can be so serious that you should never neglect the warning of increasing postpartum bleeding and clots.

The first menstruation usually occurs within six to eight weeks after childbirth. A woman who is breast-feeding often will not resume her normal menstruation pattern until she has begun to wean the baby.

☐ *Is It Normal to Lose Hair After Childbirth?*   Hormonal changes may cause hair loss in the postpartum period. Don't worry too much; the loss is usually temporary. It is almost unknown for a woman to become bald after childbearing. Begin taking extra doses of vitamins, particularly B vitamins, the antistress vitamins, and massage the scalp daily. If the hair continues to fall out, then do have your thyroid checked. A low thyroid level affects your metabolism. The body's balance can be restored by thyroid medication.

☐ *When Is It Safe to Bathe After Delivery?*   It is better to postpone taking a tub bath until you have stopped bleeding almost completely. The vaginal area has usually healed up enough to make tub bathing safe by the second or third week after childbirth, although some doctors do recommend waiting a week or two longer. There is no reason to be overcautious; just observe your body carefully for signs of healing.

Do not douche immediately after childbirth. Douching puts an undesirable pressure on the vaginal fluids, which could be pushed into the uterus. Wait until the cervix is completely healed and has closed itself. Otherwise the soap or chemicals in the douching solution may irritate the uterus. Begin douching only after your doctor has examined the vagina and the cervix to make sure that both have completely healed. After four to six weeks you can usually use tampons also, but you might check that with your obstetrician at the first visit.

☐ *The Pregnancy Mask: When Will It Disappear?*   The pregnancy mask is a distinct band of pigmentation across the nose and cheeks caused by increased hormonal activity during pregnancy. Depending on the individual, it can take months before the pregnancy mask fades away, although you can be sure it will finally disappear.

☐ **Breast Care**   You will notice a change in the shape and elasticity of the breasts after childbirth. This is normal. Pregnancy affects the tissues in the breasts and they will be softer after breast-feeding (see Chap. 32).

Watch out for cracked nipples or the beginning of a breast abscess if you are breast-feeding. Cracked nipples are often a problem in the first few days before the milk flow is well established. Try keeping the baby on the breast for a short time to begin with, and alternate breasts at each feed. Occasionally the baby's hard sucking produces a sore spot on a cracked nipple. Watch the area carefully, since the sore is open to bacteria, and you may find yourself with a painful breast abscess. Make sure to express all the milk out of the breast at the end of a feed, either by hand or with a breast pump. This precaution will keep the milk ducts open. Your doctor may prescribe an antibiotic for a few days to reduce the risk of infection.

☐ **Stretch Marks After the Birth**   Immediately postpartum, stretch marks are sometimes disturbingly prominent. Once the stomach is flatter, the loose skin may look considerably more wrinkled than it did before the birth. Don't be too concerned; you can expect to lose extra fluid in the next few weeks and the skin on the abdomen and the buttocks will tighten up as the body tissues dissolve. Cream or lotions will help keep the skin supple, and exercising and eating well will help your skin as well as the rest of your body get back into shape.

Women who are left with permanent scars can help fade them by getting out into the sun. Normally stretch marks cannot be removed surgically, although a cosmetic surgeon might operate to pull down and tuck in excessive amounts of skin left by a multiple pregnancy; this will mean moving up the navel. Women with very fair skins or young women who gain a large amount of weight are more likely to get permanent stretch marks than brunettes or women who give birth later in life. Most women hardly notice the faint permanent stretch marks left behind on the breasts or the abdomen.

☐ **Postpartum Depression—The Baby Blues**   In the weeks after childbirth, a woman can expect to experience a period of physical and emotional change. Physical changes often depend on the woman's condition prior to birth. If the pregnancy has gone smoothly and she has taken care of herself, she is usually stronger and will recover more easily than a woman who has had a difficult pregnancy or who has not been able to take care of herself adequately. A successful physical recovery will obviously affect a woman's emotional state as well. Her physical and mental condition will also be affected by the birth itself. Labor means work, and the body is put under a great deal of physical stress during a delivery. It takes time for it to rest and heal, and fatigue is only to be expected in the immediate postpartum period. Other physical symptoms may include loss of appetite, gastrointestinal symptoms, or insomnia. These symptoms can constitute a vicious circle, making the woman feel more and more tired and run down.

Along with these physical symptoms, there is often a feeling of emotional letdown in the first few days after a birth. A fairly common pattern is for the new mother to feel elated and relieved immediately after the baby is delivered, followed a few days later by fits of inexplicable crying or a general feeling of malaise. These are the "baby blues," otherwise known as the postpartum blues. A victim of the postpartum blues is sad, restless, anxious, fatigued, and emotionally hypersensitive; she experiences rapid mood changes; she has fears about the baby's safety; or she feels guilty about not enjoying her new baby. Many women realize they are experiencing the "blues," but are at a loss to know how to deal with the situation.

For most women these feelings are painful but transitory. It is natural to be scared or depressed when you consider the responsibilities of motherhood. You may either want to talk about how you feel with your mate or a close friend or you may want to be left alone for a while to deal with your emotions yourself. Remember that your needs as a new parent are legitimate, that maternal feelings grow with experience, and that many women feel guilty about their conflicting emotions in the postpartum period. Once you realize what is happening, it becomes easier to face the situation and then work your way out of the depressive phase.

☐ ***Postpartum Depression Rather than Postpartum Blues***   Psychiatrists and obstetricians make a clear distinction between the familiar "postpartum blues" and the more prolonged and debilitating postpartum depression.

Postpartum depression, like the blues, is usually caused by a combination of physical and psychological factors. In addition, the endocrine metabolic system affects a woman's emotional state. Wide mood swings can be expected as the endocrine functions return to their usual status. Disrupted dreaming may also be a contributor to postpartum depression. Severe sleep disturbances which prevent dreaming are known to increase irritability, and this inability to dream may continue for a while after giving birth.

Even when the physical adjustments have been made, psychological problems may prolong "the blues," and they may become a deep depression. Anger turned inward, for example, is a classical definition of depression. In the case of postpartum depression, even women who normally feel free to voice outrage might tend to hold back or mute their feelings about the newborn baby. It is extremely important for the new mother to get help with psychological problems, and not to remain alone with them. She may want to talk to friends or family members with whom she feels comfortable. If her depression continues, it might be wise to seek professional psychological counseling.

☐ ***Are Hormones Linked to Postpartum Emotions?***   Most people today believe the emotions women feel in the postpartum period are a combination of sudden changes after birth that are hormonal, physical, and emotional. Some, however, feel that postpartum emotional changes are the result primarily of hormonal changes. It is true that immediately after childbirth there is a great hormonal change in the body, with an increased secretion of prolactin, the hormone that stimulates milk secretion, and estrogen, and a decrease in progesterone. It is likely that this hormone fluctuation may have different effects on mood, since the hormone levels vary from one person to another.

Various theories exist about the effect of hormones on emotions, but no concrete answers exist as yet. One study from Great Britain has shown that most women who suffered from postpartum depression have a particularly high level of the female sex hormone, estrogen, and a low level of progesterone, as well as abnormal levels of other hormones. Women who suffer from premenstrual syndrome are sometimes found to have similar hormonal imbalances. Thus it is possible that premenstrual syndrome (PMS) may be linked somewhat to postpartum depression. Other studies have indicated that postpartum depression may be due to an abnormal level of thyroid hormones and that thyroid treatment might help promote healing. This approach has not been helpful in all cases, however.

☐ *Do Fathers Get Postpartum Blues?* Research about fathers has been very limited. But we know that fathers can effectively satisfy the needs of babies just as mothers can, and it appears that fathers also share the emotional highs and lows that go along with child care. It is interesting that a number of things we assume about mothers and motherhood are really typical of parenthood in general. In one study it was reported that approximately 85 to 90 percent of women had some symptoms associated with postpartum depression, and, at the same time, 62 percent of the fathers had similar symptoms. Men have also experienced anxiety and emotional problems during pregnancy, and may also experience morning sickness or weight gain along with their wives (the couvade syndrome—see Chap. 11).

Many fathers seem frustrated by their inability to help their wives cope with the new baby, or to care for the baby themselves. This may lead to the same postpartum blues described by new mothers. Both father and mother may be overwhelmed by feelings of anger or inadequacy.

The fact that men go through mood changes similar to those of women who have given birth gives weight to the argument that psychological factors may be the predominant cause of the conflicting emotions both sexes feel in the postpartum period.

☐ *How to Cope with Postpartum Depression* Although 85 to 90 percent of women experience some minor mood changes after delivery, moderate to severe postpartum depression occurs in only 10 to 12 percent of all new mothers. Surprisingly, the woman who experiences a marked postpartum depression is not always the unprepared or immature woman traditionally considered vulnerable to postpartum psychosis. A special postpartum counseling program set up in Vancouver, British Columbia,* has counseled over a thousand women experiencing postpartum depression and recognizes the following profile of a woman considered to be at risk. She is twenty-seven years old, married, middle class, college educated, with a planned pregnancy and with the father present at the delivery. In other words, the woman who becomes depressed is often the one who would be expected to make a successful transition into motherhood. (Although the Vancouver findings have been contradicted by other studies, which say that a woman is *less* likely to become depressed if she is well prepared for the birth, is in excellent health and is successfully breast-feeding.)

Strong guilt feelings and feelings of inadequacy are common among women with postpartum depression. The mother may be overconcerned about the baby,

---

* Postpartum Counseling, 923 West Eighth Avenue, Vancouver, BC, V52 1E4, Canada.

or may physically or emotionally neglect her child. Most women experience a loss of self. These women need special care, and should be urged to seek psychological counseling if the problem persists. Problems can also be discussed with the obstetrician, and a reference can often be obtained from him if further help is recommended. Many women experience fear of caring for the new child, and guidance from a professional therapist may be quite helpful in dealing with the underlying problems. Sometimes the problem exists on a family level, and the husband and/or other family members may also be asked to come in for counseling. In this way members of the family group can learn to be more open with each other about communication, and members can work together to improve the home situation.

The most effective treatment for women with postpartum depression is emotional support from spouse, family, friends, nurses, and not least, their doctors. Often, unfortunately, a woman who has given birth will find herself alone in a hospital room, without the family members she would ordinarily rely on for support. The new mother may feel unexpectedly abandoned as she senses that her needs have become secondary to those of her child; that she must now be the care-giver rather than the care-receiver. Both in the hospital and at home, a new mother needs care and attention, just as the baby does. It is interesting that in countries where people still live in closely knit communities, women are less likely to experience postpartum depression because they have the support of grandmothers and other relatives. In countries where mothers can no longer rely on relatives and neighbors, special support groups have sometimes been available to take their place. Through support groups women discover that they are not alone, that there is a way to resolve the depression. A childbirth education teacher or a therapist at the hospital might be a good source of referral.

☐ *Parents and Babies: The New Relationship* An obstetrician walking into a room on the postpartum floor often finds a new mother staring intently at her baby as if she were thinking, "Is this really mine?" Sometimes it is difficult to distinguish between the reality and the dream after the long months of pregnancy. So much happens so quickly during and after labor and delivery that new parents are often confused as well as joyful in the immediate postpartum period. Then too, postpartum emotions are often volatile; euphoria is quickly followed by anxiety or depression. This may be because the body is going through a period of change as the hormonal levels slowly return to their prepregnant state (a process that may take several months if you are breast-feeding). But once you have passed through this initial period of adjustment—a few days for some women, a few weeks for others—you will find yourself realizing that this really is your child, and you really are a mother.

If you are still pregnant, you may be surprised by the length of time it takes to form a firm parent-infant bond. While bonding may indeed take place before birth (see Chapter 14 for the new research on intrauterine bonding), it is important to remember that parents-to-be sometimes expect a dream child, not a real child. The real baby is not quite so easy to love when it spits up, cries, has a dirty diaper, or keeps its parents up all night. Be prepared for the disruptions as well as the pleasures of parenthood, and you will find it easier to cope with the inevitable difficulties of the first weeks home. The relationship between you and your

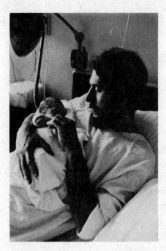

Figure 121b: Bonding Between Father and Son: Fathers who have the opportunity to bond with their children immediately after birth often develop a closer relationship with the baby that persists into later life. The love between Kenneth and his son is unmistakable from this photograph.

child is like any other relationship; it takes time to develop, but once the baby is in tune with you, both of you will begin to enjoy one another.

It is fascinating to see how the parent-infant relationship begins even before birth. Newborns have been observed in the delivery room turning toward the familiar sound of their parents' voices (again see Chapter 14). A baby whose *in utero* environment is warm and secure might be expected to bond quickly with his parents after birth. All babies, however, are social beings; that is, they are capable of responding to other human beings from the time they are born. Although the baby is physically unable to care for himself, he emerges from the womb with five finely tuned senses and the ability to make his needs felt. In fact, he can even make choices as to what he wants from his parents and shut out what he doesn't want (for instance, a newborn will prefer and turn to the smell of milk above that of water or sugar water). He uses these amazing social skills during the first hours and days with his parents to establish the close relationship we call bonding. In turn, parents instinctively develop behaviors of their own that bind them to their newborn (touching, gazing, fondling, and talking). Facial contact is a part of the natural interaction between a parent and a tiny baby. A baby put to the breast or given a bottle will often stop sucking and look up at his mother's face. It is sad to see the opportunity for pleasurable contact lost when a woman who is breast-feeding or bottle-feeding watches television or talks to friends while the baby searches for a sign of recognition from his mother. Breast-feeding or bottle-feeding should take place in a quiet environment where a mother and baby can spend the time together enjoying their new relationship. Talk to the baby, cuddle him; you will sense the baby's trust in you increasing as the weeks go on.

The stimulation of a child from the beginning enhances the growth of the infant not only emotionally but also physically and intellectually. And you will see that a child who is loved and cared for will usually develop more quickly than a child who is not as valued by his parents. Both parents have a part to play in the healthy stimulation of their baby. Fathers often complement mothers by providing the infant with a rather different form of stimulation from the touching, patting, vocalizing behavior seen in many mother-infant relationships. Mothers seem more sensitive to the baby's need for quiet stimulation. Fathers, on the other hand, often act as if they expect a playful response from their babies. Amazingly, even a tiny baby seems to enjoy his father's company in a special way; at two to three weeks of age, babies who see their fathers assume a more wide-eyed, playful expression than they do toward their mothers. The period of playful attention is short at first, but it lengthens as the child grows older. This is not to say that a father should not engage in "maternal" behavior; babies like being rocked and stroked and cuddled by a parent of either sex. Interestingly, fathers, like mothers, usually cradle their babies in the left arm, close up against the heart. A newborn listening to the soft beating of the heart is soothed by a sound familiar to him from his intrauterine life.

☐ **The Psychology of Naming; The Importance of a Child's Name**   Our name or names matter a great deal to us. Sometimes we like our given name; sometimes it embarrasses us; sometimes we hide our real identity under a nickname or a pseudonym. No one is indifferent on the subject of his or her name; how we are called is an important part of our individuality.

Finding the right name for a child is an enjoyable but delicate task. Some parents still follow a family tradition of naming, or select a given name for religious reasons. More often, though, we begin with a long list of possible names, one or two of which we hope will turn out to be exactly right for our child.

Now psychiatrists interested in naming have added another dimension to this fascinating subject: a child's name, they have concluded, is linked to the way children are viewed by others and the way they view themselves. According to this research, which was based on interviewing children and observing their behavior in and out of the classroom, having a "desirable" name such as John, Michael, or Sally, seemed related to how well a child was liked by his or her peers, and to the teacher's opinion of the child as well. The same study found the opposite among children with "undesirable" names: an Elmer or a Bertha, for instance, was less popular with contemporaries and received lower grades in class than an equally bright child named James or Susan. Is this because children behave better when they are more comfortable with their names? Think of Johnny Cash's "A Boy Named Sue," who grew up tough and mean because his father had given him that awful name.

Psychiatrists are not sure what makes one name more acceptable than another. Fashions in names do change somewhat from decade to decade. Sometimes a movie star or another celebrity inspires a fad for a particular name. Other names have always had a positive ring to them: one thinks of such ancient Hebrew names as David and Rebecca, which are still "desirable" today. Names we consider undesirable may be linked to a specific prejudice against an ethnic group or are disliked because they seem "strange." Some once popular names fall out of favor because they are associated with a notorious public figure or become the subject of too many jokes.

Nonetheless, there is no reason for a parent to get carried away with name games. Names vary in desirability from one group to another. A name, moreover, is but one factor in how a child is viewed. It is tightly interwoven with others, including appearance and economic status. Also, researchers point out that their findings indicate only what happens on the average. Some children with "strange" names are proud of them. An unusual name in politics, for instance, sometimes helps a candidate stand out ahead of his competitors.

☐ *The First Pediatric Examination*   The newborn will be evaluated within a few hours after birth by your private pediatrician or one of the hospital pediatric staff. This initial pediatric examination is scheduled as soon after birth as possible because the pediatrician wants to make sure that the baby is coping well with his new environment. These first twenty-four hours are crucial since the newborn is forced to adjust rather quickly to extrauterine life. He must begin to breathe air rather than amniotic fluid. He must learn to suck from the breast or bottle instead of receiving nutrition through the umbilical cord. Most babies, as I have said, manage this momentous transition into extrauterine life without help, but a few babies do need special care in the first hours or days of life. This is particularly true of premature infants, who are often cared for in a premature intensive-care unit.

The pediatrician's first step is to look over the baby's general appearance to make sure it has good color and is lively and responsive. Any obvious developmental abnormalities will be noted for later discussion with the parents. Next, the pediatrician will weigh and measure the baby. The average birth weight is about seven pounds, but a healthy full-term baby can weigh more or less than the average, depending on genetic factors and the individual pregnancy.

After the pediatrician has conducted his general examination, he will proceed to a more specific evaluation, beginning with the heart and lungs. It is quite common for a small dysfunctional heart murmur to show up in the initial examination because the valves of the heart are open while the baby is in the uterus. The valves close after birth to allow the bloodstream to pass through the lungs, but the process may not be completed immediately, leaving a slight dysfunction behind. Generally the symptoms will disappear soon after birth. If a structural defect is suspected (it rarely is) the pediatrician might suggest consulting a cardiologist later on.

The lungs are checked to make sure they are free of fluid and are functioning normally. Symptoms of respiratory-distress syndrome, a lung disease prevalent among prematures, develop within the first twenty-four hours, so a satisfactory report at the first examination usually rules out the presence of the disease.

Next, the pediatrician will examine the abdomen carefully to detect any enlarged organs or tumors on the kidneys or the liver. A positive finding would be followed up by a diagnostic X-ray. The doctor will also check the baby's genitalia and make sure that the rectum is open. Some babies are born with a small membrane covering the rectum, which is easily removed immediately after birth.

A baby girl's genitalia will be examined with particular care. Occasionally, unusually large female genitalia are the symptoms of a genetic abnormality or of an imbalance perhaps caused by hormone therapy during pregnancy (see Chap. 19). The pediatrician might arrange for a chromosomal analysis, or karyotype, (see Chap. 22), and call in a genetic specialist.

The pelvis is another area that will be examined carefully in this initial examination. A special brace used during infancy will correct a slight weakness of the hips before the child is old enough to learn to walk.

If any questions occur during the examination, the pediatrician will discuss them with you later. Many minor abnormalities seen in the first examination can be expected to disappear spontaneously as the baby matures. Occasionally the pediatrician finds a problem that requires his further attention or the calling in of a specialist. Again, many of these more serious problems can be solved or at least mitigated by modern medical technology. Only 9 percent of babies have some detectable newborn problem, and many of those can be corrected without surgery or prolonged therapy.

☐ *Newborn Reflexes*   The newborn exhibits a characteristic series of reflexes, many of which disappear within the first weeks or months of life. The pediatrician will check several of these reflexes to make sure that the baby's neurological system is functioning well.

The Moro Reflex The baby is placed along the doctor's forearm with the head resting in the doctor's open hand. As the doctor drops his hand suddenly, the healthy infant will immediately throw out his arms forward as if he were embracing someone. The test is also performed with the baby lying on his back. The pediatrician strikes the table on either side of the baby, who will repeat the same reflex.

The Rooting Reflex Stroking the baby's cheek near the mouth will cause the baby to turn his head and try to suck. This is the same reflex that the mother uses when she encourages the baby to "root" for the nipple before breast-feeding.

The Grasp Reflex If a finger is placed in the palm of a baby's hand, the baby should close his hand around the finger. Likewise, pressing the sole of the baby's foot at a point near the big toe should trigger a grasping movement of the foot.

The Stepping Reflex When the baby is held upright with the soles of the feet pressed gently onto a hard surface, the baby will draw up each leg in succession as if he were walking.

☐ *Newborn Screening Programs*   In many states, a screening program is provided by state departments of health to families of newborn babies. These programs are responsible for testing every infant within a few days after birth for a group of detectable disorders in the body's chemistry. Newborn screening programs identify those few babies who might have one of several rare birth defects and alert the doctor to this possibility. With early diagnosis and medical treatment, serious illness can usually be prevented.

Babies are generally screened for the rare enzyme disorder known as *phenylketonuria*, also called PKU. In this disease a component of the food protein phenylalanine cannot be broken down by the body through a lack of the proper enzyme. Brain damage inevitably results with untreated PKU, but it can be prevented by a special diet low in phenylalanine. *Hypothyroidism*, a condition caused by inadequate production of the hormone thyroxine, is another disease that can lead to mental and growth retardation. This condition occurs in one out of every 4000 newborns. Once the disease is detected, through a blood thyroid test, the newborn can be treated with thyroxine tablets to balance the body's production of thyroxine. Other rare enzyme-deficiency diseases that can be detected through a blood test and prevented early in life are *histidinemia, adenosine deaminase deficiency,* and *galactosemia.* Finally, *sickle cell disease* and the presence of the *sickle-cell trait* can be detected in the first days after birth by a simple blood test. (See Chapter 22 for more information on genetic diseases.)

You might check with your obstetrician whether these tests are routinely done in your hospital or how they can be obtained.

☐ *Born with a Birthmark*   About 60 percent of all newborns have a small, superficial birthmark, often on the nape of the neck or on the eyelids, the cheeks, or the forehead. Most of these fade away as the child grows older, or cause no real problem to the child or the parents. A very few birthmarks are of more concern because they are the symptom of a disorder in the body's structure or function.

Two major categories of birthmarks exist:

The vascular type (the hemangiomas) includes the common birthmark known as the *nevus flammeus,* or the *port-wine stain.* Probably one person in every three has a port-wine stain. Generally they are tiny or are covered by hair, but they can be large enough to cover one side of the face or a part of the arm. There is no treatment yet that will remove a port-wine stain entirely, although scientists have tried laser surgery, with some success.

A *strawberry* birthmark, another type of hemangioma, gets its distinctive appearance from a mass of tiny red capillaries, which protrude above the surface of the skin. A strawberry mark may grow in size as the child grows older, but it usually starts to fade and then disappear before the fifth birthday. It can be removed surgically if it does not fade away spontaneously. This type of birthmark is three times more common in girls than it is in boys.

The *nonvascular birthmarks* include the *pigmented nevus,* the mole. The mole is by far the most common of all birthmarks, and comes in many sizes from a pencil point to a mole large enough to cover a substantial part of an arm or a leg. Moles are usually dark brown in color and may be pigmented. They, unlike the hemangioma, do not fade with time and can be removed only surgically.

☐ *The Baby's Natural Functions*   Many babies urinate immediately after they are born. Certainly a healthy baby should begin to urinate within twenty-four hours after birth. The amount of urine passed is small initially, but once feeding is well established, you can expect to see six or more wet diapers a day. Frequent urination is a sign of good health.

The first bowel movement is commonly black because there is still meconium in the baby's bowel. The meconium will pass through the system during the first twenty-four hours of life. If the baby is breast-fed, the meconium changes to a light-yellowish stool, with a thin, almost pastelike consistency. Breast-fed babies rarely have hard stools. They often have a bowel movement after each feeding or once every few days, a variation that is quite normal from baby to baby. If the baby is bottle-fed, the stool may vary from soft to pasty, with a pale yellow or tan color. There is often a tendency to hard stools with a stronger odor than among breast-fed babies.

☐ **What Will the Navel Look Like?**   After birth the umbilical cord is clamped to about two inches away from the navel and is then left to shrink and fall off. This usually takes place within four to fourteen days after birth. Meanwhile, wash the navel carefully, keep it dry, and do not allow the area to get dirty. Any redness or other sign of infection should be reported to your pediatrician immediately. As soon as the cord falls off, the navel will start to heal and take on its permanent shape. The look of the navel is ordained by the child's genetic heritage, not, contrary to a popular misconception, by the way in which the doctor cuts the cord. Thus, if you and your mate have an "inner" navel, your baby will probably look the same.

☐ **Bathing the Newborn**   A newborn baby does not need a full bath until the umbilical cord has dropped off. You do need to wash the face and the folds of the neck and behind the ears where spit-up milk often collects and then dries up. The buttocks and genitals should also be sponged daily and after a bowel movement.

☐ **Circumcision**   Circumcision is one of the oldest of all surgical procedures. The practice of removing a part of the foreskin was performed in Egypt more than 5000 years ago, and most male mummies do indeed show signs of circumcision. Ancient peoples of many cultures used circumcision as a religious rite or as a ceremonial rite of initiation into the tribe or family.

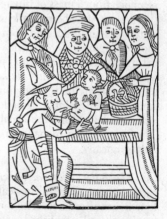

Figure 122: Circumcision of Jesus: The circumcision of Jesus has been depicted in European art since early Christian times. This is a woodcut from the fifteenth century. The circumcision, like the *bris* today, appears to be an event that is celebrated by family and friends.

Ritual circumcision among the ancient Jews may first have been adopted as a substitution for the sacrifice of the firstborn to the spirit of their ancestors. It also became a symbol of the special covenant between Jehovah and his people. According to the Old Testament, Abraham circumcised himself at the age of ninety-nine and likewise circumsised all males of his household as well as his slaves. The custom took on an added meaning after the captivity in Egypt, where the Jews were forbidden to circumcise their male offspring. Thereafter, the act of circumcision was seen as a mark of identification for the Jewish people as well as the symbol of their covenant with God. Thus, historically, circumcision was seen a religious act rather than a health measure, even though there were probably medical advantages to circumcision in the humid Middle Eastern climate.

Before the twentieth century few non-Jewish American males were circumsised. The practice became increasingly popular as "medical" texts advocated circumcision as a deterrent to masturbation and a cure for feeblemindedness, alcoholism, and lunacy. Following World War II, responsible doctors encouraged circumcision for health reasons, primarily to promote cleanliness. Circumcision was also said to reduce the chances of cancer of the penis and cancer of the cervix among the wives of circumcised men. These beliefs are still firmly held by many American parents, even though the American Academy of Pediatrics has concluded that there is no medical indication for circumcision. Surveys show that circumcision is still believed by some parents to prevent masturbation or excessive crying. Other parents believe it is simply hospital policy to circumcise all newborn males. Parents often give their consent to the procedure without discussing the pros and cons with their obstetrician. Be sure before you sign a consent form for circumcision that you are giving your *informed* consent to the procedure.

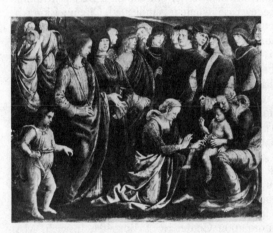

Figure 123: Circumcision of Moses' Son, Eleazar: The circumcision is being performed by Moses' wife, Zipporah. "Then Zipporah took a sharp stone and cut off the foreskin of her son and cast it at his feet and said: 'Surely a bloody bridegroom thou art to me.'" (Exodus 4:25) Although the story differs in detail from source to source, all the accounts agree that Moses had angered God by failing to circumcise his son, Eleazar. Zipporah therefore performed the circumcision for her husband and saved his life. The picture was painted by the Italian artist Pietro Perugino (1450–1524).

☐ **Why Circumcise?**　The only medical indication for circumcision is to correct phimosis, a condition in which the foreskin will not retract over the glans, the head of the penis. About 96 percent of newborns are born with phimosis but most children rapidly outgrow the condition. Only 2 percent of boys will have phimosis by the age of three. One cannot identify the child who will have permanent phimosis at birth, but a circumcision can be done later in life, if necessary.

A painful infection of the penis called balanitis sometimes afflicts uncircumcised males. Balanitis is caused when the smegma, the natural secretion that is found under the foreskin, becomes infected by bacteria. Balanitis is more likely to occur if a man is careless about hygiene and the smegma is allowed to accumulate under the foreskin. It can usually be cured with antibiotics.

☐ **Is There a Connection Between the Uncircumcised Penis and Cancer of the Cervix?**   A recent study has shown no difference in cervical cancer rates between the wives of uncircumcised men and circumcised men. A woman who has numerous sexual partners and is sexually active at an early age is at highest risk for cervical cancer, whether her partners are circumcised or not.

Smegma was once believed to be a carcinogen, but this is probably a fallacy. Smegma is a protective coating that protects the head of the penis and is identical to the protective coating produced under the clitoral foreskin. How would we regard a doctor who suggested circumcision of the clitoris?

☐ **Is the Circumcised Penis Cleaner?**   Cleanliness is one of the standard arguments in favor of routine circumcision, since a boy who is not circumcised must be particularly careful to wash himself under the foreskin. Parents may also favor circumcision because it is easier to take care of the penis when the child is young. Good penile hygiene, however, can be taught at an early age, just as a child will learn to wash behind his ears or underneath his fingernails.

☐ **Making the Decision About Circumcision**   There is no clear medical indication for circumcision. Parents who are not bound by a religious determination must therefore seriously ask themselves whether their son should undergo a potentially painful surgical procedure or whether one should leave nature alone and perform surgery only in the few cases where it is indicated. Circumcision is a relatively safe procedure, but complications do occur, including hemorrhage and wound infection. The operation also subjects the newborn to pain and psychological trauma. The foreskin is not a particularly sensitive part of the body—it contains relatively few pain fibers—but the operation is done without anesthesia to reduce the risk of complications. Many babies cry or vomit during circumcision, although babies usually recover quickly.

For most parents, the decision to perform a nonritual circumcision will finally depend on family and social considerations. A man may want his son to be circumcised because he himself is circumcised. Or parents may feel that a boy should be circumcised if he is going to go to school with other boys who are circumcised, since children are sensitive about physical differences between themselves and their peers. Of course, if fewer boys are circumcised, children will grow up accepting the differences among their friends.

Parents who want support for not circumcising their child can contact two groups: Non-Circumcision Information Center, P.O. Box 404, Ipswich, MA 01938, and Intact Capitol, Box 5, Wilbraham, MA 01095. Further information can also be found in Edward Wallerstein's book *Circumcision: An American Fallacy*, published by the Springer Publishing Company, 200 Park Avenue South, New York, NY 10003.*

☐ **The Circumcision Operation**   Surgery is usually performed on the second or third day after birth, once the baby's condition has stabilized. One advantage of doing the surgery early on is that the newborn seems to experience less pain, or at least less trauma, with the operation.

---

* For further information on ritual and nonritual circumcision, please refer to my book *It's Your Body: A Woman's Guide to Gynecology*, published by Berkley Books.

The pediatrician or obstetrician begins the procedure by placing a special clamp known as a Gomco clamp under the penis. This small clamp is squeezed tightly over the foreskin in a straight line to crush the skin and cut off the circulation in the prepuce. Once the clamp has been left in place for a couple of minutes, the foreskin is separated from the glans, along the straight line defined by the Gomco clamp. About one-third of an inch of skin is removed, thus exposing the glans. The wound is left open to the air, with Vaseline placed on it. It usually heals normally within a few days, but if anything suspicious occurs after the baby returns home, the wound must be looked at by a pediatrician. A serious infection is unlikely under sterile hospital conditions, but it does occasionally happen after a circumcision.

☐ **Infant Jaundice** A generally harmless type of jaundice known as newborn or neonatal jaundice appears rather frequently in the first days after birth (the causes and treatment of neonatal jaundice are discussed in Chapter 29). The condition is usually transitory, but a persistent case of jaundice could have serious consequences, including brain damage. Any case of neonatal jaundice must, therefore, be monitored by a pediatrician. Most babies develop jaundice in the hospital, but the condition might appear first, or become more acute, after you reach home. Although there is usually no cause for concern, your pediatrician should be alerted and the baby's condition evaluated promptly to rule out any serious problem.

☐ **Crib Death** Crib death, which is otherwise known as the sudden infant death syndrome (SIDS), is an unexplained illness that causes 8000 to 10,000 infant deaths each year. Most of its victims are apparently healthy babies between two and seven months of age who die unexpectedly while they are asleep. Rarely are any symptoms present to alert the parents or their physicians. SIDS is at least as old as the Old Testament and probably occurred as frequently in the eighteenth and nineteenth centuries as it does today. It is therefore an ancient disease whose origin was as mysterious then as it is now.

A number of tentative theories have been put forward to explain this hitherto inexplicable disease. One is hormonal. Many SIDS babies have been found to have an abnormally high level of the thyroid hormone T_3 in their bloodstream after death. Scientists still do not know if the high level of T_3 causes the syndrome or is a result of it. According to another theory, the SIDS baby may have an unsuspected immune-system deficiency that means she or he cannot combat common bacteria in such items as cow's milk or household dust. A third, and perhaps more promising theory, holds a disorder called sleep apnea responsible for many crib deaths. Sleep apnea is a prolonged cessation of breathing that occurs during sleep, commonly in middle-aged men, but also in infants. All infants stop breathing while they are asleep, but only for a few seconds, since the brain normally detects the lack of oxygen in the system and prompts the body to take action. It may be that crib death babies have some subtle physiological defect of the nervous and respiratory systems that prevents the part of the brain controlling ventilation during sleep from regulating itself. If so, it may be possible one day to identify and protect babies at high risk for SIDS. A monitoring device already exists that parents of "near miss" babies can use to detect periods of sleep apnea.

At the present moment, however, most SIDS deaths are neither predictable nor preventable by parents or pediatricians. SIDS is a tragedy that strikes the most loving and conscientious of parents. Unfortunately, a SIDS death often leads to family members' blaming themselves or others, or to a prolonged period of depression for one or both partners. A family that experiences SIDS will need help from close friends and professionals who are skilled counselors. Another essential resource is the National Foundation for Sudden Infant Death, Inc., 1501 Broadway, New York, NY 10036. Local chapter members who are themselves SIDS parents spend many hours offering consolation and advice to parents who have been recently bereaved. Consultation and help can also be obtained from the International Guild for Infant Survival, 6822 Brompton Road, Baltimore, MD 21207.

☐ *Child Care*   In the first year of life a baby triples his weight and develops new activities at an extraordinary rate. Think of the physical coordination he achieves in those first twelve months as he learns to reach out, grasp, sit, crawl, stand, and finally walk. Development proceeds so quickly you can see your baby change from month to month, sometimes even from week to week. There are a number of child-care books that you might want to consult as your child grows older. Excellent guides to the first year are *The First 12 Months of Life*, by Frank Caplan (available in paperback from Berkley Books), the revised edition of *Baby and Child Care*, by Benjamin Spock (Pocket Books, 1974) and two books by Lee Salk: *Dr. Salk: An A to Z Guide to Raising Your Child* (NAL/Signet, 1983) and *Your Child's First Year* (Simon & Schuster, 1983). The first book describes normal development month by month. The second book is the bible of child care, fully revised for a new generation of parents. Dr. Salk's two books are excellent guides to the child's emotional and physical development.

☐ *When Can You Go Home?*   Women delivering in birthing centers usually go home twenty-four hours after the birth, or as soon as the birthing center staff feel mother and baby are doing well enough to leave. The average hospital stay is longer but by only a day or two; a primipara usually stays in the hospital until the fourth postpartum day; with a second or subsequent birth, mother and baby are usually allowed to go home on the second or third postpartum day. Some women insist on going home as early as possible after a first labor, and usually there is no reason not to go home two days after an uncomplicated birth if there is adequate help at home. I try to let my healthy obstetrical patients leave the hospital as early as possible because most of them feel more comfortable at home, but this is an individual matter to be discussed between a couple and their obstetrician.

After a Cesarean birth, the usual hospital stay is from five to seven days, although it is not unusual for a Cesarean patient to go home on the fourth or fifth day postpartum. Cesarean patients tend to recover faster nowadays because hospitals encourage solid food earlier and give patients preventive antibiotics. Again, discuss your individual situation with your obstetrician well in advance of the birth. In this way you can plan ahead.

☐ *Sibling Visitation*   Many hospitals do permit sibling visits. The presence of older children on the obstetrical floor is very important in keeping the family together and alleviating jealousy among the older children. A young child is often frightened by his mother's sudden disappearance. If he is allowed to come to the hospital he will see that his mother is well and happy and still loves him. Most children are very curious about the new brother or sister and will accept the baby more easily if they see him or her in the hospital first, rather than at home.

Ask your doctor whether his hospital will allow sibling visitation. A hospital that does have this program should be one of your first choices.

☐ *Coming Home: Can You Trust Your Pets?*   A dog or cat that is used to only adults sometimes behaves strangely after a baby arrives, and many new parents worry about the possibility of their pet injuring the baby. It would depend somewhat on what type of pet you have. A normally protective dog will probably accept the baby quickly and become his or her best friend. Cats on the other hand are more unpredictable. Some cats have attacked newborns and have had to be sent away. Never leave a cat alone with the baby unless you are sure that the cat has accepted the new family situation.

Animals can be trained to recognize the baby's scent before he comes back from the hospital. It might be a good idea for your husband to bring a diaper home and leave it around the house to familiarize your pet with the baby's smell. In this way the animal will learn to recognize the baby as a part of the family rather than as an interloper.

☐ *When Can You Expect to Be in Shape Again?*   Each woman responds differently to childbirth. Normally a woman who started pregnancy with her body in good condition will find it easier to get back into shape, but even the fittest of women tire easily in the weeks and months after the baby's birth. This is partly because the body is still healing; it is also because the new responsibility of the baby depletes a woman's stamina. With a new baby your normal sleep patterns are inevitably disrupted. Lack of sleep often leads to irritability, even depression. Try to nap with the baby during the day; an afternoon nap will partly compensate for an interrupted night.

Eating well will help build up your strength. You need about 2600 calories a day when you are breast-feeding, about 500 more than before you became pregnant. Foods such as cereals, whole-grain breads, cheese, and milk are good sources of nutrition and calories. In addition, I always recommend two prenatal vitamins a day plus an iron supplement while my patients are breast-feeding, and at least one a day plus iron if they are bottle feeding. A combination of good food, extra vitamins, and exercise will bring you back into shape quickly and help you sleep better. Positive feelings and happiness naturally make recovery even faster. Every woman should be able to resume all her prepregnancy activities four to eight weeks postpartum.

☐ *Getting Back into Shape—Postpartum Exercise*   It was once customary to bind a mother's abdomen as soon as the baby was born in the belief that this would help restore muscle tone. In fact, this restrictive measure had quite the opposite effect. We know now that the only way to restore muscle tone is by exercising and *using* the muscles.

A number of books and classes include information about postpartum fitness.

One excellent book that demonstrates a comprehensive series of postpartum exercises is *Jane Fonda's Workout Book for Pregnancy, Birth and Recovery*, by Femmy DeLyser (published by Simon & Schuster).

An exercise program can usually start after the first week postpartum. Begin with some preliminary exercises to tighten your muscles. The first muscles you should exercise are the vaginal muscles.

The Kegel Exercise: This exercise can be started a week to two weeks after birth.

Lie on your back with your knees bent and your feet about a foot apart. Concentrate on the muscles between your legs, those around the bladder opening and the vagina and rectum. Begin slowly inhaling and exhaling. Then as you exhale, squeeze the muscles around the vagina, bladder, and rectum. Inhale slowly again, and then release. Gradually work up to doing the exercise twenty to thirty times daily. This exercise can also be performed sitting on the toilet. The Kegel exercise will strengthen the vaginal area so there is less chance of the uterus or vagina sagging or prolapsing in a second pregnancy or later in life. Begin the Kegel exercise as soon after delivery as possible to restore muscle tone, and continue until your body is completely back to its prepregnancy state.

☐ **The Abdominal Muscles Exercises**   You can start working on the abdominal muscles within one week after the baby is born. Lie on your back, with your head on a pillow, and bend your knees with the feet flat on the floor. Arch your back and push your arms against the floor, then push your back on the floor and raise your pelvic area. Contract the abdominal muscles, relax and then repeat four to five times. You might enjoy doing this exercise with the baby lying on your abdomen.

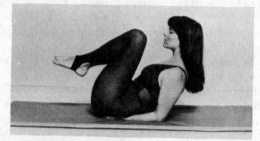

Figure 124: The Buttock Lift: Lie on the floor or on a mattress with your knees bent and your hands on the ground. Then raise your buttocks, as you keep your shoulder blades and your lower back on the floor. Lift your buttocks slightly higher and then release them slightly. This is a small movement performed by the muscles underneath the buttocks. Exhale as you lift, inhale as you release. Repeat twenty to thirty times daily.

Reproduced by permission from Jane Fonda's Workout Book for Pregnancy, Birth and Recovery, *by Femmy DeLyser, published by Simon and Schuster, New York, 1982.*

After the second or third week simple abdominal exercises can be combined with sit-ups and knee lifts. Slowly increase the number of repetitions each day to further strengthen the abdominal muscles (see figure). If you have had a Cesarean section you can perform the same exercises, but do not begin until six weeks postpartum.

The Cat Stretch: This exercise is done on your hands and knees. Keep your weight equally distributed between your arms and legs. Inhale and relax as you keep your back flat, then exhale as you drop your head and buttocks under and pull your back up. Exhale again and relax your back to the original position (see figure). Work up to twenty to thirty repetitions daily from the second or third week after childbirth.

☐ *The Buttocks Exercise* Another series of exercises are those that strengthen your buttock muscles. This exercise is known as the buttock lift. Lie on your back with your knees bent and your arms alongside your body. Breathe in and out slowly.

Keep your shoulder blades on the floor, and raise your buttocks. As you do, imagine that you are reaching with your lower back to the floor. Now lift your buttocks slightly higher and release down a little; then lift and release. This is a small movement done with the muscles underneath the buttocks. Exhale as you lift, inhale as you release. Repeat twenty-four times.

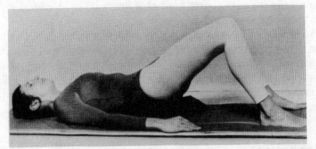

Figure 125: Abdominal Exercise: Lie on your back and place your arms alongside your body. Raise yourself into a semisitting position, supporting the upper body on your elbows with your hands underneath your buttocks. Place your feet slightly apart with bent knees. Then inhale. As you inhale, bring your knees toward your body. Keep them up until you have a slight feeling of discomfort. Then inhale again as you rest your legs on the floor. Exhale again, and repeat the exercise. Repeat twenty to thirty times daily. This exercise should help strengthen the abdominal muscles and get you back into shape. This is an initial postpartum exercise that can be combined in time with other types of exercises.
Reproduced by permission from Jane Fonda's Workout Book for Pregnancy, Birth and Recovery, *by Femmy DeLyser, published by Simon and Schuster, New York, 1982.*

Each exercise should be practiced every day. Increase the number of repetitions as you go along. A steady exercise program will slowly increase your strength and build up the various muscles in the body. Once you are four to six weeks postpartum, swimming, running, and other forms of regular exercise can be added to your individual program. It is a good idea to keep practicing the postpartum exercises until you feel your body is completely back to the way it was before childbirth.

☐ *Sex After Childbirth* How soon is it safe to resume sexual intercourse after the baby is born? Doctors usually recommend waiting at least four weeks because this is the time it generally takes for the vaginal area to heal sufficiently. Not only does the episiotomy remain stiff and painful for at least a month after birth, but the vaginal tissues are fragile and easily torn, especially if you are breast-feeding. Intercourse in the first two weeks can result in ripped stitches or damage to the delicate vaginal area. A couple may find the forced period of abstinence frustrating, but intercourse before the episiotomy has healed is really painful for many women. A couple should remember that there are many other ways to achieve mutual satisfaction—touching and holding are other ways of saying "I love you."

Once you resume a normal sex life, be prepared for some temporary changes in, for instance, your level of sexual response. It may take a few weeks before intercourse is as satisfying as it was before or during your pregnancy. Many women are surprised to find that intercourse is still uncomfortable, even painful, for up to three months after the birth. There is residual pain from the episiotomy. There are hormonal changes, which continue for many months after delivery. A lower estrogen level, which is experienced during breast-feeding, affects sexual response and makes the vaginal area drier than usual. This does not mean that you will stop enjoying intercourse, only that you will be slower to respond. It might help to use a lubricating jelly, such as Vaseline, K-Y jelly, or Surgilube, the first few times you have intercourse. A man should try to enter the vagina very gently in the beginning until his partner's fear of pain has been overcome, or the woman might prefer to be on top to control the entrance of the penis. Be patient: it is only a question of time before the vaginal tissues are fully healed and hormonal activity is back to normal. Eventually the vagina will restore itself completely and sex should be as pleasurable as or more pleasurable than it was before the birth. Sex is often more enjoyable after a woman has borne a child since childbirth matures a woman's body and heightens her sexual responsiveness. A woman also gains more self-confidence with motherhood.

Some women unfortunately believe the myth that nursing mothers have less desire for sex. It is true that nursing keeps the estrogen and steroid levels depressed longer than usual, and might therefore be expected to inhibit sexual responsiveness. Yet many women find breast-feeding itself to be a sensual experience. And according to Masters and Johnson, women who nurse report enjoying intercourse sooner than women who do not nurse. It may be that women who choose to breast-feed do so because they enjoy the intimacy of nursing as they enjoy the intimacy of sex.

Be prepared, though, to find your interest in sex diminish in the postpartum period. Most couples report a temporary loss of sexual enjoyment for a few weeks or even a few months after a birth. Fatigue is an obvious factor. Until the baby begins sleeping through the night (at two to four months of age) mothers and fathers are frequently tired a good deal of the time and may not have much energy for lovemaking. There are psychological adjustments too that make it harder for a couple to recapture their old level of sexual enjoyment. A woman may find that she is more interested in her role as a mother than in her role as a wife and lover, or an unexpectedly demanding baby may interrupt the parents' normal emotional and sexual relationship. Most people who enjoyed a good relationship before the birth work through these changes successfully, but it can take several months before a couple recapture their prepregnancy level of sexual enjoyment.

☐   *The Postpartum Checkup*   The first postpartum checkup takes place four to six weeks after delivery. Some obstetricians prefer to see their postpartum patients at four weeks; others follows the traditional six week schedule. Your obstetrician will check the episiotomy, and make sure that any lacerations in the vaginal area have healed. By now the uterus is usually back to normal and the cervix is tightly closed.

Never be afraid to call your doctor before the scheduled appointment if you think you have a problem. Even an apparently minor complication can become a major one if you wait for two to three weeks or more before discussing it with your doctor.

☐   *Contraception After Childbirth*   "What form of contraception should I use?" is a question frequently asked at the first postpartum checkup. A woman may be delighted with her baby, but in these days of carefully planned families she is unlikely to want to get pregnant again right away.

For the first few months at least, a woman who is nursing has different contraceptive needs from the woman who has decided not to nurse. When you are breast-feeding you can safely wait for a few weeks postpartum before deciding on a form of contraception, because nursing depresses your estrogen level and will therefore disrupt your normal ovulation pattern. It usually takes some time for the nursing mother to begin ovulating regularly again, sometimes as long as six months or more after the birth. Breast-feeding, nonetheless, is not a sure form of contraception, since women who are unusually fertile do become pregnant even during lactation. I usually suggest the woman's partner use a condom initially while the vaginal tissues are still tender. Inserting a diaphragm can be painful in the first couple of months after childbirth. It is also difficult for a gynecologist to fit you with the right size of diaphragm immediately after a birth because the cervix is not as tight as it will be later on. A diaphragm will fit better by the second or third month after delivery.

Birth control pills cannot be used while you are breast-feeding because the hormones from the pills will be excreted in the breast milk. You can safely resume taking the pill once the baby is weaned.

A decision on contraception must be made earlier for women who have decided not to breast-feed. Ovulation can occur within a few weeks to a month after childbearing, so an unprotected woman might find herself pregnant again almost immediately. Couples who do resume intercourse before the fourth week should use some form of protection; condoms, again, are probably the best contraceptive until a woman can use a diaphragm or go back onto the pill. Once your doctor has made sure that the vaginal tissues are well healed, you can ask him to fit you for a diaphragm or another form of barrier contraception, the cervical cap, which is popular in Europe (see Chap. 1). Usually there is no reason why you cannot go back to the pill after the postpartum checkup, unless you are one of those women who cannot tolerate the pill for medical or age reasons (again, see Chap. 1).

The IUD is a good form of contraception as long as it is tolerated without irregular bleeding or infection. You may feel that you would rather not accept an IUD if you are planning a future pregnancy because of the link between ectopic pregnancy and IUD use (see Chap. 1). This is a subject you might want to discuss with your doctor. A woman who is breast-feeding should wait several months until the uterus is completely healed before having an IUD inserted. Otherwise, studies have indicated that it is safe to have an IUD inserted four weeks after a delivery, although I prefer patients to wait for a few months, rather than a few weeks, to allow the uterus time to readjust itself.

☐ *Spacing Your Family*   Whether you decide to have more than one child and how you decide to space your family are choices that only you and your partner can make. You know your individual circumstances better than your doctor or any so-called child expert. Your relationships with your own siblings will probably affect the way you plan your family too, since our feelings about our first family ties have a strong influence on our own marriages.

No rule exists other than a warning against becoming pregnant again too quickly. Even a strong and healthy woman needs at least a year after the previous pregnancy to build up her nutritional reserves to be ready for another baby. Most couples seem to favor having a second child within two years or a second child when the first is three or four. Parents who have tightly spaced children may be older parents who don't have much time to have more children, or they may want siblings to be close in age so that they can grow up together. Sometimes it works well, especially if the family can get extra help to relieve a mother burdened by a dependent toddler and an even more dependent baby. Most child experts tend to look askance at this approach to family planning, however, even though individual families do manage successfully. They feel that most parents are too preoccupied by the physical demands of two children in diapers to have time for the children's emotional needs. In a tightly spaced family the older child in particular may be unintentionally deprived of emotional support at a critical time of development.

Once the first child is three or four years of age, child experts point out that he or she has usually developed a sense of competence and can function as an individual for at least a part of the day. An older child with friends and interests of his own is less likely to be jealous of a new baby. This is not to say that sibling rivalry is absent from families where the children are several years apart. Sibling rivalry is inevitable, it is even healthy, because the conflicts we experience as children allow us later to live and compete with people as adults. Parents can look forward to difficulties as well as pleasures however they plan their children!

☐ *IQ and Family Size*   Are the firstborn children of small families brighter than other children? Yes, according to an accumulation of empirical observations and the findings of studies on birth order and intelligence. A disproportionate number of people listed in *Who's Who*, for example, are only children or firstborn, including twenty-one out of the first twenty-three American astronauts. Firstborns predominate in such fields as business, law, and medicine, where the successful professional must combine intelligence and a will to succeed. Interestingly, a study of Californian school children has concluded that the overachieving firstborn son or daughter may score better than other children, but he or she is usually less popular among contemporaries than children born lower in the birth order.

One widely accepted explanation for the overachieving firstborn is the belief that parents spend more time with firstborns than with younger siblings. Single children especially are believed to do better than the children of larger families just because they are only children. This may be something of a misconception. According to at least one researcher, the only child generally does not do quite as well as the firstborn child of a two-child family, possibly because sibling rivalry encourages a sense of competition, or because siblings work through problems more effectively with each other than with their parents. Of course, psychologists who work with children concede that birth order is only one possible indicator of a child's future. Much depends on family circumstances and the care parents give their children, regardless of birth order.

In a family in which the children are equally loved and valued, every child has a good chance of growing up successfully and doing well in life.

Index